Cardiac Reconstructions with Allograft Tissues

Cardiac Reconstructions
with Allograft Tissues

Richard A. Hopkins, MD

Karl E. Karlson, MD, and Gloria A. Karlson, MD, Professor
and Chief, Cardiothoracic Surgery, Brown University School
of Medicine; Cardiac Surgeon-in-Chief, Rhode Island
Hospital, The Miriam Hospital, and Hasbro Children's
Hospital; and Director, Collis Cardiovascular Research
Laboratory, Providence, Rhode Island

With 437 images, 11 in Full Color

Illustrations by Thomas Xenakis

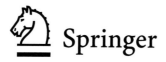 Springer

Richard A. Hopkins, MD
Karl E. Karlson, MD, and Gloria A. Karlson, MD, Professor and Chief, Cardiothoracic
Surgery, Brown University School of Medicine; Cardiac Surgeon-in-Chief, Rhode
Island Hospital, The Miriam Hospital, and Hasbro Children's Hospital; and Director,
Collis Cardiovascular Research Laboratory, Providence, RI, USA

Library of Congress Cataloging-in-Publication Data
Hopkins, R.A. (Richard A.)
    Cardiac reconstructions with allograft tissues / by Richard A. Hopkins, and 56
contributors; illustrations by Thomas Xenakis.
        p.   ;   cm.
    Cardiac reconstructions with allograft valves. c1989.
    Includes bibliographical references and index.
    ISBN 0-387-94962-3 (alk. paper)
    1. Heart valves—Surgery.   2. Homografts.   I. Hopkins, R.A. (Richard A.).
Cardiac reconstructions with allograft valves.   II. Title.
    [DNLM: 1. Heart Valves—transplantation.   2. Cryopreservation.   3. Tissue
Transplantation.   4. Transplantation, Homologous. WG 169 H795ca 2003]
    RD598. C3435 2003
    617.4′120592—dc22   2003059130

ISBN 0-387-94962-3   Printed on acid-free paper.

Printed in the United States of America.   (BS/MVY)

9 8 7 6 5 4 3 2 1   SPIN 10553102

springeronline.com

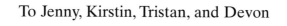
To Jenny, Kirstin, Tristan, and Devon

Preface

This volume is a follow-up to the book *Cardiac Reconstructions with Allograft Valves*, which was written with five contributors and an outstanding artist. Since its publication in 1989, the information in this field has increased dramatically, paralleling the increased clinical use of cardiovascular allograft tissues. Many new techniques have been developed and refinements of the older techniques have been published based on the experiences of many surgeons. In addition, the fundamental biology of valve transplantation and especially the use of cryopreservation to facilitate transplantation, has been a major focus of research. Thus, much more is known about these tissues than at the time of the writing of the first book. Because of this progress, a new volume seemed appropriate. Because cryopreserved cardiovascular tissues are also used without valves for many important reconstructions, I decided to expand the focus of the book, and thus the slight modification in the title. More than two-thirds of this book is new material.

The book has also undergone another fundamental change. While the first edition was predominantly written by the main author, to include much of the available knowledge in this field, this new edition mandated a contributor format. These experts explore the fundamental scientific basis of this field which is critical to an understanding of allograft tissues. Most sections have been rewritten to reflect increased clinical and research experience.

Other important additions include a special section on biochemical and morphologic studies of explanted experimental animal and clinical human valves. Because many of the fundamental clinical concepts are based on the experience of a relatively small number of centers actively transplanting homografts in the 1970s and early 1980s, I solicited summarized versions of results from the surgeons and their colleagues who contributed importantly to this early phase (Chapter 2–7). The basic cell biology of these tissues has been investigated by a number of focused laboratories (including our own), requiring complete revisions and expansions of the relevant chapters (8–30). Cryopreservation protocols have matured based on significant research, thus mandating a major rewriting of Section VIII by the authors from LifeNet Tissue Services.

The information presented firmly resolves the question of chronic interstitial leaflet cell viability following cryopreserved cardiac valve allotransplantation—the nails are driven into the coffin of the prolonged cell survival theory. An alternative theory for how and why homografts actually perform so well is presented based on significant laboratory and human data. The resolution of the conflicting theories of prolonged cell viability following cardiac valve transplantation is summarized in Chapter 20. This biology is a fascinating but constantly moving target. As biological modifications ensue with genetic, molecular and cellular manipulations of these allograft tissues, these will be an ever-expanding need for the surgical techniques of cardiac reconstructions described in this book.

Allograft tissue transplants are increasingly used by all cardiac surgeons, but are particularly important for pediatric patients as a consequence of special advantages in highly complex congenital lesions. The availability of cryopreserved allografts has initiated a wave of surgical creativity which is reflected in the marked expansion of the chapter on left ventricular outflow tract reconstructions, especially for complex neonatal problems. The growing role for autologous valve transplant procedures (e.g., Ross operations) in both children and adults has mandated marked expansion of the techniques depicted. Many new surgical methods are described, and older techniques have been refined. In addition, surgical techniques used with allografts are also applicable to unstented xenografts, so new sections have been added to depict the evolution of ventricular outflow tract reconstruction from root replacements, through "miniroots" and autografts, to the implantation methods for unstented xenografts.

As in the first edition, certain conventions are used. Half-tone or carbon dust figures are used to depict surgical techniques as viewed from the surgeon's perspective. Repetition of steps in the depiction of various surgical techniques spares the reader the need to flip pages. The terms "homograft" and "allograft" are used interchangeably as no purpose is served by a pedantic argument about which is more correct today.

All surgeons performing pediatric and/or adult valve replacements and reconstructive cardiac surgeries should be interested in these methods. Cardiothoracic residents and cardiologists will find the volume useful. Most of the surgical techniques have been used by me. When contributors' techniques vary from my own, I have noted optional variations or have noted my preferences. Refinements are based on my own personal experience exceeding 600 allograft and autograft reconstructions spanning the age spectrum of premature neonates to adults in their seventh decade, and now including shuntless valves.

Cryopreserved allograft tissues are now standard materials for the reconstructive cardiac surgeon. Surgical reconstructive methods continue to be refined and new approaches developed. Both surgical techniques and notions about the nature of this tissue we are transplanting have evolved. Putting all of this into perspective required the addition of a thirteenth section "Future Directions" with the intent of creating a critical rationale for valve replacement choice and to suggest future directions for basic and applied research, just at the start of a new era based on bioengineering which will involve decellularized and recellularized valves. For surgeons facing challenging cardiac reconstructions, an enhanced understanding of the biological/material properties of allografts and a broadening of the range of surgical techniques for which these are applicable, are the fundamental purposes of this book.

Richard A. Hopkins, MD
Spring 2004
Providence, RI

Acknowledgments

This work could not have been finished without the help of numerous people. First, the collaboration with Tom Xenakis, the illustrator, continues to be a superb intellectual exercise, and his contributions cannot be over emphasized. The clarity of his interpretation of the surgeon's manipulations is unparalleled. The 1989 allograft book garnered many compliments from colleagues on the beautiful artwork that always seemed to emphasize just the right points. The collaboration with scientists in my laboratory as well as others from around the world has been critical to furthering my own understanding of the biology of these tissues. Especially important to this process were my Georgetown PhD students who all are now accomplished surgeons: Drs. Messier, Domkowski, and Myers. Dr. Steven Hilbert and his colleague, Dr. Fred Schöen, have maintained the focus on the explant pathology of these tissues, which has contributed greatly to the understanding of allograft valve transplant biology by the surgical community. Dr. Hilbert has been a friend and colleague for 20 years and an astute collaborator, especially as we enter the era of bioengineered heart valves, the next phase of valve transplants. I acknowledge the skill and contribution of all of the surgical contributors. Many of the surgeon coauthors are members of the August Lunar Society for Congenital Cardiac Surgery, which has been a forum for the evolution of some of the techniques described. I am appreciative for the dedicated research collaboration with LifeNet, an institution of high integrity dedicated to saving lives with expertly procured and prepared tissues and organs, and especially the collegiality and professionalism of Perry Lange and Lloyd Wolfinbarger, PhD.

Dr. Arthur Bert is a cardiac anesthesiologist of world-class skill, whose superb care of our patients and talented interest in perioperative TEE for reconstructive cardiac surgical lesions has contributed greatly to the excellent outcomes enjoyed by our patients needing complex reconstructive cardiac surgery, and who's ability to image functioning allograft valves has been valuable clinically and in the laboratory.

Alan M. Gilstein and William H.D. Goddard co-chaired a cardiac fundraising campaign for our hospitals, Rhode Island Hospital, The

Miriam Hospital, and Hasbro Children's Hospital, which was remarkably and importantly successful; in appreciation, the hospitals have contributed in their names for which I now am doubly grateful for their support of our clinical and academic programs.

The family of Karl A. Karlson, MD and Gloria A. Karlson have endowed a Professorial Chair of Cardiac Surgery for Rhode Island Hospital and Brown University, in memory of their parents, which I currently, proudly, and humbly occupy. Their unselfish support for the academic commitment of the Division of Cardiac Surgery is a beautiful memorial to their father, who led the Division from 1971 to 1990, and to both parents who instilled values of respect for intellectual endeavor, service to others, integrity, philanthropy, and the virtue of lives committed to excellence.

The Roddy Foundation training grant has supported surgical resident scholars in cardiac research for seven years in the Collis Laboratory, each of whom has contributed to research reported in this volume during their tenure as Roddy Cardiac Surgical Research Scholars: Tao Hong, MD, PhD ((1998–1999), Mary Maish, MD (1999–2001), Roh Yanagida, MD (2001–2003) and Ara Ketchedjian, MD (2002–2004).

Charles and Ellen Collis have endowed the Cardiac Surgical Research Laboratory that now bears their name and which is dedicated to exploring bioengineering, biotechnology and molecular biological approaches to improved cardiac surgical solutions for our patients. The Collis laboratory research team has contributed to the success of our chronic sheep implant models, tissue culture, cell, and molecular biology of tissue engineered semilunar valves: Paula Krueger, Howard Lukoff, Gary Stearns, Jason Sousa, Elliot Robinson and Dr. James Harper, DVM.

The Children's Heart Foundation has supported portions of our heart valve basic science research from 1999 to 2002. The following companies have graciously contributed funds to defray part of the artwork costs which has enabled the publishing of this volumes affordable to the intended audience: Edwards Life Sciences LLC, Medtronic, Inc., St. Jude Medical, and Sulzer CarboMedics, Inc. I acknowledge with appreciation the ever cheerful and tireless work of our Cardiac Surgery Division Administrative Assistant, Susan Priore.

And finally, I thank my family, whose tolerance and support for many weekends and nights of work made this possible and to whom the book is dedicated.

Richard A. Hopkins, MD
Spring 2004
Providence, RI

Contents

Section XIII   Future Directions

Contributors

William W. Angell, MD
Clinical Associate Professor of Surgery, University of South Florida, Tampa, FL, USA

Robert H. Anderson, MD
Department of Surgery and Pediatrics, University of Alberta, Alberta, Canada

Erle H. Austin, III, MD
Professor of Surgery, University of Louisville, and Chief, Cardiovascular Surgery, Kosair Children's Hospital, Louisville, KY, USA

Arthur A. Bert, MD
Director of Cardiothoracic Anesthesia, Rhode Island Hospital, and Clinical Associate Professor of Anesthesiology, Brown University School of Medicine, Providence, RI, USA

Deborah A. Bishop, BS
Research Associate, Pediatric Cardiothoracic Surgery, The Children's Hospital, Denver, CO, USA

Ad Bogers, MD, PhD
Department of Thoracic Surgery, University Hospital Rotterdam, Rotterdam, The Netherlands

Scott Bottenfield, MD
Vice President for Tissue Services, LifeNet, Virginia Beach, VA, USA

J. Braun, MD
Department of Cardiothoracic Surgery, Leiden University Medical Center, Leiden, The Netherlands

Kelvin G.M. Brockbank, PhD
President, KGB Associates, Inc., Charleston, SC, USA

Scott A. Brubaker, CTBS
Director, Technical Training and Education, LifeNet, Virginia Beach, VA, USA

J.A. Bruin, MD
Department of Cardiothoracic Surgery, Leiden University Medical Center, Leiden, The Netherlands

David R. Clarke, MD
Professor of Surgery, University of Colorado Health Sciences Center, and Chairman, Pediatric Cardiothoracic Surgery, The Children's Hospital, Denver, CO, USA

A. Robert Cordell, MD
Professor of Cardiothoracic Surgery, The Bowman Gray School of Medicine, Winston-Salem, NC, USA

C.J. Cornelisse, PhD
Professor of Molecular Tumor Pathology, Department of Molecular Pathology, Leiden University Medical Center, Leiden, The Netherlands

Pedro J. del Nido, MD
Senior Associate in Cardiac Surgery, Children's Hospital, Boston, MA, USA

Margaret Deuel
Regulatory Affairs Manager, LifeNet, Virginia Beach, VA, USA

Patrick W. Domkowski, MD, PhD
Chief Resident, Surgical Training Program, Duke University School of Medicine, Durham, NC, USA

Kim F. Duncan, MD, MSc, JACS, FRCS(C)
Director, Cardiothoracic Surgery, Children's Hospital, Omaha, NE, USA

Victor J. Ferrans, MD, PhD
Pathology Section, National Heart, Lung and Blood Institute, National Institutes of Health, Bethesda, MD, USA

Y.A. Goffin, MD, PhD
Chief, European Homograft Bank, Brussels, Belgium

Frank L. Hanley, MD
Professor of Surgery and Cardiothoracic Surgery, University of California, and Chief, Cardiothoracic Surgery, Stanford University, Stanford, CA, USA

M.G. Hazekamp, MD, PhD
Chief of Pediatric Cardiac Surgery, Leiden University Medical Center, Leiden, The Netherlands

Stephen L. Hilbert, MD, PhD
Experimental Pathologist, Adjunct Professor of Surgery (Research),
Brown University School of Medicine, and Center for Devices and
Radiological Health, Office of Science and Technology, Food and Drug
Administration, Rockville, MD, USA

Franciska Hoekstra, MD
Department of Internal Medicine, University Hospital Rotterdam,
Rotterdam, The Netherlands

Diane Hoffman-Kim, PhD
Assistant Professor, Molecular Pharmacology, Physiology and
Biotechnology, Brown University School of Medicine, Providence,
RI, USA

Richard A. Hopkins, MD
Karl E. Karlson, MD, and Gloria A. Karlson, MD, Professor and Chief,
Cardiothoracic Surgery, Brown University School of Medicine; Cardiac
Surgeon-in-Chief, Rhode Island Hospital, The Miriam Hospital, and
Hasbro Childen's Hospital; and Director, Collis Cardiovascular
Research Laboratory, Providence, RI, USA

J.A. Huysmans, MD, PhD
Chief, Department of Cardiothoracic Surgery, Leiden University
Medical Center, Leiden, The Netherlands

James K. Kirklin, MD
Professor of Surgery, Director of Cardiothoracic Transplantation,
University of Alabama at Birmingham, Birmingham, AL, USA

Christiaan Knoop, Bsc
Department of Internal Medicine, University Hospital Rotterdam,
Rotterdam, The Netherlands

Neal D. Kon, MD
Associate Professor of Cardiothoracic Surgery, The Bowman Gray
School of Medicine, Winston-Salem, NC, USA

D.R. Koolbergen, MD
Department of Cardiothoracic Surgery, Leiden University Medical
Center, Leiden, The Netherlands

Perry L. Lange
Vice President, Cardiovascular Tissue Services, LifeNet, Virginia
Beach, VA, USA

R. Eric Lilly, MD
Assistant Professor, Cardiothoracic Surgery, Brown University School
of Medicine, Providence, RI, USA

Gary K. Lofland, MD
Professor of Surgery, Joseph Boon Gregg Chair, Section of Cardiac
Surgery, University of Missouri, and Chief, Cardiac Surgery, Children's
Mercy Hospital, Kansas City, MO, USA

Flavian M. Lupinetti, MD
Associate Professor of Surgery, Division of Cardiac Surgery, Children's
Hospital and Medical Center, Seattle, WA, USA

Scott F. MacKinnon, MD
Staff Anesthesiologist, Section of Cardiovascular Anesthesiology,
Rhode Island Hospital, Providence, RI, USA

Aubyn Marath, MBBS, MS, FRCSE
Department of Cardiothoracic Surgery, University of South Florida,
Tampa, FL, USA

Doff B. McElhinney, MS
Division of Cardiothoracic Surgery, University of California, San
Francisco, San Francisco, CA, USA

David C. McGiffin, MD
Associate Professor of Surgery, Director of Lung Transplantation,
Division of Cardiothoracic Surgery, University of Alabama at
Birmingham, Birmingham, AL, USA

Robert H. Messier, Jr., MD, PhD
Assistant Professor, Division of Cardiac Surgery, Duke University
School of Medicine, Durham, NC, USA

Jeff L. Myers, MD
Division of Cardiothoracic Surgery, Rainbow Babies and Children's
Hospital, Cleveland, OH, USA

John L. Myers, MD
Professor of Surgery and Pediatrics, Director, Pediatric and Congeni-
tal Cardiovascular Surgery Children's Hospital, Milton S. Hershey
Medical Center, Hershey, PA, USA

Thomas A. Orszulak, MD
Professor of Surgery, Mayo Medical School, Consultant, Division of
Cardiovascular Surgery, Mayo Clinic, Rochester, MN, USA

Patricia A. Penkoske, MD, FACC, FRCS(C)
Clinical Professor of Surgery, Cardiothoracic Surgery, St. Louis University, St. Louis, MO, USA

Ed Petrossian, MD
Division of Cardiothoracic Surgery, University of California, San
Francisco, San Francisco, CA, USA

V. Mohan Reddy, MD
Division of Cardiothoracic Surgery, University of California, San Francisco, San Francisco, CA, USA

Frederick J. Schöen, MD, PhD
Department of Pathology, Brigham and Women's Hospital, Harvard Medical School, Boston, MA, USA

Mila Stajevic-Popovic, MD, MA
Head of Department of Pediatric Cardiac Surgery, Mother and Child Health Institute of Serbia, New Belgrade, Yugoslavia

Jaroslav Stark, MD, FRCS, FACC, FACS
Consultant Cardiothoracic Surgeon, Great Ormond Street Hospital, National Health Service Trust, London, UK

James St. Louis, MD
Assistant Professor, Cardiothoracic Surgery, Brown University School of Medicine, Providence, RI, USA

Mark VanAllman, PhD
LifeNet, Virginia Beach, VA, USA

Robert B. Wallace, MD
Professor and Chairman Emeritus, Department of Surgery, Georgetown University, Washington, DC, USA

Willem Weimar, MD, PhD
Department of Internal Medicine, University Hospital Rotterdam, Rotterdam, The Netherlands

William G. Williams, MD, FRCSC
Head, Cardiac Surgery, Hospital for Sick Children; Staff Surgeon, The Toronto Hospital; Head, Cardiac Surgery, University of Toronto; and Professor, University of Toronto, Toronto, Canada

Lloyd Wolfinbarger, Jr., PhD
Director, Center for Biotechnology and Professor, Department of Biological Sciences, Old Dominion University, and Director, Research and Development, LifeNet, Virginia Beach, VA, USA

Section I
Original Principles

1
The Use of Homograft Valves: Historical Perspective

Richard A. Hopkins

In 1956 Gordon Murray reported the use of fresh aortic valve homografts transplanted into the descending thoracic aorta for amelioration of the consequences of native aortic valve insufficiency. His initial operations preceded by 5 years the availability of the Starr-Edwards mechanical aortic valve prosthesis.[1-7] Although this operation was only partially successful hemodynamically, the homograft valves had remarkable durability and performance. Four patients cited by Heimbecker had no calcification or gradient, with normal leaflet function for up to 13 years, and two patients continued to demonstrate excellent valve function for up to 20 years. Kerwin's subsequent reports support the contention that aortic leaflet homograft pliability and performance were well preserved in these early patients.[8] These clinical trials were preceded by laboratory investigations, especially that of Lam and coworkers.[9] Hemodynamic improvements were demonstrated in both stenotic and regurgitant aortic valve disease by the various early methods of reconstructing diseased aortic valves, and the results ultimately obtained with replacement utilizing the Starr-Edwards and other prostheses supported replacement treatment for ventricular outflow valvular disease, with excellent result continuing to be reported today with both mechanical and bioprosthetic valves.[10]

Professor Gunning has cited an unsuccessful operation in 1961 by Drs. Bigelow and Heimbecker as the first clinical insertion of an aortic valve homograft in the orthotopic position,[11] but the first operation with the patient surviving was by Ross, based on laboratory work reported in 1956 by Brewin.[12] In 1962, the initial clinical use of aortic valve homografts was reported independently by Donald Ross of England and Sir Brian Barratt-Boyes of New Zealand.[13-15] Duran and Gunning developed a technique in the laboratory for implanting the aortic valve homograft utilizing a single running suture line technique.[16] Interestingly, the initial homograft valve transplants were performed utilizing freshly harvested valves minimally treated and inserted into the orthotopic position relatively quickly after harvest with no attempt at ABO Blood group matching. These initial valves had remarkable performance and durability and gave great impetus to the early workers pursuing this method of aortic valve replacement.

Limitation of donor availability led to preservation attempts to increase storage time and to establish homograft valve "banks." Storage techniques included freeze-drying and antibiotic sterilization with prolonged refrigeration at 4°C. Concerns about transmission of infection led to aggressive sterilization techniques, including multiple antibiotic incubation, irradiation, and glutaraldehyde pretreatment. Unfortunately, although they increased the availability, these techniques resulted in shortened functional survival of homograft valves and caused significant disenchantment with the technique during the 1960s and early 1970s.[17]

It is the purpose of this chapter to examine in detail the earlier experiences with valve homografts and to elucidate valuable lessons pertinent to valve transplantation today.

Early Homograft Work

In 1952 Lam and his associates demonstrated that it was technically possible to transplant canine aortic valve homografts into the descending aorta of a recipient animal; however, if the cusps were not "used" and were constantly in the open position, they deteriorated. If aortic insufficiency was induced in the recipient dog, thereby "forcing" the transplanted valve to function, valve integrity was greatly enhanced.[9] This fascinating study has relevance today and was the basis on which Murray and others developed the technique for clinical use. The studies of Heimbecker and colleagues demonstrated that treatment with gamma radiation or ß-propiolactone markedly diminished the durability of transplanted homograft valves.[5] The use of radiation was confirmed by others as having deleterious effects and has been completely abandoned.[18]

Flash freezing was one of the harsher preservation methods tested, but it resulted in poor clinical results and laboratory evidence of damage to the elastic properties of the native valves.[19] Other groups found great difficulties in the durability of frozen irradiated aortic valve homografts and advised against their use because of the increased failure rates beginning around the fifth to sixth postoperative year.[20] Patient valve survival was in the 50% range at 7 years, which was equivalent to contemporaneous series of xenograft and mechanical prosthetic replacements performed during the mid-1970s.[21,22] Apart from patient survival, durability of valves prepared with the harsher methods was markedly inferior to mechanical valve replacements.

Fresh Wet-Stored Homograft Valves

During the late 1970s attention turned to the use of fresh aortic allografts in which cadaveric valves were harvested with variable ischemic times and then antibiotic-sterilized and stored at 4°C in nutrient media. Although donor cellular viability was probably not preserved, these gentler techniques improved valve and patient survival. The contrast between the use of exceedingly fresh valve tissue for transplant and the use of harsh chemical sterilization or storage techniques was stark, and thus the larger experience has been gained with the relatively gentler methods of storage: antibiotic-sterilized, "fresh wet-stored" valves.

A number of series have been reported that demonstrated good medium-term (7–10 years) results with the wet-storage technique.[23–27] Ross' group from the National Heart Hospital (London) in 1980 reported on 615 valves followed for up to 15 years, including 145 freeze-dried homografts, and 179 pulmonary autografts. The study clearly demonstrated the superiority of the autografts and fresh homografts; there were excellent clinical results with up to 90% of patients free of valve-related death at 10 years.[28] Others have also reported good results with the pulmonary autograft transplant to the aortic position.[29]

The Stanford series of 114 patients receiving fresh aortic homografts between March 1967 and March 1971 revealed ten operative deaths (8.8%): six deaths during the first year (5.8%) and then a mortality rate of 1.5% per year. Of the late deaths, only six were due to valve dysfunction, whereas 12 were due to other cardiac causes. A total of 3.2% of patients per year required re-replacement for regurgitation ($n = 20$), and only one valve developed calcific stenosis. Of 53 patients followed for 5 years or more, 47 had minimal or no disability.[24] In 1986 the Stanford group reexamined 83 patients of this original series such that 773 patient-years of follow-up were available with a maximum to 19 years.[30] For this subgroup the calculated actuarial estimate of freedom from all modes of valve failure was 83 ± 4% at 5 years, 62 ± 6% at 10 years, and 43 ± 7% at 15 years; 92 ± 3% of patients were free from endocarditis at 8 years after operation. Freedom from reoperation was 88 ± 4% at 5 years, 67 ± 6% at 10 years, and 45 ± 7% at 15 years. Interestingly, 94 ± 3% of patients were free of valve-related deaths

5 years following surgery.[25] Thus satisfactory results were achieved with the wet-stored homografts inserted with the freehand technique and were comparable to or slightly better than results with xenografts.[26]

Another pioneer in the use of allografts has been Yacoub and his group in Harefield, England, who summarized their experience in 1979–1980.[26,31,32] The homografts were procured and prepared similarly to the fresh wet-stored and antibiotic-sterilized protocol of Ross at the National Heart Hospital, with a storage time of 1–42 days, with most being used within 1 week of procurement. Yacoub's group has accepted the concept that the freshest valves function best. This remarkable series of 679 patients demonstrated a 3.9% perioperative mortality rate and actuarial patient survival rates of 87% (5 years) and 81% (8 years). Importantly, these authors noted the superb hydraulic performance of these valves, even in the smaller sizes, and suggested that they "provide almost ideal hemodynamic characteristics."[32,33]

In 1984 the Harefield group published a 10- to 13-year follow-up (mean 11 years) of 140 of their aortic valve replacements with fresh wet-stored homografts.[28] This series demonstrated 71.6% freedom from valve failure at 10 years. Valve degeneration occurred in 19.3% and endocarditis in 6.4%. In this series older age of recipient and prolonged warm ischemia time at procurement (interval between death and dissection of the homograft) were correlated with increased risk for valve degeneration ($p > 0.01$). This series had a slightly higher incidence of subacute bacterial endocarditis (SBE) than other contemporaneous homograft experiences and a significant valve degeneration rate that gradually increased from 0.8% at 3 years to 5.2% at 10 years. Patient survival (65% at 10 years) compared favorably with the 10-year survival of a classic mechanical series with Starr-Edwards valves (56%).[28,34]

Yacoub's group has also reported a very interesting analysis of reoperations for aortic valve replacement indicating that not only were better results obtained with homografts (70% freedom from valve-related deaths or reoperations at 10 years following reoperation

with homograft AVR), but the very best results were when homografts were used to replace previously inserted homografts with a probability of patient survival at 15 years of 85% ± 5% following the second homograft insertion.[35]

Prosthetic Valve Disease

With the development of the Starr and subsequent models and types of valves, prosthetic valvular disease has been substituted for native valve dysfunction despite the demonstration that patient survival is far superior with treated valve disease when indicators for surgical correction are observed.[27] The controversy of mechanical versus xenograft valves has generated a vast literature, but for adults it can be summarized as follows: Lumping morbidity/mortality and prosthetic durability together, there is an advantage for xenografts over mechanical valves for the first 5 years following replacement, but thereafter the mechanical valves' greater durability confers an advantage.[36] Specifics such as the age of the patient and valve location, e.g., left versus right ventricular outflows versus atrioventricular (AV) valve location, can favor various types or models, and the "trade-offs" of durability versus morbidity must be carefully evaluated clinically[37] (see Chapter 64 for *contemporary valve comparisons*).

Hydraulic dysfunction, to a critical degree, can occur when a small mechanical prosthesis is inserted into a small aortic annulus. This results in high gradients that worsen with exercise and result in elevated perioperative mortality rates.[38,39] Schaff and colleagues have suggested that a 19 mm Bjork-Shiley valve has satisfactory hemodynamics,[40] but otherwise most authorities recommend against placing a mechanical valve smaller than 21 mm. Valvuloplasty has not been a frequently applicable alternate solution.[41] Porcine-pericardial prostheses have the advantage of reducing the need for anticoagulation, but hydraulic performance is still limited in the smaller sizes.[42] Recent studies suggest progressive improvement in ventricular performance associated with geometric remodeling when very low gradient valves are used for reconstructions (stentless valves or allografts).

The related problems of thromboembolism and anticoagulation complications are a tremendous factor in late complications following treatment of aortic valve disease in both children and adults. After cardiac failure, thromboembolism is the leading cause of death following aortic valve replacement.[38] Potential fatal anticoagulation and complications occur at a rate of approximately 1% to 5% per year.[43]

The rapidity of calcific degeneration of xenografts in young adults has been emphasized by a number of investigators. Classical teaching has been to recommend implanting mechanical prostheses in patients younger than 60 years.[44–48] Valve replacement in children presents even greater difficulties.[49] Mechanical valves in children are associated with anticoagulation complications and hemodynamic dysfunction.[50–53] The introduction of xenograft tissue valves resulted in their enthusiastic use in young patients in the hope of avoiding anticoagulation. Their use was soon followed by widely reported high early mid-term failure rates as a consequence of calcification.[54–62] Annulus size constraints and the unsuitability of bioprostheses resulted in techniques to enlarge the aortic root, thereby allowing placement of a large mechanical prosthesis in children with aortic stenosis.[57,63] However, this solution accepts the complications associated with mechanical valves.[64] Homografts offer some solutions and improvements for the problem of prosthetic valvular disease: (1) better hydraulic performance; (2) reduced thromboembolic complications; (3) resistance to endocarditis; and (4) acceptable to superior valve durability.

The two clinical originators of the orthotopic homograft aortic valve replacement, Ross and Barratt-Boyes, have maintained a strong commitment to its use. In multiple publications their two centers have shared much of the developing knowledge. Their series warrant special attention for the many lessons on the use of "fresh wet/cold-stored" homografts.

London Homografts

Ross and colleagues have produced a number of reports over the past 20 years on the evolution of their results and techniques with aortic valve homografts.[13,21,65–70] In 1979 their group reported an 89% graft survival in the aortic position at 6 years for fresh antibiotic-sterilized allografts.[65] In this same series the frozen allograft survival rate at 6 years was reported at 79%. Although they did not claim persistent cellular viability in any of these valves, they were able to show valve functional survival far exceeding the actual native cell survival.

Although the London preservation techniques have been various over the years, the predominant one has been fresh antibiotic-sterilized valves stored at 4°C. On the basis of tritiated thymidine studies of fibroblast viability, Ross' group has shown that no donor fibroblasts are viable after 600 days in the patient when wet-stored homografts are used. Although "fresh" wet-stored homografts can appear histologically and by some metabolic tests to possess cellular viability, those that are stored for more than a few days are most likely not viable months after implantation.[71,72] Ross and coworkers have shown that valve survival following implantation is better in right-sided reconstructions than left-sided ones but that the survival has not been particularly affected by storage times or warm ischemia times.[73] This finding is not surprising, as a wet-stored valve for 6 days is probably ultimately just as nonviable as one stored for 26 days.[74] Utilizing their methods of storage and harvesting, which often included a relatively long warm ischemia time, with cadaveric recovery being delayed for up to 24–48 hours, there was only a 23 ± 6% rate of valve survival at 15 years and a rate of 50% at 12 years.[73] In their hands, this method has produced better results than those seen with prosthetic valves. Patient survival, however, has been markedly superior to valve survival, with the former averaging 75% at 15 years.

The hypothesis that cellular viability at the time of implantation is related to prolonged optimal function is suggested by the unique series of autologous transplants by Ross and colleagues.[75,76] This series demonstrated an 82% actuarial survival of the allograft valve at 14 years and an $81 \pm 5\%$ event-free survival of the concomitantly implanted aortic homograft in the right ventricular outflow tract.[69,75] However, this hypothesis assumes that viable donor and recipient cells respond similarly—an unlikely biological outcome. A subsequent study by Ross' group comparing homografts and autografts has again suggested better long-term performance by the autograft,[35] which could also be related to immunologic issues rather than peri-transplant viability.

During the early years of homograft valve use, technical factors were noted to play a significant role in early valve failure, e.g., dehiscence, prolapse, tears, and perforations.[77] The critical importance of such surgical techniques as the careful two-suture freehand technique and attention to ensuring commissural post suspension for semilunar cusp function were determined.[78]

New Zealand Homografts

The New Zealand group headed by Barratt-Boyes summarized their experience in a selected series of 252 isolated aortic homograft valve replacements with a 9- to 16.5-year follow-up (mean 10.8 years), which represents perhaps the classic summary of the fresh wet-storage era.[79] These valves were all inserted with the original freehand "subcoronary" technique. All of the valves were sterilized in antibiotic solution, stored in nutrient media at 4°C, and considered nonviable.

The results of this New Zealand series are exemplary. Their careful analysis of one of the most important series in the world has many nuggets of information. First, the results are superb, with only 20 valve-related deaths (8.4%) of which eight were due to endocarditis, seven to cusp rupture, and five to incompetence resulting in reoperation and death. Actuarial analysis demonstrated freedom from significant incompetence to be 95% at 5 years, 78% at 10 years, and 42% at 14 years. Factors increasing the risk of significant incompetence due to valve deterioration were donor valve age greater than 55 years, a young recipient age, and aortic root diameters over 30 mm. Poor results with chemical sterilization were noted by the group. Overall actuarial survival was 77% at 5 years, 57% at 10 years, and 38% at 14 years. These results are comparable to same era results with xenograft or mechanical prostheses series.

It is of note that when aortic insufficiency developed it usually progressed slowly, allowing elective reoperation for replacement at low risk of mortality. No specific embolism was proved to have originated from the valve. No stenosis occurred in any of the valves, and the authors had no difficulties with hemodynamic performance in the small valve sizes (17–19 mm). The development of aortic insufficiency was rarely due to rupture, more often being caused by either technical problems at the time of insertion, progressive dilation of an aortic root, central incompetence due to improper commissural suspension, allograft degeneration, or bacterial endocarditis.[79]

Interestingly, Barratt-Boyes and his group did not find increased valve failure related to older recipient age, longer valve salvage times (warm ischemia time), or insertion into an aortic root afflicted with stenotic disease. The New Zealand group thus recommended this valve as the valve of choice for virtually all patients and suggested the following donor characteristics: age less than 50 years, aortic valve internal diameter (ID) of 28 mm or less, a valve free of imperfections, and a valve stored no longer than 50 days when wet-stored at 4°C.[79] They believed that allografts are particularly valuable in women of childbearing age, patients unsuitable for anticoagulation, and those with small aortic roots. The resistance to endocarditis by the homograft valve, whatever its method of preservation, has been consistent in all series; although not absolute, it is most marked during the postoperative period when compared to mechanical prostheses. Risk-hazard analysis demonstrated much lower risk of prosthetic endocarditis in these valves, especially during the early postoperative phase.[80] Their listed contraindications to its use were the presence of an aortic root aneurysm, aortic root dilatation due to diffuse medial disease, cystic medial necrosis, and aortic root dilation not amenable to aortic root tailoring (see Chapter 8).[79]

Right Ventricular Outflow Tract Reconstructions

In contrast to the merely "quite good" results in the more stressful aortic position, the nonviable aortic homograft has been used with "superb" results for reconstruction of the right ventricular outflow tract, particularly in children, beginning in 1966.[81,82]

Conduit surgery revolutionized the repairs of complex congenital cardiac defects; the ability to anatomically rebuild ventricular outflow tracts has allowed repair of lesions previously not amenable to surgery.[83–89] Unfortunately, conduit malfunction has been a frustratingly frequent occurrence following initial operative successes with synthetic prostheses and is associated with significant morbidity and mortality.[90] Conduit malfunction has been due to calcification and degeneration of the xenograft valve, peel formation within the Dacron tube, and thromboembolic occurrences.[90] Hancock valve replacement in children has an optimal calculated re-replacement of 7% per year, which suggests the projected probability of a Hancock valve remaining replacement-free to be only 50% at 5 years.[58] The Stanford group reported similar pessimistic durability in studies of porcine xenografts when used as intracardiac xenografts or conduits; their linearized reoperation rates were 10% and 4% per patient-year, respectively; the rate of valve failure due to leaflet fibrocalcification was 8% per patient-year.[59] The Mayo Clinic, Toronto group, and investigators at other major centers have found that the porcine valve containing conduits fail relatively rapidly owing to both conduit peel and cumulative valve degeneration.[64] In a study from The Hospital for Sick Children (London), in which the mean age of the patients was 6.5 years, only 27% of the xenograft bioprostheses did *not* require replacement by the fifth year.[91]

One of the synthetic conduit series with representative results comes from Boston, where 201 children underwent reconstructions of the right ventricular outflow tract with porcine valve-tightly woven Dacron conduits.[92] Actuarial patient survival of perioperative survivors was 83% at 8 years. Valve durability was actuarially reported, 50% of patients being valve-replacement-free at 8 years; however, most of the late complications in these patients were due to *valve conduit* problems. Analysis suggested zero durability after 10 years.[92]

In contrast, Fontan and associates, on the basis of 103 aortic valve homograft implantations in children with complex congenital heart disease since 1968, postulated an expected graft valve survival rate of 10–15 years. Their data demonstrated an actuarial survival of 80% at 9 years.[93] The Great Ormond Street group has also demonstrated that the antibiotic-sterilized, wet-stored homografts have good durability; in 65 patients with a mean age of 6.5 years, there was 85% homograft valve survival at 5 years and 75% valve survival at 9 years.[94] Although the aortic wall calcifies with time, the valve leaflet tissue of the homografts appear to remain pliable without stenosis.[23,94–96] Kay and Ross have reported a 13% replacement (for obstruction) rate at 10 years.[97] These results with fresh antibiotic-sterilized aortic homografts contrast markedly with results with irradiated or otherwise harshly preserved homograft conduits.[17,98,99] The homograft is now the prosthesis of choice for right ventricular outflow tract reconstructions, especially for children.[73] In the latest report from Great Ormond Street on 249 right ventricular outflow tract reconstructions (72 with aortic homografts from Ross' bank at the National Heart Hospital), homograft obstructions have occurred but seemed to have often been related to the concomitant use of Dacron tubes and extensions: Only one of 29 homografts implanted without Dacron became stenotic.[100] The more common mode of failure appears to be the gradual development of insufficiency, which allows leisurely elective replacement. Immune factors may play a role in calcification of the aortic wall.[71,72,101,102]

Summary

Beginning in 1962 there have been four eras related to method of procurement, sterilization, and storage of aortic valve homografts. During the first era, *fresh aseptic harvesting with immediate transplantation* (within hours or a few days—"fresh fresh") was the rule. This method appears to have given excellent results, both initially and in terms of long-term durability. The second era consisted of a *clean harvest with harsh sterilization and storage techniques*, clearly resulting in poor durability. The third era of *clean harvest with gentle antibiotic sterilization and wet 4°C storage* for up to 6 weeks ("fresh wet-stored"), thereby preparing "nonviable" aortic homografts has had the most extensive experience with good results. The fourth technique, which is introduced in Chapter 8, involves *aseptic harvest with a short warm ischemia time, gentle antibiotic sterilization, and cryopreservation* with liquid nitrogen storage utilizing cryoprotectants ("cryopreserved").[102]

The results chronicled in this "historical" chapter relate to homografts implanted without cryopreservation. Many relevant lessons have been learned and a number of advantages of fresh wet-stored homograft valves determined.

1. These valves provide optimal hydraulic function with central nonobstructive flow resulting in excellent hemodynamic performance even in small sizes; thus a large, effective valve for a small recipient annulus can be achieved as a consequence of optimal hemodynamics.[26,31,32]
2. Thromboembolism and hemolysis rates are reduced despite no anticoagulation.
3. It is a relatively simple surgical implant.
4. Calcification rarely affects the leaflets.
5. Resistance to endocarditis is enhanced.[99]

As Kirklin and Barratt-Boyes have discussed, although there are multiple causes for prosthesis-related late deaths following aortic valve replacements, only two are relevant to homograft aortic valve replacement: incompetence and endocarditis.[99] When early technical failures are avoided and appropriate donor and recipient criteria are followed, incompetence is not an early homograft problem. Valve failure does not equate with patient mortality, the latter being far superior to that reported for most other prostheses series at medium term.

The surgical lessons from the fresh wet-storage era fall into three categories.

1. "Freehand" surgical technique must account for semilunar valve functional anatomy, thereby avoiding early technical failures, with attention to the following:
   a. Accurate sizing.
   b. Effective commissural post suspension—important for retaining semilunar function.
   c. "Normalized" aortic root geometry.
   d. Careful trimming of the allograft.
   e. Seating of the annulus without deformation.
2. Factors that have been found to lead to *decreased* durability of homografts:[81]
   a. Older donor age.
   b. Dilated aortic root (unless corrected by aortoplasty).
   c. Recipient aortic root disease, e.g., Marfan's syndrome and cystic medial necrosis.
   d. Recipient collagen vascular or immune-related diseases (e.g. rheumatoid arthritis, lupus, etc).
   e. Technically imperfect implant, causing turbulent flows.
   f. Prolonged storage of wet-stored allografts prior to use.
   g. Harsh sterilization, harvesting, or preservation techniques.
3. Conduct of aortic valve surgery has improved results of all types of aortic valve replacements and includes attention to the following.[27]
   a. Cardioplegia-myocardial protection.
   b. Coronary artery disease.
   c. Shorter cross-clamp times.
   d. Intra-operative transesophageal echocardiography.

These lessons continue to be relevant, and their applications are discussed in detail in the appropriate chapters of this book. Results of the antibiotic-sterilization/wet-storage era of homograft valve transplants proved that homografts were an important alternative with distinct advantages for certain subgroups of patients needing valve replacement.

References

1. Murray G. Homologous aortic valve segment transplants as surgical treatment for aortic and mitral insufficiency. Angiology 1956;7:466–471.
2. Murray G. Aortic valve transplants. Angiology 1960;11:99–102.
3. Daenen W. Repair of complex left ventricular outflow tract obstruction with a pulmonary autograft. J Heart Valve Dis 1995;4:364–367.
4. Heimbecker RO. The homograft cardiac valve. In Marendino KA (ed). Prosthetic valves for Cardiac Surgery. Springfield, IL; Charles C. Thomas;1961:157–159.
5. Heimbecker RO, Aldrige HE, Lemire G. The durability and fate of aortic valve grafts. An experimental study with a long term follow-up of clinical patients. J Cardiovasc Surg (Torino) 1968;9:511–517.
6. Heimbecker RO. Whither the homograft valve? Ann Thorac Surg 1970;9:487–488.
7. Heimbecker RO. Durability of fresh homograft. Ann Thorac Surg 1986;42:602–603.
8. Kerwin AG, Lenkei SC, Wilson DR. Aortic valve homograft in the treatment for aortic and mitral insufficiency. N Eng J Med 1962;266:852–857.
9. Lam CR, Aram HH, Mennell ER. An experimental study of aortic valve homografts. Surg Gynecol Obstet 1952;94:129–135.
10. Borkon A, Soule LM, Baughman KL, et al. Comparative analysis of mechanical and bioprosthetic valves after aortic valve replacement. J Thorac Cardiovasc Surg 1987;94:20–33.
11. Gunning A. Comments on Ross' first homograft replacement of the aortic valve (letter to the editor). Ann Thorac Surg 1992;54:809–810.
12. Brewin EG. The use of tissue transplants in the surgery of cardiac valve disease—an experimental study. Guy's Hospital Reports 1956; 105:328–329.
13. Ross DN. Homograft replacement of the aortic valve. Lancet 1962;2:487.
14. Hopkins RA, St. Louis J, Corcoran PC. Ross' first homograft replacement of the aortic valve. Ann Thorac Surg 1991;52:1190–1193.
15. Barratt-Boyes BG. Homograft aortic valve replacement in aortic incompetence and stenosis. Thorax 1964;19:131–150.
16. Barratt-Boyes BG. A method for preparing and inserting a homograft aortic valve. Br J Surg 1965;52:847–856.
17. Merin G, McGoon DC. Reoperation after insertion of aortic homograft-right ventricular outflow tract. Ann Thorac Surg 1973;16:122–126.
18. Malm JR, Bowman FO, Jr., Harris PD, Kowalik AT. An evaluation of aortic valve homografts sterilized by electron beam energy. J Thorac Cardiovasc Surg 1967;54:471–477.
19. Parker R, Nandakumaran K, Al-Janabi N, Ross DN. Elasticity of frozen aortic valve homografts. Cardiovasc Res 1977;11:156–159.
20. Beach PM, Jr., Bowman FO, Jr., Kaiser GA, Malm JR. Frozen irradiated aortic valve homografts. Long-term evaluation. N Y State J Med 1973;73:651–654.
21. Wain WH, Greco R, Ignegeri A, Bodnar E, Ross DN. 15 years experience with 615 homograft and autograft aortic valve replacements. Int J Artif Organs 1980;3:169–172.
22. Barratt-Boyes BG, Roche AHG, Whitlock RML. Six year review of the results of freehand aortic valve replacement using an antibiotic sterilized homograft valve. Circulation 1977;55: 353–361.
23. Saravalli OA, Somerville J, Jefferson KE. Calcification of aortic homografts used for reconstruction of the right ventricular outflow tract. J Thorac Cardiovasc Surg 1980;80:909–920.
24. Anderson ET, Hancock EW. Long-term follow-up of aortic valve replacement with the fresh aortic homograft. J Thorac Cardiovasc Surg 1976;72:150–156.
25. Barratt-Boyes BG. Cardiothoracic surgery in the antipodes. J Thor Cardiovasc Surg 1979;78: 804–822.
26. Thompson R, Yacoub M, Ahmed M, Somerville W, Towers M. The use of "fresh" unstented homograft valves for replacement of the aortic valve. J Thorac Cardiovasc Surg 1980;79:896–903.
27. Selzer A. Changing aspects of the natural history of valvular aortic stenosis. N Engl J Med 1987;317:91–98.
28. Penta A, Qureshi S, Radley-Smith R, Yacoub MH. Patient status 10 or more years after 'fresh' homograft replacement of the aortic valve. Circulation 1984;70:I182–I186.
29. Stelzer P, Elkins RC. Pulmonary autograft: An American experience. J Carciac Surg 1987;2: 429–433.

30. Miller DC, Shumway NE. "Fresh" aortic allografts: long-term results with free-hand aortic valve replacement. J Card Surg 1987;2:185–191.

31. Thompson R, Ahmed M, Seabra-Gomes R, Ilsley C, Rickards A, Towers M, Yacoub M. Influence of preoperative left ventricular function on results of homograft replacement of the aortic valve for aortic regurgitation. J Thorac Cardiovasc Surg 1979;77:411–421.

32. Thompson R, Yacoub M, Ahmed M, Seabra-Gomes R, Rickards A, Towers M. Influence of preoperative left ventricular function on results of homograft replacement of the aortic valve for aortic stenosis. Am J Cardiol 1979;43:929–938.

33. Ross D, Yacoub MH. Homograft replacement of the aortic valve. A critical review. Prog Cardiovasc Dis 1969;11:275–293.

34. Teply JF, Grunkemeier GL, D'Arch SH, et al. The ultimate prognosis after valve replacement: An assessment of twenty years. Ann Thorac Surg 1981;32:111–119.

35. Albertucci M, Wong K, Petrou M, Mitchell A, Somerville J, Theodoropoulos S, Yacoub M. The use of unstented homograft valves for aortic valve reoperations. J Thorac and Cardiovasc Surg 1994;107:152–161.

36. Hammond GL, Geha AS, Kopf GS, Hashim SW. Biological versus mechanical valves: analysis of 1,116 valves inserted in 1,012 adult patients with a 4,818 patient-year and 5,327 valve-year follow up. J Thorac Cardiovasc Surg 1987;93:182–198.

37. Schoen FJ. Cardiac valve prostheses: pathological and bioengineering considerations. J Cardiac Surg 1987;2:65–108.

38. Dale J, Levang O, Eng I. Long-term results after aortic valve replacement with four different prostheses. Amer Heart J 1980;99:155–162.

39. Bjork VO, Henze A, Homgren A. Five years' experience with the Bjork-Shiley tilting-disc valve in isolated aortic valvular disease. J Thorac Cardiovasc Surg 1974;68:393–404.

40. Schaff HV, Borkon AM, Hughes C, et al. Clinical and hemodynamic evaluation of the 19-mm Bjork-Shiley aortic valve prosthesis. Ann Thorac Surg 1981;32:50–57.

41. Mindich BP, Guarino T, Goldman ME. Aortic valvuloplasty for acquired aortic stenosis. Circulation 1986;74:I130–I135.

42. Yoganathan AP, Woo YR, Sung HW, et al. In vitro hemodynamic characteristics of tissue bioprostheses in the aortic positon. J Thorac Cardiovasc Surg 1986;92:198–209.

43. Horst-Kotte D, Korfer R, Seipel L, et al. Late complications in patients with Bjork-Shiley and St. Jude Medical Heart Valve replacements. Circulation 1983;68:II175-II184.

44. Gabbay S, Frater RWM. In vitro comparison of the newer heart valve bioprostheses in the mitral and aortic position. In Cohn LH, Gallucci V (eds). Cardiac Prostheses. New York: Yorke; 1982:457–468.

45. Villani M, Bianchi T, Vanini V, et al. Bioprosthetic valve replacement in children. In Cohn L, Gallucci V (eds). Cardiac Bioprostheses. New York: Yorke Medical Books;1982:248–255.

46. Carpentier A, Dubost C, Lane E, et al. Continuing improvements in valvular bioprostheses. J Thorac Cardiovasc Surg 1982;83:27–42.

47. Magilligan DJ, Lewis JW, Tilley B, Peterson E. The porcine bioprosthetic valve. J Thorac Cardiovasc Surg 1985;89:499–507.

48. Schaff HV, Danielson GK, DiDonato RM, et al. Late results after Starr-Edwards valve replacement in children. J Thorac Cardiovasc Surg 1984;88:583–589.

49. Milano A, Vouhe PR, Baillot-Vernant F, et al. Late results after left-sided cardiac valve replacement in children. J Thorac Cardiovasc Surg 1986;92:218–225.

50. Sade RM, Ballenger JF, Hohn HR, et al. Cardiac valve replacement in children. J Thoracic Cardiovasc Surg 1979;78:123–127.

51. William WG, Pollock JC, Geiss DM, et al. Experience with aortic and mitral valve replacement in children. J Thorac Cardiovasc Surg 1981;81:326–333.

52. Mathews RA, Park SC, Neches WH, et al. Valve replacement in children and adolescents. J Thorac Cardiovasc Surg 1977;73:872–876.

53. Klint R, Hernandez A, Weldon C, et al. Replacement of cardiac valves in children. J Pediatr 1972;80:980.

54. Berry BE, Ritter DG, Wallace RB, McGoon DC, Danielson GK. Cardiac valve replacement in children. J Thorac Cardiovasc Surg 1974;68:705–710.

55. Geha AS, Laks H, Stensel HC, et al. Late failure of porcine valve heterografts in children. J Thorac Cardiovasc Surg 1979;78:351–364.

56. Gardner TJ, Roland JMA, Neill CA, Donahoo JS. Valve replacement in children. J Thorac Cardiovasc Surg 1982;83:178–185.

57. Manouguian S, Seybold-Epting W. Patch enlargement of the aortic valve ring by extending the aortic incision into the anterior mitral

leaflet. J Thorac Cardiovasc Surg 1979;78:402–412.

58. Williams DB, Danielson GK, McGoon DC, et al. Porcine heterograft valve replacement in children. J Thorac Cardiovasc Surg 1982;84:446–450.

59. Miller DC, Stinson EB, Oyer PE, et al. The durability of porcine xenograft valves and conduits in children. Circulation 1982;66:172–185.

60. Silver MM, Pollock J, Silver MD, et al. Calcification in porcine xenograft valves in children. Am J Cardiol 1980;45:685–688.

61. Dunn JM. Porcine valve durability in children. Ann Thorac Surg 1981;32:357–368.

62. Odell JA. Calcification of porcine bioprostheses in children. In Cohn LH, Gallucci V (eds). Cardiac Bioprostheses. New York: Yorke;1982:231–237.

63. Konno S, Iai I, Iida Y, et al. A new method for prosthetic valve replacement in congenital aortic stenosis associated with hypoplasia of the aortic valve ring. J Thorac Cardiovasc Surg 1976;70:909–917.

64. Williams WG, Pollock LC, Geiss DM, et al. Experience with aortic and mitral valve replacement in children. J Thorac Cardiovasc Surg 1981;81:326–333.

65. Ross DN, Martelli V, Wain WH. Allograft and autograft valves used for aortic valve replacement. In Ionescu MI (ed). Tissue Heart Valves. Boston: Butterworth;1979:127–172.

66. Al-Janabi N, Ross DN. Long-term preservation of fresh viable aortic valve homografts by freezing. Br J Surg 1974;61:229–232.

67. Khanna SK, Ross JK, Monro JL. Homograft aortic valve replacement: seven years' experience with antibiotic-treated valves. Thorax 1981;36(5):330–337.

68. Wain WH, Pearce HM, Riddell RW, Ross DN. A re-evaluation of the antibiotic sterilization of heart valve allografts. Thorax 1977;32:740–742.

69. Bodnar E, Wain WH, Martelli V, Ross DN. Long-term performance of homograft and autograft valves. Artif Organs 1980;4:20–23.

70. Ashwood-Smith MJ, Farrant J. Low Temperature Preservation in Medicine and Biology. London: Pitman;1980.

71. Livi U, Abdulla AK, Parker R, Olsen EJ, Ross DN. Viablility and morphology of aortic and pulmonary homografts. J Thorac Cardiovasc Surg 1987;93:755–760.

72. Yankah AC, Wottge HU, Muller-Hermelink HK, Feller AC, Lange P, Wessel U, Dreyer H, Bernhard A, Müller-Ruchholtz W. Transplantation of aortic and pulmonary allografts, enhanced viability of endothelial cells by cryopreservation, importance of histocompatibility. J Card Surg 1987;2:209–220.

73. Ross DN. Application of homografts in clinical surgery. J Card Surg 1987;2:175–183.

74. Bodnar A, Ross DN. Mode of failure in 226 explanted biologic and bioprosthetic valves. In Cohn LH, Gallucci V (eds). Cardiac Bioprostheses. New York: Yorke;1982:401–407.

75. Ross DN. Replacement of the aortic and mitral valve with a pulmonary valve autograft. Lancet 1967;2:956–958.

76. Robles A, Vaughan M, Lau JK, et al. Long-Term assessment of aortic valve replacement with autologous pulmonary valve. Ann Thorac Surg 1985;39:238–242.

77. Lefrak EA, Starr A. Aortic Valve Homograft In Cardiac Valve Prosthesis. New York: Appleton-Century-Crofts;1979:283–300.

78. Moore CH, Martelli V, Al-Janabi N, Ross DN. Analysis of homograft valve failure in 311 patients followed up to 10 years. Ann Thorac Surg 1975;20:274–281.

79. Barratt-Boyes BG, Roche AH, Subramanyan R, Pemberton JR, Whitlock RM. Long-term follow-up of patients with the antibiotic-sterilized aortic homograft valve inserted free-hand in the aortic position. Circulation 1987;75:768–777.

80. Kirklin JW, Barratt-Boyes BG. Aortic valve disease. In Kirklin JW, Barratt-Boyes BG (eds). Cardiac Surgery. New York: Wiley;1986:398–416.

81. Ross DN, Somerville J. Correction of pulmonary atresia with a homograft aortic valve. Lancet 1966;2:1446–1447.

82. Ross DN, Somerville J. Use of the allograft aortic valved conduit. Ann Thorac Surg 1990;50:320–322.

83. Revuelta JM, Val F, Duran CMG. Reconstruction of right ventricular outflow and pulmonary artery with a composite pericardial monocusp patch: an experimental study. Ann Thorac Surg 1984;37:150–153.

84. Goor DA, Hoa TQ, Mohr R, Smolinsky A, Hegesh J, Neufeld HN. Pericardial-mechanical valved conduits in the management of right ventricular outflow tracts. J Thorac Cardiovasc Surg 1984;87:236–243.

85. Danielson GK. Introduction–conduit operations in surgery. In Anderson RH, Shinebourne EA (eds). Paediatric Cardiology. New York: Churchill Livingstone;1978:537–539.

86. McGoon DC. Left ventricular and biventricular extracardiac conduits. J Thorac Cardiovasc Surg 1976;72:7–14.

87. Ciaravella JM, Jr., McGoon DC, Danielson GK, Wallace RB, Mair DD, Ilstrup DM. Experience with the extracardiac conduit. J Thorac Cardiovasc Surg 1979;78:920–930.

88. McGoon DC, Danielson GK, Schaff HV, et al. Factors influencing late results of extracardiac conduit repair for congenital cardiac defects. In Cohn LH, Gallucci V (eds). Cardiac Bioprostheses. New York: Yorke;1982:217–230.

89. McGoon DC, Danielson GK, Pgua FJ, Ritter DG, Mair DD, Ilstrup DM. Late results after extracardiac conduit repair for congenital cardiac defects. Am J Cardiol 1982;49:1741–1749.

90. Agarwal KC, Edwards WD, Feldt RH, et al. Clinicopathological correlates of obstructed right-sided porcine-valved extracardiac conduits. J Thorac Cardiovasc Surg 1981;81:591–601.

91. Shore DF, deLeval MR, Stark J. Valve replacement in children: biologic versus mechanical valves. In Cohn LH, Gallucci V (eds). Cardiac Bioprostheses. New York: Yorke;1982:239–247.

92. Jonas RA, Freed MD, Mayor JE, Castaneda AR. Long term follow-up of patients with synthetic right heart conduits. Circulation 1985;72 (Suppll. 2):II77–II83.

93. Fontan F, Choussat A, DeVille C, et al. Aortic valve homografts in the surgical treatment of complex cardiac malformations. J Thorac Cardiovasc Surg 1984;87:649–657.

94. DiCarlo D, Stark J, Revignas A, deLeval MR. Conduits containing antibiotic preserved homografts in the treatment of complex congenital heart defects. In Cohn LH, Gallucci V (eds). Cardiac Bioprostheses. New York: Yorke; 1982:259–265.

95. DiCarlo D, deLeval MR, Start J. "Fresh," antibiotic sterilized aortic homografts in extracardiac valve conduits: long-term results. Thorac Cardiovasc Surg 1984;32:10–14.

96. Moore CH, Martelli V, Ross DN. Reconstruction of right ventricular outflow tracts with a valve conduit in seventy-five cases of congenital heart disease. J Thorac Cardiovasc Surg 1976;71:11–19.

97. Kay PH, Ross DN. Fifteen years' experience with the aortic homograft: the conduit of choice for right ventricular outflow tract reconstruction. Ann Thorac Surg 1985;40:360–364.

98. Castaneda AR, Norwood WI. Valved conduits: a panacea for complex congenital heart defects? In Cohn LH, Gallucci V (eds). Cardiac Bioprostheses: Proceedings of the second International Symposium. New York: Yorke; 1982: 205–216.

99. Schaff HV, DiDonato RM, Danielson GK, et al. Reoperation for obstructed pulmonary ventricle-pulmonary artery conduits: early and late results. J Cardiovasc Surg 1984;88:334–343.

100. Bull C, Macartney FJ, Horvath P, et al. Evaluation of long-term results of homograft and heterograft valves and extracardiac conduits. J Thorac Cardiovasc Surg 1987;94:12–19.

101. Bodnar E, Olsen WGJ, Florio R, et al. Heterologous antigenicity induced to human aortic homografts during preservation. Eur J Cardiothorac Surg 1988;2:43–47.

102. Angell WW, Angell JD, Oury JH, Lamberti JJ, Grehl TM. Long-term follow-up of viable frozen aortic homografts: a viable homograft valve bank. J Thorac Cardiovasc Surg 1987;93: 815–822.

Section II
Major Clinical Series of Homograft Valve Transplants: Left Ventricular Outflow Tract

2
Mayo Clinic Series

Robert B. Wallace and Thomas A. Orszulak

The use of cadaveric aortic valve homografts for the replacement of diseased aortic valves began at the Mayo Clinic in 1965. The impetus for initiating this program was concern regarding the available prosthetic valves, especially the hemodynamic characteristics and the incidence of thromboembolism, and the favorable early results achieved by Donald Ross[1] and Brian Barrett-Boyes[2] in the use of aortic valve homograft in the subcoronary position beginning in 1962. The potential of a non-thrombogenic replacement with ideal hemodynamics, and perhaps a resistance to infection was attractive.

This series consisted of 250 patients who underwent aortic valve replacement (AVR) with aortic homografts between May 1965 and October 1972. Follow up of this group of patients was reported at varying intervals. In 1991, follow up was complete in 95% of patients.[3-6]

Patients

The median age of the 250 patients operated was 48 years, (range 5–69 years). There were 186 males and 64 females. Fifteen (15) patients had had previous operations on the aortic valve. The dominant lesion was aortic stenosis in 123 patients, aortic insufficiency in 49 patients, and mixed stenosis and insufficiency in 78 patients. Seventy-nine patients required additional procedures at the time of AVR for various associated lesions; mitral valve repair in 21, mitral replacement in 21, ventricular septal

defect repair in 2, and aortic root reconstruction in 55.

Valve Preservation

The techniques of valve sterilization and preservation used in these patients have been reported in detail.[4,5] The homograft valves were obtained at autopsy in a non-sterile manner within 18 hours of death. Valves were not used when there was gross evidence of disease affecting the donor ascending aorta or the aortic or mitral valves. Valves from patients with known connective tissue disease were excluded. The valve was excised with a portion of the ascending aorta and the anterior leaflet of the mitral valve. The valve was trimmed and rinsed, and the diameter of the valve measured with a calibrated obturator. The first 92 valves used in this series were sterilized in betapropiolactone solution and incubated at 37°C for three hours. The valves was then washed in saline and stored in 250ml Hank's Solution containing penicillin, streptomycin, and tetracycline at 4 degrees centigrade. Cultures were obtained at each step of the procedure and if negative the valve was released for use after 2 weeks, and if not used, discarded after an additional 4 weeks. Following the reports of Malm and associates[7] which indicated that sterilization by irradiation better preserved aortic wall strength and valve architecture, this technique was adopted and used in the last 158 homografts in this series. After trimming, rinsing and measuring the valve it was sealed in a plastic bag and that bag sealed in two additional bags. Glass beads which turned black with irradiation were placed in the bags to verify treatment. The bags were stored in a carbon dioxide freezer at minus 70°C, and subsequently sterilized while frozen with a 6 Mev electron beam providing an absorbed dose of ionizing radiation of approximately 2.5 megarads in the 25 minutes of exposure. Valves were stored at minus 70°C until they were used or arbitrarily discarded after 12 months.

Operative Technique

All homografts were implanted freehand without the use of stents, using two rows of sutures as described by Barratt-Boyes.[2,8] The proximal suture line was of interrupted silk sutures and the distal suture line of continuous silk sutures. In 55 patients the aortic root was tailored to conform to the size of the homograft. Cardiopulmonary bypass time ranged from 63 to 295 minutes with a mean of 105 minutes. The mean cross-clamp time was 87 minutes (range 32–212 minutes). Myocardial protection was usually accomplished using moderate hypothermia, continuous direct coronary artery perfusion, and topical cooling with saline slush.

Results

Fifteen patients (6%) died within 30 days of operation or during the same hospitalization. It was not felt that the homograft *per se* was a factor in any of the deaths. Thirty-nine patients

TABLE 2.1. Reason for Reoperation After Aortic Valve Replacement with Preserved Homograft.

	Number	Percentage
AI only	121	91.7
AS only	2	1.5
AI and AS	7	5.3
Unknown	2	1.5
TOTAL	132	—

AI = aortic insufficiency; AS = aortic stenosis.

(17%) of 235 surviving patients had a diastolic murmur of aortic insufficiency at hospital dismissal. No patient required re-operation for aortic insufficiency during the initial hospitalization.

The latest follow-up of this series of patients was reported in 1991 at which time 235 patients dismissed from the hospital had been followed for a median of 11.4 years.[6]

Twelve patients were lost to follow-up prior to death or reoperation. Three patients were alive and free of re-operation at 15, 18, 20 years post operatively.

One hundred thirty-two patients underwent reoperation for replacement of the aortic homograft, and the operative mortality for this group was 4.5%. The reasons for reoperation are listed in Table 2.1. Freedom from reoperative or replacement of the aortic homograft at 15 years was only 15 ± 3 percent (Figures 2.1 and 2.2).

Ten patients developed endocarditis of the original homograft for a linearized rate of 1.0 per 100 patient years.

The pathology of 80 homograft valves removed at reoperation was not consistent. The valve cusps were usually thickened with fray-

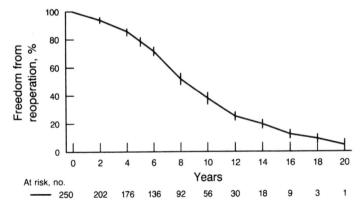

At risk, no.
—— 250   202   176   136   92   56   30   18   9   3   1

FIGURE 2.1. Actuarial estimate of freedom from reoperation for replacement of nonviable homograft aortic valve. In this and subsequent figure vertical lines represent the standard error, and zero time on abscissa represents the date of homograft implantation. Number of patients at risk is shown.

FIGURE 2.2. Actuarial estimate of freedom from reoperation by method of homograft preparation (β-propiolactone vs. irradiation).

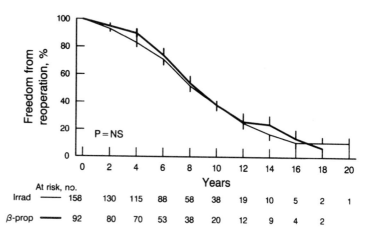

TABLE 2.2. Factors Associated with Reduced Freedom from Reoperation for Replacement of Nonviable Aortic Homograft.

	Number*	Relative Hazard	95% CI	p
Male Sex	186	1.61	1.46–2.36	0.011
Native AV insufficiency	49	1.65	1.06–1.70	0.023
Previous AV surgery	15	3.44	1.80–6.58	0.021
Previous endocarditis*	16	1.93	1.17–3.69	0.024
Decreasing age (20-year increment)	—	1.44	1.08–2.16	<0.002
Increasing homograft size (1-mm increment)	—	1.14	1.06–1.23	<0.008

* The number of patients with stated factor out of 250 patients in the study. Age and homograft size are continuous variables. CI = confidence interval; AV = aortic valve.

ing at the edges although a few cusps were described as thinner than normal. Calcification when present involved the homograft aortic valve wall and the ventricular surface of the cusps. Microscopically there was fragmentation of collagen, disruption of elastic fibers and loss of cellular nuclei.

Factors associated with an increased risk of re-operation were male sex, native aortic valve insufficiency, previous aortic valve surgery, native valve endocarditis, younger age, and larger homograft size (Table 2.2). The method of homograft preparation (Beta-propiolactone *versus* irradiation) did not effect time of re-operation.

The overall survival of patients dismissed from the hospital is shown in Figure 2.3. Factors significantly associated with decreased late

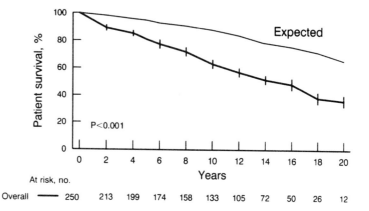

FIGURE 2.3. Actuarial estimate of patient survival after aortic valve replacement with nonviable aortic homografts. Expected survival represents that of a control group of patients matched for age and sex.

TABLE 2.3. Factors Associated with Reduced Survival After Aortic Valve Replacement with a Nonviable Homograft.

	Number*	Relative Hazard	95% CI	p
Native AV insufficiency[†]	127	1.65	1.06–2.23	0.037
Coronary artery disease	25	2.56	1.62–4.01	<0.001
Increasing age (20-year increment)	—	1.86	1.35–2.56	<0.001

* The number of patients with stated factor out of 235 operative survivors; age is a continuous variable. [†] Includes patients with mixed lesions. CI = confidence interval; AV = aortic valve.

survival were: native aortic valve insufficiency, associated coronary artery disease (no patient had concomitant coronary artery bypass grafting), and older age (Table 2.3).

Two patients had neurological events during the follow up period, both of whom were in chronic atrial fibrillation and one had had mitral valve repair at the time of homograft implantation. Patients in this series were not treated with Coumadin for long term anticoagulation.

Figure 2.4 shows survival to events of death, re-operation, thromboembolism, and endocarditis.

Discussion

This series of 250 patients underwent aortic valve replacement with a preserved aortic valve homograft between 1965 and 1972. Early results indicated excellent homodynamic performance, and a very low incidence of thromboembolic complications, despite the fact that anticoagulation therapy was not used. This experience suggested that the preserved homo-

graft might be the valve of choice for replacement of the diseased aortic valve; however, extended follow-up of these patients revealed a progressive increase in the rate of valve failure and the need for re-operation to the extent that only 3 patients were alive and free of re-operation 15, 18, and 20 years postoperatively.

Despite the need for re-operation, patient survival was similar to that in the series using other prostheses (Figure 2.5). The relatively low operative mortality of re-operation and the low incidence of serious valve-related complications contributed to the survival rate.

O'Brien's experience with cryopreserved homografts suggests a longer durability of homografts treated in this manner (Figure 2.6). The increased durability has been attributed to increased cell viability with cryopreservation.[9,10] However, long-term cellular viability has not been proven nor correlated with graft durability.[11] It is quite likely that cryopreservation is less damaging to the tissues than the preservation techniques used in this series and this may be a factor in durability.

Current techniques of homograft insertion,[12–16] including root replacement and inser-

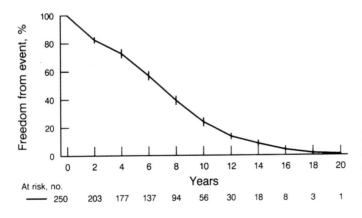

FIGURE 2.4. Actuarial estimate of freedom from events of death, re-operation, thromboembolism, or endocarditis after aortic valve replacement with nonviable aortic homografts.

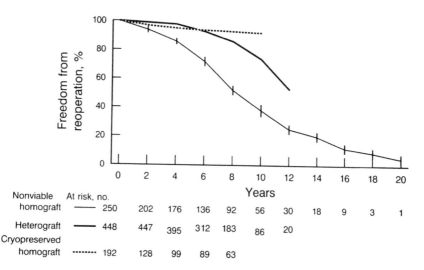

FIGURE 2.5. Actuarial estimate of freedom from reoperation after aortic valve replacement with cryopreserved aortic homografts ($n = 192$),[9] porcine heterografts ($n = 448$) (Jones et al), and nonviable aortic homografts (this series, $n = 250$). Number of patients at risk is shown for each series.

tion of the graft as a cylinder within the aorta reduced the incidence of malalignment of the commissures and preserves the sino-tubular portion of the graft, thus reducing the incidence of early aortic insufficiency which was a factor leading to early reoperation.

The decreased survival in older patients with coronary artery disease may be improved by preoperative recognition and concomitant revascularization which was not done in this group of patients. Failure due to endocarditis may be reduced by antibiotic prophylaxis which was not carried out in most of the patients in this series.

The hemodynamic performance, better means of preservation and sterilization which has improved durability, improved techniques of insertion which reduces the incidence of early aortic insufficiency and the low incidence of serious complications would support the use

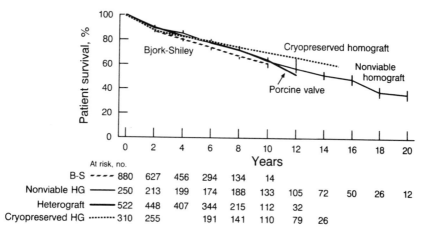

FIGURE 2.6. Actuarial estimate of patient survival after aortic valve replacement with cryopreserved aortic homografts ($n = 310$),[9] porcine heterografts ($n = 522$) (Jones et al.), Björk-Shiley mechanical valves ($n = 880$) and nonviable aortic homografts (this series, $n = 250$). Number of patients at risk is shown for each series.

of an aortic valve homograft as an option for aortic valve replacement, certainly in selected groups of patients.

References

1. Ross DN. Homograft replacement of the aortic valve. Lancet 1962;2:487.
2. Barratt-Boyes BG. Homograft aortic valve replacement in aortic incompetence and stenosis. Thorax 1964;19:131–150.
3. Hoeksema TD, Titus JL, Giuliani ER, Kirklin JW. Early results of use of homografts for replacement of the aortic valve in man. Circulation 1967;35:I9–14.
4. Wallace RB, Giuliani ER, Titus JL. Use of aortic valve homografts for aortic valve replacement. Circulation 1971;43:365–373.
5. Wallace RB, Londe SP, Titus JL. Aortic valve replacement with preserved aortic valve homografts. J Thorac Cardiovasc Surg 1974;67:44–52.
6. Daly RC, Orszulak TA, Schaff HV, McGovern E, Wallace RB. Long-term results of aortic valve replacement with nonviable homografts. Circulation 1991;84:III81–III88.
7. Malm JR, Bowman FO, Jr., Harris PD, Kowalik AT. An evaluation of aortic valve homografts sterilized by electron beam energy. J Thorac Cardiovasc Surg 1967;54:471–477.
8. Barratt-Boyes BG. A method for preparing and inserting a homograft aortic valve. Br J Surg 1965;52:847–856.
9. O'Brien MF, Stafford EG, Gardner MA, Pohlner PG, McGiffin DC. A comparison of aortic valve replacement with viable cryopreserved and fresh allograft valves, with a note on chromosomal studies. J Thorac Cardiovasc Surg 1987;94:812–823.
10. Yacoub M, Rasmi NRH, Sundt TM, Lund O, et al. Fourteen-year experience with homovital homografts for aortic valve replacement. J Thorac Cardiovasc Surg 1995;110:186–194.
11. Bodnar E, Matsuki O, Parker R, Ross DN. Viable and nonviable aortic homografts in the subcoronary position: a comparative study. Ann Thorac Surg 1989;47:799–805.
12. Somerville J, Ross D. Homograft replacement of aortic root with reimplantation of coronary arteries. Results after one to five years. British Heart Journal 1982;47:473–482.
13. Okita Y, Franciosi G, Matsuki O, Robles A, Ross DN. Early and late results of aortic root replacement with antibiotic-sterilized aortic homograft. J Thorac Cardiovasc Surg 1988;95:696–704.
14. McGiffin DC, O'Brien MF. A technique for aortic root replacement by an aortic allograft. Ann Thorac Surg 1989;47:625–627.
15. Knott-Craig CJ, Elkins RC, Stelzer PL, et al. Homograft replacement of the aortic valve and root as a functional unit. Ann Thorac Surg 1994;57:1501–1506.
16. Rubay JE, Raphael D, Sluysmans T, et al. Aortic valve replacement with allograft/autograft: subcoronary versus intraluminal cylinder or root. Ann Thorac Surg 1995;S78–S82.

3
University of Alabama at Birmingham Series

David C. McGiffin and James K. Kirklin

Homograft valves have proved a useful replacement device in the management of aortic valve and aortic root pathology. Since the first insertion by Ross,[1] in 1962, a number of different methods of homograft valve collection, sterilization, storage and insertion have been used. Consequently, this has made comparison of results between the centers that have achieved considerable experience with this valve difficult.

The purpose of this section is to present the clinical experience with the homograft aortic valve at the University of Alabama at Birmingham (UAB). However, this clinical experience will be used as a backdrop to discuss a number of aspects of the homograft valve, including survival after homograft valve replacement, valve durability, mechanisms of homograft valve failure, the concept of competing risk as it applies to the probability of homograft valve re-replacement, and other morbid event such as thromboembolism and endocarditis.

The UAB[2] series comprises a total of 178 patients undergoing implantation of a cryopreserved aortic valve homograft between 1981 and January 1991. The valve was placed in the infracoronary position by the freehand implantation technique in 155 patients and was part of a combined aortic valve replacement and ascending aortic replacement in 23 patients. During this ten year period, 13 of these underwent homograft reoperation with 12 patients requiring explantation. The study group included 124 males and 54 female patients, age 9 months to 80 years (median age 46 years).

Indications for homograft aortic regurgitation in 16 patients, native or prosthetic valve endocarditis in 41 patients, congenital aortic stenosis in 80 patients, aortic dissection in 9 patients, aortic aneurysm in 3 patients and bioprosthetic valve degeneration in 9 patients. All homograft valves which were obtained under sterile operating conditions from multi-organ donors or tissue donors, were sterilized by low dose antibiotics and stored by cryopreservation.

Survival: The actuarial survival of all patients was 92% at one month, 91% at one year and 85% at eight years (Figure 3.1). By multivariable analysis of the entire group of 178 patients, risk factors identified for early mortality were advanced preoperative New York Heart Association Class and where the operation incorporated replacement of the ascending aorta.

For the patients undergoing isolated aortic valve replacement using the infracoronary technique, the early mortality rate was particularly low (1%) and long-term survival was excellent attesting to the safety of this procedure. However, there is evidence to suggest that survival after aortic valve replacement is independent of the type of valve prosthesis used where the device is of contemporary design. In a study by McGiffin and colleagues,[3] examining risk factors for death in 2100 patients undergoing aortic valve replacement with xenograft, mechanical or homograft valves, by multivariable analysis, no contemporary valve replacement device was identified as a risk factor for early or late death. It is very likely in this UAB series that the low early mortality and excellent

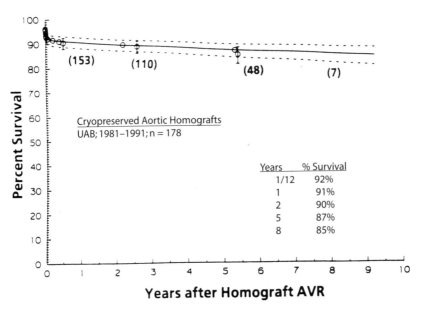

Years after Homograft AVR

FIGURE 3.1. Actuarial (Kaplan-Meier) and parametric survival for all 178 patients receiving cryopreserved aortic homograft valves at the University of Alabama at Birmingham from 1981 to 1991. Open circles indicate individual patient deaths and vertical bars represent plus and minus one standard error. The solid line represents the parametric survival estimate with 70% confidence limits (dashed lines). Reproduced from Kirklin with permission.

long-term survival in these patients may be explained by variables other than the device implanted.

Homograft valve durability: Homograft valve failure resulting in the development of progressive aortic regurgitation is usually regarded as resulting from the mutually exclusive mechanisms of geometric distortion, leaflet degeneration and progressive aortic root dilatation and is usually reported by the use of the endpoints of reoperation and development of progressive aortic regurgitation (so called presumed leaflet failure).

The actuarial freedom from valve reoperation for the 155 patients undergoing aortic valve replacement using the infracoronary technique was 77% at eight years and for the 23 patients undergoing aortic valve replacement combined with an ascending aortic replacement was 100% at eight years (Figure 3.2).[2] There were two intraoperative valve removals for "obstruction" in both cases for patients with congenital left ventricular outflow tract obstruction with accompanying aortic

stenosis. An estimate of primary leaflet failure was obtained by considering both explantation information (reoperation or autopsy) and follow-up echocardiographic data. Patients were considered to have *presumed leaflet failure* if there was evidence of cusp rupture or degeneration at explantation, or severe or moderately severe (3 out of 4 or greater) aortic regurgitation on follow-up echocardiography. The freedom from presumed leaflet failure was 94% at 5 years and 85% at 8 years (Figure 3.3).[2] Hazard function analysis demonstrated a slowly rising late risk of leaflet failure (Figure 3.4)[2] It should be mentioned that this estimate of presumed leaflet failure did not include explanted valves that, to the surgeon, had normally appearing leaflets in the presence of central incompetence or leaflet malalignment.

When published homograft valve series, which may have undergone different preservation protocols and insertion techniques, are compared it is usual to invoke common unifying theories to explain differences in durability such as the presence or absence of leaflet via-

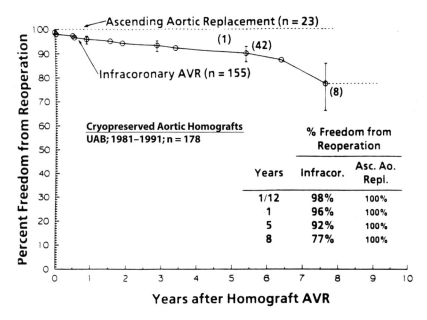

FIGURE 3.2. Actuarial (Kaplan-Meier) freedom from valve reoperation for patients undergoing ascending aortic replacement (upper dashed line) and infra-coronary aortic valve replacement (circles). Reproduced from Kirklin with permission.

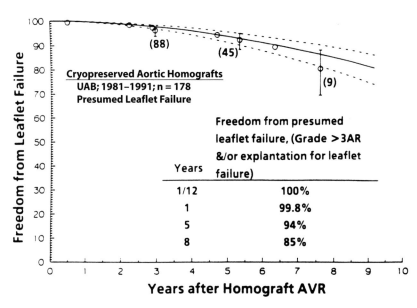

FIGURE 3.3. Actuarial and parametric freedom from presumed leaflet failure. This includes patients with aortic regurgitation by echo grade 3 or 4 (n = 4), patients undergoing explantation for leaflet failure (n = 4), or leaflet degeneration found at autopsy (n = 0), AR, aortic regurgitation. Reproduced from Kirklin with permission.

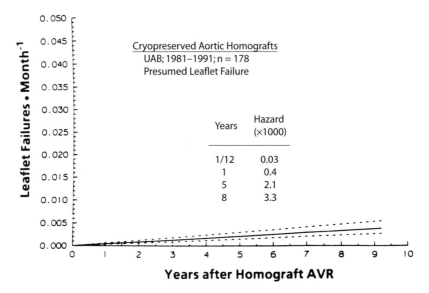

FIGURE 3.4. Hazard function (instantaneous risk) for presumed leaflet failure. Reproduced from Kirklin with permission.

bility or the technique with which the valve has been inserted. This ignores the complex way in which homograft valves may fail. Homograft valve endocarditis and paravalvular leak are uncommon occurrences and, although they may result in aortic regurgitation that may be progressive and severe enough to necessitate reoperation, they will not be considered here as mechanisms of homograft valve failure.

There are a number of important mechanisms of homograft valve failure and of equal importance is the way in which these mechanisms may interact. Christie and Barratt-Boyes[4] by using mathematical modeling demonstrated the progressive development of aortic regurgitation after insertion of a homograft as a result of the change in mechanical properties of the leaflets over time. This change in mechanical properties of the leaflets is characterized by *progressive loss of leaflet extensibility in the radial direction* which is an exaggeration of the normal change in the mechanical properties of leaflet tissue resulting from the aging process. Although this modeling was performed by incorporating the mechanical properties derived from antibiotic-sterilized leaflet tissue, the finding of progressive loss of leaflet coaption caused by reduction of radial extensibility

is almost certainly a feature observed in explanted cryopreserved homograft leaflets.

Cryopreserved homograft valves may also fail due to a *degenerative process of the leaflets* characterized by leaflet thinning, tearing and perforation.[2] Leaflet calcification may also occur.[5]

Geometric distortion after insertion of a homograft valve is an important mechanism of valve failure. Although the subcoronary technique has been the traditional method of insertion, distortion with progressive aortic regurgitation may be less likely with the cylindrical or the aortic root replacement techniques.[6–8]

Homograft valves may also fail as a result of progressive *dilatation of the aortic root*, and this has been reflected in the finding by multivariable analysis of larger aortic root size as a risk factor for the development of aortic regurgitation.[9]

These mechanisms of homograft valve failure are, of course, interrelated and their impact is influenced by a number of known risk factors. Figure 3.5[10] represents an attempt to depict the interrelationship between these mechanisms of homograft valve failure and their risk factors. For example, older donor age[11] as a risk factor for homograft valve failure may be explained by preimplantation loss of radial extensibility. If this older donor valve was implanted by subcoronary technique rather than the cylindrical method, then any geometric distortion, exacerbated by further loss of radial extensibility may quite significantly reduce the likelihood of adequate long-term leaflet coaption. There are many other combinations of mechanisms of homograft valve failure and their risk factors. Homograft valve failure is complex and multifactorial and not amenable to oversimplified explanations such as presence or absence of viable leaflet cells or the type of insertion technique.

The Homograft valve failure and competing risk: Usual means of depicting homograft valve failure is by the use of the Kaplan-Meier estimate of freedom of homograft valve re-replacement (or other endpoints such as valve degeneration). However, many patients, particularly elderly patients, die before a homograft valve requires re-replacement. In the setting of competing risks (in this context valve re-replacement before death and death before re-replacement) the Kaplan-Meier curve for freedom from valve re-replacement is conditional that no patient dies since the censoring process is used at the time of each death that occurs before re-replacement. In other words, the Kaplan-Meier estimate assumes that all patients are immortal. However, the information that is perhaps more important for the patient and the surgeon in the decision making process regarding the use of the homograft valve is that probability of re-replacement of a biological valve *before death* which takes into account the competing risks of death and re-replacement. This concept of competing risk has been previously applied by Grunkemeier

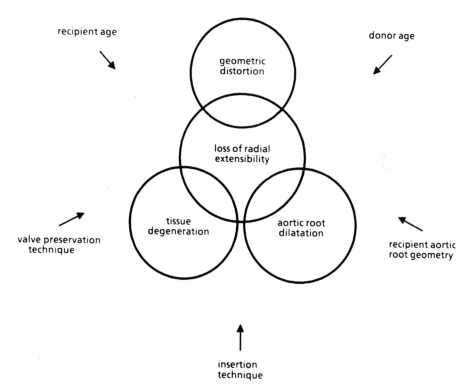

FIGURE 3.5. A depiction of the interrelationships between the overlapping mechanisms of allograft valve failure influenced by known risk factors—(younger) recipient age, (older) donor age, (larger) aortic root diameter, insertion technique, and valve preservation technique. Although compiled from a series of cryopreserved and antibiotic sterilized valves, these risk factors may play a role in failure of either type of valve. Reproduced from Kirklin with permission.

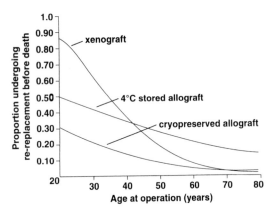

FIGURE 3.6. Nomogram of the time-related proportion of patients with cryopreserved allograft valves (94 patients, 28 re-replacements) who will actually require valve re-replacement for any reason *before death* according to the age of the patient. The solid lines are the parametric estimates. Reprinted from *Journal of Thoracic and Cardiovascular Surgery*. vol 113, McGiffin et al. "An Analysis of Valve Re-replacement after Aortic Valve Replacement," 315. © 1997, with permission from Elsevier.

and colleagues[12] to a group of patients undergoing valve replacement with xenograft prostheses to determine both *actuarial* valve failure (conditional that no patient dies) and *actual* valve failure (probability of failure before death). In a similar study by McGiffin and colleagues[13] using the concept of competing risk, the probability of re-replacement of xenograft, 4°C stored homograft and cryopreserved homograft valves *before death of the patient* was determined. (Figure 3.6) From this analysis it appears that the probability of requiring re-replacement before death for patients over the age of 60 years is no different receiving cryopreserved homografts or xenograft valves.

The use of a competing risk analysis appears to be a useful method of providing information regarding biological valve failure that is complimentary to the usual Kaplan-Meier estimate.

Thromboembolism: In this series,[2] there was only one identified thromboembolic episode which occurred six months after operation. This supports the very low thromboembolic risk of homograft valves found in other studies.[9,14]

Homograft valve endocarditis: In this series,[2] three episodes of probable endocarditis were identified at 1.2, 31 and 56 months after operation, each being successfully managed with intravenous antibiotic therapy. It appears that the homograft valve does have some intrinsic resistance to infection and for that reason is the valve replacement device of choice for patients with active aortic valve endocarditis.[15,16]

In summary, the UAB cryopreserved homograft valve experience supports the concept that the homograft aortic valve offers a number of special features that make it an attractive replacement device for many patients with aortic valve and aortic root disease.

References

1. Ross DN. Homograft replacement of the aortic valve. Lancet 1962;2:487.
2. Kirklin JK, Smith D, Novick W, et al. Long-term function of cryopreserved aortic homografts: a ten year study. J Thorac Cardiovasc Surg 1993; 106:154–166.
3. McGiffin D, OBrien M, Galbraith A. An analysis of risk factors for death and mode specific death after aortic valve replacement with allograft, xenograft, and mechanical valves. J Thorac Cardiovasc Surg 1993;106:895–911.
4. Christie GW, Barratt-Boyes BG. Identification of a failure mode of the antibiotic sterilized aortic allograft after 10 years: implications for their long-term survival. J Card Surg 1991;6: 462–467.
5. Clarke D, Campbell D, Hayward A, et al. Degeneration of aortic valve allografts in young recipients. J Thorac Cardiovasc Surg 1993;105: 934–942.
6. Vural KM, Sener E, Tasdemir O, Bayazit K. Approach to sinus of Valsalva aneurysms: a review of 53 cases. EJCTS 2001;20:71–76.
7. Luciani GB, Casali G, Tomezzoli A, Mazzucco A. Recurrence of aortic insufficiency after aortic root remodeling with valve preservation. Ann Thorac Surg 1999;67:1849–1852.
8. O'Brien M. Aortic valve implantation techniques —Should they be any different for the pulmonary autograft and the aortic homograft? J Heart Valve Dis 1993;2:385–387.
9. Barratt-Boyes BG, Roche AH, Subramanyan R, Pemberton JR, Whitlock RM. Long-term follow-up of patients with the antibiotic-sterilized aortic

homograft valve inserted freehand in the aortic position. Circulation 1987;75:768–777.

10. McGiffin D. Invited Letter: Leaflet viability and the durability of the allograft aortic valve. J Thorac Cardiovasc Surg 1994;108:988–990.

11. O'Brien MF, Stafford EG, Gardner MA, Pohlner PG, McGiffin DC. A comparison of aortic valve replacement with viable cryopreserved and fresh allograft valves, with a note on chromosomal studies. J Thorac Cardiovasc Surg 1987;94: 812–823.

12. Grunkemeier GL, Jamieson W, Miller D, Starr A. Actuarial vs. actual risk of porcine structural valve deterioration. J Thorac Cardiovasc Surg 1994;108: 709–718.

13. McGiffin D, Galbraith A, O'Brien M, et al. An analysis of valve re-replacement following aortic

valve replacement with biological devices. J Thorac Cardiovasc Surg 1997.

14. O'Brien MF, Stafford G, Gardner M, Pohlner P, McGiffin D, Johnston N, Brosnan A, Duffy P. The viable cryopreserved allograft aortic valve. J Card Surg 1987;2:153–167.

15. McGiffin D, Galbraith A, McLachlan G, et al. Aortic valve infection: risk factors for death and recurrent endocarditis after aortic valve replacement. J Thorac Cardiovasc Surg 1992;104:511–520.

16. Haydock D, Barratt-Boyes B, Macedo T, Kirklin JW, Blackstone E. Aortic valve replacement for active infectious endocarditis in 108 patients. A comparison of freehand allograft valves with mechanical prostheses and bioprostheses. J Thorac Cardiovasc Surg 1992;103:130–139.

4

Modified Root Replacement Concept: Influence of Implant Technique on Allograft Durability

William W. Angell and Aubyn Marath

Allograft Durability

Indications for the use of allografts for aortic valve replacement should be built upon an appreciation that this is non-viable collagen tissue, which will be subjected to a slow, variable but relentless immunological response, destined for eventual deterioration. Allograft durability and the performance characteristics which relate to durability depend upon several factors. These include donor age, procurement and preservation techniques, as well as immunogenicity. A primary issue, is that the integrity of allograft tissue is mostly influenced by the physical orientation and configuring of the valve leaflets after implantation in the recipient.

Allograft are the best, longest used, and most proven valve commercially available to us. Despite this, less than 1% of aortic valve replacements are performed using the allograft. In part, this is due to a reluctance by surgeons to use more complex surgical methods for aortic valve replacement, even in young people where longevity and complication-free intervals are critical. Other often proffered reasons for infrequent use relate to the perceptions of availability, and the surgical experience or expertise required, as well as what may be an inherent reluctance by surgeons to alter or destroy a normal aortic root in order to replace it with an allograft substitute. Allograft root implantation, however, unlike the original techniques for scalloped subcoronary methods,

can be taught and learned easily. There is little requirement for extensive experience or an unusual talent for determining the correct size and fit of the allograft.

In this chapter, popular issues of contention regarding aortic valve replacement are discussed and our technique of allograft replacement is described. With modern methods of myocardial protection, it is a technique which adequately serves the needs of a variety of clinical presentations; not only can it be easily accomplished with a standard step-wise approach, but it also permits the surgeon to leave the patient's own aortic root intact.

Disputed Concept

Scalloped Subcoronary vs. Root Replacement

Conceptually, the aortic valve leaflet can be perceived as a smooth membrane covering a series of guy-ropes anchored at perfectly aligned geometric positions on the leaflet. Together with the other leaflets, this results in full hydraulic competence. Re-creation of the coaptive surface by surgical maneuvers is performed to try to achieve appropriate support, both at the upper portion of the commissure, and along the leaflet edge to the corpora arantii (those bodies in the central portion of the leaflet which coapt for about 4 mm under normal physiological conditions).

Using calculated stress/strain curves to provide a computer model of the aortic leaflet, Christie[1] emphasized the critical importance of the coaptive surfaces and the configuration of the aortic leaflets individually and with each other. The surgical objective must, therefore, aspire to imitate the normal human aortic anatomy, so that 50% of the aortic leaflet surface coapts with the adjacent leaflet. Achieving this geometric profile reduces each leaflet's strain at the commissure and at the corpora arantii. The pressure on each side of the leaflet neutralizes or transfers all the forces to the belly of the leaflet where the major collagenous bundles are located. These forces primarily act along the lower half of the commissure, as coaptive surfaces extend downwards, due to their shape *and* the forces of inertia provided by the column of blood above and beyond the valve. Thus, whether stent-mounted porcine xenografts or approximately orientated allografts are being considered as the surgical option, competence and optimal performance over an extended period of time is likely to be best achieved if the natural anatomy is re-created. The original method of implanting freehand infra-coronary allografts was sometimes compromised by the creation of left ventricular/aortic gradients.[2] This method resulted in an incidence of aortic incompetence which was difficult to predict and probably, in retrospect, too great for continued clinical use. In taking advice from those who apply general engineering principles regularly, it is agreed that the best mechanical advantage obtained for a structure which does not have regenerative ability is to try to place the stresses whenever possible, where they belong.

Reconstruction of the valve cylinder is, therefore, probably more likely to achieve the long-lasting result if it is accomplished by implantation as one congruous unit in which the "natural" architecture and bio-mechanical components are not altered. This presumes that careful handling and minimal manipulation of the leaflet mechanism is undertaken. In our experience, use of the aortic allograft root implantation technique results in markedly improved overall performance with no significant gradient or aortic incompetence early *or* late following implantation.

Viable vs. Non-Viable Leaflets

Whichever valve concept and implantation technique are adopted, it must be appreciated that while the leaflets are potentially viable at the time of thawing, they are clearly non-viable after implantation. Some postimplantation reaction may occur immediately[1] and this may influence the long-term function of the valve. Two events may occur: indigenous fibroblasts may be re-activated following implantation, or instead, a deposition of a secondary population from the patient's own cell line may slowly inflict a chronic rejection effect over several years. These fibroblasts appear to be non-functional, and the implanted valve is, essentially, an elaborate collagen matrix in which some "preserved" cellular elements of uncertain significance are seen.[1] It *is* clear that allografts elicit an antigenic response from the patient and to some extent, this is suppressed by antibiotic sterilization and cryopreservation.[3] This early reaction may be due to endothelial and myocyte cells which are immunologically more active than fibroblasts. Tissue-typed matching or immunosuppressive therapy fail, however, to reduce the temporally related degenerative process, which is probably less forceful in older age groups.[3] Irrespective of these viability and immunogenicity issues, the allograft root replacement does offer a better long-term option than other currently available techniques.

Stented vs. Unstented Configurations

Each of the proponents who have promulgated the stenting of valve tissue for surgical implantation, have also helped define and clarify the optimal configuration and orientation of the valve leaflets by their individual contributions. In the early development of the xenograft, stent support was developed to achieve hemodynamic competence and, initially, appeared superior to any other concept tried at the time, because it immediately eliminated valvular insufficiency. Additionally, stents offered both the obvious advantage of versatility of clinical application accompanied by standardization of the insertion technique.

Subsequent clinical experience, however, suggests that the stent adversely impacts on durability.[4] *In vitro* evaluation of hydraulic performance analyses was performed by valve manufacturers using pulsed *in-vitro* valve testing apparatus, and offered convincing evidence of the overall competence and efficiency of stented valves. Though this experimental design has many shortcomings, it also showed that the degree of commissural flexibility and stressful turbulent flow are limiting factors common to all stent designs.

Whichever type of valve is considered, the issues relating to valvular support, surgical implantation technique, and the resultant three-dimensional geometric configuration of the implanted allograft within the aorta, are crucial to minimizing leaflet stress. They will each directly influence bio-mechanical durability. The stentless homograft and the development of the stentless xenograft tissue valve (which grew out of that concept) both appear to be more durable than the stented valves currently available. Creating a more natural valve configuration and new methods of fixation of porcine leaflet tissue[4] have also contributed to improved medium-term durability with the unstented porcine bioprosthesis.[5]

Both the manufacturer and the surgeon have learned that mimicking the natural valve configuration as far as possible, is paramount in optimizing the result. Unlike fixed porcine tissue, the allograft retains leaflet flexibility and orifice size as long as it is not deformed. Leaflet compliance is normal and gradients are considerably less than those found with porcine tissue valves.[1] The utilization of an allograft conduit, in which the valve mechanism is retained in perfect position, has obvious advantages.

Root Replacement

Measurement/Sizing

If it is accepted that the well-preserved, but non-viable, unstented root replacement is the best choice, surgeons are still left with the question of precisely how the root replacement should be optimally accomplished with a standardized technique.

Conceptually, the allograft must fit at three levels:

1. Annular (sub-annular or left ventricular outflow tract region),
2. the Sinuses of Valsalva
3. the Sino-tubular junction

In clinical practice, the anatomy and dimensions of these three regions in disease presentation, are often quite disparate. This may be due to dysgenesis, distorting mechanisms produced by hydraulic forces, infection or previous surgical intervention. Normally, the sinus occupies the largest dimension followed by the annulus which is a 10% to 15% larger than that sino-tubular junction may be totally expanded from post-stenotic dilatation or through mural weakening due to medial cystic pathology. Congenital or surgical deformities may also substantially alter that relationship between these three dimensions.

The measurement of the annulus can be easily carried out by transesophageal echocardiography (TEE), with accuracy to within a millimeter if appropriate imaging is done.[2] Annular dimensions greater than 28 mm in diameter and/or a root dimension 3 mm larger than any easily available allograft may preclude allograft implantation or else require a preliminary annular reduction technique. The obturator measurement of the aortic root at the time of surgery should therefore be regarded as only a confirmatory procedure; the allograft will have already been chosen, thawed and ready for implantation when the annulus size is finally checked. To optimize root implantation, careful planning is required to obtain, preoperatively, information about sizing and correct choice of the appropriate allograft available; with this strategy, it is possible to achieve a predictable result in the majority of presentations.

Modification of Total Root Excision and Replacement

Orientation of allograft valve is essential in order to ensure optimal leaflet dynamics, and this is best accomplished by reconstructing the valve cylinder in its natural anatomical configuration. Such reconstruction, by root replacement, preserves the natural profile of the implanted allograft as a "valved cylinder." The technique of modified rather than extended root replacement has been used consistently in our last 70 cases and is also applicable to the autograft and xenograft.

Several advantages—

a) Root replacement with native root preservation

Combination of root replacement by the implanted allograft, but with native root preservation by careful trimming, leaves the patient with an almost normal aortic valve cylinder. This technique provides minimal manipulation of the valve and permits implantation with greater predictability and a smaller margin of error than with other techniques.

b) Avoidance of extensive resection

This modified root replacement method avoids an extensive resection and leaves most of the native aortic root intact. The anatomy of the aortic valve ring and root is such that removing part of the aortic wall or sub-annular tissue becomes unnecessary; it is simply displaced when the aortotomy is performed and the allograft is sewn into position. Suture line bleeding into residual "potential secondary cavities" between the suture line and native aortic tissue may be initially difficult to identify when the technique is being learned, but usually resolves with revision of the sewing technique.

c) Application to pulmonary artery autograft transfer (Ross procedure)

When this method is applied to the pulmonary autograft transfer (Ross procedure), the same familiar step-wise approach is used, and thus, the learning curves have mutually complementary procedural steps. In performing the Ross operation, the viable muscle tissue of the autograft is easier to handle and sew, as it is less friable than cryopreserved allograft muscle. Except when performing a preliminary annular reduction, we avoid reconstruction with pledgets, Teflon buttresses or circumferential retaining collars as these may later distort the valvular mechanism and reduce coaptation. In

our opinion, prosthetic material is best avoided in the presence of infection.

d) Re-replacement

In the event of re-replacement after previous modified allograft root replacement, use of alternative techniques are made much easier if, at the first operation, there has not been extensive root dissection, and the aortic root is still intact. Now, several surgical operative management choices are made available. Several options may be considered depending on the age and clinical presentation.

A Ross Procedure

i. Re-replacement with allograft. If necessary, suturing to the sub-aortic curtain and ventricular septum can be performed to accomplish this. This is then followed by concomitant coronary reimplantation.

ii. A standard prosthetic aortic valve/conduit replacement.

iii. Preservation of the allograft cylinder, excising just the allograft leaflets and replacing with a bioprosthetic or mechanical valve.

Options When Accompanied by Subacute Bacterial Endocarditis

In this difficult management scenario, the native aorta may have been disrupted by infection, dilatation or abscess formation, with resultant hemodynamic insufficiency or systemic embolization. Some patients may have had previous aortic valve surgery and have indwelling prosthetic valve. In our experience, full clearance of necrotic and infected tissue following by reconstruction is required, ensuring minimal distortion of the valvular mechanism. An allograft or autograft works well using the modified aortic root replacement approach and produces immediate hemodynamically acceptable results. A cryopreserved allograft or transposed pulmonary autograft will be least likely to produce reinfection even in the presence of abscess reaction. Allograft implantation has a low constant reinfection risk rate, whereas mechanical or biological valve prostheses have an increased risk of early infection.[6,7]

Interestingly, Hvass et al. have managed the infected aortic valve with a Bravo (Bravo Cardiovascular, Inc. USA) xenograft supra-annular fixation technique in subacute endocarditis and also found no reinfection in their series.

Our Recommended Intra-Operative Technique

Our step-wise operative procedure consists of the following:

General Operative Approach

We have found that the operation is easily performed through a median sternotomy, under hypothermic cardiopulmonary bypass, using interval anterograde and retrograde cardioplegia and topical cooling of the myocardium. Following cross-clamping of the aorta, a transverse aortotomy 2 cm above the sino-tubular junction is made, extending across three-fourths of the circumference of the aorta, leaving a relatively narrow band or "tongue" of intact posterior aortic wall. (Preserving this posterior aspect of the aortic wall helps stabilize the aortic longitudinal dimension during retraction, so that the distal allograft-aorta anastomosis is sized well, once the inferior and coronary anastomoses have been completed.)

Aortotomy

Following the transverse aortotomy described above, vertical caudal extension of the aortotomy is then carried all the way to the base of the non-coronary sinus. Traction sutures on the aortic wall open the aortic root further and expose it for sizing and suture placement. It also allows the anterior non-coronary sinus and its adjacent commissure to float more freely, achieving an unstressed position for accurate positioning of the new left coronary ostium (Figure 4.1).

Coronary Ostial Identification

Inspection of the coronary ostia is then performed, and their orientation noted, for determination of their optimal location when the valve cylinder is placed in position. If mal-alignment of the right coronary ostium results, this is easily resolved once the cylinder is in position by attaching it as a free button, or as a tongued pedicle. The situations which may cause concern in making this assessment, are dilated aortic root (with diameters consistent with 28 mm or greater), a constricted root with a diameter of less than 21 mm, destruction of the aortic root, or marked congenital or acquired deformations. In these special circumstances, preservation of the recipient root may be neither feasible nor desirable. The decision about how much remnant of the aortic valve to leave intact varies according to the size and configuration of the allograft. For a very large dilated root, it is better to leave some of the old valvular tissue in place as a neatly described ring, which will make up the difference between the size of the allograft and the recipient root. If necessary, annular reduction should be carried out now.

Orientation During Implantation

The allograft should be oriented anatomically as one unit. Displacement of the cusps from their normal radial orientation may result in disruption of the configuration of the commissure and leaflets, and thereby produce aortic incompetence secondarily to malalignment. In positioning the allograft for suture alignment, we recommend that it is hand held (without forceps) oriented about 10 cm above in the implanting position (aligning the allograft also for best placement of the new left coronary ostium.

Preparation of the Allograft

Septal muscle is inspected and should be trimmed to produce optimal shape for alignment with the aortic root and maximum hemostatic control. This measure is less likely to provoke suture loosening, as compressed or non-viable allograft tissue is resorbed over time. Great care should be taken during this procedure to avoid damaging the allograft valve cusps, and the assistant should display the allograft in such a way that, throughout this

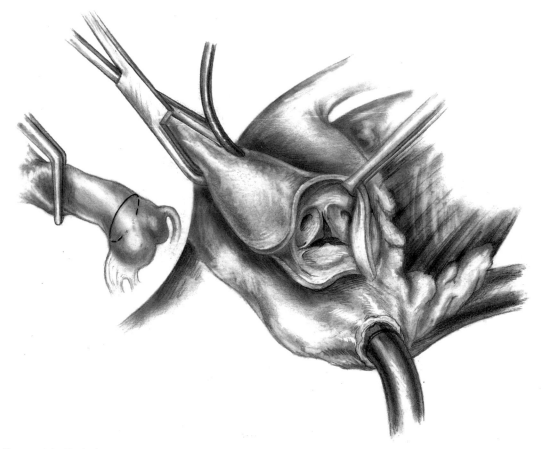

FIGURE 4.1. Technique of transverse aortotomy to achieve full exposure of the aortic root. Posterior wall of aorta is left intact.

resection, the allograft valve cusps can be continually check from within (Figure 4.2).

We recommend 3-0 running Prolene suture with a large needle is used, beginning below and approximately 2 mm beneath the left coronary ostium, so that the middle of the left coronary cusp of the allograft and the left coronary ostium of the native aorta are aligned perfectly. The suture commences at the midpoint of the left coronary cusp of the allograft (from inside-out) and then continues in a clockwise fashion beneath the left coronary ostium and circumferentially around towards the right coronary ostium. Several loops of suture can be achieved before trailing on with the next suture. The needle should penetrate deep to the residual allograft tissue and anchor to the adjacent fibrous tissue of the aortic root. Again, the assis-

tant holds the allograft so as to resist the downward traction effect of serial loops on the allograft, and thereby prevent it tightening too early and spoil perfect suture placement. Great care should be taken to avoid distortion, tearing or entrapment of the allograft valve cusps. Passing the needle at an oblique angle from inside the allograft to outside (rising slightly up the allograft cylinder) gives greater strength without distortion than a direct transverse suture placement (Figure 4.3).

Inspecting the Suture Line

It is best to inspect the inferior suture line from the side, above and within the allograft cylinder with a nerve hook before proceeding to pull the suture lines tight. Next, the tagged lower suture

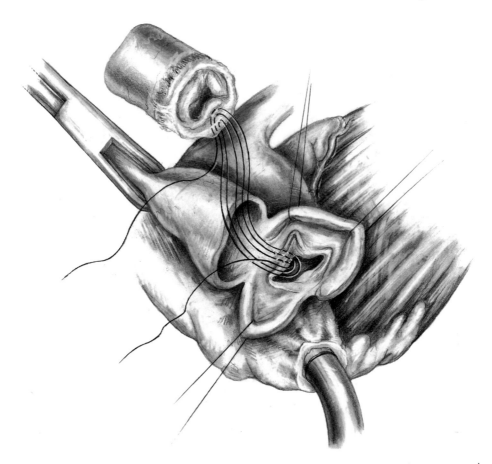

FIGURE 4.2. Inferior suture line anastomosis, with complete visual access to both suture margins

ends are now knotted down in place, resulting in 9–12 suture ties which produces a partial intermittent/running suture technique.

Coronary Ostial Attachment

The allograft left coronary sinus and left coronary artery stub are then approximately with the left coronary ostium, and a standard anastomosis completing with a running suture. This fixes the allograft in place, but since it is only fixed circumferentially at the annular level, the rest of the valve can be allowed to orient itself in a normal manner. This permits unstressed reimplantation of the left coronary ostium. If this cannot be achieved without distortion of the allograft commissures, the existing allograft coronary stub is further tied off, and a fresh circular aortotomy made at a convenient place

in the supra-annular position which will facilitate unstressed approximation.

Distal Allograft/Aortic Anastomosis

End-to-end approximation between the distal aorta and the allograft is now carried out, being sure to adjust the length of the allograft appropriately, so that the valvular mechanism, commissural geometry and left coronary attachment are not stretched or distorted. Though this requires judgment, this is usually quite obvious. This task may appear easier if the native aorta is now transected, but we prefer to leave a posterior "tongue" of aortic tissue behind (as mentioned in 1.) to ensure that the axial orientation and length are preserved—as "normal" as possible. As with extended root replacement, the orientation of the leaflets to each other is a critical feature in the concept of root replacement. When the distal running suture line has been completed, the aortic root is essentially reconstructed, however at this stage, it is helpful to pass the ties through a Rummel tourniquet so that a second internal observation can be made later, if necessary.

Testing the Anastomosis and Valvular Mechanism

Blood cardioplegia is now instilled into the aortic root. This simple test not only provides further myocardial protection, but also confirms valve competence, non-entrapment of the leaflets, and tests the left coronary ostial anastomosis before this becomes inaccessible. Blood cardioplegia given under the cross-clamp will close the aortic valve, so the integrity of the inferior suture line is not properly tested until the left ventricle is pressurized and blood passes through the aortic lumen under pressure. It does identify left coronary bleeding as distinct from that due to the proximal suture line—so helps separate these two adjacent areas in situations of posterior hemorrhage. If posterior bleeding cannot be visualized exteriorly, the distal anastomosis can be easily reopened. This can be accomplished by careful retraction with a copper blade or narrow retractor. If TEE is already available intraoperatively, the valve mechanism can also be viewed in the static state, with the root distended to confirm that leaflet coaptation is adequate. In special circumstances, using crystalloid cardioplegia, the valve can be viewed directly, with a pediatric nephroscope/bronchoscope or similar sterile telescope. *Although this would not be applicable routinely, it can resolve uncertainty about valvular competence and*

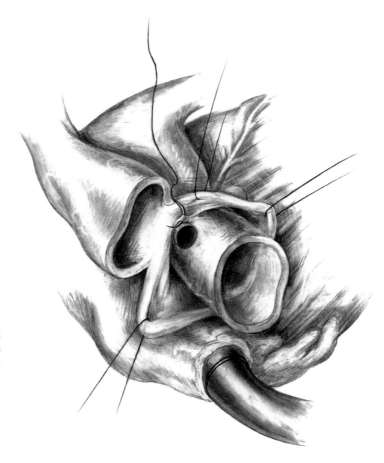

FIGURE 4.3. Completing the left coronary ostial anastomosis to the allograft. Posterior wall is left intact. Left main coronary native orifice is difficult to see from this angle but "button" is sutured to a large oval defect in homograft root.

evenly distributed suture placement, before continuing, when faced with a very difficult implantation or unsatisfactory operative situation.

Right Coronary Ostial Implantation

Next, the right coronary artery ostium is freed as a button or "tongue" of aortic wall, and anastomosed side-to-side into the right coronary sinus. This may be conveniently line up with the allograft's right coronary stub, but if not, an opening can be made in the allograft at any point that does not interfere with the commissure. Further instillation of cardioplegia may help define optimal orientation and alignment.

Intra-Operative Assessment of Valvular Hemodynamics

On weaning from cardiopulmonary bypass support, TEE should again be used to assess valve competence and gradient. It is not uncommon to see a trace of regurgitation which may persist with even perfect alignment. Initially, this seems a worrisome finding as it cannot be readily separated from malalignment aortic incompetence. Provided, however, that the steps of operative implantation have been followed carefully, a trace of regurgitation is most likely due to asynchrony of closure rather than malalignment or poor coaptation. In our experience, this is of no consequence and does not affect valve durability or hemodynamic function.

Discussion

The different technical issues that relate to certain methods of implantation of allografts/ xenografts are discussed in the relevant chapters of this book, and all are critical determinants of a satisfactory result for the particular method described. They should not be lightly transposed from one operative technique to another.

We regard that scalloped, subcoronary or totally inclusive aortic root methods of insertion are intrinsically compromised because of their requirement for great precision in access-

ing the aortic dimensions. The subcoronary suturing of scalloped allograft has to be very carefully performed to achieve perfect coaptation. In the intra-operative scenario of an open aortic root of a collapsed hypothermic heart, this may be very difficult to estimate. In contrast, the modified root replacement technique allows the surgeon to avoid these operative issues, offers minimal intrusion into the valve mechanism, a better step-wise learning curve, and serially reproducible and satisfactory hemodynamic results for a range of presentations.

Based on our long personal experience (W. A.), and those of others, the concept with the most appeal is one which is easy to do and supports reconstruction of the natural allograft aortic root and valve—as an integral unit. Single center data from O'Brien's longer-term experience (reaching a second decade evaluation) with optimally selected and treated frozen allografts (personal communication) suggests that this approach is well supported.

All surgeons developing their own valve experience would like to be able to tell their patients that they have an 80% chance of an implanted allograft lasting 20 years. The sine-qua-non of aortic allograft surgery is that "less than optimal coaptation" will negatively influence the structural integrity of the collagen matrix and reduce the durability of the allograft. We know that allografts are capable of functioning for 20 years or longer. It is therefore reasonable that if proper selection, good preservation and appropriate implantation can be carried out, a consistently achievable result with success rates of 80% can reasonably be expected. A reproducible step-wise approach utilizing a valve cylinder concept, as described above, makes this aspiration plausible. We regard the implantation of the aortic allograft non-inclusion cylinder maximizes the operative options. The procedure does not require a long "learning curve," and can be accomplished by a "less experienced surgeon." Native tissue is saved, and other salvage procedures left open, if, during the operation, or later, it is discovered that allograft root replacement cannot be accomplished. Education of the surgeons about the merits and disadvantages of each technological advance and product line is therefore critical in order to offer the best option to the patient. Provided that there are no substantial advances in either the use of glutaraldehyde-treated animal tissue or mechanical prostheses, the incidence of use of allografts around the world should increase several-fold and be a logical best option for most young patients undergoing aortic valve replacement in whom an autograft is not considered appropriate (or as an option, is deferred until they are older). In view of the low mortality of reoperations performed in established centers, there is much appeal to the strategy of utilizing allograft implantation until that point in a patient's life is reached, when the "one time-Ross procedure" can be most appropriately performed. One should be able to offer availability of allograft valves for virtually all patients with isolated aortic valve disease under the age of 70 years. Clearly across the nation and around the world we have come nowhere near achieving that goal.

References

1. Christie GW. Age dependent changes in the radial stretch of human aortic valve leaflets determined by bi-axial testing. Ann Thorac Surg 1995;60: S156–S158.

2. Elkins RC. Editorial: Pulmonary Autograft: Expanding indications & increasing utilizations. J Heart Valve Dis 1994;3:356–357.

3. O'Brien M. Aortic valve implantation techniques—Should they be any different for the pulmonary autograft and the aortic homograft? J Heart Valve Dis 1993;2:385–387.

4. Kon ND, Westaby S, Pillae R, Amaresena N, Cordell R. Comparison of implant techniques using freestyle stentless porcine aortic valve. Ann Thorac Surg 1995;59:857–862.

5. David TE, Feindel CM, Bos J, Sun Z, Scully HE, Rakowski H. Aortic valve replacement with a stentless porcine aortic valve. A six year experience. J Thorac Cardiovasc Surg 1994;108:1030–1036.

6. Oswalt J. Management of Aortic Infective Endocarditis by Autograft Valve Replacement. J Heart Valve Dis 1994;3:377–379.

7. Kirklin JW, Barratt-Boyes BG. Aortic valve disease. In Kirklin JW, Barratt-Boyes BG (eds). Cardiac Surgery. New York: Wiley; 1986:398–416.

8. Hvass U, Chatel D, Assayag P, Juliard JM, Laperche T, Caliani J, Oroudji M, Pansard Y. The stentless Bravo 300 aortic porcine xenograft: supra-annular versus annular implantations. Cardiovascular Surgeon 1997;5:220–224.

Section III
Major Clinical Series of Homograft Valve Transplants: Right Ventricular Outflow Tract

5
Great Ormond Street Series

Jaroslav Stark and Mila Stajevic-Popovic

Homograft conduits implanted between the subpulmonary ventricle and pulmonary artery have made possible the repair of many complex congenital heart defects. Since the first homograft was used in a patient with pulmonary atresia and ventricular septal defect by Ross in 1966,[1] the operative mortality has declined steadily. However, problems with longevity of homografts were soon acknowledged. Homografts presented by radiation calcified and stenosed early.[2] The introduction of porcine valves used in Dacron conduits[3] was an important new development. Unfortunately, porcine valves showed accelerated degeneration when used in children.[4] In addition, Dacron conduits developed neo-intimal peel which contributed to the development of severe obstruction. Thus, the Boston group reported in 1985 that all their heterograft conduits had to be replaced within ten years of implantation.[5]

In recent years, the new developments in homograft harvesting, storage and use included cryopreservation, use of fresh homografts obtained at the time of heart and heart-lung transplantation, and use of pulmonary in addition to aortic homografts.[6,7]

Currently, aortic and pulmonary homografts, cryopreserved or preserved in nutrient/antibiotic solution are used, and both cadaveric and "transplant" donors are used. In addition, commercially available heterografts as well as "home-made" valved conduits[8,9] are being used. We have recently reviewed the long-term results of a series of homograft conduits used in our institution between 1971–1993.[10]

Materials and Methods

Between 1971 and 1993, we implanted 656 conduits between the subpulmonary ventricle and the pulmonary artery. We have evaluated 293 aortic and 94 pulmonary homografts. In 18 patients, our records did not show whether aortic or pulmonary homograft was used. We have excluded all heterografts and valveless conduits. We have also excluded patients dying within 90 days of operation. The diagnoses of patients are shown on Table 5.1.

Follow up data were obtained from our own cardiology clinics and from the referring physicians. Where follow up was incomplete, the last contact with our department was entered as the last information available. We have collected the following data: diagnosis, age at operation and at the last follow-up visit, date of reintervention or death, type of conduit, size of conduit, mode of preservation, ABO and Rhesus compatibility between donor and recipient, material used for extension of the conduit, and surgeon. In patients in whom a conduit was replaced, the number of conduits previously used was recorded. It was not possible to identify retrospectively the exact mechanism of failure. We have therefore decided that replacement of conduits for whatever reason (conduit valve stenosis/incompetence, stenosis of proximal, distal anastomosis or conduit itself, endocarditis, aneurysm or pseudoaneurysm, conduit compression by sternum) were all included as conduit failures.

TABLE 5.1. Diagnoses of Patients Who Received Homograft Conduits in Subpulmonary Position.

Transposition of the great arteries plus ventricular septal defect plus left ventricular outflow tract obstruction	108
Pulmonary atresia plus ventricular septal defect	90
Truncus arteriosus	78
Fallot's Tetralogy	53
Atrioventricular discordance	31
Absent pulmonary valve plus ventricular septal defect	16
Other	29
TOTAL	405

Statistical Methods

The end points for analysis of conduit survival were conduit replacement for any reason, reintervention (operation or balloon dilatation) on the conduit, or death of the patient with conduit in place. Survival curves were prepared using Kaplan-Meier methodology. Univariate and multivariate analysis of risk factors for conduit survival was performed using a Cox proportional hazards method. Factors for the final model were chosen using statistical as well as clinical criteria.

Results

Follow up was 3 months to 22.8 years (mean 5.4 years). Mean age at operation was 6.8 (2 days—28 years). The longest surviving conduit has been in place for 22.8 years. There were 13 balloon dilatations. Sixty patients had one, 11 had two, 1 had three and 1 had four conduit replacements. There were 15 deaths not associated with reoperation. Freedom from conduit replacement was 84%, 58%, and 31%; and 5, 10, and 15 years. (Figure 5.1) In univariate analysis, the following factors appeared irrelevant to conduit longevity: size of the conduit, ABO and Rhesus compatibility, diagnosis of truncus arteriosus (compared to patients with other diagnoses), or material used for extension of the conduit. We were rather surprised, that unlike other studies, we failed to show significance of conduit size (Figure 5.2) and the diagnosis of truncus (Figure 5.3).

Factors considered relevant for freedom from conduit replacement were: replacement conduits, order number, age at operation, type of homograft, mode of preservation and surgeon.

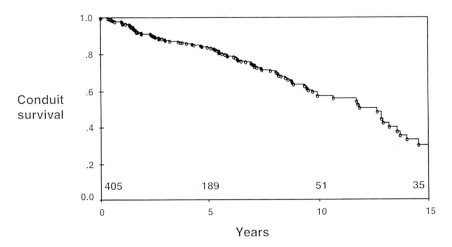

FIGURE 5.1. Survival of homograft conduits at 5, 10, and 15 years. Numbers on this and subsequent figures show number of patients at risk.

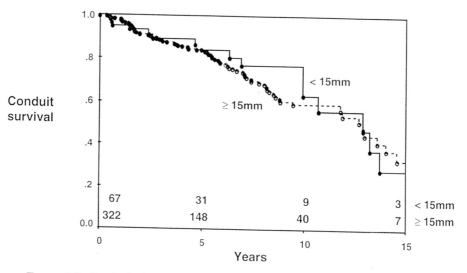

FIGURE 5.2. Survival of small (<15 mm) and large (>15 mm) homograft conduits.

Conduit Replacement

A small conduit has to be placed when an operation is required in infancy. At reoperation, such conduits could be replaced with adult-size conduits and it has been generally accepted that such a conduit should last much longer—possibly a lifetime. However, we were rather surprised to find in our own series that replacement conduits did not last as long as first time placed conduits (Figure 5.4). We can only speculate about the reasons for this finding. It may be that adhesions and calcifications of the tissues around the conduit may be the reason why it is more difficult to obtain an ideal fit of the conduit which would result in suboptimal flow characteristics. There may be other more subtle technical details which we have been as yet unable to identify. We believe that details of operative technique have relevance to

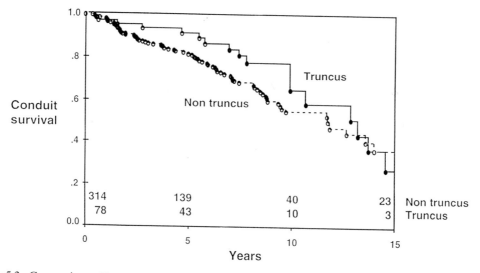

FIGURE 5.3. Comparison of homograft conduit survival between patients with truncus arteriosus and patients with other diagnoses.

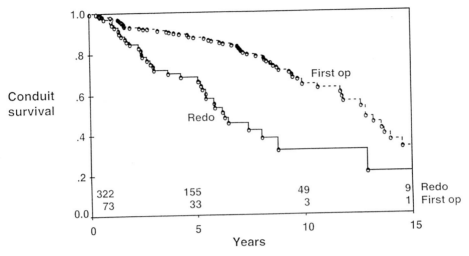

FIGURE 5.4. Survival of first conduits compared to survival of replacement conduits.

conduit longevity, as shown in the studies by Heinemann[11] and Razzouk.[12] Because of our own finding that replacement conduits require re-replacement earlier, we believe that we should further explore techniques of repair of congenital heart defects which avoid the use of conduits.[13–15]

Order Number

Although we have objective information about some aspects of management of patients with valved conduits which have changed over the years, other aspects, such as indications for conduit replacement, are more subtle. Recognizing that these subtle trends in practice might also influence survival of conduits in our patients, we have introduced the concept of "order number" in our analysis. The first conduit inserted in 1971 was thus number 1 and the last in the series in 1993 was number 405.

Again, we were surprised to find that conduits placed earlier in the series lasted longer than conduits inserted more recently. This was not explained by the fact that in earlier years we tried to use larger conduits in infants nor by the increasing prevalence of reoperation with time. When we looked at patients' survival as opposed to conduit survival, we found that patients' survival in recent years was better

than in the earlier years. (Figure 5.5) The experience of other authors[14,15] and our own increasing experience showed that overall risk of conduit replacement is low. It also showed that decreased ventricular function may determine the patient's outcome after conduit replacement. It may well be that we now indicate conduit replacement earlier than in the past. Shorter survival of conduits in our analysis may therefore be appropriate as this pattern is associated with improved overall survival of patients.

Age at Operation

Conduits implanted in younger patients survived better than conduits implanted in older children. This finding contrasts with the data of Clarke,[16] Schorn et al.,[17] and Bando et al. (1995).[18]

Five year freedom from reoperation was 43% in Clarke's series and 48% in Schorn's. In our experience, 5 and 10 year survival was 91% and 77% for infants, and 83% and 50% for children older than 3 years at the time of operation (Figure 5.6). Univariate analysis favored aortic versus pulmonary homograft and antibiotic preserved versus cryopreserved homografts. However, in multivariate analysis both these factors, as well as that of surgeon, were not significant. (Table 5.2)

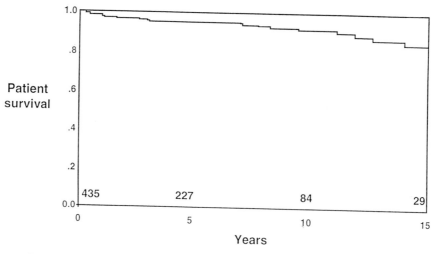

FIGURE 5.5. Long-term survival of patients (who survived 90 days after conduit insertion).

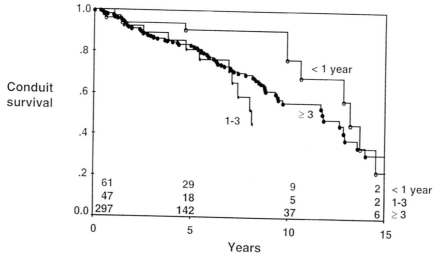

FIGURE 5.6. Survival of homograft conduits in three age groups (<1, 1–3, >3 years).

TABLE 5.2. Univariate and Multivariate Analysis of Risk Factors for Conduit Failure.

	Univariate				Multivariate		
Factor	Worse	B	p	Factor	Worse	B	p
First conduit or redo	redo	1.08	0.00001	First conduit or redo	redo	1.06	0.00001
Order number	recent	.0065	0.00001	Order number	recent	.005	0.003
Age at operation	older	.65	0.002	Age at operation		.01	0.64
Aortic or pulmonary	pulmonary	.46	0.04	Aortic or pulmonary		.57	0.06
Preservation	cryo	.05	0.05	Preservation		−0.19	0.55
Conduit Size (mm)		.03	0.35	Conduit size (mm)		0.002	0.97
Surgeon	Surgeon 3	.474	0.004				
Conduit size for age		.044	0.80				
ABO Match		.21	0.45				
Rh match		−.05	0.90				
Conduit extension		−.13	0.08				
Diagnosis		−.31	0.24				

Information about pulmonary versus aortic homografts is somewhat controversial in the literature. Longer freedom from reoperation of pulmonary compared to aortic homografts was observed by Bando, Heinemann, and Schorn.[11,17,18] Cleveland[19] and Hawkins[20] failed to show difference between the two, while in Clarke's series pulmonary homograft degenerated earlier.

Homograft Preservation

The original technique of homograft preservation in nutrient/antibiotic solution produced excellent results as reported by Kay and Ross[21] and Tam.[22] In our series, cryopreserved homografts performed somewhat worse than those preserved in antibiotic/nutrient solution but the difference could be accounted for by association with recent patient number and with earlier reintervention in recent years. We therefore feel that the use of both cryopreserved homografts and homografts preserved in antibiotic/nutrient solution is currently justified.

Immunological Response

Several studies have suggested that immunological response may be a factor in homograft deterioration.[15,23] Baskett[24] demonstrated that a short interval from retrieval to cryopreservation was a risk factor in homograft failure. The authors therefore inferred that fresher homografts are more likely to react immunologically and therefore deteriorate earlier. In our series, "fresh" homografts were used in a very few patients. ABO and Rhesus compatibility between the donor and the recipient appeared to confer no advantage.

Conclusions

1. Homograft conduits enable us to repair many complex congenital heart defects.

2. 31% of conduits were functional at 15 years after insertion. However, longevity of the homograft conduits is limited. Some patients will need one or even more replacements during their lifetime.

3. Currently, both aortic and pulmonary homografts preserved either in nutrient/antibiotic solution or cryopreserved can be used.

4. In view of less than optimal performance of second and subsequent conduits, we should continue exploring techniques of repair of complex congenital heart defects which avoid the use of conduits.

References

1. Ross DN, Somerville J. Correction of pulmonary atresia with a homograft aortic valve. Lancet 1966;2:1446–1447.
2. Merin G, McGoon DC. Reoperation after insertion of aortic homograft-right ventricular outflow tract. Ann Thorac Surg 1973;16:122–126.
3. Bowman FO, Jr., Hancock WD, Malm JR. A valve-containing Dacron prosthesis: Its use in restoring pulmonary artery-right ventricular continuity. Arch Surg 1973;107:724.
4. Bissett GS III, Schwartz DC, Benzing G, Helmsworth JA, Schreiber JT, Kaplan S. Late results of reconstruction of right ventricular outflow tract with procine xenografts in children. Ann Thorac Surg 1981;31:437–443.
5. Jonas RA, Freed MD, Mayor JE, Castaneda AR. Long term follow-up of patients with synthetic right heart conduits. Circulation 1985;72 (Suppll. 2):II77–II83.
6. McNally R, Barwick R, Morse BS, Rhodes P. Actuarial analysis of a uniform and reliable preservation method for viable heart valve allografts. Ann Thorac Surg 1989;48:S82–S84.
7. Santini F, Faggian G, Chiominto B, Bertolini P, Stellin G, Mazzucco A. Application of fresh and cryopreserved homografts harvested from transplant patients for correction of complex congenital heart disease. Jour Card Surg 1993;8:453–458.
8. Imai Y, Takanashi Y, Hoshino S, Nakata S. The equine pericardial valved conduit and current strategies for pulmonary reconstruction. Sem in Thor and Card Surg, No 3 1995;7:157–161.
9. David TE, Armstrong S, Ivanov J, Feindel CM, Omran A, Webb G. Results of valve-sparing

operations. J Thorac Cardiovasc Surg 2001;122: 39–46.

10. Stark J, Bull C, Stajevic M, Jothi M, Elliott M, De Leval MR. Fate of subpulmonary homograft conduits: determinants of late homograft failure. J Thorac Cardiovasc Surg 1997.

11. Heinemann MK, Hanley FL, Fenton KN, Jonas RA, Mayer JE, Castaneda AR. Fate of small homograft conduits after early repair in truncus arteriosus. Ann Thorac Surg 1993;55:1409–1412.

12. Razzouk AJ, Williams WG, Cleveland DC, Coles JG, Rebeyka IM, Trustler GA, Freedom RM. Surgical connections from ventricle to pulmonary artery: comparison of four types of valved implants. Circulation 1992;86, No 5 (Suppl. 2):II-154–II-158.

13. LeCompte Y, Zannini L, Hazan E, Jarreau MM. Anatomic correction of transposition of the great arteries: new technique without the use of a prosthetic conduit. J Thorac Cardiovasc Surg 1981;82:629–631.

14. Danielson GK, Downing TP, Schaff HV, Puga FJ, DiDonato RM, Ritter DG. Replacement of obstructed extracardiac conduits with autogenous tissue reconstructions. JTVCS 1987;93:555–559.

15. Sano S, Karl TR, Mee RB. Extracardiac valved conduits in the pulmonary circuit. Ann Thorac Surg 1991;52:285–290.

16. Clarke DR. Extended aortic root replacement with cryopreserved allografts: do they hold up? Ann Thorac Surg 1991;52:669–673.

17. Schorn K, Yankah AC, Alexi-Meskhishvili VA, Weng Y, Lange PE, Hetzer R. Risk factors for early degeneration of allografts in pulmonary circulation. European Journal of Cardiothoracic Surgery 1997;11:62–69.

18. Bando K, Danielson GK, Schaff HV. Outcome of pulmonary and aortic homografts for right ventricular outflow tract reconstruction. J Thorac Cardiovasc Surg 1995;109:509–518.

19. Cleveland DC, Williams WG, Razzouk AJ. Failure of cryopreserved homograft valved conduits in the pulmonary circulation. Circulation 1992;86 (suppl II):II-150–II-153.

20. Hawkins JA, Bailey WW, Dillon T, Schwartz DC. Midterm results with cryopreserved allograft valved conduits from the right ventricle to the pulmonary arteries. J Thorac Cardiovasc Surg 1992;104:910–916.

21. Kay PH, Ross DN. Fifteen years' experience with the aortic homograft: the conduit of choice for right ventricular outflow tract reconstruction. Ann Thorac Surg 1985;40:360–364.

22. Tam RK, Tolan MJ, Zamvar VY, Slavik Z, Pickering R, Keeton BR, Salmon AP, Webber SA, Tsang V, Lamb RK, Monro JL. Use of larger sized aortic homograft conduits in right ventricular outflow tract reconstruction. J Heart Valve Dis 1995;4:660–664.

23. Lupinetti FM, Cobb S, Kioschos HC, Thompson SA, Walters KS, Moore KC. Effect of immunological differences on rat aortic valve allograft calcification. J Card Surg 1992;7:65–70.

24. Baskett RJ, Ross DB, Nanton MA, Murphy DA. Factors in the early failure of cryopreserved homograft pulmonary valves in children: preserved immunogenicity? J Thorac Cardiovasc Surg 1996;112:1170–1179.

6
Denver Series

David R. Clarke and Deborah A. Bishop

The history of right ventricular outflow tract reconstruction in pediatric patients at The Children's Hospital and the University of Colorado Health Sciences Center in Denver is a small-scale reflection of the world experience. Since Ross and Somerville first attempted right ventricular outflow tract reconstruction with an extra-cardiac valved conduit in 1966,[1] the ability to reconstruct right ventricle to pulmonary artery continuity has been of benefit to pediatric cardiac surgery. The Denver experience chronicles the surgical phases of development and illustrates the rationale behind the evolution of current concepts in the treatment of complex right ventricular outflow tract anomalies in children.

The original valve conduit used by Ross and Somerville was an aortic allograft, although prosthetic alternatives were explored when aortic allograft calcification and degeneration were reported as early as 1968.[2] Originally, allografts were processed with antibiotic solutions and stored at 4°C resulting in inconsistent cell viability and variable but overall poor conduit survival.[3] Structural deterioration of the valve and conduit were also common with other methods of preservation such as gamma radiation and freeze drying, or fixation with beta-propriolactone or ethylene oxide.[4,5] Mechanical prostheses were implanted in some pediatric patients but their use was limited to children who were physically large enough to receive an 18 or 20 mm external diameter valve. In addition, most pediatric cardiac surgeons avoided the use of mechanical valves secondary to risk factors associated with anticoagulation and thromboembolism. The search for long-lasting options for replacement of the right ventricular outflow tract then began in earnest.

Use of Porcine Valved Conduits

Background

In the early 1970s, porcine bioprostheses, that had been implanted in adults with good results, were used for right ventricular outflow tract repairs in children. By the early 1980s in the Denver experience as well as elsewhere, the popularity of porcine valve conduits declined rapidly as early and late postoperative complications became evident.[6] Inherent graft rigidity and large conduit to patient size resulted in early conduit complications,[3] late conduit obstruction or valve insufficiency resulted from formation of intimal peel or valve degeneration.[7]

Denver Patient Population

From May of 1979 through July of 1984, 24 children underwent right ventricular outflow tract reconstruction with the Carpentier-Edwards porcine valved conduit. There were 14 females (58%) and 10 males (42%). Patient age and weight at operation ranged from one month to 13 years (mean age: 4.2 years) and

TABLE 6.1. Preoperative Diagnosis.

Diagnosis	Type of Right Ventricular Outflow Tract Reconstruction			
	Porcine	Aortic	Patch	Pulmonary
Complex Tetralogy of Fallot	NA	7	10	47
Tetralogy of Fallot	6	2	19	35
Pulmonary atresia	2	4	2	34
Conduit replacement	NA	2	NA	40
Truncus arteriosus	1	11	NA	23
Transposition of the great arteries	9	4	NA	20
Double outlet ventricle	5	4	NA	13
Pulmonary stenosis	NA	NA	4	NA
Aortic insufficiency with or without aortic stenosis	NA	NA	NA	12
Hypoplastic left heart	1	NA	NA	NA
Aortic atresia, hypoplastic transverse arch, VSD	NA	1	NA	NA
Ebstein's Anomaly, pulmonary stenosis, VSD, ASD	NA	NA	NA	1
Total Procedures	24	35	35	225

VSD = ventricular septal defect; ASD = atrial septal defect.

3.5 kg to 35 kg (mean weight: 14.3 kg) respectively. Preoperative diagnoses are listed in Table 6.1. Seventeen children (71%) had undergone previous cardiac surgeries; four failed complete repairs and 12 palliative procedures.

Surgical Technique

Appropriate porcine valve conduit size was estimated before surgery on the basis of patient weight. Operations were performed through a median sternotomy with cardiopulmonary bypass and in smaller patients, hypothermic circulatory arrest. Existing shunts were double ligated and divided during preparation for cardiopulmonary bypass. Vertical right ventriculotomy was performed and if present, a previously placed conduit was excised. Associated septal defects were repaired. A standard circular anastomosis of running suture was performed distally from prosthetic conduit to native main pulmonary artery. Proximally, the porcine valved conduit was anastomosed directly to the right ventricular outflow tract with running suture. The aortic cross-clamp was removed during completion of the proximal connection and the patient weaned from cardiopulmonary bypass in standard fashion. Conduit annulus external diameters ranged from 12 mm to 25 mm (mean diameter: 20 mm).

Results

Nine of the porcine valved conduit recipients (38%) died within 30 days of operation and are detailed in Table 6.2. As depicted in Table 6.3, 87% of all patients who received a porcine valved conduit experienced significant postoperative complications. Fifteen operative survivors have been followed for three months to 12.2 years (mean follow up: 6.4 years). Two children were clinically well when they were lost to follow up at 6.8 and 6.9 years after implantation of their xenograft. Three of 13 remaining patients (23%) experienced late deaths. Two sudden deaths at ten and 35 months postoperative, were attributed to porcine valve conduit obstruction. One infant died of pneumonia four months after heterograft placement. Nine porcine valve conduit explants (69%) have been performed because of conduit stenosis from 3.2 to 11.3 years (mean: 7.4 years) post operatively. One teenager (4%) remains alive and cardiovascularly well at the 12.6 years of follow-up.

TABLE 6.2. Early Postoperative Mortality.

Cause of Death	Porcine	Aortic	Patch	Pulmonary
Intraoperative cardiac failure	6	3	1	5
Right ventricular failure	1	1	3	9
Sepsis	NA	1	NA	4
Myocardial failure	NA	3	NA	1
Cardiac tamponade	1	NA	1	NA
Arrhythmia	1	NA	NA	1
Myocardial infarct right ventricular failure	NA	1	NA	1
Metabolic derangement cardiopulmonary failure	NA	NA	NA	2
Poor coronary artery flow multiple organ failure	NA	NA	1	NA
LVOT allograft dehiscence expired at reoperation	NA	NA	NA	1
Pulmonary vascular disease	NA	NA	NA	1
Total Deaths	9 (38%)	9 (26%)	6 (17%)	25 (11%)

LVOT = left ventricular outflow tract.

Use of Aortic Allografts

Background

As enthusiasm for synthetic porcine valved conduits declined, interest in aortic valve allografts resurfaced. In the middle 1970s, Angell and associates[8] resurrected the use of aortic allografts for cardiac reconstruction. Their innovative method of tissue cryopreservation and super-cold storage resulted in increased cellular viability and implied increased durability.[9] In addition, the allografts could be stored for long periods, thus increasing availability. In 1984, these cryopreserved allografts were made readily available in the United States by CryoLife®, Inc. and thereafter by others. Aortic valve allografts were again used to reconstruct the right ventricular outflow tract in children.[10]

Patient Population

Between February 1985, and December 1996, 35 children received a cryopreserved aortic valve allograft to repair or replace their right ventricular outflow tract. The patient group was comprised of 22 females (63%) and 12 males (37%). Age at operation ranged from nine days

TABLE 6.3. Early Postoperative Morbidity.

Complication	Type of Right Ventricular Outflow Tract Reconstruction			
	Porcine	Aortic	Patch	Pulmonary
Pulmonary	7	10	8	55
Sepsis, mediastinitis or endocarditis	3	7	6	32
Hemorrhage	3	2	NA	24
Arrhythmia or heart block	2	4	4	22
Right ventricular failure	NA	8	3	13
Neurologic impairment	4	5	NA	23
Postpericardiotomy syndrome	1	3	NA	18
Renal insufficiency or failure	2	1	NA	6
Diaphragm paralysis	NA	3	NA	9
Delayed sternal closure	NA	1	NA	7
Balloon angioplasty distal pulmonary arteries	NA	NA	NA	3
Extracorporeal membrane oxygenator	NA	NA	NA	2
Cardiac transplant	NA	NA	NA	1
Revise allograft repair	NA	NA	NA	1
No complication	2 (13%)	4 (15%)	9 (31%)	83 (41%)

to 8.7 years (mean age: 1.5 years) and operative weights were 2.5 kg to 18.5 kg (mean weight: 7.4 kg). Preoperative diagnoses, the most prevalent being truncus arteriosus, are listed in Table 6.1. Sixteen children (46%) had undergone no previous cardiac surgeries. Nineteen patients had previous surgery including seven unilateral and two bilateral Blalock-Taussig shunts, six allograft right ventricular outflow tract reconstructions, three pulmonary artery bands, two transannular patch repairs of Tetralogy of Fallot, one Senning procedure and one aortic coarctation repair.

Surgical Technique

Standard surgical approach was through a median sternotomy. All operations were performed with the use of cardiopulmonary bypass and moderate hypothermia from 24°C to 26°C. When cardiac arrest was necessary to accomplish internal cardiac repairs such as ventricular septal defect closure or infundibular muscle resection, cold blood cardioplegia was administered in bolus doses every 20 to 30 minutes throughout that portion of the surgery. Deep hypothermia with circulatory arrest was used with or without cardioplegia in infants less than 6 kg. A vertical right ventriculotomy was extended through the pulmonary artery, which was transected and the distal allograft to native pulmonary artery anastomosis was performed first. The proximal anastomosis connected the allograft into the right ventricular outflow tract or onto the surface of the right ventricle. A polytetrafluoroethylene patch was used to complete the connection from the anterior portion of the allograft to the ventriculotomy and rewarming was initiated. When the patient was normothermic, bypass was weaned and the procedure completed in standard fashion. Aortic valve allografts of 10 mm to 25 mm internal diameter (mean: 17 mm) were implanted.

Results

There were nine hospital deaths (26%) that are identified in Table 6.2. Twenty-two of 26 operative survivors (85%) encountered a variety of early postoperative complications (Table 6.3). Follow up of the 26 remaining children ranged from 1 month to 11.2 years (mean follow up: 4.8 years). Four late deaths (15%) occurred from 1.7 months to 5.9 years after aortic allograft surgery. A female with double outlet right ventricle and pulmonary atresia who had undergone a previous Blalock-Taussig shunt, received an aortic allograft at two years of age and died 1.7 months postoperatively due to an arrhythmia. A second female underwent pulmonary valve allograft repair of truncus arteriosus as a neonate. Mediastinitis led to infection of the pulmonary allograft which was replaced by an aortic valve allograft two months after the initial surgery. The child succumbed to severe right ventricular dysfunction four months after reoperation. A three year old girl with pulmonary atresia underwent primary aortic allograft repair. She expired 16 months postoperatively with hemoptysis and massive pulmonary hemorrhage. The final death occurred in a female child born with Tetralogy of Fallot and absent pulmonary valve who presented at eight years of age with prosthetic pulmonary valve insufficiency. An aortic valve allograft was used to replace the prosthesis and the child died five years following aortic allograft implantation from complications of human immunodeficiency virus acquired prior to her allograft surgery.

Nine children (35%) experienced allograft fibrocalcification and degeneration that required aortic replacement from 2.7 to 10.2 years after implantation of the valve conduit. A synopsis of each child's experience is presented in Table 6.4. Thirteen remaining patients are clinically well.

Use of Transannular Patch

Background

Because in the pediatric population, synthetic porcine valved conduits suffered from unacceptably high early failure rates and aortic valve allografts although fairing better, seemed never-the-less doomed to degeneration and eventual failure, many surgeons returned to

TABLE 6.4. Allograft Replacement in Aortic Allograft Recipients.

Patient	Diagnosis at First Allograft Repair	Age at First Allograft Repair	Complication	Reoperation	Months After First Allograft Repair	Outcome
SH	Aortic atresia, hypoplastic aortic arch (s/p Damus-Kaye-Stansel)	9 days	Allograft valvar stenosis	Pulmonary allograft RVOTR	38	Well 3.3 years postop
TB	Truncus arteriosus type II	2 months	Allograft insufficiency, distal PA stenosis	Pulmonary allograft RVOTR	33	Expired @ ARR 2.5 years postop
DH	Truncus arteriosus type I	2.5 months	Allograft calcification and stenosis	Pulmonary allograft RVOTR	45	Well 2 years postop
MC	Truncus arteriosus type I	7 months	Allograft stenosis and insufficiency	Pulmonary allograft RVOTR	95	Well 4.2 years postop
JK	Tetralogy of Fallot	7 months	Allograft stenosis and insufficiency	Pulmonary allograft RVOTR	83	Well 4.7 years postop
MM	Pulmonary atresia, ventricular septal defect	9 months	Allograft conduit and left PA stenosis	Pulmonary allograft RVOTR	48	Well 6.2 years postop
MS	Pulmonary atresia, ventricular septal defect	1.6 years	Allograft stenosis and insufficiency	Pulmonary allograft RVOTR	122	Well 1.7 years postop
AR	Tetralogy of Fallot	1.8 years	Allograft valvar stenosis	Pulmonary allograft RVOTR	77	Well 5.6 years postop
LS	Pulmonary atresia, ventricular septal defect	3.5 years	Allograft stenosis and insufficiency	Pulmonary allograft RVOTR	113	Well 9 months postop

increased usage of transannular patching for right ventricular outflow reconstruction. Because of poor previous results with the use of large transannular patches, application of the technique was limited to relatively mild cases of Tetralogy of Fallot, pulmonary valvar stenosis, or pulmonary atresia and the technique itself was modified to minimize production of pulmonary valve regurgitation.

Patient Population

From September of 1984 through December of 1996, 35 children underwent right ventricular outflow tract reconstruction with a transannular patch. The patient group was comprised of 19 boys (54%) and 16 girls (46%). At the time of surgery, patient age ranged from two days to 4.8 years (mean age: 1.3 years). Operative weights ranged from 2.5 kg to 16.9 kg (mean weight: 8.2 kg). Tetralogy of Fallot was the pre-operative diagnosis for the majority of patient (Table 6.1). Ten of the transannular patch patients (29%) had undergone previous unilateral Blalock-Taussig shunt procedures. Twenty-five children (71%) had undergone no prior cardiac surgery but balloon pulmonary valvotomy had been performed in 11 of them.

Surgical Technique

Transannular patch repair of the right ventricular outflow tract was performed through a median sternotomy using cardiopulmonary bypass. Hypothermic circulatory arrest was utilized only in the presence of complicating cardiac anomalies such as large aortopulmonary collaterals. After isolating the pulmonary arteries, a vertical right ventriculotomy was performed and extended across the pulmonary annulus, taking care to preserve pulmonary valve leaflet tissue. Septal defects were repaired if present. An approximately sized piece of polytetrafluoroethylene patch was inserted into the outflow tract with continuous suture. Widening of the annulus was limited to the minimum necessary to achieve relief of obstruction. The patient was weaned from cardiopulmonary bypass and the procedure completed in routine manner.

Results

Six transannular patch recipients (17%) died in the early perioperative period and the cause of mortality is shown in Table 6.2. One early death that requires elaboration occurred in a three month old male. Intraoperatively, the transannular patch was placed under an aberrant left anterior descending coronary artery and resulted in compromised flow to the coronaries and eventual multiple organ failure. Of the 29 remaining patients, 20 (69%) experienced post-operative complications; primarily pulmonary sequelae, sepsis, arrhythmias and right heart failure (Table 6.3).

Twenty-nine operative survivors have been followed clinically for two months to 12.6 years (mean follow up: 3.5). One child was cardio-vascularly well when she was lost to follow up nine months after transannular repair. The single late death (4%) occurred in a boy who was 18 months old at the time of repair for Tetralogy of Fallot. His sudden death two months after surgery was attributed to an arrhythmia. One child (4%) with Tetralogy of Fallot and right ventricular outflow tract hypoplasia underwent transannular patch repair at eight months of age. Twenty-one months later, pulmonary due to severe pulmonary insufficiency. The 26 remaining patients clinically are well. Mild to moderate pulmonary insufficiency detected by echocardiography is universally present.

Use of the Pulmonary Allografts

Background

Intuitively, it seemed that a pulmonary allograft would be the ideal option for reconstitution of right ventricle to pulmonary artery continuity because it represented the most complete restoration of native structure and function. In addition, it was postulated that pulmonary allografts should not calcify as quickly as aortic allografts that have an intrinsically greater elastin and calcium content in their conduit walls (1904). As demand for aortic allografts for left ventricular outflow tract reconstruction increased in the mid 1980s, surgeons began to opt for the more available pulmonary allografts to repair the right ventricular outflow tract. The advantage of having intact branch pulmonary arteries with which to reconstruct distal arterial anomalies was appreciated.

Patient Population

From April 1985 through December 1996, 225 children underwent right ventricular outflow tract reconstruction using a cryopreserved pulmonary valve allograft. There are 126 males (56%) and 99 females (44%) who ranged in age from six days to 18 years at operation (mean age: 4.5 years). Mean weight at the time of surgery was 16.3 kg and ranged from 1.2 kg to 82.3 kg. Preoperative diagnoses are listed in Table 6.1. The primary diagnosis in 12 children was aortic insufficiency with or without aortic stenosis; all had undergone prior surgical procedures to the left ventricular outflow tract. Right ventricular outflow tract reconstruction was performed as part of a pulmonary autograft procedure (Ross procedure) that is described in detail in Section X. The other 213 patients received pulmonary allografts due to obstruction or complete discontinuity between the right ventricle and pulmonary artery system or as treatment for pulmonary valvar regurgitation. Forty-nine patients (22%) had undergone no previous cardiac surgeries. In the other 176 children, 114 systemic to pulmonary artery shunts constituted the most prevalent previous procedure. The most common prior definitive repairs included 45 ventricle to pulmonary artery conduits, 28 complete Tetralogy of Fallot repairs, 21 of which were transannular patch repairs, and 18 pulmonary valvotomies or outflow tract patches that were not transannular.

Surgical Technique

Preparatory phases of pulmonary valve allograft right ventricular outflow tract reconstruction including median sternotomy and implementation of cardiopulmonary bypass with moderate or deep hypothermia were iden-tical to that used with the previously described aortic allograft technique. Because pulmonary valve allografts offered the advantage of left and right pulmonary artery branch reconstruction, the distal anastomosis was accomplished in one of three ways; standard circular anastomosis to the main pulmonary artery, unilateral allograft conduit flap to one distal branch, or use of a bifurcated pulmonary allograft independently to left and right pulmonary arteries. Pulmonary allografts of 9 mm to 27 mm internal diameter (mean: 20 mm) were implanted.

Results

Twenty-five of 225 children (11%) suffered early postoperative deaths. Five patients expired intraoperatively in cardiac failure. Right ventricular failure resulted in nine hospital deaths. Four early deaths were attributed to sepsis and two deaths to cardiopulmonary failure induced by metabolic derangements. One death each occurred as a result of myocardial failure, pulmonary vascular disease, and arrhythmia and acute myocardial infarct that produced right ventricular failure. One child received aortic and pulmonary allografts for left and right ventricular outflow tract reconstructions respectively. Sudden cardiac arrest on postoperative day number two led to emergent reoperation that revealed aortic allograft dehiscence which was repaired but the patient expired in the operating room. Massive hemorrhage was the cause of death for one patient who required tricuspid and reoperative pulmonary valve replacement. The child was emergently returned to the operating room where a completely dehisced distal allograft suture line was discovered.

Pulmonary sequelae, infection, and bleeding that required reoperation were the most frequently encountered early postoperative complications although 83 of 200 surviving children (41%) experienced a completely benign hospital course. Early postoperative allograft-related events occurred in four patients. Three children underwent balloon dilation of stenotic allograft to distal pulmonary artery anastomoses and one insufficient pulmonary autograft was replaced by an aortic allograft.

Cardiac transplantation was the outcome for a female with the primary diagnosis of Tetralogy of Fallot who underwent transannular patch repair at three years of age followed by pulmonary allograft reconstruction at five years old. Six years later, tricuspid regurgitation and severe pulmonary insufficiency developed and she was reoperated. The original allograft was excised, a second pulmonary allograft was implanted, and a bidirectional Glenn shunt and tricuspid annuloplasty were performed. The child was placed on extracorporeal membrane oxygenation when she could not be weaned from cardiopulmonary bypass and she underwent cardiac transplantation 48 hours later.

In one month to 11.9 years of follow up (mean follow up: 5.1 years) of 199 pulmonary allograft recipients, two children have been lost to follow up. Among 197 remaining children, there were 21 late deaths (11%), two late cardiac transplants (1%), and 19 operations to replace the original pulmonary allograft valve conduit (10%).

The 21 late deaths occurred from 35 days to 10.8 years postoperative (mean: 13.2 months). Four children died within the first five to eight weeks following pulmonary allograft surgery. A neonate with Tetralogy of Fallot and absent pulmonary valve suffered death due to hepatic and pulmonary cytomegalovirus. Postoperative seizures with neurologic dysfunction was the cause of death in a one year old female with double outlet right ventricle. Two 2.5 year old males, one diagnosed with Tetralogy of Fallot and atrioventricular canal and the other with pulmonary atresia, ventricular septal defect and multiple aortopulmonary collaterals, succumbed to cardiopulmonary failure and pulmonary hemorrhage respectively. Two neonates died between ten and twelve weeks postoperatively; an infant who underwent allograft implantation to repair truncus arteriosus with truncal valve insufficiency died of a pulmonary embolus and another who presented with Tetralogy of Fallot and absent pulmonary valve expired in right ventricular failure aggravated by increased pulmonary vascular resistance and pulmonary infection. Sepsis was the cause of death at three months after allograft insertion for a twelve day old and a four month old child.

The neonate underwent pulmonary and aortic allograft valve reconstruction of the right and left ventricular outflow tracts respectively to correct type I truncus arteriosus with an insufficient truncal valve and succumbed to sepsis that resulted in renal and liver failure. The four month old experienced poor perfusion after allograft surgery to repair pulmonary atresia and ventricular septal defect and died with overwhelming sepsis. Four children, a 14 month old and three year old with Tetralogy of Fallot, a six month old with transposition of the great vessels status post complete repair, and an infant with pulmonary atresia and ventricular septal defect experienced sudden death at home three to 24 months after allograft surgery.

Each incident was attributed to probable arrhythmia. Three children expired after subsequent hospital admissions to replace an additional cardiac valve. A two year old female with transposition of the great arteries and a 15 year old female with Tetralogy of Fallot and atrioventricular canal who was status post complete repair, each had experienced a benign postoperative course. At five months and 11.1 respectively following implantation of their pulmonary allograft, both children requiring mitral valve replacement and both died perioperatively. A three year old female with truncus arteriosus type II underwent aortic root replacement 2.5 years after pulmonary allograft right ventricular outflow tract reconstruction and experienced a postoperative myocardial infarction that resulted in death. Two infants who were two months of age at the time of allograft implantation succumbed to pneumonia.

One child expired four months after surgery to repair Tetralogy of Fallot with absent pulmonary valve and the second patient died eight months after complete pulmonary allograft repair of type II truncus arteriosus. Three patients died secondarily to chronic congestive heart failure. A four week of age infant with type I truncus arteriosus and a six week old child with pulmonary atresia each expired ten months after allograft placement A three month old female with type I truncus arteriosus, ventricular septal defect and DiGeorge syndrome died four months postoperatively. Lastly, an asymptomatic teenager died in an automobile accident 18 months following pulmonary allograft replacement of a stenotic prosthetic valve.

Two children ultimately required cardiac transplantation. A twelve year old boy with double outlet left ventricle and aortic valvar insufficiency underwent aortic allograft left and pulmonary allograft right ventricular outflow tract reconstructions. Myocardial dysfunction prompted his cardiac transplantation 3.7 years after double allograft placement. Both allografts were functional upon explant. A seven year old male with double outlet right ventricle, atrioventricular canal, single atrium and pulmonary stenosis underwent pulmonary right ventricular outflow tract reconstruction. One month later, he required placement of a prosthetic mitral valve due to severe insufficiency. Secondary to development of a cardiomyopathy that resulted in chronic congestive heart failure, he underwent cardiac transplantation 7.5 years after allograft insertion. The explanted

valve conduit was calcified with severe cusp degeneration.

Nineteen children (10%) required replacement of their pulmonary allograft from nine days to 8.9 years after the initial allograft surgery. Each incident is chronicled in Tables 6.5 and 6.6. Pathology results were unavailable for two infant allograft recipients. Pathologic examination of 17 explanted allografts revealed all were calcified and seven contained mild cellular infiltrates. Reoperation resulted in a favorable outcome in 13 children. Four children died intraoperatively to four months postoperatively. One child with poor ventricular function underwent cardiac transplantation in the early postoperative period. Another patient required replacement of a third pulmonary allograft when the second developed kinking in the conduit that was attributed to technical error.

One hundred and fifty five pulmonary valve allograft recipients (69%) are alive with their

TABLE 6.5. Allograft Replacement in Pulmonary Allograft Recipients.

Patient	Diagnosis at First Allograft Repair	Age at First Allograft Repair	Complication
CW	Truncus arteriosus type I	9 days	Mediastinitis, allograft infection
JS	Truncus arteriosus type I	2 months	Allograft insufficiency
TJ	Truncus arteriosus type I	2.5 months	LPA and RPA stenosis
JE	Truncus arteriosus type I	3 months	Allograft stenosis and insufficiency
PF	Truncus arteriosus type I	4 months	Allograft compression of LCA
AG	Truncus arteriosus type I	7 months	Allograft stenosis and insufficiency
CD	TGA, RVOT obstruction	10 months	Allograft stenosis
WM	ToF, Pulmonary Atresia	1.1 years	Allograft insufficiency
DT	Pulmonary Atresia, VSD, small RPA	1.2 years	Allograft insufficiency
TSM	ToF	2 years	Allograft insufficiency, LPA stenosis
AJ	DORV	2 years	Allograft stenosis and insufficiency
TK	Pulmonary atresia, VSD, hypoplastic LPA & RPA	2.9 years	Allograft insufficiency
TT	ToF	3 years	Allograft insufficiency, kinked distal allograft anastomosis
TS	ToF	3.2 years	Allograft insufficiency, LPA & RPA stenoses
HE	ToF	4.9 years	Allograft insufficiency, TR, cardiomyopathy
SG	ToF	5 years	Allograft insufficiency
TWM	Critical PS	5 years	Allograft insufficiency, kinked distal allograft conduit
LG	ToF	8.1 years	Allograft stenosis & insufficiency, LPA stenosis
TMS	Absent pulmonary valve, TR	8.9 years	Allograft stenosis and insufficiency

VSD = ventricular septal defect; LPA = left pulmonary artery; RPA = right pulmonary artery; LCA = left coronary artery; TGA = transposition of the great arteries; RVOT = right ventricular outflow tract; ToF = Tetralogy of Fallot; DORV = double outlet right ventricle; PS = pulmonary stenosis; TR = tricuspid regurgitation.

original allograft at 6.0 months to 11.9 years after surgery (mean: 5.8 years). Echocardiographic evidence of mild to moderate pulmonary insufficiency is common.

Upon review of follow up data in the latter patient group who underwent right ventricular outflow reconstruction with a pulmonary allograft, it is obvious that allograft fibrocalcification and degeneration that requires reoperation occurs at an increased rate in infants when compared to older allograft recipients. In children greater than one year of age at operation, interval to explant ranges from 13 months to 9.8 years after primary allograft repair (mean interval: 4.9 years). Interval to allograft replacement ranges from two months to 7.5 years (mean interval: 2.3 years) in children one year of age and younger at the time of initial allograft placement. Table 6.7 documents the statistical difference in incidences of early and late mortality and of allograft replacement between older and younger patient groups. The percentage of patients who experienced each adverse event is significantly higher in every category for children who are 12 months of age or younger at the time of pulmonary allograft right ventricular outflow tract reconstruction. Figure 6.1 is an actuarial event-free curve that illustrates freedom from hospital death, allograft-related death, or allograft replacement. By nine years of follow up, 80 percent of the older children are alive with the original allograft while only 52 percent of the younger children remain event-free. While the patient count becomes extremely small by ten years postoperatively especially in the infant group, event-free percentages remain significantly different. It is noteworthy that a large percentage of the difference between the two curves can be attributed to early postoperative mortality. Beyond the perioperative period, the curves run roughly parallel.

TABLE 6.6. Allograft Replacement in Pulmonary Allograft Recipients (Continued).

Patient	Reoperation	Months After First Allograft Repair	Outcome After Redo RVOTR
CW	Aortic allograft RVOTR	2	Expired 4 months postop RV failure
JS	Redo pulmonary allograft RVOTR	42	Well 3.7 years postop
TJ	Aortic allograft RVOTR	2	Expired intraoperatively Biventricular failure
JE	Redo pulmonary allograft RVOTR	31	Well 5.7 years postop
PF	Aortic allograft RVOTR	4	Expired 4 days postop Myocardial failure
AG	Redo pulmonary allograft RVOTR	21	Well 6.1 years postop
CD	Redo pulmonary allograft RVOTR	90	Well 16 months postop
WM	Redo pulmonary allograft RVOTR	13	Well 5 months postop
DT	Aortic allograft RVOTR	29	Well 3 months postop
TSM	Redo pulmonary allograft RVOTR	38	Well 5.4 years postop
AJ	Redo pulmonary allograft RVOTR	118	Well 1.8 months postop
TK	Redo pulmonary allograft RVOTR	18	Expired hours postop Distal allograft anastomotic hemorrhage
TT	Redo pulmonary allograft RVOTR	36	Well 1.6 years postop
TS	Redo pulmonary allograft RVOTR	15	Well 10.2 years postop
HE	Redo pulmonary allograft RVOTR	74	Cardiac transplant 2 days postop expired
SG	Redo pulmonary allograft RVOTR	111	Well 1.4 years postop
TWM	Redo pulmonary allograft RVOTR	69	Reop 15 months postop Kinked allograft conduit
LG	Redo pulmonary allograft RVOTR	105	Well 1.4 years postop
TMS	Carpentier-Edwards	83	Well 7 months postop

RVOTR = right ventricular outflow tract reconstruction; RV = right ventricular.

TABLE 6.7. Comparison of Older and Younger Pulmonary Allograft Recipients in Early and Late Postoperative Follow-Up.

Patient Age Group	Early Mortality	Late Mortality	Allograft Explant
>12 months	15/179 (8%)	5/163 (5%)	6/163 (7%)
12 months	9/40 (22%)	12/36 (33%)	7/36 (19%)
Combined	24/225 (11%)	21/199 (11%)	19/199 (9%)
p value (>12 mo vs. 12 mo)	$p < 0.05$*	$p < 0.001$*	$p < 0.10$*

* χ^2 for independent samples.

Discussion

Comparative review of follow up for all surgical repair groups incites a few pertinent observations. Early and late mortality as well as late morbidity in the form of allograft explant are depicted numerically in Table 6.8 and graphically in Figure 6.2 to compare each of the four right ventricular outflow tract reconstructive methods presented herein. Per Table 6.8, the incidences of early mortality, late mortality and allograft explant are consistently lower in patients who underwent transannular patch or pulmonary allograft procedures than those who had a porcine or aortic allograft valve implanted. Better results in the transannular patch patient group might appear intuitively appropriate considering the selective simplicity of the anomalies being treated. Specifically, none of the transannular patch children needed complete outflow tract reconstruction whereas a percentage of patients in each of the porcine, aortic allograft and pulmonary allograft valve groups did require surgery that would provide them with a previously nonexistent outflow tract. However, when valve placement or replacement is necessary in more complex anomalies, pulmonary valve allograft reconstruction of the right ventricular outflow tract appears to be the method of choice.

In the actuarial curves (Figure 6.2) which illustrate freedom from hospital death, valve related death or valve failure that required reoperation, the poor early postoperative results experienced by porcine valve conduit recipients is immediately evident. Almost 40% of the children who receive a porcine bioprostheses died in the perioperative period. Some

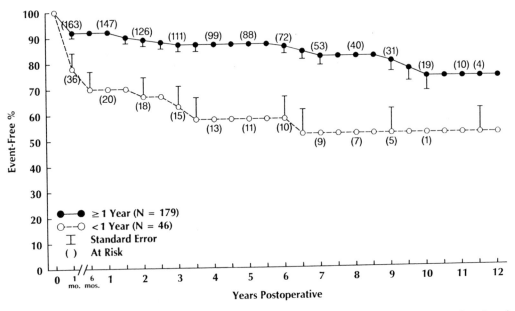

FIGURE 6.1. Actuarial curves for older and younger pulmonary allograft recipients to illustrate freedom from hospital death, valve replaced death, or valve explant.

TABLE 6.8. Comparative Morbidity and Mortality.

Result	Type of Right Ventricular Outflow Tract Reconstruction			
	Porcine	Aortic	Patch	Pulmonary
Early mortality	9/24	9/35	6/35	25/225
	(38%)	(26%)	(17%)	(11%)
Late mortality	3/13	4/26	1/28	21/197
	(24%)	(15%)	(4%)	(11%)
RVOT	9/13	1/28	1/28	19/197
	(69%)	(35%)	(4%)	(10%)
Lost to follow up	2	0	1	5*
Alive without additional operation	1/24	13/35	26/35	155/255

* Includes three children who underwent cardiac transplantation in the late follow-up period.

of this mortality is related to the state of the art at the time, but a portion is also attributable to implantation difficulties associated with these rigid prostheses. Late follow-up continues to be dismal as evidenced by a consistent decline in event-free percentages that is reduced to almost zero by 11.5 years after surgery. Early postoperative failures for aortic allograft, transannular patch and pulmonary allograft recipients are not statistically different. By three years of follow-up, the aortic allograft curve begins to drop rather steeply reflective of the accelerated rate of calcification that has been documented for aortic versus pulmonary valve allografts when used to reconstruct the right ventricular outflow tract.[11,12] At eleven years of follow-up, less than 40% of children who received an aortic allograft are alive with the valve conduit in place. From three to eight years postoperatively, follow-up of transannular patch and pulmonary allograft children remains promising with relatively few adverse

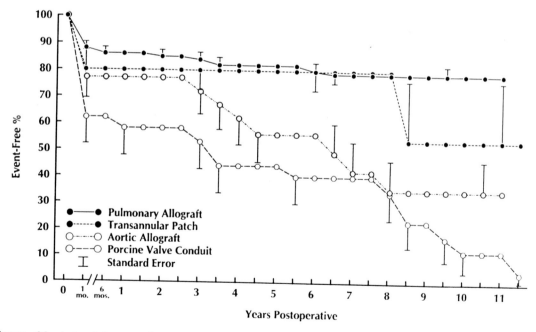

FIGURE 6.2. Actuarial curves for recipients of pulmonary valve allografts, aortic valve allografts, porcine bioprostheses and transannular patches for repair of the right ventricular outflow tract to illustrate freedom from hospital death, valve related death, or reoperation on the right ventricular outflow tract.

events. The transannular patch curve takes a significant dip at 8.5 years that is not significant due to the small number of patients who have been followed for that length of time. By 11.5 years after pulmonary allograft implantation, almost 70 percent of the children are event-free.

Conclusion

Reconstruction of the right ventricular outflow tract in the pediatric population remains a challenge. As the Denver experience reflects, lessons in the surgical treatment of right sided cardiac lesions are learned slowly but consistently. The pulmonary allograft has proven superior performance and endurance over its porcine bioprosthetic and aortic allograft competitors but the ideal valve conduit replacement has not been found. For less severe anomalies of the right ventricular outflow tract that do not require valve replacement, the transannular patch is a reasonable option.

References

1. Ross DN, Somerville J. Correction of pulmonary atresia with a homograft aortic valve. Lancet 1966;2:1446.
2. Brock L. Long-term degenerative changes in aortic segment homografts, with particular reference to calcification. Thorax 1968;23:249–255.
3. Yankah AC, Hetzer R. Procurement and viability of cardiac valve allografts. In Yankah AC, Hetzer R, Miller DC, Ross DN, Somerville J, Yacoub MH (eds). Cardiac Valve Allografts 1962–1987. New York: Springer-Verlag;1988:23–34.
4. Gavin JB, Herdson PB, Barratt-Boyes BG. The pathology of chemically-sterilized human heart valve allografts. Pathology 1972;4:175–183.
5. Moore CH, Martelli V, Al-Janabi N, Ross DN. Analysis of homograft valve failure in 311 patients followed up to 10 years. Ann Thorac Surg 1975;20:274–281.
6. Jonas RA, Freed MD, Mayor JE, Castaneda AR. Long term follow-up of patients with synthetic right heart conduits. Circulation 1985;72 (Suppll. 2):II77–II83.
7. Agarwal KC, Edwards WD, Feldt RH, et al. Clinicopathological correlates of obstructed right-sided porcine-valved extracardiac conduits. J Thorac Cardiovasc Surg 1981;81:591–601.
8. Angell JD, Christopher BS, Hawtrey O, Angell WM. A fresh viable human heart valve bank-sterilization sterility testing and cryogenic preservation. Transplant Proc 1976;8 (Suppl 1): 127–141.
9. Brockbank KG, Bank HL. Measurement of post-cryopreservation viability. J Card Surg 1987;2 (supp I):145–151.
10. O'Brien MF, Stafford EG, Gardner MAH, Phaler PG, McGiffin DC, Kirklin JW. A comparison of aortic valve replacement with viable cryopreserved and fresh allograft valves with a note on chromosomal studies. J Thorac Cardiovasc Surg 1987;94:812–823.
11. Livi U, Abdulla AK, Parker R, Olsen EJ, Ross DN. Viability and morphology of aortic and pulmonary homografts. J Thorac Cardiovasc Surg 1987;93:755–760.
12. Al-Janabi N, Ross DN. Enhanced viability of fresh aortic homografts stored in nutrient medium. Cardiovasc Res 1973;7:817–822.

7
Toronto Series

William G. Williams

There are a number of congenital cardiac defects (Table 7.1) in which connection from the heart to the pulmonary arteries is absent or inadequate. Repair of these defects requires construction of an unobstructed pathway from the heart to the pulmonary arteries, preferably with a competent valve.

Whenever possible, the connection should be made with the patient's own tissue, to provide growth potential. For example, most children with tetralogy are repaired with a longitudinal patch enlargement of the pulmonary artery, which may be transannular. The posterior wall of the reconstructed outflow tract is native tissue and therefore has the potential for growth. The need for further intervention in the intermediate term is minimal and related primarily to pulmonary valve incompetence (PI).[1]

Inferences from Natural History and Surgical Experience

Survival without a pulmonary valve is possible. Shimazaki and coworkers[2] gathered data from the literature on 72 patients with isolated PI. These individuals were symptom-free, with survival not different from the normal population for the first 20 to 30 years of life. After age 30, however, a rapid increase in the onset of symptoms was documented. Three of the 72 patients died, at an average of 39 months after developing symptoms.

It is probable that individuals with PI *and* congenital heart disease will develop symptoms of right-heart decompensation earlier in life than PI patients with otherwise normal hearts, such as those reported by Shimazaki et al. (Figure 7.1).

Follow up data from patients after repair of Tetralogy of Fallot demonstrate that PI is well tolerated for many years. In the absence of right ventricular outflow tract obstruction, Tetralogy patients with a transannular patch have only a 7% chance of reintervention for PI within 20 years of repair.[3] The coexistence of important right ventricular outflow tract obstruction increases that risk to 28%. Gatzoulis and associates[4] demonstrated that post repair Tetralogy patients with reduced right ventricular compliance were protected from the late homodynamic burden of pulmonary valve insufficiency.

The late sequelae of pulmonary valve insufficiency after Tetralogy repair include fatigue and dyspnea with increasing right heart size, and the development of tricuspid valve insufficiency. Atrial and ventricular arrhythmias will develop in some patients and account for an increasing incidence of late sudden death.[5–10]

To lessen the burden of pulmonary valve insufficiency caused by a transannular patch of the right ventricular outflow tract, my associates and I have fashioned a free-hand pericardial cusp on the inside of the patch as described by Asano and Eguchi.[11] Others have used a homograft patch containing one or two valve leaflets. Gundry and associates[12] modified the

TABLE 7.1. Congenital Cardiac Defects.

Absent connection from ventricle to pulmonary artery

- Pulmonary atresia with ventricular septal defect (VSD)
- Truncus arteriosus

Inadequate connection from ventricle to pulmonary artery

- Complete transposition with VSD and pulmonary stenosis (PS)
- Congenitally corrected transposition with PS

and in selected situations:

- Tetralogy of Fallot
- Double-outlet ventricle
- Isolated PS or pulmonary valve incompetence

technique is used, the pulmonary "valve" becomes incompetent within a few weeks. Fortunately, the monocusp almost never becomes obstructive.[13]

The concept of a direct tissue connection has been extended to more complex lesions, such as complete transposition and congenitally corrected transposition. Le Compte et al.[14] pioneered this approach in patients with transposition, thereby avoiding the use of a valved conduit. While this operation is more extensive, and at first was associated with a high mortality rate, recent experience has been more favorable. The avoidance of a conduit may improve late survival.

outflow patch leaflet concept by making an oversized monocusp of pericardium or polytetrafluoroethylene (PTFE). Their technique allows accurate determination of the pulmonary valve orifice, and I believe it provides better early valve function than the smaller leaflet patch we have used. However, whichever

Recommendations

Whenever possible, reconstruction of the connection from the heart to the pulmonary arteries should be made with the patient's own tissue.

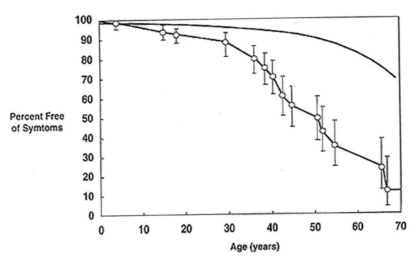

FIGURE 7.1. Data from Shimaziki et al.[2] illustrate the favorable early course of 72 patients with isolated pulmonary valve insufficiency collected from the literature. The comparison group (upper line) was made up of the age-matched normal individuals. After the age of 30, the rate of development of symptoms among patients with isolated pulmonary

incompetence accelerates. Three deaths occurred an average of 39 months after developing symptoms. It is probable that patients with pulmonary valve incompetence *and* associated congenital heart disease, such as Tetralogy of Fallot, will develop symptoms at a earlier age than those with pulmonary insufficiency and a normal heart.

The addition of a monocusp to the outflow tract is probably helpful in the patient's early recovery, and unlikely to be detrimental in the long term.

Late hemodynamic deterioration from isolated pulmonary valve insufficiency should be anticipated, but will not usually occur within 20 years of surgery. If there are other residual lesions, such as increased pulmonary artery resistance from any cause, pulmonary valve insufficiency will be poorly tolerated.

Pulmonary Valves and Tubular Conduits

There are situations where insertion of tubular conduit, containing or not containing a valve prosthesis, is required to connect the heart to the pulmonary arteries. Historically, patients with pulmonary valve atresia and ventricular septal defect (VSD) were the first to undergo repair with the pulmonary conduits. The technique was soon adapted to the treatment of pulmonary stenosis (PS) in patients with complete transposition or congenitally corrected transposition, and to the treatment of truncus arteriosus and other lesions (Table 7.1).

In the cases of Tetralogy of Fallot, a pulmonary valve or conduit is indicated in cases of:

- Anomalous origin of the left coronary from the right coronary artery when the outflow tract cannot be adequately relieved of obstruction
- Absent pulmonary valve syndrome (usually a valve can be implanted in the outflow tract, thereby avoiding the tubular conduit)
- Some cases of increased pulmonary resistance from inaccessible branch pulmonary artery stenosis, hypoplastic pulmonary arteries, or increased arteriolar resistance
- Low output syndrome early after Tetralogy repair in patients with PI
- Right heart failure, progressive tricuspid insufficiency, or ventricular arrhythmias, late after Tetralogy repair

Brief Historical Overview

The first successful construction of a pulmonary conduit was reported in 1965 by Kirklin and coworkers,[15] who fashioned a tube of pericardium in the operating room for a patient with pulmonary valve atresia. Klinner and Zenker[16] in the same year reported the use of a Teflon tube to bypass the obstruction in patients with Tetralogy; Ross and Somerville[17] published their experience the following year. In their patients, who had pulmonary atresia, they utilized an aortic homograft as a valved conduit.[17]

Difficulty in procuring homograft material in North America led to the commercial production of Dacron tubular grafts containing a porcine vale. These prostheses were widely adopted into clinical practice. The orifice of the porcine valve is 5 to 6mm smaller than the diameter of the Dacron tube; this relative stenosis led to the incorporation of a pericardial valve within the conduit to reduce the transconduit pressure gradients. Other, less commonly used devices were also devised, including mechanical valves.

From these beginnings, there has evolved a variety of prosthetic devices with few, if any, comparisons of their long term efficacy. With the publication[18] of reports of valve calcification leading to stenosis and insufficiency, and of fibrous obstruction within the Dacron leading to reoperation to replace a stenotic or, less frequently, incompetent prostheses, it soon became apparent that durability was a problem. Reports of satisfactory durability of the homograft conduit from Ross's patients by Saravalli and coworkers[19] renewed interest in allograft material. They demonstrated important differences in durability because of different allograft preservation techniques, but also noted rapid deterioration in young patients and in those with associated congenital heart disease. A subsequent publication[20] demonstrated superior durability in pulmonary as opposed to aortic homograft conduits. In our earlier publication,[21] we did not demonstrate a significant difference in long-term valve survival; but with further follow-up, a significant difference is evident.

Experience with Pulmonary Valve Replacement—Toronto

Our total experience with pulmonary valve replacement at The Hospital for Sick Children and the Toronto Congenital Cardiac Centre for Adults to the end of 1995 consisted of 661 patients. Of these, 160 (30%) have undergone 200 reoperations to replace the prosthetic pulmonary devices.

In a recent analysis of our experience from 1966 to 1994, my associates and I reviewed the first 606 patients to determine the importance of various factors in predicting long term outcome. A multivariate analysis examined the following risk factors: diagnosis; age at operation; year of operation; patient weight and surface area at operation; type of device—valved conduit or pulmonary valve orthotopic implant (PVI); size of prosthetic valve; location of proximal anatomic correction (from morphologic right or left ventricle); and source of homograft (commercial or "in-house" preservation). The outcome variables were survival of the patient and reoperation for valve failure. The causes of valve failure were not analyzed in detail; but although there were many mechanisms of failure, the great majority were calcific stenosis of the valve or the conduit, with a rising right ventricular pressure (Table 7.2).

Factors Affecting Patient Survival

Patient survival (Figure 7.2) was not affected by the type of prosthesis. Valve size did affect sur-

TABLE 7.2. Summary of Toronto Experience with Replacement of Pulmonary Valves, 1966–1994.

	Number (%)
Patients	606
Operative mortality	112 (18.5%)
Operative survivors	494
Reoperations	143 (29%)
Late deaths	45 (9.1%)
Prosthetic Valves	
Initial Valves	606
Valved conduits	453 (75%)
Homograft	236
Porcine/Dacron	153
Polystan	61
Other	3
Valve implants	153 (25%)
Pericardial	93
Porcine	35
Homograft	18
Other	7
Reoperations	178
Valve conduits	148
PVIs	30

vival: Operative survival is better in patients receiving larger valves. In addition, more recent year of operation and the diagnosis of Tetralogy had a favorable influence on patient survival (odds ratio, 0.5). Patients with truncus arteriosus had a higher operative risk (odds ratio, 1.14).

During the period of follow-up, which averaged 5.4 years per patient, 143 patients (29% of the 494 hospital survivors) required reoperation to replace the pulmonary valve. The fre-

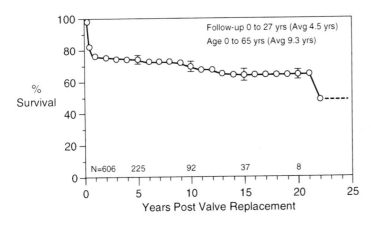

FIGURE 7.2. Survival of 606 patients who underwent pulmonary valve replacement. All patients operated upon from 1966 to 1994 are included. Survival at 20 years after pulmonary valve replacement is 62%.

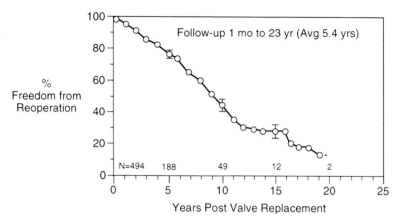

FIGURE 7.3. Freedom from reoperation for all 494 patients discharged from hospital after pulmonary valve replacement.

quency of reoperation is 5% per year during the first 10 years of observation (Figure 7.3).

Factors Affecting Valve Survival

By univariate analysis, freedom from reoperation is better for the 140 patients who received an orthotopically implanted pulmonary valve (PVI), in comparison to the 354 who received a pulmonary valve conduit (Figure 7.4).

Pulmonary Valve Orthotopic Implants Patients

Among the 140 patients receiving an orthotopic pulmonary valve without a conduit, only the size of the valve had a statistically important effect upon the interval free of valve reoperation. Valve size is an important determinant of valve durability for all types of prosthetic pulmonary valves (Figure 7.5).

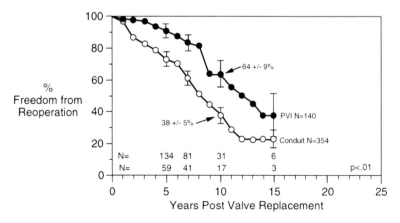

FIGURE 7.4. There is a greater chance of being free of pulmonary valve reoperation with an orthotopic implant (PVI, n = 140 at operation) than with a valved conduit (n = 354 at operation, p < 0.01). Ten years after operation, 64% (±9%) of the PVI group (n = 31, 10 years post valve replacement) were free from reoperation, compared to only 38% (±5%) of the conduit group (n = 17).

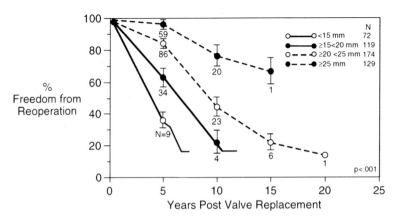

FIGURE 7.5. Only prosthetic valve size had a statistically significant effect upon survival of the pulmonary valve implants. The data illustrate the effect of valve size upon the interval to reoperation for all 494 patients surviving an initial pulmonary valve replacement (p < 0.001).

Although the type of valve (porcine vs. pericardial) did not affect the interval free of reoperation, 83% of patients with porcine valves were free of reoperation at 10 years, compared to only 64% with pericardial valves. I expect this difference to become statistically significant with longer follow-up.

Conduit Patients

Multivariate analysis of the 453 patients with a valved conduit demonstrated that age at operation, year of operation, valve size and valve type are important predictors for reoperation. The risk of reoperation increases with younger age and with smaller prosthesis. Paradoxical to patient survival (which has improved in recent years), the risk of reoperation is increased in patients operated upon more recently.

Valve type does have an effect upon the interval to reoperation. Porcine conduits survive longer than homograft conduits, although the interval free of reoperation is not significantly different. Analysis of all 255 patients with homograft conduits who were discharged from hospital after an initial valve replacement or a valve reoperation demonstrated a statistically important improvement in survival free of reoperation for the group with pulmonary homografts. Both porcine valve conduits and the pulmonary homograft conduits offer better long-term valve survival free of reoperation than aortic-valve conduits. Figure 7.6 attempts to illustrate the complex interaction between the age of the patient and the type of conduit used.

The influence of the size and type of valve on valve survival (data now shown) is virtually identical to that seen in Figure 7.6.

Conclusions: Factors Affecting Survival

Patient survival 15 years after an operation that includes pulmonary valve replacement is 65% (±3%) and is:

- Improving in recent years
- Better for larger valve sizes
- Affecting by diagnosis (better in patients with Tetralogy; worse among patients with truncus arteriosus)

Valve survival (interval free of reoperation) is only 45% at 10 years after valve replacement. Results are improved by:

- Larger valve size
- Older age of the patient at valve replacement
- Valve type
  — PVI results are better than those for valve conduits

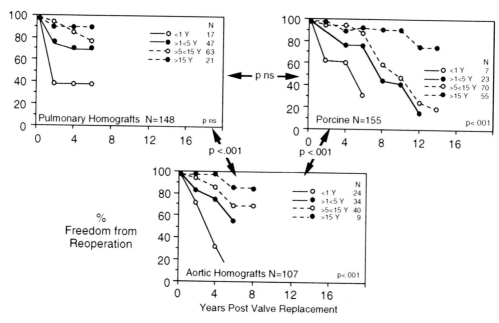

FIGURE 7.6. The effect of age on the interval free of reoperation is evident for each type of valved conduits. Younger patients are at risk of earlier reoperation irrespective of the type of conduit. There is no statistically important difference between pulmonary homograft and porcine conduits, by each provided durability significantly superior to that of aortic homografts (p < 0.001).

— Porcine conduits and pulmonary homograft conduits do better than aortic homograft conduits

Discussion

Our data are useful in explaining some of the confusion and controversy evident in the literature.

Valve Type

Homograft valved conduits have handling characteristics superior to synthetic materials. They are more easily sutured, bleed less, mold to fit complex configurations, and can be less expensive. However, their long-term durability is a disappointment—especially in smaller sizes, in younger patients and in the aortic homograft conduit.

The long-term results reported in the large series from the Mayo clinic are similar to our experience.[22,23] Of 326 patients with homograft conduits, the 5-year survival rate free of valve failure as 94% for pulmonary and 70% for aortic homograft. Failure of the valve was more likely in young patients (under 4 years old) with an aortic homograft. In an earlier paper from that clinic,[24] an analysis of 352 patients with an extracardiac conduit placed before 1977 showed that patients with a heterograft conduit were less likely to require reoperation within 5 years than those with an aortic homograft (6% vs. 28%); however, this was in an area when chemical "preservation" of the homograft was used.

In contrast, in Kay and Ross's experience[25] using fresh aortic homografts in 97 patients with pulmonary valve atresia, only 13% required reinterventions for valve failure within 10 years of operation. The youngest patient in his series was 2 years old (mean age, 11 years). Another report from Ross's series by Saravalli and associates[19] described less favorable results in younger patients and in patients with cyanotic heart disease. However, a comparison of different prosthesis in the pulmonary position from The Hospital for Sick Children in London showed no difference in performance of homografts or heterograft conduits: Only 20% of patients with either prosthesis were free of reoperation 10 years after implantation. Interestingly, the authors of that report used fresh antibiotic homografts from the same source as those used by Ross. The younger age of the patients (18 years at most, with 25% under 4 years old) may explain some of these differences.[26]

There is general agreement that young age increases the risk of early reoperation for valve failure, even with a homograft conduit.[27-30] In our analysis, aortic homografts fared substantially less well than pulmonary homografts in the younger patients (Figure 7.6).

The mechanism or mechanisms of homograft failure have not been clearly defined. Salim et al.[31] demonstrated that some homografts shrink after implantation. Explanted conduits had dense fibrous tissue with calcification of the media and chronic mononuclear cell infiltration. We have seen this dramatic reduction of conduit diameter several times.

Evidence for immunologic rejection leading to valve failure is inconclusive as yet, but is a probable mechanism.[32] Yacoub and co-workers[33] summarized the current state of knowledge and concluded that further study, including controlled trials, is necessary before specific recommendations for changes in clinical management of patients with homograft valves can be offered. Gonzalis-Lavin et al.[34] demonstrated that viable fresh aortic homografts placed in puppies deteriorate more when they came from unrelated donors. We[21] and others[35] have failed to show a correlation with graft destruction and donor/recipient blood type.

Whether fresh antibiotic preservation or cryopreservation techniques results in better long term performance of homografts is unclear. Kirklin and associates[36] demonstrated excellent short-term function of cryopreserved homografts ($n = 128$) grouped with fresh homografts

($n = 19$), with 94% freedom from reoperation at 3.5 years. The data of O'Brien and associates for aortic valve replacement with homografts show no significant difference between fresh and cryopreserved preservation techniques for the first 10 years of follow-up. Similar data for the presence of valves in the pulmonary circuit have not been reported.

There is general agreement that the long term performance of pulmonary homografts is superior to that of aortic conduits. In our previous publication,[21] we did not demonstrate a difference; but as these patients were followed longer, the difference became evident. Livi et al.[37] showed that the normal pulmonary arterial wall has less calcium and elastic tissue than the aorta and proposed that these features would make the pulmonary graft less prone to calcification. In clinical practice, pulmonary grafts seldom calcify, whereas aortic homografts become heavily, and often rapidly, calcified.

Mechanical Valves

Little has been reported regarding the use of mechanical valves in the pulmonary position. The requisite life-long anticoagulation and higher intrinsic pressure gradients have precluded wide acceptance into clinical practice. Goor and coworkers[38] reported 7 patients with mechanical valves and no complications with a short follow up, although 3 had pressure gradients >40mmHg. Ilbawi and associates[39] noted a high incidence of valve thrombosis among 16 children with pulmonary (or tricuspid) bileaflet mechanical valves. At 2 years after replacement, freedom from reoperation was only 70% for right sided valves, compared to 100% for aortic/mitral valves. He recommended that these mechanical valves not to be used in the pulmonary position. Other anecdotal reports[40,41] of mechanical pulmonary valve malfunction also discourage the use of these devices.

Tubular Prostheses

The additional synthetic material, either as a hood or as a tubular extension to a homograft, has been found to increase the risk of late stenosis.[26,42] Pericardial patches or discarded pieces of the homograft are less prone to develop the intimal fibrous peel that usually forms with Dacron and leads to obstruction. Molina et al.[43] studied a number of synthetic materials implanted in the right heart of 100 lambs; they concluded that PTFE conduits have substantially better long term performance, similar to that of allografts. Various fabrics with different pore sizes had no favorable long-term advantage. Clinical use of PTFE is limited by difficulty in controlling bleeding from suture lines, and in fitting the material to a curve.

Barbero-Marcial and associates[44] reported on the use of bovine pericardial valved conduits with crimped walls in 29 patients. In a short follow up period (44 months at most), results were satisfactory, with low pressure gradients and no reoperations. Hand made equine pericardial valved conduits (n = 143) performed better than Dacron heterograft conduits in a series reported by Imai and coworkers,[45] but were inferior to a direct tissue connection.

Conclusions

There is not yet an ideal substitute for the natural pulmonary valve and its artery. In cardiac anomalies requiring construction of a connection between the right heart and the pulmonary arteries, reoperation may be inevitable.

Consideration of the long term outlook for the patient should be made at the initial and at each subsequent operation. Recognizing that the absence of a pulmonary valve is well tolerated in otherwise healthy individuals for many years, the surgeon should first consider, whenever feasible, avoiding a prosthetic valve and tube. In the absence of distal pulmonary artery obstruction, where left heart function is normal and the tricuspid valve is competent, a pulmonary valve may not be necessary. By mobilizing distal pulmonary arteries, a direct tissue connection to the right heart (augmented by autologous pericardium, with or without a monocusp leaflet) may be a satisfactory long-term solution.

In situations where a valved conduit is required (such as where there is a discontinuity between the right heart and the pulmonary arteries, increased pulmonary resistance, inadequate left heart function, or tricuspid valve insufficiency), none of the currently available devices is ideal. In infants, a pulmonary homograft is technically easier to use and is the valve of choice; however, replacement should be anticipated within 2 to 5 years.

In situations where a homograft would required a tubular extension to bridge the gap between pulmonary arteries and the right heart, such as complete transposition or congenitally corrected transposition, a Dacron tube containing a heterograft valve should provide durability equal to a homograft conduit, particularly in older patients, who can accommodate a larger valve. In this circumstance my preference is a Dacron heterograft prosthesis.

When a conduit is replaced, one should anticipate a more hazardous operation and risk of bleeding in the presence of a previous homograft conduit. If the patient's size does not permit a large conduit (>20 mm), I recommend implanting another homograft, preferably pulmonary. Otherwise replace the homograft with a Dacron heterograft conduit, which has longevity equal to that of a homograft and is safer to reoperate upon.

When reoperating upon a Dacron heterograft conduit, consideration should be given to removing the old prosthesis from its fibrous sheath and using the sheath by patching its anterior wall with pericardium, as describing by Danielson et al.[46] If necessary, a porcine valve may be sewn into the bed of the fibrous sheath and covered with the pericardial patch.

In future, newer developments in transplant immunology may offer substantial improvements in long-term durability of both allograft and xenograft tissue. Techniques to construct connections with native tissue, which provides the advantage of growth potential, will also improve. Advances should focus upon treatment of the young child, for whom durability of current technology is particularly inadequate.

References

1. Kirklin JK, Kirklin JW, Blackstone EH, Milano A, Pacifico AD. Effect of transannular patching on outcome after repair of tetralogy of Fallot. Ann Thorac Surg 1989;48:783–791.
2. Shimazaki Y, Blackstone EH, Kirklin JW. The natural history of isolated congenital pulmonary valve incompetence: Surgical implications. Thorac Cardiovasc Surg 1984;32:257–259.
3. Murphy JC, Gersh BJ, Mair DD, Fuster V, McGoon MD, Ilstrup DM, McGoon DC, Kirklin JW, Danielson GK. Long-term outcome in patients undergoing surgical repair of tetralogy of Fallot. New Eng Journ Med 1994;329(9): 593–599.
4. Gatzoulis MA, Clark AL, Cullen S, Newman CG, Redington AN. Right ventricular diastolic function 15 to 35 years after repair of tetralogy of Fallot. Circulation 1995;91:1775–1781.
5. Quattlebaum TB, Varghese J, Neill CA, Donahue JS. Sudden death among postoperative patients with tetralogy of Fallot. Circulation 1976;54: 289–293.
6. Rocchini AP, Rosenthal A, Freed M. Chronic congestive heart failure after repair of tetralogy of Fallot. Circulation 1977;56:305–310.
7. Warner KB, Anderson JE, Fulton DR, Payne DD, Geggel RL, Marx GR. Restoration of the pulmonary valve reduces right ventricular volume overload after previous repair of tetralogy of Fallot. Circulation 1993;88(5 Pt 2):II-189–II-197.
8. Burns RJ, Liu PP, Druck MN, Seawright SJ, Williams WG, McLaughlin PR. Analysis of adults with and without complex ventricular arrhythmias after repair of tetralogy of Fallot. J Am Coll Cardiol 1984;4:226–233.
9. Gatzoulis MA, Till JA, Somerville J, Redinton AN. Mechanoelectrical interaction in tetralogy of Fallot: QRS prolongation relates to right ventricular size and predicts malignant ventricular arrhythmias and sudden death. Circulation 1995; 92:231–237.
10. Dietl CA, Gazzaniga ME, Dubner SJ, Perez-Balino NA, Torres AR, Favaloro RG. Life-threatening arrhythmias and RV dysfunction after surgical repair of tetralogy of Fallot. Circulation 1994;90:7–12.
11. Asano K, Eguchi S. A new method of right ventricular outflow reconstruction in corrective surgery for tetralogy of Fallot. J Thorac Cardiovasc Surg 1970;59:512–517.
12. Gundry SR, Razzouk AJ, Boskind JF. Fate of the pericardial monocusp pulmonary valve for right

ventricular outflow tract reconstruction: Early function, late failure without obstruction. J Thorac Cardiovasc Surg 1994;107:908–913.
13. Kirklin JK, Smith D, Novick W, et al. Long-term function of cryopreserved aortic homografts: a ten year study. J Thorac Cardiovasc Surg 1993;106:154–166.
14. Le Compte Y, Neveux JY, Leca F. Reconstruction of the pulmonary outflow tract without prosthetic conduit. J Thorac Cardiovasc Surg 1982;84:727.
15. Rastelli GC, Ongley PA, Davis GD, Kirklin JW. Surgical repair for pulmonary valve atresia with coronary-pulmonary artery fistula: Report of a case. Mayo Clin Proc 1965;40:521–727.
16. Klinner W, Zenker R. Experience with correction of Fallot's tetralogy in 178 cases. Surgery 1965;57:353–357.
17. Ross DN, Somerville J. Correction of pulmonary atresia with a homograft aortic valve. Lancet 1966;2:1446–1447.
18. Ciaravella JM, Jr., McGoon DC, Danielson GK, Wallace RB, Mair DD, Ilstrup DM. Experience with the extracardiac conduit. J Thorac Cardiovasc Surg 1979;78:920–930.
19. Saravalli OA, Somerville J, Jefferson KE. Calcification of aortic homografts used for reconstruction of the right ventricular outflow tract. J Thorac Cardiovasc Surg 1980;80:909–920.
20. Albert JD, Bishop DA, Fullerton DA, Campbell DN, Clarke DR. Conduit reconstruction of the right ventricular outflow tract. J Thorac Cardiovasc Surg 1993;106:228–236.
21. Cleveland DC, Williams WG, Razzouk AJ. Failure of cryopreserved homograft valved conduits in the pulmonary circulation. Circulation 1992;86(suppl II):II-150–II-153.
22. Danielson GK, Anderson BJ, Schleck CD, Ilstrup DM. Late results of pulmonary ventricle to pulmonary artery conduits. Sem in Thor and Card Surg, No 3 1995;7:162–167.
23. Bando K, Danielson GK, Schaff HV. Outcome of pulmonary and aortic homografts for right ventricular outflow tract reconstruction. J Thorac Cardiovasc Surg 1995;109:509–518.
24. McGoon DC, Danielson GK, Pgua FJ, Ritter DG, Mair DD, Ilstrup DM. Late results after extracardiac conduit repair for congenital cardiac defects. Am J Cardiol 1982;49:1741–1749.
25. Kay PH, Ross DN. Fifteen years' experience with the aortic homograft: the conduit of choice for right ventricular outflow tract reconstruction. Ann Thorac Surg 1985;40:360–364.

26. Bull C, Macartney FJ, Horvath P, et al. Evaluation of long-term results of homograft and heterograft valves and extracardiac conduits. J Thorac Cardiovasc Surg 1987;94:12–19.

27. Heinemann MK, Hanley FL, Fenton KN, Jonas RA, Mayer JE, Castaneda AR. Fate of small homograft conduits after early repair in truncus arteriosus. Ann Thorac Surg 1993;55:1409–1412.

28. Clarke D, Campbell D, Hayward A, et al. Degeneration of aortic valve allografts in young recipients. J Thorac Cardiovasc Surg 1993;105:934–942.

29. Chan KC, Fyfe DA, McKay CA. Right ventricular outflow tract reconstruction with cryopreserved homografts in pediatric patients: intermediate-term follow-up with serial echocardiographic assessment. J Am Coll Cardiol 1994;24:483–489.

30. Sano S, Karl TR, Mee RB. Extracardiac valved conduits in the pulmonary circuit. Ann Thorac Surg 1991;52:285–290.

31. Salim MA, DiSessa TG, Alpert BS, Arheart KL, Novick WM, Watson DC. The fate of homograft conduits in chilren with congenital heart disease: An angiographic study. Ann Thorac Surg 1995;59:67–73.

32. Muller-Hermelink HK. Immunohistopathology of cardiac valve allograft explants. In Ross, Somerville J, Yacoub MH (eds). Proceedings of the Symposium on Cardiac Valve Allografts 1962–1987: Current Concepts on the Use of Aortic and Pulmonary Allografts for Heart Valve Substitutes. Berlin: Springer-Verlag; 1987: 89–94.

33. Yacoub M. Applications and limitations of histocompatibility in clinical cardiac valve allograft surgery. In Ross, Somerville J, Yacoub MH (eds). Proceedings of the Symposium on Cardiac Valve Allografts 1962–1987: Current Concepts on the Use of Aortic and Pulmonary Allografts for Heart Valve Substitutes. Berlin: Springer-Verlag; 1987.

34. Gonzalez-Lavin L, Bianchi J, Graf D, Amini S, Gordon CI. Homograft valve calcification: Evidence for an immunological influence. In Ross, Somerville J, Yacoub MH (eds). Proceedings of the Symposium on Cardiac Valve Allografts 1962–1987: Current Concepts on the Use of Aortic and Pulmonary Allografts for Heart Valve Substitutes. Berlin: Springer-Verlag; 1987: 69–74.

35. Shaddy RE, Tani LY, Sturtevant JE, Lambert LM, McGough EC. Effects of homograft blood type and anatomic type on stenosis, regurgitation and calcium in homografts in the pulmonary position. Am J Cardiol 1992;70:392–393.

36. Kirklin JW, Blackstone EH, Maehara T, Pacifico AD, Kirklin JK, Pollock S, Stewart RW. Intermediate-term fate of cryopreserved allograft and xenograft valved conduits. Ann Thorac Surg 1987;44:598–606.

37. Livi U, Abdulla AK, Parker R, Olsen EJ, Ross DN. Viability and morphology of aortic and pulmonary homografts. J Thorac Cardiovasc Surg 1987;93:755–760.

38. Goor DA, Hoa TQ, Mohr R, Smolinsky A, Hegesh J, Neufeld HN. Pericardial-mechanical valved conduits in the management of right ventricular outflow tracts. J Thorac Cardiovasc Surg 1984;87:236–243.

39. Ilbawi MN, Lockhart G, Idriss FS, et al. Experience with St. Jude medical valve prosthesis in children: A word of caution regarding right-sided placement. J Thorac Cardiovasc Surg 1987;93: 73–79.

40. Hartzler GO, Diehl AM, Reed WA. Nonsurgical correction of a "frozen" disc valve prosthesis using a catheter technique and intracardiac streptokinase infusion. J Am Cardiol 1984;4: 779–783.

41. Fleming WH, Sarafian LB, Moulton AL, Robinson LA, Kugler JD. Valve Replacement in the Right Side of the Heart in Children: Long-Term Follow-up. The Society of Thoracic Surgeons 1989;48:404–408.

42. Kabayashi J, Backer CL, Zales VR, Crawford SE, Muster AJ, Mavroudis C. Failure of the Hemashield extension in right ventricle-to-pulmonary artery conduits. Ann Thorac Surg 1993;56:277–281.

43. Molina JE, Edwards JE, Bianco RW, Clack RW, Lang G, Molina JP. Composite and plain tubular synthetic graft conduits in right ventricular-pulmonary artery position: Fate in growing lambs. J Thorac Cardiovasc Surg 1995;110:427–435.

44. Barbero-Marcial M, Baucia JA, Jatene A. Valved conduits of bovine pericardium for right ventricle to pulmonary artery connections. Sem in Thor and Card Surg, No 3 1995;7:148–153.

45. Imai Y, Takanashi Y, Hoshino S, Nakata S. The equine pericardial valved conduit and current strategies for pulmonary reconstruction. Sem in Thor and Card Surg, No 3 1995;7:157–161.

46. Downing TP, Danielson GK, Schaff HV, Puga FJ, Edwards WD, Driscoll DJ. Replacement of obstructed right ventricular-pulmonary arterial valved conduits with non-valved conduits in children. Circulation 1985;72(Suppl II):II-84–II-87.

Section IV
Cryopreserved Allograft Tissue for Cardiac Reconstruction

8
Cryopreserved Cardiac Valves: Initial Experiences and Theories

Richard A. Hopkins

As outlined in Chapter 1, definite advantages were realized with the use of "fresh" wet-stored antibiotic-sterilized human homograft valves for the reconstruction of left and right ventricular outflow tracts. However, problems with availability and lack of certainty concerning preservation and storage techniques limited their widespread use. The combination of their apparent resistance to infection, excellent hydraulic function, absence of need for anticoagulation, and versatility in difficult outflow reconstructions made them optimal choices for many categories of patients, beyond the single issue of durability. The durability of the nonviable but gently preserved homografts was certainly as good as xenografts in adults and even better than xenografts in children. For the past 15 to 20 years, the theoretical hope has been that, if durability could be improved, a homograft would combine the superior attributes of xenografts with the superior attributes of mechanical prostheses and thus be the valve of choice for large numbers of patients.

Evaluation of data from the fresh, wet-stored series suggested that tissue viability at the time of transplantation was associated with increased durability.[1-3] This impression that short, warm ischemia times and shorter, cold storage periods contributed to prolonged graft durability has been difficult to prove with retrospective analyses. Attention to such issues was not what it is today in the era of multiple-organ donor retrievals.[4] Nevertheless, there does appear to be some suggestion that it has indeed been the case when looking at the larger series from the 1960s and 1970s. For example, many of the original recipients of homografts had prolonged durability of their prostheses, and these patients were the very ones in whom prolonged cold storage did not precede the implant. Also, comparing the Harefield series with the National Heart Hospital series of Ross suggested better durability in the former series.[5] The techniques of preservation and harvesting were essentially the same, with the primary difference being that the Harefield group tended to use homografts sooner following procurement; they reported their 8-year actuarial patient survival at 72%, with homograft valve failure occurring in only 19.3% of their patients by 13 years.[6-10] The Harefield group suggested by logistic analysis a significant negative contribution ($p < 0.01$) of warm ischemia time (defined by them as the death-to-dissection interval) to valve durability.[10] Thus these intriguing tidbits plus the teleological thinking that transplanting a viable fibroblast that can remodel and repair by synthesizing structural proteins would confer greater durability led to cryopreservation techniques and alterations in retrieval protocols designed to enhance cellular viability.[11]

Beginning in June 1975, O'Brien from Brisbane, Australia began a series of valve replacements utilizing allograft valves that had undergone gentle antibiotic sterilization after retrieval, with attention to short, warm ischemia times; these were then cryopreserved with a dimethylsulfoxide (DMSO) controlled-rate freezing technique with storage in liquid nitrogen at −190°C. His group has published histologic as well as biochemical data suggesting viability.[1,4] In addition the Brisbane center recovered cryopreserved valves from patients dying of unrelated causes 2 months to 9.5 years following implant; the tissue culture results from these valves suggested some residual "fibroblast" viability, and chromosomal analysis confirmed donor origin of the "fibroblasts." Origin of these cells have subsequently been questioned.

Angell and associates have reported on their early use of DMSO cryopreserved aortic allografts inserted between 1973 and 1975. Thirty-two such valves were placed, some of which were mounted on stents and 23 sewn freehand. At 10 years' follow-up, 80% of the freehand valves were functional in alive patients.[11] This early clinical application of the cryopreservation process was followed by an intensive and consistent effort by the Brisbane group under the direction of O'Brien. His group has reported on 192 valves placed between June 1975 and December 1986. A number of important points are made in review of the data in these early reports.[1,4] For the cryopreserved aortic valves, they reported a 100% freedom from reoperation for valve degeneration at 10 years. There was minimal thromboembolism and a 4% prosthetic endocarditis rate. Ninety-two percent of patients were free of reoperation (actuarial) at 10 years for viable cryopreserved valves. The reason for reoperation was usually technical malalignment leading to insufficiency, not a consequence of allograft valve degeneration. Incremental risk factor analysis demonstrated that the combination of young recipient age and old donor age were associated with a greater risk of degeneration of fresh, wet-stored allograft valves, but it was not applicable to the cryopreserved valves. The resistance to prosthetic endocarditis and the pattern of its occurrence, being primarily late rather than early, was demonstrated not only in the O'Brien series but also in the experience of the Alabama and New Zealand groups.[12,13] The role of the pulmonary valve implanted in the aortic position is still being defined. Although technically it can be implanted easily, as proved by the autotransplant series of Ross, the pulmonary valve is structurally different and has yet to be proved a suitable allograft replacement in the aortic position[14,15] (see Chapter 8).

Combining what was learned from the use of fresh wet-stored valves with the notions which emerged from the early stages of the cryopreservation era of ventricular outflow tract reconstructions with allograft valve transplants, the emerging role for the use of cryopreserved valves is affected by the following concepts:[16]

1. In certain patient subgroups allograft durability may be superior to any other available biological valve except autotransplants.

2. Optimal hydraulic function due to central non-obstructed flow minimizes the problem of small aortic roots.

3. Optimal hydraulic function improves ventricular performance which may continue to improve with time as left ventricular hypertrophy regresses.

4. Allografts have low thromboembolism rates without anticoagulation. This suggests an advantage for cryopreserved allografts in patients for whom anticoagulation is contraindicated, e.g., children, young women, workers with traumatic occupations, athletes, etc.

5. Allografts may have some resistance to prosthetic bacterial endocarditis.

6. From a material properties standpoint, an allograft is a flexible prosthesis for complex ventricular outflow tract reconstructions.

Left Ventricular Outflow Tract Reconstructions with Cryopreserved Allografts

In the 1990s, emphasis had been placed on the role of viability in the durability of cryopreserved aortic allografts and the refinement in surgical techniques to optimize their early to mid-term performance. The role of cryopreservation and viability is discussed elsewhere in this volume. Implantation techniques have been evaluated by many authors, which in general have shown that in experienced hands, all techniques can be used effectively. However, in less experienced hands, perivalvular leaks and postoperative regurgitation have been consistently higher with the original subcoronary implantation technique than with either root replacement or modified techniques such as the flange or scallop technique.[17] In a very important study by Doty and colleagues from Salt Lake City, 117 patients receiving cryopreserved aortic allograft replacement between 1985 and 1996 were analyzed.[18] This series demonstrated that four different techniques, including 120° rotation, freehand aortic placement with intact non-coronary sinus, aortic root enlargement with intact non-coronary sinus and total aortic root replacements have relatively equivalent results although the 120° rotation technique was abandoned. They, like us, have noted the advantage of leaving the noncoronary sinus intact and the relative ease of the root replacement with or without enlargement.[19-27] This series of adult patients confirmed excellent outcomes which were achieved with the addition of intra-operative echocardiography: operative mortality equaled 3% and freedom from valve-related mortality at 10 years was 9% ± 5%, only four patients required valve explantation for structural deterioration with a 10 year freedom from reoperation for allograft-related causes of 92% ± 3.5%. There was very low incidence of thromboembolism, but like other series, there was a definite incidence of endocarditis (2.5%).

Thus, with the enhanced accessibility to homografts by the availability of cryopreservation vapor phase liquid nitrogen storage and with relatively consistent results obtained in adult left ventricular outflow tract reconstructions surgeons have used allografts more frequently. As in the right-sided conduits, durability in the younger patients appears to be less good. However, the other advantages of homografts make them attractive prosthetic choices for children. The aortic homograft remains an excellent choice for aortic valve replacement in patients who cannot, or do not wish to have anticoagulation and for whom the Ross operation is not appropriate or desired. It is clearly indicated in infectious destruction of the left ventricular outflow tract as the replacement of choice. It is a very reasonable alternative in younger patients, although in patients with more than a 20 year life expectancy, there is at least a 50% chance that a second operation will be required. Technical facility with the implantation techniques remains critical to their success and is a major theme of this book.[28] Surgical techniques which minimize distortion, turbulence and obstruction will result in less energy dissipation across the homograft and thus less stimulus for fibrosis, calcification or deposition of blood-borne microbes. Every effort must be made by the implanting surgeon to obtain the most hemodynamically advantageous reconstruction.

Right Ventricular Outflow Reconstructions with Cryopreserved Allografts

As has been clearly demonstrated in a number of centers, human tissue is superior material for reconstructions of the right ventricular outflow tract.[29-33] Fontan and associates[29] have reported 103 homograft reconstructions between 1968 and 1983 with no episodes of valvular dysfunction, thromboembolism, or hemolysis, although one-third of the patients died either early or late. None of these deaths was due to the aortic valve allograft itself, and only one replacement was required for the development of obstruction. The Alabama group has reported a significant series of 128 patients with cryopreserved aortic allograft reconstructions of the pulmonary outflow tract.[34] This important series demonstrated excellent short-term results, with a 94% actuarial freedom from reoperation at 3.5 years.

Most authorities agree that right-sided valve-Dacron conduits have limited durability, with obstruction inevitably developing and progression resulting in ultimate failure. Such failure can occur as quickly as 18–24 months, although, to be fair, excellent palliation may be achieved. The Mayo Clinic series of approximately 1,100 patients led Danielson to cite a failure-free rate of 94% at 5 years and to estimate a 10-year rate of approximately 75%.[34] Kirklin and colleagues cited a 15-year replacement-free rate of only 11%.[35]

The San Francisco group has reported good short-term palliation with the small Hancock prosthesis (12 mm) in infant reconstructions for up to 44 months.[36] Valve survival is not equivalent to patient survival (which is better), or to a complication-free life (which is often worse). Allografts are easier to place in small infants and do not become obstructive as rapidly.

When utilizing a valve for reconstruction of the right ventricular outflow tract in young children, evidence to date suggests that a porcine valve conduit might have a projected useful life to the patient for as little as 4 years as a consequence of poor hemodynamic function and limited durability, whereas homograft reconstruction could last 10 years.[10,34]

Ross and others have noted that the right-sided position is less stressful than the left-sided position for transplanted valve tissues. If the encouraging results with aortic valve replacements utilizing cryopreserved allografts have a similar contribution to right-sided reconstructions, valve durability approaching 20 years might very well be achievable. Initially, most groups used aortic allografts for right-sided reconstructions, but pulmonary allografts appear to have significant advantages and are increasingly preferentially used.[37]

Although it has long been known that a normal right ventricle can dispense with a pulmonary valve and pulmonary regurgitation is a lesion that is well tolerated for many years, there is increasing evidence that valved reconstructions are superior. Thus an argument can be made for using valves in reconstructions of the right ventricular tract because: (1) the long-term effects of pulmonary insufficiency lead to right ventricular dysfunction and right ventricular dilatation; (2) right ventricular outflow tract reconstructions must not be obstructive; (3) allografts have superior hemodynamic performance; (4) protection of the compromised right ventricle from pulmonary insufficiency helps prevent tricuspid regurgitation, and tricuspid incompetence clearly adds to the hemodynamic compromise of pulmonary regurgitation, leading to rapid and persistent right ventricular failure, which is often difficult to manage medically; and (5) many patients presenting for right ventricular outflow tract reconstructions already have less than normal right ventricular function (e.g. pulmonary atresia).[38]

All 13 patients in the San Francisco series of right ventricular outflow tract patches with preoperative tricuspid regurgitation required attention to the tricuspid valve.[39] In addition, right-sided prosthetic valves of either mechanical or xenograft materials are notoriously prone to calcification and failure. These factors, coupled with the increased durability of the cryopreserved allograft valves, presently mandate their use in such reconstructions in both adults and children.

Valve replacements in children tend to magnify problems with prostheses, and in these younger age groups xenograft durability is known to be poor.[40,41] Size constraints are exaggerated.[42] Thromboembolic/anticoagulation problems may be more difficult to manage, although the risk of emboli from the aortic position appears to be significantly less than the mitral position.[43–45]

Ilbawi and associates have reported that porcine prostheses have fared better in right-sided applications in young patients than on the systemic side, but with reduced durability compared to that in older adults.[46] Thus the xenograft is preferable to a mechanical valve for the right-sided atrioventricular (AV) valve position, but allografts are superior in the pulmonary outflow tract position. It is technically easier to insert, is probably more resistant to subacute bacterial endocarditis (SBE), has superior hemodynamic performance, has longer durability when Dacron extensions are avoided, and does not require anticoagulation.[47] Ilbawi's group, as others, have demonstrated excellent performance by the St. Jude prosthesis in the aortic position, with 88.7% actuarial freedom from prosthesis-related complications at 5 years in that position in the pediatric age group.[48] In comparison, the allograft appears to be as good and avoids the problem of anticoagulation in children.[48]

Stark and colleagues from the Great Ormond Street Hospital for Children in London, England have published an important series of 405 homografts inserted between 1971 and 1993 for pulmonary outflow reconstruction.[49] While their longest surviving homograft conduit lasted 23 years, their series documented an overall homograft durability of over 80% at 5 years, falling to 50% at 10 years and 30% at 15 years. Best results were obtained with the first conduit and decreasing durability achieved with subsequent reoperative conduits in the same patient, suggesting perhaps immune factors might intensify in subsequent reoperations. They also found that older patients did less well than younger patients in terms of conduit durability in contradistinction to the findings by others as exemplified by the report of Clarke and Bishop.[50] Interestingly, they also noted that conduits implanted earlier in their series seemed to have longer durability, suggesting that prolonged wet storage (fresh) might produce a homograft with better durability that cryopreserved. However, multifactorial analysis seemed to indicate that this was not a major factor. While other authorities have suggested that small homograft conduits perform less effectively, in this Great Ormond Street Series this was not an important factor.[51] The series from Nova Scotia by Baskett is in agreement with the Great Ormond Street data indicating that the type of donor valve (pulmonic or aortic), donor age and blood group mismatch are not associated with decreased conduit durability, but did suggest that short periods between homograft retrieval and cryopreservation was associated with *worse* durability outcome suggesting that enhanced viability might go hand-in-hand with increased antigenicity and an aggressive immune response, especially in younger recipients.[52]

There has been significant controversy about the effect of the size of the conduit. Some authorities suggest that a larger conduit improves the durability of allografts especially in infants and small children,[53] while in the Great Ormond Street data no effect on durability by conduit size was demonstrated. The Melbourne, Australia data suggest that a strategy in which the conduit is matched to patient is best since other factors lead to early re-replacement in the smaller children and thus risking anatomical distortion simply to get the largest conduit possible into the patient is unrewarding.[54] Their strategy is to plan a second operation with a larger prosthesis.

The controversy concerning cell viability has been significant with various authorities advocating one end of the spectrum—homovital (very fresh homografts) while others recommended prolonged storage of fresh wet homografts presumably to decrease antigenicity.[33] The Mayo Clinic data presented in 1995 compared 230 aortic and 118 pulmonary cryopreserved homografts placed in the right ventricular outflow tract with a five year freedom from homograft failure for pulmonary homografts at 94% versus 70% for the aortic homografts. The Mayo Clinic group found that aortic homografts became calcified more rapidly and to a greater extent. This characteristic was aggravated by age of recipient being younger than 4 years, especially in the aortic homograft recipients. Thus, their recommendation of a preference for the pulmonary homograft on the basis of durability for right ventricular outflow tract reconstructions.[51,52,55–59] Other groups have suggested that the type of preimplantation processing his significant effects as related to cell viability.[60] This issue is discussed extensively elsewhere in this text.

For balance, it should be mentioned that there are published studies which have indicated that homografts perform less well in the pulmonary circulation than bioprostheses.[61] In particular, the Toronto Group published a conduit-related failure of 45% at five years in their pediatric series. In this particular group, the average age of operation was approximately 7 years and no difference was noted between aortic and pulmonary homografts. But their analysis suggested that the durability of cryopreserved homograft conduits in children was disappointingly short and clearly different from other authorities.[33,54] However, even those centers reporting less favorable results often prefer homografts in the right ventricular outflow tract because of their other advantages and characteristics. It is not a permanent replacement and may be viewed as a staging procedure, that when containing a valve helps to protect the medium and long term right ventricular function, even at the cost of a second operation.

Allograft tissues are the optimal choice for all right ventricular outflow reconstructions in children for the reasons defined in this chapter and in Chapter 1, and probably for many complex left ventricular outflow tract repairs as well. Presently, the only apparent reasons not to use allografts are lack of availability and the rare instance in which a rigid conduit offers an advantage against compression or distortion.

The allograft is the replacement of choice for right ventricular outflow tract reconstructions in children and adults. It is also probably one logical choice for complex left ventricular outflow reconstructions: (1) aortoventriculo-plasty; (2) small aortic roots; (3) aortic root replacements for multilevel and complex left ventricular outflow tract abnormalities that cannot be otherwise repaired/remodeled; and (4) valve or root replacements for highly destructive bacterial endocarditis. For aortic valve replacements in other situations it is considered competitive or superior to the porcine graft in young patients and those with contraindications to anticoagulation, where life expectancy exceeds the expected durability of xenograft options. Its role in routine aortic valve replacement has yet to be defined and may be inappropriate owing to limited availability, which may limit use to specific patient and indication categories in which major advantages have been demonstrated. Both the autograft operation and the stentless porcine valves may further narrow the indications in adults for left ventricular outflow reconstructions with allograft valves.

References

1. O'Brien MF, Stafford G, Gardner M, Pohlner P, McGiffin D, Johnston N, Brosnan A, Duffy P. The viable cryopreserved allograft aortic valve. J Card Surg 1987;2:153–167.
2. Barratt-Boyes BG. Long-term follow-up of aortic valve grafts. Br Heart J 1971;33:Suppl:60–Suppl:65.
3. Kosek JC, Iben AB, Shumway NE, et al. Morphology of fresh heart valve homografts. Surgery 1969;66:269–277.
4. O'Brien MF, Stafford EG, Gardner MA, Pohlner PG, McGiffin DC. A comparison of aortic valve replacement with viable cryopreserved and fresh allograft valves, with a note on chromosomal studies. J Thorac Cardiovasc Surg 1987;94:812–823.
5. Penta A, Qureshi S, Radley-Smith R, Yacoub MH. Patient status 10 or more years after "fresh" homograft replacement of the aortic valve. Circulation 1984;70:I182–I186.
6. Thompson R, Yacoub M, Ahmed M, Somerville W, Towers M. The use of "fresh" unstented homograft valves for replacement of the aortic valve. J Thorac Cardiovasc Surg 1980;79:896–903.
7. Thompson R, Ahmed M, Seabra-Gomes R, Ilsley C, Rickards A, Towers M, Yacoub M. Influence of preoperative left ventricular function on results of homograft replacement of the aortic valve for aortic regurgitation. J Thorac Cardiovasc Surg 1979;77:411–421.
8. Thompson R, Yacoub M, Ahmed M, Seabra-Gomes R, Rickards A, Towers M. Influence of preoperative left ventricular function on results of homograft replacement of the aortic valve for aortic stenosis. Am J Cardiol 1979;43:929–938.
9. Ross D, Yacoub MH. Homograft replacement of the aortic valve. A critical review. Prog Cardiovasc Dis 1969;11:275–293.
10. Jonas RA, Freed MD, Mayor JE, Castaneda AR. Long term follow-up of patients with synthetic right heart conduits. Circulation 1985;72 (Suppl. 2):II77–II83.
11. Angell WW, Angell JD, Oury JH, Lamberti JJ, Grehl TM. Long-term follow-up of viable frozen aortic homografts: a viable homograft valve bank. J Thorac Cardiovasc Surg 1987;93:815–822.
12. Kirklin JW, Barratt-Boyes BG. Aortic valve disease. In Kirklin JW, Barratt-Boyes BG (eds). Cardiac Surgery. New York: Wiley;1986:398–416.
13. Matsuki O, Okita Y, Almeida RS. Two decades' experience with aortic valve replacement with pulmonary autograft. J Thorac Cardiovasc Surg 1988;95:705–711.
14. O'Brien MF, Stafford EG, Gardner AH, Pohlner P, McGiffin DC, Johnston N, Tesar P, Brosnan A, Duffy P. Cryopreserved viable allograft valves. In Yonkah AC, Hetzer R, Miller DCea (eds). Cardiac valve allografts 1962–1987. New York: Springer Verlag;1988:311–321.
15. Livi U, Abdulla AK, Parker R, Olsen EJ, Ross DN. Viability and morphology of aortic and pulmonary homografts. J Thorac Cardiovasc Surg 1987;93:755–760.

16. Barratt-Boyes BG, Roche AH, Subramanyan R, Pemberton JR, Whitlock RM. Long-term follow-up of patients with the antibiotic-sterilized aortic homograft valve inserted freehand in the aortic position. Circulation 1987;75:768–777.

17. Williams TP, Van Herwerden LA, Taams MA, Kleyburg-Kinger VE, Roelandt JR, Bos E. Aortic allograft implantation techniques: Pathomorphology and regurgitant jet patterns by Doppler echocardiographic studies. Ann Thorac Surg 1998;66:412–416.

18. Doty JR, Salazar JD, Liddicoat JR, Flores JE, Doty DB. Aortic valve replacement with cryopreserved aortic allograft: ten year experience. J Thorac Cardiovasc Surg 1998;115:371–380.

19. Doty DB, Michielon G, Wang N. Replacement of the aortic valve with cryopreserved aortic allograft. Ann Thorac Surg 1993;56:228–236.

20. O'Brien MF, Stafford EG, Gardner MA, et al. Allograft aortic valve replacement: Long term follow-up. Ann Thorac Surg 1995;60:S65–S70.

21. Doty DB. Replacement of the aortic valve with cryopreserved aortic allograft: the procedure of choice for young patients. Jour Card Surg 1994;9 (suppl):192–195.

22. Jones EL, Shah VB, Shanewise, et al. Should the freehand allograft be abandoned as a reliable alternative for aortic valve replacement? Ann Thorac Surg 1995;59:1397–1404.

23. Rubay JE, Raphael D, Sluysmans T, et al. Aortic valve replacement with allograft/autograft: subcoronary versus intraluminal cylinder or root. Ann Thorac Surg 1995;S78–S82.

24. Barratt-Boyes BG. Aortic allograft valve implantation: freehand or root replacement? Jour Card Surg 1994;9 (suppl):196–197.

25. O'Brien MF, Finney RS, Stafford EG, et al. Root replacement for all allograft aortic valves: Preferred technique or too radical? Ann Thorac Surg 1995;60:S87–S91.

26. Willems TP, Herwerden LA, Steyerberg EW, Taams MA, Kleyburg VE, Hokken RB, et al. Subcoronary implantation or aortic root replacement for human tissue valves: Sufficient data to prefer either technique? Ann Thorac Surg 1995; 60:583–586.

27. Yankah AC, Weng Y, Hofmeister J, Alexi-Meskhishvilli V, Siniawski H, Lange PE, et al. Freehand subcoronary aortic valve and aortic root replacement with cryopreserved homografts: intermediate term results. J Heart Valve Dis 1996;5:498–504.

28. Hopkins RA, Reyes A, Carpenter GA, Imperato DA, Myers JL, Murphy KA. Ventricular outflow tract reconstructions with cryopreserved cardiac valved homografts—A single surgeon's ten-year experience. Ann Surg 1995;223:544–554.

29. Fontan F, Choussat A, DeVille C, et al. Aortic valve homografts in the surgical treatment of complex cardiac malformations. J Thorac Cardiovasc Surg 1984;87:649–657.

30. Shabbo FB, Wain WH, Ross DN. Right ventricular outflow reconstructions with aortic homograft: analysis of long-term results. Thorac Cardiovasc Surg 1981;29:21–27.

31. Saravalli OA, Somerville J, Jefferson KE. Calcification of aortic homografts used for reconstruction of the right ventricular outflow tract. J Thorac Cardiovasc Surg 1980;80:909–920.

32. DiCarlo D, Stark J, Revignas A, deLeval MR. Conduits containing antibiotic preserved homografts in the treatment of complex congenital heart defects. In Cohn LH, Gallucci V (eds). Cardiac Bioprostheses. New York: Yorke;1982: 259–265.

33. Kay PH, Ross DN. Fifteen years' experience with the aortic homograft: the conduit of choice for right ventricular outflow tract reconstruction. Ann Thorac Surg 1985;40:360–364.

34. Danielson DK, Jr. Discussion of Kay, P.H., Ross D.N.: Fifteen years' experience with aortic homografts: the conduit of choice for right ventricular outflow tract reconstructions. Ann Thorac Surg 1985;40:360–364.

35. Kirklin JW, Blackstone EH, Maehara T, Pacifico AD, Kirklin JK, Pollock S, Stewart RW. Intermediate-term fate of cryopreserved allograft and xenograft valved conduits. Ann Thorac Surg 1987;44:598–606.

36. Boyce SW, Turley K, Yee ES, et al. The fate of the 12 mm porcine valved conduit from the right ventricle to the pulmonary artery: a ten year experience. J Thorac Cardiovasc Surg 1988;95:201–207.

37. McGrath LB, Gonzalez-Lavin L, Graf D. Pulmonary homograft implantation for ventricular outflow tract reconstruction: early phase results. Ann Thorac Surg 1988;45:273–277.

38. Ebert PA. Second operations for pulmonary stenosis or insufficiency after repair of tetralogy of Fallot. Am J Cardiol 1982;50:637–640.

39. Ebert PA. Second operations for pulmonary stenosis or insufficiency after repair of tetralogy of Fallot. In Engle MA, Perloff JK (eds). Congenital heart disease after surgery: Benefits, residua, sequela. New York: Yorke;1983:202–209.

40. Iyer KS, Reddy KS, Rao IM, et al. Valve replacement in children under twenty years of age. J Thorac Cardiovasc Surg 1984;88:217–224.

41. Williams DB, Danielson GK, McGoon DC, et al. Porcine heterograft valve replacement in children. J Thorac Cardiovasc Surg 1982;84:446–450.

42. Williams WG, Pollock LC, Geiss DM, et al. Experience with aortic and mitral valve replacement in children. J Thorac Cardiovasc Surg 1981;81:326–333.

43. Makhlouf AE, Friedli B, Oberhansli I, et al. Prosthetic heart valve replacement in children. J Thorac Cardiovasc Surg 1987;93:80–85.

44. Edmonds LH. Thrombotic and bleeding complications of prosthetic heart valves. Ann Thorac Surg 1987;44:430–445.

45. Robbins RC, Bowman FO, Jr., Malm JR. Cardiac valve replacement in children: a twenty year series. Ann Thorac Surg 1988;45:56–61.

46. Ilbawi MN, Idriss FS, DeLeon SY, et al. Valve replacement in children: guidelines for selection of prosthesis and timing of surgical intervention. Ann Thorac Surg 1987;44:398–403.

47. Hopkins RA. Right ventricular outflow tract reconstructions: the role of valves in the viable allograft era. Ann Thorac Surg 1988;45:593–594.

48. Pass HI, Sade RM, Crawford RA, Hohn AR. Cardiac valve prostheses in children without anticoagulation. J Thorac Cardiovasc Surg 1984;87:832–835.

49. Stark J, Bull C, Stajevic M, Jothi M, Elliott M, De Leval MR. Fate of subpulmonary homograft conduits: determinants of late homograft failure. J Thorac Cardiovasc Surg 1997.

50. Clarke DR, Bishop DA. Allograft degeneration in infant pulmonary valve allograft recipients. EJCTS 1993;7:365–370.

51. Heinemann MK, Hanley FL, Fenton KN, Jonas RA, Mayer JE, Castaneda AR. Fate of small homograft conduits after early repair in truncus arteriosus. Ann Thorac Surg 1993;55:1409–1412.

52. Baskett RJ, Ross DB, Nanton MA, Murphy DA. Factors in the early failure of cryopreserved homograft pulmonary valves in children: preserved immunogenicity? J Thorac Cardiovasc Surg 1996;112:1170–1179.

53. Tam RK, Tolan MJ, Zamvar VY, Slavik Z, Pickering R, Keeton BR, Salmon AP, Webber SA, Tsang V, Lamb RK, Monro JL. Use of larger sized aortic homograft conduits in right ventricular outflow tract reconstruction. J Heart Valve Dis 1995;4:660–664.

54. Sano S, Karl TR, Mee RB. Extracardiac valved conduits in the pulmonary circuit. Ann Thorac Surg 1991;52:285–290.

55. Bando K, Danielson GK, Schaff HV. Outcome of pulmonary and aortic homografts for right ventricular outflow tract reconstruction. J Thorac Cardiovasc Surg 1995;109:509–518.

56. McGoon DC, Danielson GK, Puga FJ, et al. Late results after extracardiac conduit repair for congenital cardiac defects. Am J Cardiol 1982;49:1741–1749.

57. Schaff HV, DiDonato RM, Danielson GK, et al. Reoperation for obstructed pulmonary ventricle-pulmonary artery conduits: early and late results. J Cardiovasc Surg 1984;88:334–343.

58. Cochran RP, Kunzelman KS. Cryopreservation does not alter antigenic expression of aortic allografts. J Surg Res 1989;46:597–599.

59. Albert JD, Bishop DA, Fullerton DA, Campbell DN, Clarke DR. Conduit reconstruction of the right ventricular outflow tract: lessons learned in a twelve-year experience. J Thorac Cardiovasc Surg 1993;106:228–236.

60. Gall KL, Smith SE, Willmette EN, O'Brien MF. Allograft Heart Valve Viability and Valve-Processing Variables. Ann Thorac Surg 1998;65:1032–1038.

61. Cleveland DC, Williams WG, Razzouk AJ. Failure of cryopreserved homograft valved conduits in the pulmonary circulation. Circulation 1992;86 (suppl II):II-150–II-153.

9
Surgery for Infections

David C. McGiffin and James K. Kirklin

Infective endocarditis, both native and prosthetic, is ultimately a fatal illness without therapy, reflecting the inability of innate defenses to importantly influence the course of the disease. Following the diagnosis, the therapy of this illness depends on identification of the organism, administration of bactericidal antibiotics and the use of timely cardiac surgical intervention in patients with complications such as heart failure from valvular destruction, annular abscess formation, uncontrolled sepsis and embolization.

This chapter deals with one aspect of the therapy of infective endocarditis, namely the role of homograft valves in the reconstruction of the infected aortic root and will only deal with the pathology of the infected aortic root and surgical details that are of relevance to the insertion of homograft valves.

Pathology of aortic root infection: The rapidity of the infection and, to some extent the extensiveness of valve destruction is, in part of a reflection of the responsible organism. Organisms such as Staphylococcus aureus and Streptococcus pneumoniae[1] may cause rapid valve destruction as opposed to a more indolent process due to organisms such as the viridans streptococci or enterococci. Acute and subacute infective endocarditis are anachronistic terms that reflect fulminant and indolent infection respectively and are reminders of a much earlier era when the natural history of infective endocarditis was played out due to the lack of effective therapy.

Native valve endocarditis (NVE), which in approximately 50% of cases occurs without obvious predisposing valve disease,[2] causes leaflet destruction and perforation. Aortic obstruction due to large vegetations may rarely occur. Aortic valve infection frequently involves adjacent structures such as the annulus and other components of the fibrous skeleton of the heart. In patients dying with native aortic valve endocarditis[3] or patients undergoing operation for this disease,[4,5] at least one third will have aortic root abscess formation. Annular abscesses may erode into the left ventricular myocardium, and rarely cause aortic wall invasion and false aneurysms of the sinuses of Valsalva or aortic wall and fistulerazation to adjacent chambers.[6] Circumferential annular infection may result in aorto-left ventricular discontinuity. Based on a number of surgical series[7] Staphylococcus aureus and viridans streptococci are most frequently isolated from aortic root abscesses.

Prosthetic valve endocarditis (PVE) is arbitrarily categorized[8] into "early" (with 60 days of valve replacement) and "late" PVE (beyond 60 days from valve replacement) since "early" and "late" PVE tend to have different microbiological and clinical characteristics. An alternative way to express "early" versus "late" PVE is by the use of hazard function which depicts the instantaneous risk of PVE (Figure 9.1).[9,10] The early peaking phase of risk, which corresponds to "early" PVE, transitions to a constant risk corresponding to "late" PVE at approximately 6 months after valve replacement. Organism

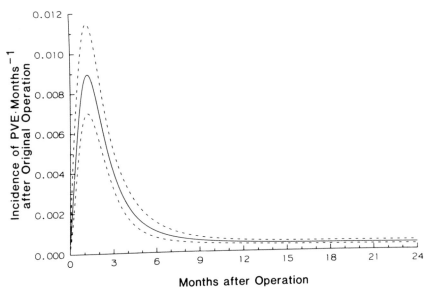

FIGURE 9.1. Hazard function for the development of PVE after a primary valve replacement operation. The depiction is the parametric estimate of the hazard function (or instantaneous risk) of developing PVE (solid line), surrounding by the 70% confidence limits (dashed lines). The initial peak phase of risk merges with constant phase approximately 6 months after operation. Reprinted from *Cardiac Surgery*, 2e, Vol 1, Kirklin JW, Barratt-Boyes BG, © 1993, with permission from Elsevier.

specific hazard of PVE after aortic valve replacement (Figure 9.2)[11] indicates that staphylococcal infection (Staphylococcus epidermidis, Staphylococcus aureus and methicillin-resistant Staphylococcus aureus), which are responsible for up to 50% of episodes of PVE[8,12,13] is most likely to occur early after aortic valve replacement, probably related to intra- or perioperative contamination. Other organisms that may result in early PVE include gram-negative aerobic organisms, streptococci, diphtheroids and fungi. The microbiological profile of late PVE resembles that seen in NVE. Late PVE is characterized by a constant risk of both streptococcal and staphylococcal infection.

PVE may involve mechanical and xenograft prostheses and homograft valves. Mechanical PVE is characterized by annular abscess formation, paravalvular leak and prosthesis dehiscence. Based on a number of studies,[14] annular abscesses may occur in approximately 60% of patients with mechanical PVE and is more likely to occur in the aortic than the mitral position.[15] Early PVE of a xenograft valve is morel likely to result in periannular infection than late PVE in which the infection is more likely to involve the leaflet.[16] Homograft valve infection usually results in leaflet involvement with destruction resulting in incompetence, but extension into the annulus is unusual.[17]

Infection of the aortic valve may involve the mitral valve by either the jet effect from aortic regurgitation or by direct extension. The jet of aortic regurgitation due to aortic valve infection strikes the anterior leaflet of the mitral valve and embeds organisms in the leaflet resulting in a perforation (so called "drop lesion"). The mitral valve may also be involved by direct extension from aortic valve infection, and may result in abscess formation in the aortico-mitral septum with eventual separation of the continuity between aortic valve and anterior leaflet of the mitral valve.

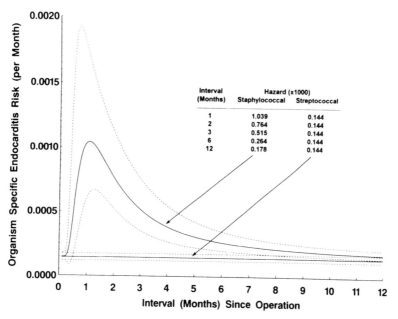

FIGURE 9.2. Hazard function for Staphylococcal and Streptococcal PVE after aortic valve replacement. Solid lines represent the hazard estimates and the corresponding dashed lines enclose 70% confidence limits. The risk of Staphylococcal endocarditis is increased early after aortic valve replacement and the constant phase risk is similar for Staphylococcal and Streptococcal endocarditis. Reprinted from *Journal of Thoracic and Cardiovascular Surgery*, Vol 110, Agnihotri et al, "Prevalence of infective endocarditis after aortic valve replacement." 1708–1724. © 1995, with permission from Elsevier.

The role of Homograft Valves in the Treatment of Endocarditis

The value of surgical intervention in patients with NVE who develop heart failure, uncontrolled infection and aortic root abscess formation has been previously demonstrated.[18] Similarly, surgical therapy for some patients with PVE[18,19] has improved the high mortality associated with this condition. Patients with PVE and heart failure, uncontrolled sepsis, prosthesis dehiscence, prosthesis obstruction and fungal etiology are the ones most likely to benefit from valve replacement.

One of the concerns regarding valve replacement for endocarditis is the placement of prosthetic valves in a potential site of active infection with the possibility of recurrent PVE. Although the probability of developing PVE following valve replacement for NVE is relatively low, the risk is approximately 5 times that for patients undergoing valve replacement for reasons other than endocarditis. By hazard function analysis, this risk is highest within the first 6 months of operation.[10] In a series of patients[20] undergoing valve replacement for active or remote aortic NVE or PVE, the actuarial freedom from recurrent endocarditis at 10 years was 79% (70% confidence limits), 75% to 83%, the greatest risk being in the first 3 months after operation. The mechanism of recurrent endocarditis in this setting may not just be reinfection from the contaminated aortic root, but also perhaps a biological predisposition in some patients to recurrent valve infection.

When choosing a valve replacement device in a patient with aortic valve infection, consideration must be given to minimizing the risk of recurrent valve infection. The traditional approach to valve replacement in the setting of endocarditis has been the insertion of mechanical or xenograft prosthesis. Patients with extensive aortic root infection have been managed by methods such as patch closure of abscess cavities and aortic valve replacement,[21] and composite prosthetic aortic root replacement.[22] Aorto-left ventricular discontinuity has been managed by cephalad translocation of the implanted aortic valve prosthesis and closure of the native coronary ostia and saphenous vein bypass grafts.[23] All of these methods carry a low, but not insignificant risk of recurrent valve infection.

A number of reports appeared describing the use of the homograft valve in patients with NVE and PVE, often in association with extensive aortic destruction. In one report,[24] thirty patients with active PVE underwent aortic root replacement with a homograft, with 2 of the 21 survivors developing recurrent endocarditis, one at 9 months and the other at 5 years after operation. A number of other reports described the use of the homograft valve for NVE[25–27] and PVE[28] and extensive aortic root infection with subsequent freedom from recurrent endocarditis, suggesting that the homograft valve had an intrinsic resistance to infection. Further evidence of this resistance to infection became available with the demonstration[8] that after aortic valve replacement (for any reason) the risk of PVE for mechanical and xenograft valves was higher early after operation, whereas the homograft valve did not have this early phase of risk (Figure 9.3). Note that in this study xenograft and mechanical valve groups were combined to produce a single estimate of the hazard for PVE.

More substantial evidence to support the homograft's putative resistance to infection became available from two publications in 1982. A study by McGiffin and colleagues[20] analyzed a series of patients undergoing aortic valve replacement with homograft, mechanical and xenograft valves for NVE or PVE (which may have been active or healed). The risk of recurring endocarditis with mechanical and xenograft valves (early peaking hazard phase) was higher than with homografts, which had a constant and low risk (Figure 9.4A,B). The other study, by Haydock and colleagues[31] analyzed a group of patients with active NVE or PVE to determine the probability of recur-

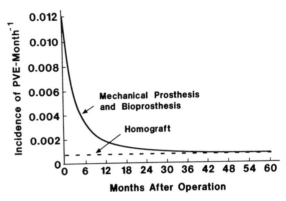

FIGURE 9.3. Hazard function for PVE after valve replacement with mechanical and xenograft valves (solid line) and with homografts aortic valves (dashed line). There is an early high risk of PVE for mechanical and xenograft that is absent with homograft valves. Reprinted from *Cardiac Surgery*, 2e, Vol 1, Kirklin JW, Barratt-Boyes BG. © 1993, with permission from Elsevier.

rent endocarditis after aortic valve replacement, and the findings were identical to McGiffin's study. Haydock's study also found a late phase of risk of PVE with mechanical and xenograft valves but not with homograft valves, and this late phase commenced at about 10 years (Figure 9.5). It should be noted that in both studies, multivariable analyses to determine risk factors associated with recurrent endocarditis did not identify non-use of a homograft to be independently associated with recurrent endocarditis. The inference from both of these studies that the homograft valve is the device of choice for endocarditis is based on qualitative difference in the hazard function for recurrent endocarditis with mechanical, xenograft and homograft valves. Although this represents a difference based on a univariate comparison, the data does suggest that for active endocarditis the homograft valve is the preferred replacement device. It is interesting to note that in a study by Agnihotri and colleagues,[11] use of the homograft valve reduced the risk of PVE in patients with active endocarditis within the first few months after valve replacement. However, in patients undergoing valve replacement for reasons other than endocarditis, use of the homograft did not offer any

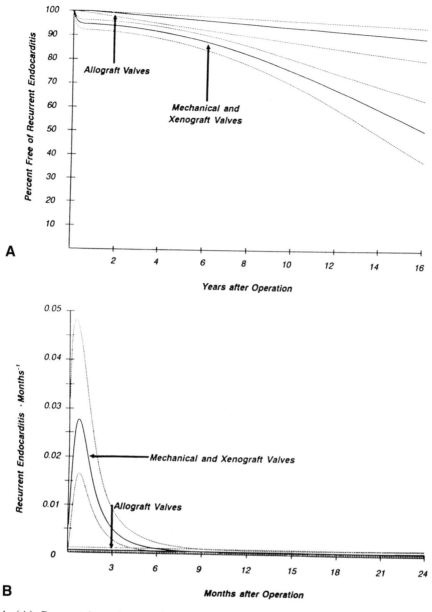

FIGURE 9.4. (A) Parametric estimate of freedom from recurrent endocarditis (solid lines) for mechanical and xenograft valves and allograft (homograft) valves after aortic valve replacement for NVE or PVE. The 70% confidence limits are indicated by the dotted lines. (B) Corresponding hazard function. The depiction is the same as in part A. Reprinted from *Journal of Thoracic and Cardiovascular Surgery*, Vol 105, Sett S et al, "Prosthetic valve endocarditis: experience with porcine bioprosthesis." 428–434. © 1993, with permission from Elsevier.

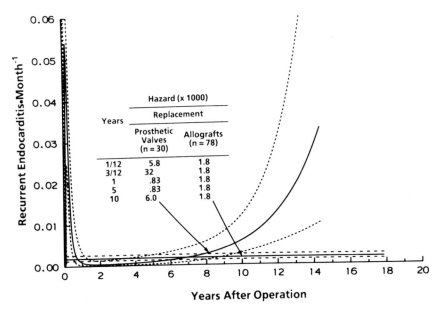

FIGURE 9.5. Hazard function for recurrent endo-carditis in patients receiving allograft (homograft) valves compared with those receiving mechanical or bioprosthetic valves in the aortic position. The depiction is the same as in Figure 9.1. Reprinted from *Journal of Thoracic and Cardiovascular Surgery*, Vol 103, Haydock et al, "Aortic valve replacement for active infectious endocarditis in 108 patients: a comparison of freehand allograft valves with mechanical prostheses and bioprostheses," 130–139. © 1992, with permission from Elsevier.

long-term advantage over xenograft or mechanical valve devices in terms of freedom from PVE. Perhaps the known morphologic changes that occur in homograft valve leaflets with time may reduce its resistance to infection.

Homograft Valve Insertion for Endocarditis

The general principles of the surgical management of endocarditis include a) timely valve surgery in the setting of appropriate bactericidal antibiotics, b) debridement of all infected tissue including abscess cavities and the infected fibrous skeleton of the heart, c) removal of all prosthetic material in PVE, d) reconstruction including valve replacement, annular reconstruction and closure of any holes between chambers. Abscess cavities are not specifically closed unless required for the integrity of the reconstruction or for the anchoring of the valve replacement device. Autologous pericardium is probably the material of chose for reconstruction[6] although bovine pericardium can also be used. A maneuver that has been described is to fill abscess cavities prior to closure with a mixture of antibiotics and fibrin glue in an attempt to reduce the likelihood of recurrent infection.[29,30]

The homograft valve is a flexible replacement device that can be inserted using methods such as the subcoronary and cylindrical techniques and as an aortic root replacement. The homograft valve can be used to bridge over abscess cavities and can be inserted in patients with the most extensive destruction such as aorto-left ventricular discontinuity. For example, the anterior leaflet of the mitral valve of the aortic homograft can be used to bridge over an annular defect created by debridement of an abscess cavity. (Figure 9.6)

For extensive aortic root destruction that may be associated with PVE (Figure 9.7), aortic

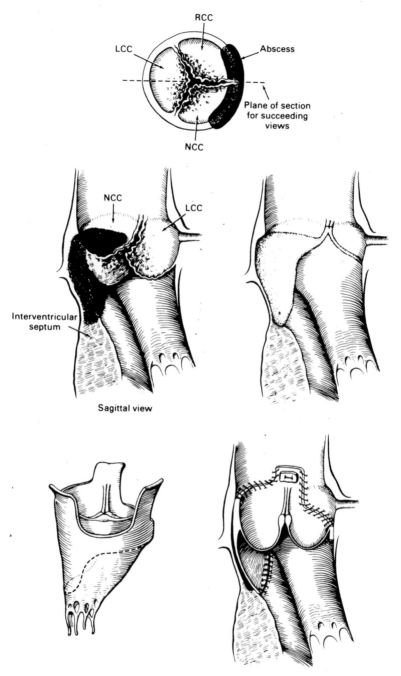

Transverse Section at Aortic Anulus

FIGURE 9.6. A technique of homograft aortic valve replacement to bridge an annular defect due to debridement of an abscess, using the anterior leaflet of the mitral valve of the homograft. Reprinted from *Annals of Thoracic Surgery*, Vol 48, Zeischenberger et al, "Viable cryopreserved aortic homograft for aortic valve endocarditis and annular abcesses," 365–370. © 1989, with permission from Elsevier.

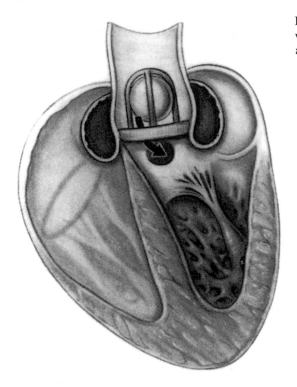

FIGURE 9.7. Illustration of extensive aortic PVE with abscess cavities involving the aortic annulus and mitral valve. Reprinted with permission.[32]

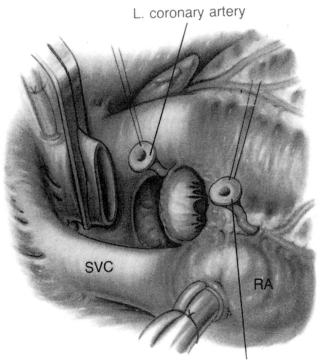

FIGURE 9.8. The aortic root is excised and the coronary ostia mobilized on the buttons of aorta. Reprinted with permission.[32]

FIGURE 9.9. The proximal anastomosis and coronary anastomoses are performed. Reprinted with permission.[32]

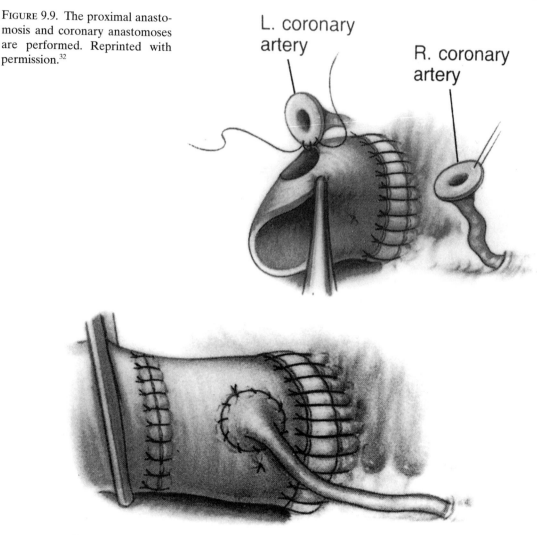

FIGURE 9.9. The proximal anastomosis and coronary anastomoses are performed. Reprinted with permission.[32]

FIGURE 9.10. The distal anastomosis is coupled. Reprinted with permission.[32]

root replacement may be required. This technique involves excision of the aortic root, debridement of the abscess cavities and mobilization of the coronary ostia on aortic buttons (Figure 9.8). The proximal anastomosis is performed, followed by anastomosis of the coronary buttons to the homograft (Figure 9.9), then the distal anastomosis (Figure 9.10).

References

1. Wilson W, Thandroyen F. Infective endocarditis. In Willerson J, Cohn J (eds). Infective Endocarditis Cardiovascular Medicine. New York: Churchill Livingstone 1995:240–255.
2. Garvey G, Neu H. Infective endocarditis—an evolving disease. A review of endocarditis at the Columbia-Presbyterian Medical Center, 1968–1973. Medicine 1978;57:105–127.
3. Arnett E, Roberts W. Valve ring abscess in active infective endocarditis: Frequency, location, and clues to clinical diagnosis from the study of 95 necropsy patients. Circulation 1976;54:140–145.
4. D'Agostino R, Miller D, Stinson E, et al. Valve replacement in patients with native valve endocarditis: What really determines operative outcome? Ann Thorac Surg 1985;40:429–438.

5. David T, Bos J, Christakis G, Wong D, et al. Heart valve surgery in patients with active infective endocarditis. Annals of Thoracic Surgery 1997.

6. David T, Komeda M, Brofman P. Surgical treatment of aortic root abscess. Circulation 1989;80 (Suppl I):269–274.

7. David T. Aortic root abscess. In Emery R, Arom K (eds). The Aortic Valve. Philadelphia: Hanley & Belfus, Inc. 1991:289–294.

8. Dismukes W, Karchmer A, Buckely M, Austen W, Swartz M. Prosthetic valve endocarditis: analysis of 38 cases. Circulation 1973;48:365–377.

9. Kirklin JW, Barratt-Boyes BG. Cardiac Surgery, Second Edition: Volume 1. New York: Churchill Livingstone, Inc. 1993.

10. Ivert T, Dismukes W, Cobbs C, Blackstone E, Kirklin J, Bergdahl L. Prosthetic vlave endocarditis. Circulation 1984;69:223–232.

11. Agnihotri A, McGiffin D, Galbraith A, O'Brien M. Prevalence of infective endocarditis after aortic valve replacement. J Thorac Cardiovasc Surg 1995;110:1708–1724.

12. Gardner TJ, Roland JMA, Neill CA, Donahoo JS. Valve replacement in children. J Thorac Cardiovasc Surg 1982;83:178–185.

13. Masur H, Johnson W. Prosthetic valve endocarditis. J Thorac Cardiovasc Surg 1980;80:31–37.

14. Gnann J, Cobbs C. Infections of prosthetic valves and intravascular devices. In Mandell G, Douglas R, Bennett J (eds). Principles and Practice of Infectious Disease, 2nd Edition. New York: John Wiley & Sons 1984:530–539.

15. Mayer K, Schoenbaum S. Evaluation and management of prosthetic valve endocarditis. Prog Cardiovasc Dis 1982;25:43–54.

16. David T. The surgical treatment of patients with prosthetic valve endocarditis. Sem in Thor and Card Surg 1995;7:47–53.

17. Clarkson PM, Barratt-Boyes BG. Bacterial endocarditis following homograft replacement of the aortic valve. Circulation 1970;42:987–991.

18. Croft C, Woodward W, Elliott A, Commerford P, Barnard C, Beck W. Analysis of surgical versus medical therapy in active complicated native valve infective enodcarditis. Am J Cardiol 1983; 51:1650–1655.

19. Sett S, Hudon M, Jamieson W, Chow A. Prosthetic valve endocarditis: experience with porcine bioprostheses. J Thorac Cardiovasc Surg 1993;105:428–434.

20. McGiffin D, Galbraith A, McLachlan G, et al. Aortic valve infection: risk factors for death and recurrent endocarditis after aortic valve replacement. J Thorac Cardiovasc Surg 1992;104:511–520.

21. Symbas P, Vlasis S, Zacharopoulos L, Lutz J. Acute endocarditis: surgical treatment of aortic regurgitiation and aortico-left ventricular discontinuity. J Thorac Cardiovasc Surg 1982;84: 291–296.

22. VanHooser D, Johnson R, Hein R, Elkins R. Successful management of aortic valve endocarditis with associated periannular abscess and aneurysm. Ann Thorac Surg 1986;42:148–151.

23. Reitz B, Stinson E, Wtason D, Baumgartner W, Jamieson S. Translocation of the aortic valve for prosthetic valve endocarditis. J Thorac Cardiovasc Surg 1981;81:212–218.

24. Glazier J, Verwilghen J, Donaldson R, Ross D. Treatment of complicated prosthetic aortic valve endocarditis with annular abscess formation by homograft aortic root replacement. J Am Coll Cardiol 1991;17:1177–1182.

25. Tuna I, Orszulak T, Schaff H, Danielson G. Results of homograft aortic valve replacement for active endocarditis. Ann Thorac Surg 1990;49: 619–624.

26. Zwischenberger J, Shalaby T, Conti V. Viable cryopreserved aortic homograft for aortic valve endocarditis and annular abscesses. Ann Thorac Surg 1989;48:365–370.

27. Kirklin J, Pacifico A. Aortic valve endocarditis with aortic root abscess cavity: surgical treatment with aortic valve homograft. Ann Thorac Surg 1988;45:674–677.

28. Bedi H, Farnsworth A. Homograft aortic root replacement for destructive prosthetic endocarditis. Ann Thorac Surg 1993;55:386–388.

29. Watanabe G, Haverich A, Speier R, Dresler C, Borst H. Surgical treatment of active infective endocarditis with paravalvular involvement. J Thorac Cardiovasc Surg 1994;107:171–177.

30. McGiffin D, Galbraith A, Wong M, Burstow D. Non-toxigenic corynebacterium diptheriae var gravis endocarditis of the aortic valve. Asia Pacific J Thorac Cardiovasc Surg 1990.

31. Haydock D, Barratt-Boyes B, Macado T, Kirklin J, Blackstone E. Aortic valve replacement for active infectious endocarditis in 108 patients: a comparison of freehand allograft valves with mechanical prostheses and bioprostheses. J Thorac Cardiovasc Surg 1992;103:130–139.

32. Ross D, McKay R. Aortic root replacement. In Stark J, Pacifico A (eds). Reoperations in Cardiac Surgery. London: Springer-Verlag 1989: 259–270.

10
Pulmonary Valve Autotransplant Procedure: Clinical Results Compared with Other Methods for Aortic Valve Replacement

Erle H. Austin, III

When aortic valve replacement is required and long-term anticoagulation is to be avoided, a tissue valve is generally selected. Limited durability, however is a recognized disadvantage of this approach. Long-term follow-up now exists for four tissue valve options. The first and more commonly applied option is the stented porcine bioprostheses. A stented pericardial bioprosthesis is a second option. A third option is the aortic allograft. More recently there has been renewed interest in the pulmonary autograft technique in which the patient's own pulmonary valve is transferred to the aortic position with the pulmonary valve being replaced with a pulmonary valve allograft. When deciding which of these four operations should be applied for aortic valve replacement, it is appropriate to carefully compare the techniques and devices. The comparison should include ease of implantation, cross-clamp time required, operation mortality, the hemodynamic result and long-term durability.

Porcine Bioprosthesis

In the case of the stented porcine bioprostheses, implantation is straightforward and low risk. The majority of surgeons can successfully implant a stented porcine bioprosthesis in less than 60 minutes of cross-clamp time. Operation mortality is commonly less than 5% and often less than 2%. When large size stented porcine bioprostheses are implanted hemodymanics are generally good, but in sizes of 21 millimeters in diameter or less, an outflow tract gradient is common. In terms of durability, early failure is rare for stented porcine bioprostheses. There is, however, a well documented failure curve of porcine bioprostheses in the aortic position with failures beginning at 7 years and a 50% failure rate at 12 years. Figure 10.1 is a complication of actuarial durability curves for stented porcine valves. Grunkemeier and Bodnar[1] collected all of the published results and superimposed them on a single graph. A probability distribution (Weibull limits) was derived to provide a reliable generalization for the expected long-term outlook of a porcine valve placed in the aortic position.

Pericardial Bioprosthesis

In the case of the pericardial prosthesis, implantation is also straightforward and low risk with cross-clamp times similar to those observed for the porcine bioprosthesis. The operative mortality is also similarly low. In small sizes, a mild gradient may exist across this valve although it might be slightly less than a porcine valve. In terms of durability, the first generation of stented pericardial valves (Ionescu-Shiley) began to fail at three to four years. However, currently available valves (Carpentier-Edwards, Mitroflow) have demonstrated superior long-term results, which may, in fact, surpass the porcine bioprosthesis. Figure 10.2 is

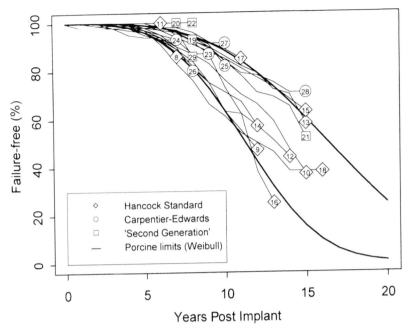

FIGURE 10.1. Reported actuarial durability curves for stented porcine valves. Each line represents a single series. The shape of the symbol at the end of each line corresponds to the type of valve. The number within the symbol indicates the reference as reported in Grunkemeier GL, Bodnar E: Compara-tive Assessment of Bioprosthesis Durability in the Aortic Position. *The Journal of Heart Valve Disease* 4:49, 1995 The two heavy lines describe the Weibull probability distribution of the curves depicted. Reproduced with permission.

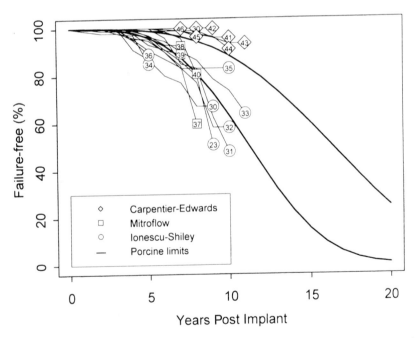

FIGURE 10.2. Reported actuarial durability curves for pericardial valves. Symbols at the end of each line correspond to the model of pericardial valve, and the numbers within the symbols refer to the reference number cited in Grunkemeier GL, Bodnar E: Com-parative Assessment of Bioprosthesis Durability in the Aortic Position. *The Journal of Heart Valve Disease* 4:49, 1995 the Weibull limits derived from the stented porcine valve experience (Figure 10.1) are superimposed for comparison. Reproduced with permission.

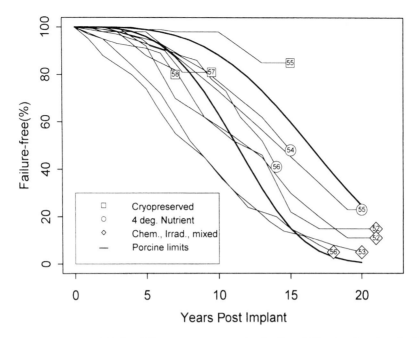

FIGURE 10.3. Reported actuarial durability curves for homograft aortic valve replacement. The symbols at the end of each line correspond to the type of preservation and sterilization with numbers referring to the specific references cited in Grunkemeier GL, Bodnar E: Comparative Assessment of Bio-prosthesis Durability in the Aortic Position. *The Journal of Heart Valve Disease* 4:49, 1995 (Chem = chemically sterilized; Irrad = sterilized by irradiation; mixed = irradiation and antibiotic valves combined). Reproduced with permission.

another depiction from Grunkemeier and Bodnar[1] showing the published durability curves for stented pericardial valves. The length of follow up is, of course, shorter than that for many of the porcine valve series.

Aortic Allograft

When an aortic allograft is utilized to replace the aortic valve the complexity of the operation increases. If a freehand subcoronary technique is utilized, implantation time is increased and valve misalignment may occur. If a root replacement technique is utilized, the technical aspects of the implantation may be simplified and problems with misalignment avoided, but the risk of bleeding is increased and imperfect reimplantation of the coronaries may result in myocardial ischemia. The cross-clamp time for insertion of an aortic allograft is typically longer than that for insertion of stented tissue valves. For many surgeons, the cross-clamp time is likely to exceed 60 minutes. As such, operation mortality can be expected to be somewhat higher, probably within the 5 to 10% range. In most cases, however, there is no hemodynamic gradient across an aortic allograft. This is one of the benefits of the technique, especially for implantation into a small aortic root. In terms of durability, early failures begin before 5 years. Figure 10.3 shows the published actuarial durability curves for allograft valves. With the exception of the experience of O'Brien and colleagues,[3] the majority of experiences are no better than those reported using stented porcine or pericardial valves.

Pulmonary Valve Autograft

For the pulmonary valve autograft (Ross procedure) the implantation can be performed with a freehand coronary or a root replacement

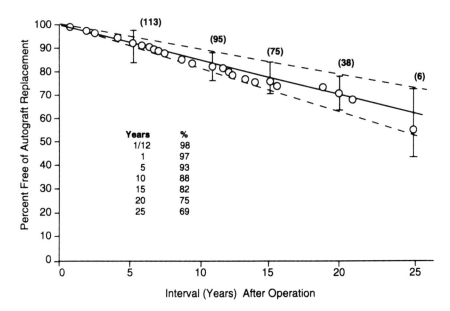

FIGURE 10.4. Actuarial durability of the pulmonary autograft in the series of Ross at the National Heart Hospital, London. This data is derived from 131 consecutive patients from 1967 to 1984 with a minimum follow up of 9 years and an average follow up of 21 years. Reprinted from *Seminars in Thoracic and Cardiovascular Surgery*, Vol 8, Ross, D, "The pulmonary autograft: history and basic techniques," 354. © 1996, with permission from Elsevier.

technique. The cross-clamp time is typically longer than for simple allograft insertion, being at least 90 minutes and occasionally exceeding two hours. Operative mortality is in the 3 to 10% range.[4-6] As with the allograft, there is no hemodynamic gradient with this technique, Early failures have been noted with the pulmonary autograft but, based on a single series,[7] long term reoperation rates appear to be the lowest among biological valves. Figure 10.4 shows the actuarial rate free from reoperation on the pulmonary autograft from Mr. Ross' series. Whether other surgeons can duplicate Ross' long term results remains to be seen.

Other Factors

Other factors must be considered in choosing among the devices and techniques for aortic valve replacement. Thromboembolism, of course, is important. For the stented porcine bioprosthesis, the thromboembolic rate ranges from 0.5 to 2% per patient-year.[8] For the allograft valve, the incidence of thromboembolism

appears to be rare and is essentially unreported for the Ross procedure.

Endocarditis is another potential complication of any aortic valve replacement. For the stented porcine bioprosthesis, it occurs at 0.5% per patient-year.[8] It appears to be the same for the pericardial valve[8] as well as the pulmonary autograft.[4-6] Interestingly, most reports for the aortic allograft show an endocarditis rate of less than 0.5% per patient-year.[3]

Summary

In summary, easily inserted porcine and pericardial bioprostheses demonstrated durability that is as good as or better than that achieved using aortic allografts. Recent interest and experience with stentless versions of the porcine valve[9] may, in fact, extend durability further. The most recent reports with the pericardial bioprosthesis suggest a major improvement over all heterograft types of replacement.[1] In view of the complexity of technique and its mediocre durability, the aortic allograft is unwarranted as a routine form of the aortic valve replacement. However, there may be some uncommon circumstances such as endocarditis with an aortic root abscess where allograft root replacement is the best technique. Of all of the devices and techniques discussed, it appears that the pulmonary autograft (Ross procedure) provides the best event-free survival for aortic valve replacement. It does present a technical challenge and imposes a greater risk. Unfortunately, data regarding long term follow up is essentially limited to the single experience of Dr. Ross. With further time results from other centers should shed further light on what happens to be a promising approach for aortic valve replacement.

References

1. Grunkemeier GL, Bodnar E. Comparative Assessment of Bioprosthesis Durability in the Aortic Position. J Heart Valve Dis 1991;6:534.
2. Tam RK, Tolan MJ, Zamvar VY, Slavik Z, Pickering R, Keeton BR, Salmon AP, Webber SA, Tsang V, Lamb RK, Monro JL. Use of larger sized aortic homograft conduits in right ventricular outflow tract reconstruction. J Heart Valve Dis 1995;4: 660–664.
3. O'Brien MF, McGiffin DC, Stafford EG, Gardner MA, Pohlner PF, McLachlan GJ, Gall K, Smith S, Murphy E. Allograft aortic valve replacement: long-term comparative clinical analysis of the viable cryopreserved and antibiotic 4 degrees C stored valves. J Card Surg 1991;6:534–543.
4. Matsuki O, Okita Y, Almeida RS. Two decades' experience with aortic valve replacement with pulmonary autograft. J Thorac Cardiovasc Surg 1988;95:705–711.
5. Ross Procedure International Registry. Summary: The Ross Procedure International Registry at St. Patrick Hospital. Ross Procedurel International Registry. [April 1993 to April 1996]. 1009. Missoula, Montana.
6. Elkins RC, Santangelo K, Stelzer P, et al. Pulmonary autograft replacement of the aortic valve: An evolution of technique. J Cardiac Surg 1992; 7:108.
7. Ross D. The Pulmonary autograft: History and Basic Techniques. Sem in Thor and Card Surg 1996;8:350.
8. Grunkemeier GL, Starr A, Rahimtoola SH. Prosthetic heart valve performance: long-term follow-up. Curr Prob Cardiol 1992;17:329.
9. Konertz W. Aortic valve replacement with stentless xenografts. J Heart Valve Dis 1992;1:249.

11
In Vivo Pulsatile Hemodynamics of Homografts

Jeff L. Myers and Richard A. Hopkins

Historically, comparative studies between valves have centered on the measurement of life expectancy of patients and failure rates of the valves. Difficulties in obtaining reproducible hemodynamic data in the postoperative, closed chest patient have resulted in a reliance on relatively crude measures of function such as the assessment of valve gradients with correlation to subsequent regression of left ventricular hypertrophy. The hemodynamic characteristics of individual valves as they function *in vivo* are critical since failure rates of the valve are likely related to these properties. Our own *in vivo* data regarding the energy dissipation of homograft valves in the sheep model demonstrates not only a comprehensive laboratory method for quantifying differences in valves, but also shows critical differences between fresh and cryopreserved valves that may effect long-term results.

The ideal valve would be biological and require no anti-coagulation, with a durability that equals or exceeds mechanical valves. Ricou et al. compared first and second generation (zero-pressure fixation) porcine prosthetic valves to St. Jude mechanical valves.[1] The negligible differences in pressure gradients across the mechanical valves were mostly accounted for by annulus size. Zero-pressure fixation (Medtronic Intact and Freestyle) may prove to be a more durable process since this retains the natural collagen crimp of the valve cusp and maintains the tissue's shock absorbing capacity which aids in resisting cyclic fatigue. The zero pressure fixation method is also thought to

increase leaflet compliance and extensibility, improvements that may extend valve life. This study also pointed out discrepancies that may arise when studies are not standardized to cardiac output. Cardiac output across a given valve size may be of critical importance in smaller mechanical valves. The favorable hemodynamics of the smaller valve were demonstrated by Rashtian who demonstrated a resting mean gradient of 5 mm Hg and a peak gradient of less than 15 mm Hg in the 19 mm St. Jude bileaflet valves.[2] Some studies have suggested that the gradients across the 19 mm St. Jude valve are small and acceptable only in patients with a body surface area (BSA) less than 1.7 m.[2,3] Others found that the valve functioned well regardless of BSA.[4]

O'Brien[5] notes that the switch from formaldehyde to glutaraldehyde preservation occurred at the same time as the advent of stents. It is possible that the adverse effects of the stents were initially obscured by improvements in preservation methods. David's work with the unstented porcine valve has shown a number of beneficial aspects in short-term follow-up.[6] These valves showed regression of left ventricular hypertrophy and a reduction in residual gradient. It was shown in a separate study[7] that the stentless porcine valve in the aortic position is associated with a greater decrease in left ventricular systolic wall stress, a decrease in transvalvular pressure gradient, and a decrease in valvular energy loss, when compared to the stented biological valve. Presence of a rigid stent contributes to a poor hemodynamic profile secondary to a reduction in the valve orifice area. Use of the stentless xenograft by Westaby[8] revealed excellent hemodynamics over the next several months. In fact, echocardiography showed the hemodynamic function at 6 months to be "directly equivalent to an aortic homograft." Additionally, the cylinder within a cylinder technique they employed resulted in less regurgitation than with the homograft.

The homograft valve remains the most difficult in which to obtain good comparative *in vivo* hemodynamic data, primarily due to small study series and the heterogeneity of both the patients and the implanted valves. A postoperative study by Jin et al. using Doppler and M-mode ECHO showed a clear hemodynamic advantage as well as a greater decrease in left ventricular mass with both homografts and unstented porcine valves when compared to stented valves or mechanical valves.[9] They not only document a hemodynamic advantage with these valves, but show a clinically significant effect of the superior hemodynamics. It should be pointed out that clinical studies using Doppler estimates of valve stenosis have well-recognized limitations. Peak velocity across a stenotic valve is a measure of peak pressure drop, not the peak-to-peak value measured by cardiac catheterization. These estimates are based on the simplified Bernoulli equation and may be appropriate for an aortic prosthesis since resistive flow across the valve exists. However, flow across the normal valve (and aortic homograft) is dominantly inertial and the simplified Bernoulli equation may not apply. Kirklin's 10-year experience with cryopreserved valves showed a transvalvular gradients of less than 10 mm Hg in 77% of patients and less than 20 in 94% of patients with follow-up of 8.7 years.[10] Their analysis indicates that cryopreserved homografts are similar in long-term performance to fresh homografts for the first 8–10 years, despite several theoretic disadvantages that include more complex insertion, limited availability, and limited durability.[11] Methods other than cryopreservation, such as chemical preservation, irradiation, and freeze drying have been shown to have a profound deleterious effect on long-term performance of the valve.[10]

As the hemodynamic profile of all prosthetic valves continues to improve, it will become necessary to have a model sensitive enough to measure the very small differences between them. Doppler and ECHO have been shown not to be sufficiently sensitive. In addition, as in any pulsatile system, measurement of mean pressure and flow alone will not fully account for the energy losses across the valves. Studies have shown that as much as 50% of ventricular work may be contained within the pulsatile components of the pressure and flow waveforms.[12] Since invasive monitoring of pressure and flow in the left ventricle and ascending aorta is unlikely to be accomplished in the postoperative patient, it would be desirable to construct an *in vivo* animal model. In our acute sheep model all valves were implanted in the descending aorta with a aorto-left atrial shunt proximal to the valves to ensure complete coaptation of the leaflets. Assessment of leaflet coaptation was obtained by open-chest echocardiography. High fidelity pressure and flow transducers were placed equidistant from the valve proximally and distally. Cardiac output was manipulated to a level of 3.0 L/min to eliminate differences related to left ventricular function. Fourier analysis of the pressure and flow waveforms was then performed to calculate the oscillatory power (W_o, reflecting aortic elasticity and geometry) mean power (W_m, energy converted to forward blood flow) and total power (W_t, oscillatory + mean) on each side of the valve.

Modeling the circulation in terms of pulsatile (waveforms) flow, pressure and impedance allows calculation of energy losses (or gains) in the pulsatile (oscillatory) components which are ignored when modeling in terms of mean (and peak) flow, pressure and resistance.[12–14]

The analysis that we performed accounts for the mean and oscillatory components of both pressure and flow. Energy lost as blood passes through the valve must be considered a result of the inherent properties of the valve such as the valve profile (both the amount of projection into the vessel as well as the shape of the projection), leaflet mobility and opposition to flow, and in the case of the bioprosthetic valves, the effects of cryopreservation. Gorlin and Gorlin[15]

TABLE 11.1. Cryopreserved versus Fresh Homografts.

	W_m/W_t	$\%W_o$ loss	$\%W_m$ loss	$\%W_t$ loss
Fresh homografts $n = 5$	89.8 ± 0.07	41.5 ± 7.0	8.5 ± 0.5	9.1 ± 0.9
Cryopreserved $n = 5$	$91.6 \pm 0.06*$	46.2 ± 0.6	$18.2 \pm 1.5*$	$19.2 \pm 4.2*$
St. Jude 19mm $n = 5$	$94.3 \pm 0.04*$	44.4 ± 6.1	$21.0 \pm 9.2*$	$21.3 \pm 9.4*$

* $p < 0.05$ vs. fresh homografts. Seventy-five heartbeats were measured for each group. W_o/W_t is the proportion of total power lost across the valve that is oscillatory power. $\%W_o$, $\%W_m$, and $\%W_t$ loss are the percentages of those components lost across the valves.

were the first to derive discharge coefficients from measurements of flow and pressure and apply them to diseased valves. These equations relied on a number of assumptions that made them highly inaccurate. So much so that the differences between calculated and measured orifices ranged from −27% to +33%. While later reports state the differences were much smaller, in general these calculations are most useful in distinguishing between moderately and severely diseased valves. This illustrates the difficulties inherent in measuring very small difference in the hemodynamics of normal valves. Our model calculates the energy within the pulsatile component of blood flow, not normally calculated when mean terms are used, and therefore accurately documents energy losses across the various valves. These calculations provide a precise and accurate measurement of the efficiency of the valve that is only approximated by current *in vivo* studies.

As the data in the Table 11.1 shows, the cryopreserved valves exhibit a hemodynamic disadvantage and appear to be stiffer than the fresh homografts. The remarkable amount of oscillatory power dissipated ($\%W_o$ loss) is similar in the three valve groups and demonstrates reproducible study conditions in our model. The fact that it is unchanged regardless of the valve studied is also consistent with the understanding that the pulsatile component is determined by the dimensions and elasticity of the native aorta, rather than the valve.[16] Since mean power makes up 89.8–94.3% of the total power dissipated in the three groups (W_m/W_t), mean power loss ($\%W_m$ loss) closely reflects the total power loss ($\%W_t$ loss). The mean power loss across the cryopreserved valves is nearly twice that seen across the fresh valves

and is the same as that across the rigid St. Jude valves. This increased rigidity represents kinetic energy absorbed by the valve and is consistent with previous studies that demonstrated decreased leaflet compliance and collagen crimp associated with cryopreservation.

These previously undocumented hemodynamic consequences of cryopreservation may affect durability over the life of the valve and may contribute to eventual valve failure. The freshly implanted valves (harvested from a living donor and implanted immediately) were associated with minimal energy losses and most closely approximate the normal *in situ* valve. Methods such as zero-pressure fixation may preserve the structural integrity of the valve and result in an energy profile that more closely resembles the native valve. This may in turn result in improvements in valve durability. As previously stated, oscillatory energy accounts for only 5–10% of the total power and the majority of the energy loss is in the mean terms across all valves studied. This indicates that while the mean terms do not provide a complete hydraulic power performance analysis, they do give a good indication of valve performance. As differences in valve performance become more difficult to quantify, a pulsatile hemodynamic analysis such as the one described provides a sensitive and reliable measure for the future evaluation of bioprosthetic valves.

References

1. Ricou F, Brun A, Lerch R. Hemodynamic comparison of Medtronic intact bioprostheses and bileaflet mechanical prostheses in aortic position. Cardiology 1996;87:212–215.

2. Rashtian MY, Stevenson DM, Allen DT, Yoganathan AP, et al. Flow characteristics of four commonly used mechanical heart valves. Am J Cardiol 1986;58:743–752.

3. Gonzalez-Juanatey JR, Garcia-Acuna JM, Vega Fernandez M, et al. Influence of the size of aortic valve prostheses on hemodynamics and change in left ventricular mass: implications for the surgical management of aortic stenosis. J Thorac Cardiovasc Surg 1996;112:273–280.

4. Sawant D, Singh AK, Feng WC, Bert AA, Rotenberg F. Nineteen-millimeter aortic St. Jude Medical heart valve prosthesis: Up to sixteen years follow up. Ann Thorac Surg 1997;63:964–970.

5. O'Brien MF. Composite stentless xenograft for aortic valve replacement: clinical evaluation of function. Ann Thorac Surg 1995;60:S406–S409.

6. Del Rizzo DF, Goldman BS, Christakis GT, David TE. Hemodynamic benefits of the Toronto stentless valve. J Thorac Cardiovasc Surg 1996;112:1431–1446.

7. Jin XY, Gibson DG, Yacoub MH, Pepper JR. Perioperative assessment of aortic homograft, Toronto stentless valve, and stented valve in the aortic position. Annals of Thoracic Surgery 1995;60:Suppl-401.

8. Westaby S, Amarasena N, Long V, Prothero A, Amarasena GA, Banning AP, Pillai R, Ormerod O. Time-related hemodynamic changes after aortic replacement with the freestyle stentless xenograft. Annals of Thoracic Surgery 1995;60: 1633–1638.

9. Jin XY, Zhang Z, Gibson DG, Yacoub MH, Pepper JR. Effects of valve substitute on changes in left ventricular function and hypertrophy after aortic valve replacement. Ann Thorac Surg 1996;62:683–690.

10. Kirklin JK, Smith D, Novick W, et al. Long-term function of cryopreserved aortic homografts: a ten year study. J Thorac Cardiovasc Surg 1993; 106:154–166.

11. Yacoub M, Rasmi NRH, Sundt TM, Lund Oea. Fourteen-year experience with homovital homografts for aortic valve replacement. J Thorac Cardiovasc Surg 1995;110:186–194.

12. Milnor WR, Bergel DH, Bargainer JD. Hydraulic power associated with pulmonary blood flow and its relation to heart rate. Circ Res 1966; XIX (No. 3):467–480.

13. Hopkins RA, Hammon JW, Jr., McHale PA, Smith PK, Anderson RW. Pulmonary vascular impedance analysis of adaptation to chronically elevated blood flow in the awake dog. Circ Res 1979;45:267–274.

14. Hopkins RA, Hammon JW, Jr., McHale PA, Smith PK, Anderson RW. An analysis of the pulsatile hemodynamic responses of the pulmonary circulation to acute and chronic pulmonary venous hypertension in the awake dog. Circ Res 1980;47:902–910.

15. Gorlin R, Gorlin SG. Hydraulic formula for calculation of the area of the stenotic mitral valve, other cardiac valve and central circulatory shunts. Am Heart J 1951;41:1–29.

16. Milnor WR. Hemodynamics. Baltimore: Williams & Wilkins 1989.

Section V
Cell Biology of Heart Valve Leaflets

12
Leaflet Endothelium

Flavian M. Lupinetti

The endothelium is a component of the allograft valve that has received far less attention from investigators than have the fibroblasts. The endothelium composes a far smaller proportion of the allograft mass and is less important in terms of structural integrity and valve competence. The endothelium is of considerably greater importance, however, in determining properties of immunogenicity and resistance to thrombus formation. The endothelium also plays an important role in mediating vascular smooth muscle tome, providing nutrition to fibroblasts, and preventing calcification. This chapter reviews the characteristics of vascular endothelial cells with particular reference to their role in cardiac valves. The functions of the endothelium will be considered, and the preservation or loss of these functions in both fresh and cryopreserved allograft valves will be addressed. Finally, the implications of these characteristics for long term fate of the allograft will be explored.

Anatomy of the Endothelium

The vascular endothelium is a nearly perfect monolayer in the absence of disease. Any defects occurring in the endothelial lining of the vascular system are rapidly repaired by migration and proliferation. When any discontinuity in the endothelial lining is observed, it is usually attributable either to artifacts of specimen preparation or to a pathologic process.[1] Therefore, one of the most important questions

to be answered regarding the endothelium of the allograft valve is whether it is present, and if so, under what conditions.

The ability to study this tissue must rely on positive identification of the cells as uniquely endothelial. Much of what is known or suspected about properties of cardiac valve endothelium is based on observations of endothelial cells obtained from blood vessels remote from the valves themselves. For most properties thus far examined, valvar endothelium has not differed dramatically from vascular endothelial cells elsewhere. however, a study by Simon and associates has shown that human aortic and mitral valve endothelium does not constitutively express factor VII,[2] These endothelial cell did express factor VIII weakly in response to interferon-γ. This suggests that a degree of caution should be exercised in extrapolating observations regarding other vascular endothelium to valve endothelium. More specifically, it calls into question studies that depend on immunocytochemical stains directed at factor VIII for identification of endothelium.

The preservation of endothelial cell function in allograft may be negatively affected by immunologic differences between donor and recipient, surgical manipulation, ischemia and reperfusion, and other influences. In human allograft valves subjected to contemporary methods of cryopreservation, it appears doubtful whether endothelium is preserved in most cases. A study from this laboratory examined 131 specimens from cryopreserved allografts,

TABLE 12.1. Prevalence of Endothelial Cells in Cryopreserved Allograft Valve Tissues.

	Number Positive/Total Samples (%)
All specimens	34/134 (25%)
Site of specimen	
Aortic valve	0/2 (0%)
Aortic wall	6/33 (18%)
Pulmonary wall	18/35 (51%)*
Pulmonary artery wall	10/64 (16%)
Donor Sex	
Male	28/87 (32%)**
Female	6/47 (13%)
Cause of death	
Blunt trauma	7/38 (18%)
Penetrating trauma	4/13 (31%)
Cardiovascular event	4/13 (31%)
Cerebrovascular event	12/41 (29%)
Other	7/29 (24%)

* $p = 0.0001$; ** $p = 0.02$.

both valve leaflets and arterial walls, using an immunocytochemical stain specific for human endothelium.[3] Only 21, or 16% of these tissues had any detectable endothelium. By contrast, examination of native valve leaflets and arterial walls from specimens removed at operation found endothelial cells present in 70 of 90 cases or 78%. These findings indicate that cryopreservation methods, at least as carried out in routine clinical practice by the largest processor of human valves, result in the complete loss of endothelium in the overwhelming majority of cases.

A subsequent study from this laboratory performed a multivariable analysis to determine what factors, if any, correlate with endothelial cell presence on cryopreserved allograft tissues.[4] As shown in Table 12.1, site of tissue examined (pulmonary valve leaflet vs. other components of the allograft) correlate with presence of endothelial cells. Male sex of the donor was the only other significant predictor of the presence of endothelial cells. these factors were predictive in a multiple logistic model as well, although the overall predictive value was limited. In a stepwise logistic analysis, the pulmonary valve leaflet was the best predictor of endothelial cell presence. This finding raises the interesting question of why

endothelial cells are so well preserved on the pulmonary valve leaflet while being poorly preserved elsewhere. Mechanical characteristics of the tissue may play a role, as may the relatively lower pressure environment to which the pulmonary valve is subjected. It must be cautioned, however, that examinations of endothelial cell presence in unimplanted tissue may have limited importance in determining the fate of these cells after implantation.

Viability

The demonstration of endothelial cells presence on allograft valves must not be considered equivalent to proof of cell viability. *Viability* is a property that has been imputed to allograft valve tissues, often with little evidence to support it. Viability has many dimensions, including the ability of the cell to replicate, synthesize essential proteins, and effect changes on other cells. These properties may be symmetrically or asymmetrically affected by storage protocols, implant techniques and host response. Ideally, statements regarding endothelial cell viability should be limited to those properties specifically tested, and findings should not be inappropriately extrapolated to other indicators of cell survival or function.

A commonly used method for evaluating endothelial cell viability is the dye exclusion technique. This was first employed to demonstrate endothelial viability in aortic valve grafts by Yankah and associates.[5] These authors studied rat aortic valves harvested after varying periods of time following the death of the animal and after varying temperature exposures. Alcian blue dye, a dye that cannot cross intact cell membranes, was used as a marker of cell death. Warmer temperatures and delay in carrying out cold storage were associated with a progressive decline in endothelial cell viability. Furthermore, regardless of the variables before storage, viability declined over a 10 day period at storage at 4°C. Yankah performed this work using the model of heterotopic valve transplantation into the abdominal aorta of rats, a model that has since become widely used for studying characteristics of these tissues.[6] In their initial investigations, these authors used Alcian blue dye exclusion as a marker of cell viability. They showed that fresh grafts were characterized by the presence of endothelial cells normal in appearance and with a high degree of viability by dye exclusion. Surprisingly, cryopreserved grafts showed a decrease of only 8–20% in the percentage of viable cells compared to fresh tissues. Grafts stored at 4°C in an antibiotic solution had a much higher degree of endothelial cell death. Yankah and associates extended this technique to human tissues.[7] Once again, cryopreserved grafts showed a 70–80% endothelial cell viability, compared to 0–8% viability in grafts stored at 4°C.

An investigation by Christy and coworkers examined the presence and viability of endothelial cells in rat aortic grafts stored at 4°C in a nutrient medium.[8] Cells were identified as endothelial by labeling with fluresceinated *Griffonia simplicifolia*, a lectin with high affinity for the α-D-galactopyranosyl residues of rat endothelial cell membranes. Cells were assessed for viability based on exclusion of propidium iodide, a fluorescent dye that binds to nucleic acids but is unable to penetrate the intact cell membrane. Flow cytometry was used to evaluate thousands of cells and precisely identify viable and non-viable endothelium. This study found that 95% of endothelial cells were viable immediately after harvest. With storage at 4°C, percentage viability declined in linear fashion to 92% at three days, 86% at seven and ten days, 83% at 14 days and 64% at 21 days. This study demonstrated the ability of this storage technique to preserve endothelial cell viability but also showed that preservation is probably limited to a relatively short time. A subsequent study attempted to use these same techniques to quantitate endothelial viability in cryopreserved tissues. No cells identifiable as endothelium were recovered, however (unpublished reference). Whether this finding is due to the absence of endothelium in cryopreserved allografts or the inapplicability of the method to cryopreserved tissues was not known at the time. The examination of cryopreserved human tissues cited above[3,4] suggests the former explanation is more likely correct.

Despite the general usefulness of dye exclusion as a marker for endothelial cell viability, there are limitations to this technique. Some cells that are incapable of protein synthesis or replication appear to retain the ability to exclude large molecule dyes for a certain period of time. Thus, quantitation of cellular viability by dye exclusion may represent an upper limit estimate. Dye exclusion by its very nature is based on the absence of a marker of cell death, rather than on affirmative evidence of life. Accordingly, a more rigorous test of endothelial cell viability may provide more clinically relevant observations. One such test is the ability of endothelial cells to replicate. This issue was addressed in this rat model of aortic valve transplantation.[9] In this study, rats that had undergone heterotopic aortic valve allografting into the abdominal aorta were administered radiolabeled thymidine. Because actively replicating cells incorporate thymidine, autoradiography was then used to examine the endothelial cells of the grafts and determine which cells contained the radiolabel. The presence of sufficient quantities of labeled thymidine constituted evidence of cellular replication. All tissues were excised for study three days after implant, the earliest interval at which thymidine uptake can be practically employed. The endothelium of the native aorta demonstrated 0.3 to 2/3% replicating cells, a normal finding for rats of this age and size. Freshly implanted aortic allografts, whether syngeneic or strongly allogeneic, demonstrated an endothelial replication frequency of over 12%. Allografts implanted after cryopreservation, regardless of histocompatibility, exhibited few endothelial cells, none of which were replicating. This study suggests that in the earliest observable period after allograft valve transplantation, fresh grafts show an increased replication rate that is not affected by immunologic differences between donor and recipient. Cryopreserved valve grafts, however, show no evidence of endothelial cell viability. This also leads to speculation that any endothelium found on allograft valves subsequently is more likely to be of recipient origin.

Resistance to Thrombus Formation

The normal endothelium is a powerful inhibitor of thrombus formation. Some of the properties of the endothelium that contribute to its thromboresistance include a strongly negative electrical charge, production of prostacyclin, binding of thrombin by synthesis of antithrombin III, elaboration of tissue plasminogen activator, and production of plasminogen-activator-inhibitors.[10] This listing of potentially important antithrombotic properties does not suffice as a complete explanation for why thrombosis does not occur on the normal, much less the abnormal or injured, endothelium. Perhaps the most impressive evidence for the thromboresistance of the endothelium is the thrombosis that occurs when endothelial injury is severe or persistent.

In allograft valves, the thrombogenicity of the luminal surface of the graft has not been well characterized. The experimental evidence cited above showing that endothelium is seldom present in cryopreserved allografts at the time of implant might raise concerns that thrombus formation would be a common occurrence. Clinical evidence, however, is nearly uniform in observing that allograft valves are quite seldom associated with thromboembolic complications despite the lack of anticoagulant therapy. This suggests that the surface of the allograft tissue retains some important thromboresistant capacity.

Antigen Expression

The vascular endothelium exhibits constitutive expression of class I antigens, which in the human includes HLA-A, -B and -C antigens. Class II antigens, in humans HLA-DP, -DQ and -DR, are expressed in response to stimuli, such as transplantation into an allogenic recipient. Yacoub and co-investigators studied human aortic valves for expression of these antigens.[11] In valves studied immediately after harvest, class I antigens were expressed but class II antigens were not. After 48 hours of storage at 4°C, valves expressed neither class I nor class II antigens.

Similar observations were obtained in studies of rat aortic valves.[12] Fresh grafts and grafts sterilized and stored at 4°C for 24 hours expressed class I antigens. All grafts were negative for class II antigens. These studies suggest that antigen expression by allograft valves is easily disrupted by sterilization and storage techniques.

Expression of Inflammatory Mediators

Endothelial cells express numerous mediators of the inflammatory response. One important class of mediators are the leukocyte adhesion molecules (LAMs). LAMs are involved in a wide variety of inflammatory conditions, including sepsis, autoimmune disorders, and response to allogenic tissues. Leukocytes have specific ligands for different LAMs, which are expressed by endothelial cells in response to cytokines such as interleukin-1 and tumor necrosis factor α. Thus, expression of LAMs leads to leukocyte adhesion, diapedesis, and inflammation. Mulligan and colleagues examined experimental aortic valve grafts in the rat heterotopic transplant model for the presence of LAMs E-selectin (formerly known as endothelial-leukocyte adhesion molecule-1).[13] This investigation included both syngeneic and strongly allogeneic grafts. Grafts were implanted in the fresh state, following cryopreservation, or after storage at 4°C in a nutrient medium for one to 21 days. Grafts were retrieved from four hours to 21 days after transplant. Tissues were then stained with monoclonal antibodies directed at each of the three LAMs. Syngeneic grafts, regardless of storage methods, in all cases failed to express any LAM. This indicates that surgical trauma, ischemia and reperfusion, cryopreservation, and cold storage are insufficient stimuli to elicit LAM expression. For the fresh allogeneic grafts, expression of all three LAMs was intense, immediate (present within four hours after implantation), and persistent (evident as much as 21 days after implant). In the cryopreserved grafts, LAM expression was absent at four hours and two days implant but was present, although weak, at 10 and 21 days after implant. Grafts stored at 4°C showed similarly weak expression at four hours and two days but somewhat stronger expression at 10 days and definite expression at 21 days. In a general fashion, the intensity of adhesion molecule expression correlated with the degree of leukocytic infiltrate in the allograft tissue. These findings suggest that allograft storage methods clinically in use result in delayed and diminished LAM expression. It further suggests that storage methods reduce endothelial preservation and function, perhaps in a way that reduces allograft injury and improves longevity.

Recipient Sensitization

The endothelium is perhaps the most immunologically potent component of allografted tissues.[14] Endothelial cells in a mixed lymphocyte cell culture reaction have been shown to be two to three fold more stimulatory than peripheral blood lymphocytes.[2] Recipient sensitization, therefore, might be expected to be predictable based on antigenic properties of the endothelium, mass of endothelium present, and viability of donor cells.

One of the earliest studies of allograft immunogenicity in the rat concluded that allograft valve immunogenicity was primarily related to the cardiac muscle component.[15] Subsequent investigations have demonstrated recipient sensitization by allograft valve implantation, irrespective of the nature of the implant, subcutaneous[16] or intravascular.[17–19] Furthermore, these latter studies observed similar recipient sensitization resulting from both fresh and cryopreserved valve grafts.

Clinical observations support this interpretation. Studies by Schutz[20] and Smith[21] and associates have demonstrated recipient sensitization by cytoimmunologic monitoring and formation of panel-reactive antibodies in human recipients of allograft valves. In the latter study, the degree of sensitization was greater in recipients of grafts not subjected to antibiotic preservation and presumably containing greater numbers of viable endothelium. In addition, the sensitization was shown to be donor-specific in many cases.

The balance of evidence, therefore, suggests that endothelium contributes to recipient sensitization, but that the reduction or elimination of endothelial cells from the valve does not achieve an immunologically inert graft. It is clear that other components of the graft are sufficient to elicit a host immune response.

Elaboration of Vasoactive Substances

One function of endothelium that may be important in vascular physiology is the ability to mediate relation of the underlying smooth muscle in response to appropriate stimuli. Endothelial-dependent relaxation is now recognized as resulting from release of nitric oxide, which is synthesized by endothelial cells in response to shear forces and various pharmacologic agents. Sjoberg and his co-investigators evaluated the ability of the transplanted aorta to mediate endothelial-dependent relaxation in the rat.[22] This study used syngeneic donors and recipients, and the vascular grafts were transplanted with a mean ischemic time of 41 minutes. Thus, this study considered the best case situation of a graft transplanted with minimal possibility of immunologic response or adverse consequences of harvest, sterilization and storage. These grafts exhibited excellent preservation of endothelia-mediated relaxation at both three and 60 days after implant. Although this experimental protocol is markedly different from the clinical situation of allogeneic tissue subjected to complicated storage methods, it provides evidence that endothelial cell function can be retained under some circumstances. It also indicates that brief ischemic injury and surgical trauma are not sufficient to eliminate or even substantially reduce this capacity of endothelial cells.

Altering the techniques of cryopreservation may allow improvements to be made to endothelial cell preservation. Feng and colleagues reported marked improvement in endothelial cell preservation in experimental porcine aortic valves, primarily resulting from an alteration in their controlled freezing program.[23] They used a bioassay of endothelial cell viability based on prostacyclin release, both in an unstimulated state and in response to bradykinin. The authors' newer cryopreservation methods resulted in significant increases in prostacyclin production compared to the older methods used. Furthermore, when the newer method was used, the presence or absence of fetal calf serum in the preservation media did not affect prostacyclin production. These findings suggest that in cryopreserved valves, endothelial cell persistence and function can be maintained at least until the time of implantation if the preservation methodology is optimal.

Summary

The endothelium of cardiac valve grafts is a complex and dynamic tissue. It is highly vulnerable to commonly employed methods of sterilization and storage. When it survives, it may have profound effects on the immunologic characteristics of the graft. It is intriguing to speculate that some degree of endothelial injury may in fact be advantageous to the overall pathologic fate of the allograft.

References

1. Gotlieb AI. The role of endothelial cells in vascular integrity and repair. Cardiovasc Pathol 1992;1:253–257.
2. Simon A, Zavazava N, Sievers H, et al. In vitro cultivation and immunogenicity of human cardiac valve endothelium. J Card Surg 1993;8:656–665.
3. Lupinetti FM, Tsai T, Kneebone J, et al. Effect of cryopreservation on the presence of endothelial cells on human valve allografts. J Thorac Cardiovasc Surg 1993;106:912–917.
4. Lewis CF, Tsai TT, Kneebone JM, et al. Determinants of endothelial cell presence in cryopreserved human allograft valves. Surgical Forum 1993;44:228–230.
5. Yankah AC, Randzio G, Wottge HU, et al. Factors influencing endothelial-cell viability during procurement and preservation of valve allografts. In Thiede A (ed). Microsurgical models in rats for transplantation research. Heidelberg: Springer-Verlag Berlin 1985:107–111.
6. Yankah AC, Dreyer W, Wottge HU, et al. Kinetics of endothelial cells of preserved aortic valve allografts used for heterotopic transplantation in inbred rat strains. In Bodnar E, Yacoub M (eds). Biologic and bioprosthetic valves. New York: York Medical Books 1986:73–84.
7. Yankah AC, Wottge HU, Muller-Hermelink HK, Feller AC, Lange P, Wessel U, Dreyer H, Bernhard A, Muller-Ruchholtz W. Transplantation of aortic and pulmonary allografts, enhanced viability of endothelial cells by cryopreservation, importance of histocompatibility. J Card Surg 1987;2:209–220.
8. Christy JP, Lupinetti FM, Mardan AH, Thompson SA. Endothelial cell viability in the rat aortic wall. Ann Thorac Surg 1991;51:204–207.
9. Lupinetti FM, Tsai TT, Kneebone JM. Endothelial cell replication in an in vivo model of aortic allografts. Ann Thorac Surg 1993;56:237–241.
10. Zilla P, von Oppell U, Deutsch M. The Endothelium: A Key to the Future. J Card Surg 1993;8:32–60.
11. Yacoub M, Suitters A, Khaghani A, et al. Localization of major histocompatability complex (HLA, ABC, and DR) antigens in aortic homografts. In Bodnar E, Yacoub M (eds). Biologic and bioprosthetic valves. New York: Yorke Medical Books 1986:65–72.
12. Lupinetti FM, Christy JP, King DM, el Khatib H, Thompson SA. Immunogenicity, antigenicity, and endothelial viability of aortic valves preserved at 4 degrees C in a nutrient medium. J Card Surg 1991;6:454–461.
13. Mulligan MS, Tsai TT, Kneebone JM, et al. Effects of preservation techniques on in vivo expression of adhesion molecules by aortic valve allografts. J Thorac Cardiovasc Surg 1994;107:717–723.
14. Pober JS, Collins T, Gimbrone MAJr, et al. Inducible expression of class II major histocompatability complex antigens and the immunogenicity of vascular endothelium. Transplantation 1986;41:141–146.
15. Heslop BF, Wilson SE, Hardy BE. Antigenicity of aortic valve allografts. Ann Surg 1973;177:301–306.

16. Cochran RP, Kunzelman KS. Cryopreservation does not alter antigenic expression of aortic allografts. J Surg Res 1989;46:597–599.

17. el Khatib H, Lupinetti FM. Antigenicity of fresh and cryopreserved rat valve allografts. Transplantation 1990;49:765–767.

18. el Khatib H, Thompson SA, Lupinetti FM. Effect of storage at 4 C in a nutrient medium on antigenic properties of rat aortic valve allografts. Ann Thorac Surg 1990;49:792–796.

19. Zhao X, Green M, Frazer IH, et al. Donor-specific immune response after aortic valve allografting in the rat. Ann Thorac Surg 1994;57: 1158–1163.

20. Schutz A, Fischlein T, Breuer M, et al. Cytoimmunological monitoring after homograft valve replacement. Eur J Cardio-thorac Surg 1994;8: 609–612.

21. Smith JD, Ogino H, Hunt D, et al. Humoral immune response to human aortic valve homografts. Ann Thorac Surg 1995;60:S127–S130.

22. Sjoberg T, Massa G, Steen S. Endothelium-mediated relaxation in transplanted aorta. Ann Thorac Surg 1992;53:1068–1073.

23. Feng X-J, van Hove CE, Mohan R, et al. Improved endothelial viability of heart valves cryopreserved by a new technique. Eur J Cardio-thorac Surg 1992;6:251–255.

13
Leaflet Interstitial Cells

Robert H. Messier, Jr., Patrick W. Domkowski, and Richard A. Hopkins

Leaflet interstitial cells (LIC) are the major cellular components of cardiac valves. Historically they have been referred to as fibroblasts,[1] fibrocytes,[2] interstitial cells,[3] matrix cells,[4] myofibroblasts[5] and stromal cells.[4] LIC reside throughout the valve layers, though they are more dense in the lamina spongiosa than the lamina fibrosa. Because they resemble fibroblasts in structure and participate in extracellular matrix turnover, their major function was originally thought to be valve matrix synthesis. Recently these cells have been found to possess characteristics of both synthetic, fibroblast-like cells and contractile, smooth muscle-like cells. This chapter will focus on studies of atrioventricular and aortic valve LIC in pig, rabbit, hamster, rat, mouse, and human, and the structural and functional characteristics of these cells.

Morphology

LIC are elongated cells with long cytoplasmic processes that connect to each other in a network throughout the valve. They can be grown in tissue culture, and in culture they reproduce their cell-cell connections and form patterns of a mixed population of cells, with most cells elongated, and others cobblestone-like.[6,7] As LIC reach confluence, different studies have documented a variety of cellular patterns: Johnson et al. observe ridges resembling those seen in smooth muscle cell cultures,[8] while others report whorl-like patterns lacking the "hills and valleys" that are typical of smooth muscle cells.[6,7,9] Messier et al. note the lack of "cobblestones" in the cultures; in contrast, Zacks et al. see cobblestone morphology in a sub-population of cells. These variations in cell types may arise from distinctions in the cell culture methods, which include explant cultures and dissociated cell cultures.

Ultrastructure

LIC have adherens junctions, extensive desmosomal complex junctions, and intercellular communicative gap junctions, similar to those present in smooth muscle bundles.[6,7,10,11] Like fibroblasts, LIC associate closely with extracellular matrix components, and they are rich in cellular organelles. Some cells possess prominent microfilaments and intermediate filaments, others have more prominent rough endoplasmic reticulum and Golgi apparatus, and many display both types of ultrastructural organelles.[7,11–13] Microfilaments are typically oriented parallel to the long axis of the cell, and likely serve a contractile function. Many of these cells with more filamentous organelles also contain an incomplete basal lamina. Together, these characteristics suggest that LIC are contractile cells, but are distinct from smooth muscle cells, which typically are surrounded by an intact basal lamina.

Cytoskeleton

The cytoskeleton of LIC has been characterized further by histology and immunocytochemistry. The presence of actin filaments in LIC has been demonstrated by immunocytochemistry with various antibodies and by rhodamine phalloidin staining, which selectively labels F-actin in a stoichiometric manner. Since the various forms of actin are present in different cell types, the particular antibody employed for identification has been important to note. Recent studies have utilized anti-smooth muscle actin, an antibody directed against an amino acid sequence found in smooth muscle cells but not homologous with the actin in stress fibers of fibroblasts and other non-smooth muscle cell types, and HHF35, an antibody that recognizes muscle-specific alpha- and gamma-actin isotopes.[14] The co-localization of anti-myosin with rhodamine phalloidin on stress fibers further supports a contractile function of these cells.[14] LIC also show immunoreactivity for a number of cytoskeletal markers typically found in fibroblasts and smooth muscle cells, including diffuse desmin and tubulin staining, and a characteristic web-like pattern of vimentin staining, with some concentration around the nucleus.[7,14]

Extracellular Matrix

Historically, a synthetic function has been ascribed to LIC. In support of this, Messier et al. have shown immunoreactivity for fibronectin and chondroitin sulfate in close association with cultured porcine aortic valve LIC, suggesting that these cells synthesize extracellular matrix components in vitro. In addition, labeling of a subpopulation of LIC for the procollagen hydroxylating enzyme, prolyl-4-hydroxylase, gives evidence that LIC carry out post-translational modification of collagen.[7]

Contractile Function

LIC have several properties in common with smooth muscle cells; actin and myosin are co-localized, well-developed microfilament networks and cyoskeletons are present, the cells stain positive for the smooth muscle cell marker anti-GMP-dependent protein kinase, and motor nerve terminals are closely apposed to the cells.[10] Two groups have explored these cellular characteristics further and asked directly if LIC possess another property of smooth muscle cells—the ability to contract. For these studies, LIC are cultured on a flexible substratum of polydimethyl siloxane and incubated with different stimuli. When the cells encounter a stimulus to contract, their cell bodies shrink, cytoplasmic extensions shorten, and wrinkles are generated on the substrate surface. The opposite effect is seen in response to a relaxation stimulus. LIC contract following stimulation with epinephrine,[7,10] carbachol, angiotensin II, KCl, and bradykinin.[7] They relax in response to isoproterenol.[7] In these experiments, most LIC exhibited a baseline tonus, characteristic of cells with contractile function. Those that did not demonstrate this tonus failed to respond to the drugs.

Conclusion: The Leaflet Interstitial Cell as Myofibroblast

Table 13.1 provides a summary of the phenotypic characteristics of LIC, as demonstrated by the work of our group and others. The results of these studies together indicate that the cardiac valve LIC can be designated a myofibroblast, that is, a cell that possesses properties of both connective tissue fibroblasts and smooth muscle cells. LIC are not alone in this designation. In other tissues, interstitial cells that resemble fibroblasts have also been found to have contractile properties.[15,16] The name myofibroblast has been given to interstitial cells that exhibit smooth muscle cell characteristics and function in wound contraction.[16] It is of interest to consider the dual function of the myofibroblast LIC in the context of cardiac valve function. Matrix production is essential for flexibility and strength in the cardiac valve throughout its cyclic motion. The significant and increasing amounts of extracellular matrix components in cardiac valves in association with LIC suggest that these cells have a robust

TABLE 13.1. Phenotypic Characteristics of Leaflet Interstitial Cells.

Characteristic	Observation	Assay	References
Morphology	Elongated	Light microscopy	7,10
	Cobblestone/Cuboidal		12,14
	Lack of cobblestones		7
	Ridged patterns		8
	Whorl patterns		6,7,9
Ultrastructure	Adherens junctions	Electron microscopy	7,10,14
	Desmosomes		7
	Gap junctions		10,14
	Microfilaments		7,12,14
	Intermediate filaments		7,12,14
	Rough endoplasmic reticulum		7,12,14
	Golgi apparatus		7,12,14
Cytoskeleton	Actin	Electron microscopy	10
		Rhodamine phalloidin	14
		Alpha smooth muscle actin	7
		HHF35	14
	Myosin	Anti light chain myosin	7,14
	Desmin	Polyclonal Ab	7
	Tubulin	Monoclonal Ab	7
	Vimentin	Monoclonal Ab	7,14
Extracellular matrix	Fibronectin	Monoclonal Ab	7
	Chondroitin sulfate	Monoclonal Ab	7
	Collagen	Anti prolyl 4 hydroxylase	7
Contractile function	Response to epinephrine, angiotensin II	Culture on silicone substrate	7,10
	Response to carbachol, bradykinin, isoproterenol, KCl		7

synthetic capacity. Increasing amounts of these molecules over time in cultures of LIC provide further evidence of this capability. The role of LIC contraction is not well-defined currently, since valve leaflets were historically thought to respond to forces passively. It has been suggested that a cytoskeleton capable of responding to cyclic forces may actively anchor collagen fibrils as valve leaflets appose each other in diastole.[17,18] It may be that, as in the case of other tissues that undergo continuous physical force, the cells that perceive mechanical stress respond biochemically. For example, in response to the load born by the articular long bone cartilage, chondrocytes modulate their matrix secretory rates.[19] In the case of cardiac valve leaflets, the stimulus-response effect may involve the interaction between endothelial cells and LIC; the degree of vascular shear stress has been found to influence endothelial cells' production of endothelin I, which can stimulate the contraction of LIC in vitro.[20] In the non-endothelial cell layers, the rate of pro-

teoglycan synthesis is higher in leaflet attachment regions than in the middle of the leaflet, whereas in contrast, collagen synthesis is more rapid in the leaflet mid-section. These differences in extracellular matrix production may arise from LIC responses to differing forces in these regions. The matrix composition of particular subregions may, in turn, contribute to the leaflets' dual characteristics of flexibility and strength. Thus structure and function at the cellular level underlie the impressive abilities of the cardiac valve to open and close efficiently in continuous cycles throughout life.

References

1. DeBiasi S, Vittellaro-Zuccarello L, Blum I. Histochemical and ultrastructural study of the innervation of human and porcine atrio-ventricular valves. Anat Embryol 1984;169:159.
2. Kosek JC, Iben AB, Shumway NE, et al. Morphology of fresh heart valve homografts. Surgery 1969;66:269–277.

3. Hibbs RG, Ellison JP. Atrioventricular valves of the guinea pig. II. An ultrastructural study. American Journal of Anatomy 1973;138:347.

4. Crescenzo DG, Hilbert SL, Messier JrRH, Domkowski PW, Barrick MK, Lange PL, Ferrans V, Wallace RB, Hopkins RA. Human cryopreserved allografts: Electron microscopic analysis of cellular injury. Ann Thorac Surg 1993;55: 25–31.

5. Bairati A, DeBiasi S. Presence of a Smooth Muscle System in Aortic Valve Leaflets. Anatomy and Embryology 1981;161:329–340.

6. Lester W, Rosenthal A, Granton B, Gotlieb AI. Porcine Mitral Valve Interstitial Cells in Culture. Laboratory Investigation 1988;59:710–719.

7. Messier RH, Bass BL, Aly HM. Dual structural and functional phenotypes of the porcine aortic valve interstitial characteristics of the leaflet myofibroblast. J Surg Res 1994;57:1–21.

8. Johnson CM, Nyberg Hanson M, Helgeson SC. Porcine cardiac valvular endothelial cells in culture: cell isolation and growth characteristics. J Mol Cell Cardiol 1987;19:1185–1193.

9. Gotlieb AI, Spector W. Migration into an in vitro experimental wound: a comparison of porcine aortic endothelial and smooth muscle cells and the effect of culture irradiation. American Journal of Pathology 1981;103:271–282.

10. Filip DA, Radu A, Simionescu M. Interstitial Cells of the Heart Valves Possess Characteristics Similar to Smooth Muscle Cells. Circulation Research 1986;59:310–319.

11. Lester WM, Gotlieb AI. In vitro repair of the wounded porcine mitral valve. Circ Res 1988;62: 833–845.

12. Zacks S, Rosenthal A, Granton B, Havenith M, Opas M, Gotlieb AI. Characteristic of cobblestone mitral valve interstitial cells. Archives of Pathology & Laboratory Medicine 1991;115: 774–779.

13. Romeo MG, Distefano G, Di Bella D, Mangiagli A, Caltabiano L, Roccaro S, Mollica F. Familial Jarcho-Levin syndrome. Clin Genet 1991;39:253–259.

14. Lester WM, Damji AA, Gedeon I, Tanaka M. Interstitial cells from the atrial and ventricular sides of the bovine mitral valve respond differently to denuding endocardial injury. In Vitro Cellular and Developmental Biology 1993;29A: 41–50.

15. Kapanci Y, Assimacopoulos A, Irle C, Zwahlen A, Gabbianni G. Contractile interstitial cells in pulmonary alveolar septa: A possible regulator of ventilation/perfusion ratio. J Cell Biol 1974; 60:375–392.

16. Majno G. The story of myofibroblasts. American Journal of Surgical Pathology 1979;3:535–542.

17. Deck JD. Histology and cytology of the aortic valve. In Thubrikar M (ed). The Aortic Valve. Boca Raton, FL: CRC Press 1990:21–38.

18. Crescenzo DG, Hilbert SL, Barrick MK, Corcoran PC, St.Louis JD, Messier RH, Ferrans VJ, Wallace RB, Hopkins RA. Donor heart valves: electron microscopic and morphometric assessment of cellular injury induced by warm ischemia. J Thorac Cardiovasc Surg 1992;103: 253–257.

19. Pytela R, Pierschbacker MD, Ruoslahti E. Identification and isolation of a 140kd cell surface glycoprotein with properties of a fibronectin receptor. Cell 1985;16:675.

20. Inerot S, Heineg~ard D, Olsson SE, Telhag H, Audell L. Proteoglycan alterations during developing experimental osteoarthritis in a novel hip joint model. Journal of Orthopedic Research 1991;9:658.

14
Leaflet Interstitial Cell Growth and Recovery

Robert H. Messier, Jr., Diane Hoffman-Kim, and Richard A. Hopkins

Cardiac valve leaflet interstitial cells (LIC) provide the essential synthetic means of continuous matrix production and remodeling within the valve and possess contractile functions that likely contribute to the valve's enormous capacity for endurance. In light of their importance, the present chapter focuses on these cells' capacity to maintain a viable, functional population, both in culture and after typical post-harvest processing.

LIC Growth

Two studies have looked at the responses of LIC to isolation and cell culture, including their characteristics at different passages and in response to growth factors and serum. While the studies are complimentary and together provide an interesting study of LIC growth, their methodologies differ somewhat and are worth noting. Messier et al. have evaluated LIC isolated enzymatically from porcine aortic valves,[1] and Lester et al. have examined LIC derived from explant cultures of porcine mitral valves.[2] For enzymatic isolation, endothelial cells were removed by scraping, and the central one-third of the left cusps were dissected and treated with collagenase overnight. The resulting single-cell suspension was plated and reached confluence in 7 days. The characteristics of the LIC were assessed with cells from passages 1–3. For explant cultures, following similar scraping removal of the endothelium, the distal one-third of anterior mitral valve were cut into pieces, covered with glass coverslips, and cultured for 3–5 weeks. At that point, the cells that had emerged from the explants were subcultured for up to 22 passages.

In the case of the enzymatically isolated cells, a 3-day experiment focused on the initial proliferative capacity of first passage LIC after isolation and culture. Second passage cells from explant cultures were examined over a 13-day period, testing their ability to reach confluence. Both groups concluded that less than 5% serum is not conducive to mitotic stimulation, and that 15–20% serum is optimal for cell proliferation to confluence. Passage number showed no effect on the growth rates of explant-derived cells from passages 1–22 cultured in 10% serum. The effects of a variety of growth factors on the growth of enzymatically isolated LIC were examined. While a number of factors suboptimally influenced cell growth, and basic fibroblast growth factor (bFGF) and platelet derived growth factor (PDGF) were found to stimulate mitosis. Each factor showed this effect when added individually, and when combined, they act in a synergistic manner, suggesting that they may work at different points in the cell cycle. Of interest for "resuscitation studies" (see below) was the observation that when compared to all the growth factors tested, 15% fetal bovine serum was found to be the best stimulus of cell proliferation. Taken together, these studies of LIC growth suggest that cultured LIC are not in a condition of stasis and terminal differentiation, but rather retain proliferative capacities (Figures 14.1 and 14.2).

FIGURE 14.1. Growth curves of enzymatically isolated aortic valve leaflet interstitial cells in response to serum concentration. Cell counts were performed at 24, 48, 72 and 96 hours after serum administration in ascending concentrations. Each curve represents cells cultured with a specific concentration of serum. At baseline and 24 hours, counts are without significant change. 0.1% and 1.0% FBS do not stimulate mitosis throughout 96 hours of culture. By 48 hours, 10%, 15%, and 20% FMS have markedly increased growth rates. This pattern is maintained at 72 hours. Similarly, at 96 hours, 20% FBS has the greatest mitogenic effect (20% > 15%, 10 > 5%, 0.1%. $p < 0.05$, ANOVA).

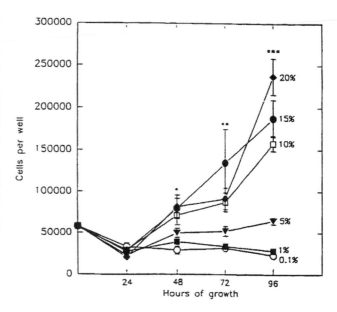

Within this chapter, we have separated the various experiments into examinations of cell "growth" and "recovery"; however, it is important to note that all cultured cells must undergo a period of "recovery" from the physical and/or enzymatic treatments used to generate single-cell cultures.

LIC Recovery

When human cardiac valves are procured and prepared for use as allografts, they undergo a series of processing stages. These include pre-harvest ischemia (less than 24 hours in the US),

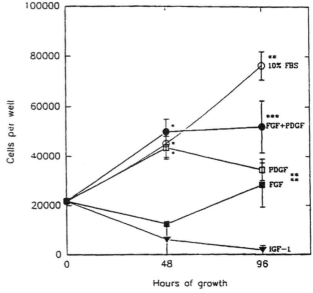

FIGURE 14.2. Serum growth factor responses of enzymatically isolated aortic valve leaflet interstitial cells. Cells were counted at 48 and 96 hours of growth. By 96 hours, 10% FBS appears more capable of stimulating growth than any single growth factor or the bFGF+PDGF-BB combination, however, the latter remains more effective than bFGF, PDGF-BB and IGF-1 alone ($p < 0.05$, ANOVA).

disinfection (24 hours), and cryopreservation. This section of the chapter will review a recent study in which valves were harvested, and the post-explant treatment conditions were designed to mimic the clinical processing which occurs in the course of organ donation, valve harvest, and cryogenic storage. It has previously been shown that this process leads to a reduction in cell metabolism (for review see Section VI). The observation of this depletion in ATP gave rise to the idea that although harvested valves contain cells, those cells may be functionally impaired or "stunned". Messier et al. have examined the characteristics of LIC following processing which approximates clinical conditions, and have assessed the cells' abilities to recover.[3] They evaluated this capacity by examining cell ultrastructure, cell surface, matrix and cytoskeletal markers, and contractile function. The hypothesis of this work is that since LIC retain a proliferative capacity in vitro, perhaps they can be treated following valve harvest in such a way as to maximize their ability to proliferate before and/or after transplantation, thus ensuring a valve replacement which has maximal functional capacity.

In the process of valve procurement, there is a typical ischemic period of 2–24 hours in the donor while the body cools prior to harvest. This period of ischemia alone led to no change in LIC number as assessed by vital dye exclusion. However, the cell state appeared more complex than dye exclusion could reveal; leaflets exhibited sparse cellularity with toluidine blue staining, as well as other ultrastructural changes. While plasma membranes remained intact, there was separation of nuclear membrane layers and nuclei appeared crescent-shaped, possibly due to osmotic imbalances. All cells appeared somewhat injured in this way. Examination of cytoskeletal components revealed sparse vimentin immunostaining, and smooth muscle actin immunoreactivity only in one, interrupted row of cells (as compared to positive actin staining throughout the layers in normal leaflets). Evaluation of extracellular matrix showed a severe reduction in chondroitin sulfate immunostaining and a slight decrease in fibronectin staining as compared to normal leaflets. Thus although LIC retained

intact cell membranes that could exclude trypan blue dye following ischemia, a number of significant subcellular and matrix changes suggest that the cells were functionally impaired.

Following ischemia, disinfection, and cryopreservation, LIC were in a worse state. Cell numbers were reduced, with fewer intact cells and more pyknotic nuclei seen by toluidine blue staining. Under electron microscopy, increases in the number of necrotic cells, myelin figures, intracellular lipid droplets, and cells with halos (most likely due to dissolved extracellular matrix) were observed, and only a few cells with normal ultrastructure were present. Both vimentin and smooth muscle actin immunoreactivity were minimal. In the extracellular matrix, a decrease in fibronectin immunostaining was clearly observed, and no chondroitin sulfate could be seen with immunohistochemistry. After these processing steps, the leaflet composition was substantially changed, with a cell population of diminished number and functional capacity, and a matrix lacking many essential soluble components.

To "resuscitate" the LIC, dissociated cells or individual leaflets were placed in culture media with 15% fetal bovine serum and incubated at 37C for 8 days. The serum concentration was selected based on previous work showing its optimal mitogenic capacity for cultured LIC.[3] When leaflets underwent ischemia, disinfection, and cryopreservation, followed by resuscitation, LIC numbers remained the same as in normal leaflets, with round nuclei. Ultrastructural examination showed evidence of normal cell states, as demonstrated by mitosis, cytokinesis, and intercellular junctions. Some remnants of necrotic cells could be observed, but most cells appeared healthy. Vimentin staining was evenly distributed, and smooth muscle actin immunoreactivity was intense throughout the layers. Homogenous chondroitin sulfate immunostaining was present, and an increase in fibronectin staining indicated fibronectin synthesis in the leaflet tissue, presumably by LIC. Cultures of LIC dissociated from cryopreserved valves and subsequently resuscitated showed normal proliferation capacity, positive immunoreactivity for the above

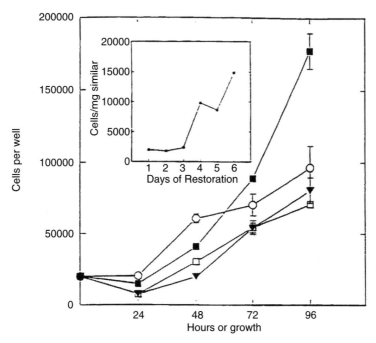

FIGURE 14.3. Cellular Restoration. Growth curves and *in situ* repopulation (inset). Parent graft depicts growth rates of cells released from aortic valve leaflets at each interval (○ = 2 hours preharvest ischemia only [2hr Group I]; ■ = 24hrs preharvest ischemia only [24hr Group I]; □ = 2hrs preharvest ischemia and fully processed [2hr Group II]; ▲ = 24hrs preharvest ischemia and fully processed [24hr Group II]). Regardless of ischemia or processing aortic valve leaflet interstitial cells (AoLIC's) retain the ability to respond mitogenically to media sup-plemented with 15% FBS. These retained capabilities were used to bioengineer the residual population surviving completed processing, and restore the leaflet to normal AoLIC density. The inset depicts the pattern of this repopulation. On each of the six days of "restoration," a single leaflet was weighted and digested in 0.08% *collagenase*. After release of cells, viable numbers were derived by hemacytometer and trypan blue exclusion, and plotted on the graph. These data suggest the rate of repopulation is similar to the native growth rates in 15% FBS.

markers, and contractile capabilities. When assessed in terms of cell numbers and functionality, and matrix composition, the resuscitation process as performed seems to have been successful (Figure 14.3).

Native cardiac valve leaflets possess impressive strength, flexibility, and durability, characteristics due in part to their component cells' abilities to synthesize extracellular matrix proteins in response to stress-strain stimuli. Following the stresses of harvesting, processing, and cryopreservation, small numbers of residual surviving cells provide enough genetic capacity to respond to mitotic stimuli, proliferate, and restore leaflet cellularity and function.

Currently used processing methods result in allograft cardiac valves which are composed of a substantially altered matrix, containing reduced numbers of cells, most of which exhibit decreased functionality. However, even the most severely damaged leaflets possess small numbers of normal cells. These retain the capacities for proliferation, synthesis, and contractile function. By mitogenic stimulation of the remaining surviving cell population, the reduction in the number of healthy cells and depletion of matrix proteins can be reversed to normal levels in the intact leaflets. Post-harvest processing that includes a period of resuscitation can result in a cardiac valve with leaflets that have the biological cellular capacity to continue the important functions of growth, repair, remodeling, and responding to varying stimuli within the recipient, as long as an immune response is avoided.

Development of the technique to manipulate these cells *in vitro* both as cell suspensions and within the matrix environment of intact leaflets is an important development that portends the ability to maintain not just cellular viability but also retained appropriate phenotypic expression.

References

1. Messier RH, Bass BL, Aly HM. Dual structural and functional phenotypes of the porcine aortic valve interstitial characteristics of the leaflet myofibroblast. J Surg Res 1994;57:1–21.
2. Lester W, Rosenthal A, Granton B, Gotlieb AI. Porcine Mitral Valve Interstitial Cells in Culture. Laboratory Investigation 1988;59:710–719.
3. Messier R, Bass BL, Domkowski PW, Hopkins RA. Interstitial Cellular Matrix Restoration of Cardiac Valves Following Cryopreservation. J Thorac Cardiovasc Surg 1999;118:36–49.

15
Activation of the Immune System by Cardiac Valve Allografts

Franciska Hoekstra, Christiaan Knoop, Ad Bogers, and Willem Weimar

The antigenicity of valve allografts has been a matter of debate since their introduction for clinical use. Fresh and cryopreserved valve allografts have classically been regarded as tissues with low antigenicity. Indeed, long-term follow-up studies after implantation of cryopreserved valves showed good clinical results, especially in adults.[1,2] Nevertheless, valve allograft deterioration, resulting from an intrinsic abnormality (structural valve damage) is frequently seen, although these findings do not necessarily lead to valve dysfunction.[3-5]

Early valve allograft failure is especially observed in young recipients.[6-9] This structural failure may have an immunologic basis, because valve donor and acceptor are not matched for the Major Histocompatibility Complex (MHC) antigens, which immunosuppressive therapy is not routinely administered to valve recipients.

In this chapter, we discuss the immunological aspects of cardiac valve transplantation in animal studies (sensitization of the recipients, histological and immunohistochemical findings *in vivo*), the immunogenicity of human cardiac valve allografts *in vivo* and *in vitro*, the effect of the ABO blood group compatibility on graft survival, some aspects of immunomodulation and immunosuppression, and the potential use of cross-match procedures, especially for patients who receive second allografts, to avoid antibody-mediated graft destruction.

Immunogenicity of Valves in Animal Studies

To analyze the antigenicity of fresh and cryopreserved allogeneic cardiac valves *in vivo*, various animal models have been used to study histological signs of rejection after implantation of allogeneic valves and on the possible correlation between immunological activity in the graft and valve insufficiency.

Mohri et al. showed that allogeneic skin grafts were rapidly rejected when dogs were sensitized by subcutaneous implantation of a valve of the same donor.[10] In contrast, when a valve instead of a skin graft was transplanted in the orthotopic position in these sensitized animals, no acute rejection was observed. Histology showed only few polymorphonuclear leukocytes and mononuclear cells in an intact valve stroma. No significant differences were found in the functional durability of orthotopically transplanted leaflets in either sensitized or non-sensitized dogs. However, plasma cells and lymphocytes infiltrating the allogeneic implants were observed more than 2 months after transplantation. The authors suggested that this late cellular rejection could be the result of the low antigenicity of the aortic valve. This conclusion is however, not in line with their findings that these valves are able to sensitize their experimental animals as they showed by the rapid rejection of skin grafts. An alternative explanation could be that these transplanted valves are not instantly recognized, not even by a sensitized immune system, suggesting that their implantation procedure temporarily affected the antigenicity of the valve. The relative lack in immune response is, however, not a uniform finding. Baue et al. examined the immunologic response to heterotopic fresh aortic valve transplants in nonsensitized calves and animals presensitized with donor skin.[11] Destruction of the allogeneic valves after 7 days of transplantation was found in all instances. No histological differences in the explanted valve allografts was found between the presensitized and nonsensitized animals. In this study, the histological findings were comparable to that of rejecting organ transplants, although the acute rejection process did not result in dysfunction of the transplanted valves.

Buch et al. examined the histological differences between fresh transplanted allogeneic valves and autologous valve allografts in dogs after various months after implantation.[12] In the allogeneic explanted valves, structural alterations were observed already 5 days after implantation. Absence of endothelium and a superficial zone of acellularity was found, while autologous grafts retained the normal endothelial lining. Three months, 6 months and 1 year after implantation, both homologous and autologous were moderately thickened due to hypercellularity. The explanted homografts showed fibroblast hyperplasia and areas of acellularity, but infiltrates were not detected. Despite the histological evidence for valve damage, these valves remained well functioning during this experimental study.[12]

In a study on rats, Thiede et al. examined the level of sensitization after transplantation of one versus two allogeneic valve leaflets implanted intravascularly. One heart valve leaflet caused strong sensitization, resulting in accelerated skin rejection. There was no statistically significant difference in the moment of rejection between rats that received one or two valve leaflets, showing that an overload valve antigen was not able to either enhance or suppress the antigeneic process. In this report, the degree of sensitization varied significantly according to the degree of histoincompatibil-ity,[13] which was also observed by el Khatib et al.[14] Lupinetti et al. examined the effect of immunological different rat strains on aortic valve allograft calcification.[15] Immunogenetic factors were also of importance in a study by Gonzalez-Lavin et al., who showed that transplantation of valves between genetically related dog combinations was associated with significantly less degenerative changes compared to histological findings in valves transplanted between genetically different dogs.[16]

Zhao et al. examined the immune response to MHC antigens after implantation of an allogeneic valve in different rat strains.[17] The proliferative response of acceptor lymphocytes against donor-spleen cells was measured before and after implantation of the allogeneic valve using mixed lymphocyte cultures. The authors demonstrated a donor-specific stimulation one month after implantation. The same group also observed an increase of donor specific cytotoxic T-lymphocyte frequencies in a limiting dilution analysis assay of splenocytes, accompanied by an increase in the level of anti-donor antibodies.[17]

In conclusion, these experimental animal studies show that implantation of allogeneic valves is followed by a specific donor-directed immunological response. Histological signs of acute and chronic rejection, especially in the allogeneic grafts are generally observed, although these findings do not correlate with valve dysfunction. Autologous valves show less signs of inflammation than allogeneic valves, and the degree of the immune response is related to the degree of histoincompatibility in some animal models presented. These results suggest that matching for Major Histochemical Complex (MHC) antigens can result in a decreased immune response against the donor valve compared to valve donors and acceptors who are not matched for MHC antigens.

Immunogenicity of Human Valves

Target Antigens

The effect of compatibility for the ABO blood group antigens between valve donor and acceptor on graft-survival has sparsely been reported in the literature. In the only available study, Balch et al. showed that there was no relationship between ABO compatibility and long term valve allograft survival.[18] In this study, the majority of the patients with valve failure (130/188) were ABO compatible. Regardless of this finding, the authors mentioned the presence of denuded endothelium, fibrin deposits, calcification and mononuclear infiltrates in unsuccessful aortic valve transplants, suggesting a role for other antigens than the ABO system in evoking an immune response. The cell surface antigens coded by the Major Histocompatibility Complex (MHC) are obvious candidates. The presence of these so-called transplantation antigens is a prerequisite for the initiation of an immune response against foreign tissue. In valve transplantation, the viability of fibroblasts and endothelial cells is considered an important factor contributing to immunostimulation, because both fibroblasts and endothelial cells cultured from valve allografts have shown to be able to express HLA class I and class II antigens. Salomon et al. examined the expression of HLA class II on fibroblasts cultured from cryopreserved aortic valves after incubation with interferon-gamma.[19] The authors observed an upregulation of class II antigens on the majority of fibroblasts. Yacoub et al. also examined the presence of HLA-antigens. Different components of human cardiac valves were studied by staining with monoclonal antibodies and the influence of sterilization procedures was investigated.[20] Before storage, valve allografts showed weak staining for class I on endothelial cells, which gradually disappeared within 48 hours during storage in Hartmann's solution. Within the matrix, class I positive leucocytes were observed that had also disappeared within 48 hours. Class II staining of endothelium was negative both before and after storage, but positive for cells just below the endothelium, possibly representing the presence of leukocytes or dendritic cells.

As endothelial cells form the first barrier between the allo-reactive immune system and the donor valve, these cells could play an important role in the initial immune response

against the donor valve. To analyze the immunogenicity of valve endothelium in vitro, both Simon and Hoekstra et al. cultured endothelial cells from fresh valve leaflets,[21,22] according to the isolation method of Johnson and Fass.[23] Mixed cell cultures with valve endothelium as stimulator and lymphocytes as responder cells resulted in high proliferative responses when lymphocytes were mismatched for HLA-A, B, C and DR with the valve donor.[22,24] Schoen et al. examined cryopreserved valve allografts which had to be explanted because of growth-related conduit or valve stenosis.[25] They concluded that the function of cryopreserved valves is not related to the presence of viable cells, but to preserve collagen.[26] Immunohistochemical studies of these explants showed that inflammatory cells, primarily T-lymphocytes, were present in only one valve (out of 20, while viable fibroblasts or endothelial cells could not be detected).

Immunological Response

Yankah et al. identified activated complement (C3C) and immunoglobulins by staining with monoclonal antibodies on the surface of explanted allogeneic valves 4 weeks after implantation.[26,27] The immunological findings were again not related to valve failure in these cases. In a comparable study by Lupinetti et al., comparable results were reached.[28] Our group detected anti-HLA class I antibodies in 23/31 (74%) patients in the first year after implantation of an allograft valve. The HLA-type of the valve donor was available in 17 patients from whom blood samples taken 4 or more weeks after transplantation were available. From these 17 patients, 14 (83%) showed antibodies specifically directed against HLA class I of the donor. Among the patients examined, significant valve insufficieny has not been observed within 13 months after valve transplantation.

To follow the immunologic process after allogeneic valve implantation, cytoimmunological monitoring has been used by Schutz et al.[29] This group examined 16 patients that had received ABO compatible (n = 9) or ABO incompatible ($n = 7$) cryopreserved aortic valves. An immunological reaction could be detected in all patients after 5 days of implantation. The increased activation index spontaneously disappeared 7 days after implantation without the use of immunosuppression, but in the ABO compatible group, a prolonged activation was observed. Echocardiography as postoperative function control 3 months after implantation showed hemodynamically irrelevant valve insufficiency in both groups. The authors conclude that allogeneic cryopreserved valve transplantation leads to an immunological reaction in the early postoperative course due to T-cell activation, which is reversible and that ABO incompatibility does not affect the echocardiographic outcome after 3 months. Although we think for the diagnosis of rejection after organ transplantation,[30] cytoimmunological monitoring is an aspecific method, it certainly reflects immunological reactivity in peripheral blood after transplantation.

In allograft valves explanted because of dysfunction after 6 months to 6 years of implantation, Hoekstra et al. examined the presence of graft-infiltrating cells by culturing small pieces of valve in an interleukin 2 containing culture medium. The donor specific cytotoxic capacity of the cell cultures obtained was measured in a cell-mediated lympholysis assay.[31] Indeed lymphocyte cultures could be obtained in 5/6 explants. One culture consisted of CD4 positive lymphocytes only and lacked cytotoxic capacity. The HLA-type of the donor was not available in another case. 3/4 cultures from valves of patients with available HLA-type of the donor contained CD8 positive cells with donor specific reactivity. These data suggest that immunologic activity against the transplanted valve may persist more than 6 months after implantation implicating that valve donor cells, capable of expressing transplantation antigens remain present.

Modulation of Valve Antigenicity

A reduction of the antigenicity of the transplant could lead to a less aggressive immune response of the acceptor. Reducing the number of cells expressing transplantation antigens, as mentioned on the preceding pages could be an option, provided the function of the valve leaflets remains unaffected. Preservation methods could therefore be considered as a form of immunomodulation, because this process disturbs the composition of the cells in the valve allograft. It has been reported by el Khatib et al. that fresh aortic valve allografts contain more viable endothelial cells than allografts stored at 4°C in an antibiotic solution, leading to the loss of antigenicity.[32] Transplantation of allogeneic valves between rats resulted in a shorter time to skin graft rejection in rats when fresh valves were transplanted, compared to rats that received an allograft preserved for 21 days in a nutrient medium.[32] Lang et al. detected viable endothelial cells on cryopreserved valves (and no viable fibroblast),[33] while VanDerKamp et al. reported the presence of viable fibroblasts and an electron microscopic intact structure of collagen fibrils after sterilization and controlled freezing of aortic valves.[34] Lupinetti et al. found by immunofluorescence staining techniques that endothelial cells were present on 16% of 131 cryopreserved aortic valve allografts.[35] Also Yankah et al. demonstrated the presence of viable endothelial cells after cryopreservation, while these cells were absent on fresh sterilized valves.[36] These studies show that the presence of endothelium on cryopreserved valves may vary. We think this can be explained by the use of different freezing techniques and antibiotic sterilization procedures. Nevertheless, the presence of endothelial cells is an important factor to explain the immunologic processes, because in studies on the immunogenicity of vascular endothelium, these cells have shown to be a major target of cell mediated immune injury.[37-41] Moreover, allo-antibodies specific for endothelial cell surface molecules have also been detected in explanted rejected organs.[42,43]

Long-term follow-up studies in the clinic show a marked improvement with transplantation of cryopreserved versus fresh valves,[1] suggesting that the antigenicity of valve allografts is altered by cryopreservation. Cochran used Fisher rats to study the effect of cryopreservation on antigenic expression of aortic allografts.[44] Allogeneic aortic valves were implanted subcutaneously and the rejection times of skin grafts (first and second set reaction) was compared between recipients of fresh and cryopreserved valves, but no statistical difference was found for first and second rejection phenomena, indicating no effect of cryopreservation.

Calhoun examined the difference between survival of fresh and cryopreserved venous allografts in genetically characterized dogs.[45] In contrast to Fisher, he detected early deterioration of the intima of cryopreserved veins while fresh vein transplants were histologically normal. It remained unclear why cryopreservation was associated with early thrombosis and transplant failure in this study.

Jonas et al. compared the hemodynamic, angiographic and histological findings in long-term sheep model after implantation of a cryopreserved versus an antibiotic sterilized aortic valve allograft.[46] The authors found no significant difference in transconduit gradient or histological findings 9 months after transplantation, but calcification was prominent within the conduit wall of all animals. Hoekstra et al. examined the proliferative response *in vitro* of lymphocytes incubated with fresh versus cryopreserved human valve pieces.[47] In this study, cryopreservation was associated with lower lymphoproliferation, although cryopreserved valves were still able to stimulate immune-competent cells. Matching for HLA-DR between valve donor and responder cells resulted in a lower immune response compared to the HLA-DR mismatched responders.

Modulation of alloreactivity by phenotypic manipulation of donor endothelium has been performed on heart allografts in rats.[48] Therefore, host endothelium was isolated and perfused into donor allografts. Allografts pretreated with host endothelium survived for 12 days while untreated heart allografts survived 7 days. This method could be an alternative method to reduce the immunogenicity of valve allografts because endothelial cells can be easily isolated[49] and valve allografts could remain *ex vivo* for more extended periods than heart transplants to allow attachment of the donor endothelium on the graft. Another alter-native would be pretreatment of allografts with cyclosporine, which has been earlier performed on venous allografts in dogs. This treatment resulted in an improved survival of the graft and also less degenerative changes on scanning electron microscopic findings.[50]

Immunosuppression

Immunosuppressive therapy is not routinely given to recipients of human cardiac valves in contrast to patients receiving organ transplantation, although donor and recipient are not matched for MHC antigens in cardiac valve transplantation. The effect of immunosuppression on histologic findings of valve rejection could be compared in patients who received heart transplants (with immunosuppressive therapy) and patients who received valve allografts (no immunosuppression). Schoen et al. and the group of Melo found as a most striking factor that there was a marked decrease in cellularity (fibroblasts) in the valve replacement group, and T-cells were especially present in valve allografts.[25,51,52]

Cyclosporine, a highly potent immunosuppressive drug, has been used in individual cases in the clinic.[6] The general opinion of the use of this drug after valve implantation is to use this drug with caution because of it's serious side effects. There are no reports in the literature on controlled follow-up studies of patients with an allogeneic valve treated with cyclosporin or other immunosuppressive drugs and the effect on valve function. However, Augelli et al. examined dogs receiving venous allografts with or without cyclosporin treatment. Dogs treated with cyclosporin showed improved graft survival compared to dogs receiving no treatment.[53]

Conclusion

Many experimental animal studies and studies on human valve allografting *in vitro* and *in vivo* show findings of early and late allogeneic reactions with deterioration of the valve leaflets. The immunologic activity against valve allografts is comparable to that of organ transplantation. Despite the evidence of rejection, a correlation between these immunologic processes and clinical valve function remains absent in the majority of studies. Long-term follow-up studies comparing groups of patients with or without HLA-DR matched valves and/or ABO compatible valve transplants could help to understand the clinical role of immune reactivity against the donor valve. Methods to reduce the immunogenicity of valve allografts should be further examined. Meanwhile, cross-matching should seriously be considered in patients operated for repeat allograft implantation, to anticipate acute antibody-mediated tissue destruction in sensitized patients. Low-dose immunosuppressive drugs or induction therapy should only be considered in high risk patients, in case of second allogeneic transplants and young recipients, although the potential side-effects of these drugs may not outweigh its benefits.

References

1. O'Brien MF, Stafford EG, Gardner MA, Pohlner PG, McGiffin DC. A comparison of aortic valve replacement with viable cryopreserved and fresh allograft valves, with a note on chromosomal studies. J Thorac Cardiovasc Surg 1987;94:812–823.
2. Angell WW, Angell JD, Oury JH, Lamberti JJ, Grehl TM. Long-term follow-up of viable frozen aortic homografts: a viable homograft valve bank. J Thorac Cardiovasc Surg 1987;93:815–822.
3. Hammermeister KE, Sethi GK, Henderson WG. A comparison of outcomes in men 11 years after heart-valve replacement with a mechanical valve or bioprosthesis. N Engl J Med 1993;328(18):1289–1296.
4. Jones EL, Shah VB, Shanewise, et al. Should the freehand allograft be abandoned as a reliable alternative for aortic valve replacement? Ann Thorac Surg 1995;59:1397–1404.
5. Doty DB, Michielon G, Wang N. Replacement of the aortic valve with cryopreserved aortic allograft. Ann Thorac Surg 1993;56:228–236.
6. Clarke D, Campbell D, Hayward A, et al. Degeneration of aortic valve allografts in young recipients. J Thorac Cardiovasc Surg 1993;105:934–942.
7. Clarke DR, Bishop DA. Allograft degeneration in infant pulmonary valve allograft recipients. EJCTS 1993;7:365–370.
8. Kirklin JK, Smith D, Novick W, et al. Long-term function of cryopreserved aortic homografts: a ten year study. J Thorac Cardiovasc Surg 1993;106:154–166.
9. Clarke DR. Extended aortic root replacement with cryopreserved allografts: do they hold up? Ann Thorac Surg 1991;52:669–673; discus.
10. Mohri H, Reichenbach DD, Barnes RW, Nelson RJ, Merendino KA. Studies of antigenicity of the homologous aortic valve. J Thorac Cardiovasc Surg 1967;54:564–572.
11. Baue AE, Donawick WJ, Blakemore WS. The immunologic response to heterotopic allovital aortic valve transplants in presensitized and nonsensitized recipients. J Thorac Cardiovasc Surg 1968;56:775–789.
12. Buch WS, Kosek JC, Angell WW. The role of rejection and mechanical trauma on valve graft viability. J Thorac Cardiovasc Surg 1971;5:696–706.
13. Thiede A, Timm C, Burnhard A, et al. Studies on the antigenicity of vital allogeneic valve leaflet transplants in immunogenetically controlled strain combinations. Transplantation 1978;26:391–395.
14. el Khatib H, Lupinetti FM. Antigenicity of fresh and cryopreserved rat valve allografts. Transplantation 1990;49:765–767.
15. Lupinetti FM, Cobb S, Kioschos HC, Thompson SA, Walters KS, Moore KC. Effect of immunological differences on rat aortic valve allograft calcification. J Card Surg 1992;7:65–70.
16. Gonzales-Lavin L, Bianchi J, Graf D, Amini S, Gordon CL. Degenerative changes in fresh aortic root homografts in a canine model: evidence of an immunologic influence. Transplant Proc 1988;20:815–819.
17. Zhao X, Green M, Frazer IH, et al. Donor-specific immune response after aortic valve allografting in the rat. Ann Thorac Surg 1994;57:1158–1163.
18. Balch CM, Karp RB. Blood group compatibility and aortic valve allotransplantation in man. J Thorac Cardiovasc Surg 1975;70:256–259.
19. Salomon RN, Friedman GB, Callow AD, et al. Cryopreserved aortic homografts contain viable smooth muscle cells capable of expressing transplantation antigens. J Thorac Cardiovasc Surg 1993;106:1173–1180.
20. Yacoub M, Suitters A, Khaghani A, et al. Localization of major histocompatability complex

(HLA, ABC, and DR) antigens in aortic homografts. In Bodnar E, Yacoub M (eds). Biologic and bioprosthetic valves. New York: Yorke Medical Books; 1986:65–72.

21. Simon A, Zavazava N, Sievers H, et al. In vitro cultivation and immunogenicity of human cardiac valve endothelium. J Card Surg 1993;8: 656–665.

22. Hoekstra F, Knoop C, Aghai Z, et al. Stimulation of immune-competent cells in vitro by human cardiac valve-derived endothelial cells. Ann Thorac Surg 1995;60:S131-S134.

23. Johnson CM, Fass DN. Porcine cardiac valvular endothelial cells in culture. A relative deficiency of fibronectin synthesis in vitro. Lab Invest 1983; 49:589–597.

24. Lupinetti FM, Tsai TT, Kneebone JM. Endothelial cell replication in an in vivo model of aortic allografts. Ann Thorac Surg 1993;56:237–241.

25. Schoen FJ, Mitchell RN, Jonas RA. Pathological considerations in cryopreserved allograft heart valves. J Heart Valve Dis 1995;4:S72–S76.

26. Yankah AC, Muller-Hermelink HK, Muller-Ruchholtz W, et al. Antigenitat allogener Herzklappen. Z Herz Thorax GefaBchir 1992;6:41–47.

27. Muller-Hermelink HK, Muller-Ruchholtz W, et al. Antigentat allograft explants. In Yankah AC, Hetzer R, Miller DC, Ross DN, Sommerville J, Yacoub HM (eds). Cardiac valve allografts 1962–1987. New York: Steinkopff, Darmstadt, Springer; 1989.

28. Lupinetti FM, King DM, Khatib HE, et al. Immunogenicity of aortic valve allografts does not correlate with presence of antigen. J Am Coll Cardiol 1991;17:213A.

29. Schutz A, Fischlein T, Breuer M, et al. Cytoimmunological monitoring after homograft valve replacement. Eur J Cardio-thorac Surg 1994;8: 609–612.

30. Jutte NHPM, Hop WCJ, Daane R, et al. Cytoimmunological monitoring of heart transplant recipients. Clin Trans 1990;4:297–300.

31. Hoekstra F, Knoop C, Vaessen L, et al. Donor-specific immune response against human cardiac valve allografts. J Thorac Cardiovasc Surg 1997; in press.

32. Khatib HE, Thompson SA, Lupinetti FM. Effect of Storage at 4C in a Nutrient Medium on Antigenic Properties of Rat Aortic Valve Allografts. The Society of Thoracic Surgeons 1990;49:792–796.

33. Lang SJ, Giordano MS, Cardon-Cardo C, et al. Biochemical and cellular characterization of cardiac valve tissue after cryopreservation or antibiotic preservation. J Thorac Cardiovasc Surg 1994;108:63–67.

34. VanDerKamp AWM, Visser WJ, van Dongan JM, Nauta J, Galjaard H. Preservation of aortic heart valves with maintenance of cell viability. J Surg Res 1981;30:47.

35. Lupinetti FM, Tsai T, Kneebone J, et al. Effect of cryopreservation on the presence of endothelial cells on human valve allografts. J Thorac Cardiovasc Surg 1993;106:912–917.

36. Yankah AC, Wottge HU, Muller-Hermelink HK, Feller AC, Lange P, Wessel U, Dreyer H, Bernhard A, Müller-Ruchholtz W. Transplantation of aortic and pulmonary allografts, enhanced viability of endothelial cells by cryopreservation, importance of histocompatibility. J Card Surg 1987;2:209–220.

37. Pober JS, Collins T, Gimbrone MAJr, et al. Inducible expression of class II major histocompatability complex antigens and the immunogenicity of vascular endothelium. Transplantation 1986;41:141–146.

38. Lodge PA, Haisch CE. T-cell subset responses to allogenic endothelium. Transplantation 1993;56: 656–661.

39. Hengstenberg C, Rose ML, Page C, et al. Immunocytochemical changes suggestive of damage to endothelial cells during rejection of human cardiac allografts. Transplantation 1993; 49:895–899.

40. Theobald VA, Lauer JD, Kaplan FA, et al. "Neutral allografts"—lack of allogeneic stimulation by cultured human cells expressing MHC Class I and Class II antigens. Transplantation 1993;55:128–133.

41. Jutte NHPM, Heijse P, Van Batenburg, et al. Donor heart endothelial cells as targets for graft infiltrating lymphocytes after clinical cardiac transplantation. Transplant Immuno 1993;1:39–44.

42. Moraes JR, Stastney P. A new antigen system expressed in endothelial cells. J Clin Invest 1977; 60:449–453.

43. Claas FHJ, Paul LC, van Es LA, et al. Antibodies against donor antigens on endothelial cells and monocytes in eluates of rejected kidney allografts. Tissue Antigens 1980;15:19–25.

44. Cochran RP, Kunzelman KS. Cryopreservation does not alter antigenic expression of aortic allografts. J Surg Res 1989;46:597–599.

45. Douglas Calhoun A, Baur GM, Porter JM, et al. Fresh and cryopreserved venous allografts in genetically characterized dogs. J Surg Res 1977; 22:687–696.

46. Jonas RA, Ziemer G, Britton L, Armiger LC. Cryopreserved and fresh antibiotic-sterilized valved aortic homograft conduits in a long-term sheep model. Hemodynamic, angiographic, and histologic comparisons. J Thorac Cardiovasc Surg 1988;96:746–755.

47. Hoekstra F, Knoop C, Jutte, et al. Effect of cryopreservation and HLA-DR matching on the cellular immunogenicity of human cardiac valve allografts. J Heart Lung Transplant 1994; 13:1095–1098.

48. Quigly RL, Switzer SS, Victor A, et al. Modulation of alloreactivity in transplant recipients by phenotypic manipulation of donor endothelium. J Thorac Cardiovasc Surg 1995;109:905–909.

49. Johnson CM, Nyberg Hanson M, Helgeson SC. Porcine cardiac valvular endothelial cells in culture: cell isolation and growth characteristics. J Mol Cell Cardiol 1987;19:1185–1193.

50. Bandlien KO, Toledo-Pereyra LH, Barnhart MI, et al. Improved survival of venous allografts in dogs following graft pretreatment with cyclosporine. Transplant Proc 1983;4:3084–3091.

51. Young WP, Rowe GG. A study of aortic regurgitation in aortic-valve homografts. Ann Thorac Surg 1968;6:11–15.

52. Neves J, Monteiro C, Santos R, et al. Histologic and genetic assessment of explanted allograft valves. Ann Thorac Surg 1995;60:141–145.

53. Augelli NV, Lupinetti FM, Khatib H, Sanofsky SJ, Rossi NP. Allograft vein patency in a canine model. Additive effects of cryopreservation and cyclosporine. Transplantation 1991;52:466–470.

Section VI
Cryobiology of Heart Valve Preservation

16
Application of Cryopreservation to Heart Valves

Lloyd Wolfinbarger, Jr., Kelvin G.M. Brockbank, and Richard A. Hopkins

The intention of this chapter is to deal with the issues associated with the cryopreservation of heart valves and to review some of the approaches taken to resolve these issues. Cryopreservation protocols have been developed empirically, based upon knowledge gained from the cryobiology of single-cell suspensions, and these protocols have consistently provided valves that perform adequately for extended periods of time.[1] It now becomes important to find out why cryopreserved allogeneic valves perform so well and to develop methods which may lead to even better performance.

Great advances have been made in the cryopreservation of living cells since the pivotal publication of Polge, Smith and Parkes in 1949.[2] In this article the cryoprotective properties of glycerol for biological materials was first described. Subsequently, in 1959, Lovelock and Bishop reported that dimethyl sulfoxide (DMSO) was also a cryoprotectant. Since then a variety of cryoprotective agents have been reported and other advances have occurred including development of controlled cooling rate freezing equipment and cryogenic storage freezers.

Historically, most research and technological development has focused on the preservation of single cell suspensions such as gametes, red blood cells and dispersed cell suspensions. Multicellular tissues are orders of magnitude more complex than single cells both structurally and in the requirements for cryopreservation. Some cell systems such as platelets, sperm, and embryos may be subject to thermal or cold shock upon cooling without freezing. Heart valves are not known to be sensitive to cold shock. However, due to concerns that the cryoprotectant DMSO may increase tissue sensitivity to cold shock and DMSO toxicity, DMSO is usually added to cells and tissues, including heart valves, after an initial cooling and prior to freezing. Frozen tissues have extensive extracellular and interstitial ice formation following use of tissue bank cryopreservation procedures which, however, result in excellent cell viability. After thawing, it is usually not possible to detect where the ice was present by routine histopathology methods. Freeze substitution techniques which reveal where ice was present in tissues have, however, demonstrated significant extracellular tissue matrix distortion and damage.[3] The extent of freezing damage depends upon the amount of free water in the system and the ability of that water to crystallize during freezing.

Other factors, in addition to ice formation, have biological consequences during freezing: the inhibitory effects of low temperatures on chemical and physical processes and, perhaps most important, the physiochemical effects of rising solute concentrations as the volume of liquid water decreases during crystallization. The latter process results in cell volume decreases, pH changes and the risk of solute precipitation. There have been several hypotheses on mechanisms of freezing-induced injury based upon such factors.[3,4] Cryopreserved tissue properties can also be modified by events prior to cryopreservation and by the

TABLE 16.1. Factors that Affect Heart Valve Quality.

1. Donor related factors
2. Harvesting and transport of the donor heart
3. Valve preparation, low temperature-compatible pH buffers and antibiotic sterilization
4. Selection of cryoprotectants and cooling protocol
5. Tissue storage and transportation conditions
6. Processing steps and valve handling performed in the surgical suite

final processing steps in the surgical suite leading up to transplantation.

Although many types of isolated cells and small aggregates of cells can be frozen by simply following published procedures, obtaining adequate and reproducible results for most tissues requires an understanding of the major variables involve in tissue processing and cryopreservation (Table 16.1). Optimization of these variables must be derived for each tissue by experimentation guided by an understanding of the chemistry, physics and toxicology of cryobiology.

Before discussing the factors affecting heart valve quality in detail it is necessary to consider the meaning of "viability" with respect to heart valve function *in vivo*. Viability may simply be defined as the ability of frozen and thawed cells or tissues to perform their normal functions. Tissues such as heart valves may lack cellular viability yet remain viable with respect to performance of their normal functions post-transplantation. Historically, however, a viable heart valve has been a valve which retains some level of metabolically active (viable) cell population at the time of transplantation. Many means of assessing cell viability have been described including amino acid uptake, protein synthesis, contractility, dye uptake, ribonucleic acid synthesis, and 2-deoxyglucose phosphorylation.[5–10] The assay(s) used to determine cellular viability should be a clear indication that the cells are alive and preferably should report on functions relating to activities important for long-term valve durability. Most such assays attempt to measure some plasma membrane associated function such as metabolite (i.e. proline, glycine, 2-deoxyglucose uptake and phosphorylation, due uptake, etc.) transport via

a membrane localized transport system. Alternatively, the assays(s) may measure post-transport accumulation of some metabolite (proline, glycine, etc.) into proteins or similar macromolecular form. These latter assays, of course, actually measure multiple functions associated with a metabolically viable cell such as plasma membrane associated active transport, charging of the amino acid onto a transfer RNA, and the incorporation of this amino acid into proteins.

In addition, it is important that the assay contribute some information as to the metabolic viability of the total cell population of the tissue and/or the metabolic viability of individual cells in that total cell population. For example, representative tissue samples, usually leaflet tissue, may be incubated in a radiolabeled amino acid such as proline or glycine and then either solubilized for direct scintillation counting or the tissue may be fixed, embedded, sectioned, and then subjected to autoradiography. The former method tends to measure the metabolic viability of the total cell population whereas the latter method tends to measure the metabolic viability of individual cells in that total population. With the former method it is difficult to determine whether a 50% reduction in metabolite transport means that half of the cells are totally "dead" or all of the cells are half "dead." With the latter method, it is possible to determine a percentage of cells that are metabolically active, but not how active they are without considerable attention to the degree of film darkening associated with each cell after autoradiography. Ideally, both types of assays should be used in assessment of cellular viability of heart valves. It is also important to ascertain the appropriateness of radiolabeled metabolite used in the assessment of cellular viability. Radiolabeled proline has traditionally been the metabolite of choice in that it is transported across the plasma membrane of metabolically viable cells via an active amino acid carrier that is not affected by the presence of other amino acids in the transport solution.

Metabolites such as glycine and 2-deoxyglucose, however, are transported across the plasma membrane via a general amino acid and glucose transport mechanism, respectively, and it becomes important to control for the presence of potentially competitive molecules such as other amino acids or glucose in the transport solution. In addition, for 2-deoxyglucose transport, catabolite repression of glucose transport can occur without a long-term reduction in metabolic viability of the cell population. The idea that cell viability is important for clinical function is based on the observation that fibroblasts are responsible for maintenance of the valve matrix[11] and thus by extrapolation they must be important for long-term transplant durability. O'Brien and his colleagues[1] contributed to this concept by demonstrating persistence of donor cells in explanted human allograft valve leaflets. Subsequently there has not been much support for donor fibroblast survival in human explants and it has even been suggested that "viable" valves may have immunological consequences in neonates and/or that as these viable cells die due to induced apoptosis they release hydrolytic enzymes which contribute to matrix degradation and subsequent calcification of the valve tissues.[12,13] Cell viability was assessed in aortic and pulmonic allografts in a growing sheep model.[14] Viable donor cells were observed in zero and 43% of leaflets at 8–15 months post transplantation from aortic and pulmonary valves, respectively. Observations such as these cast doubt on the importance of cell viability for long term valve durability and lead to the suggestion that the link between the extended performance of cryopreserved valves and variability is not persistence of donor cells *in vivo*, *per se*, but rather that viability correlates with gentle treatment of the valves *in vitro* resulting in better *in vivo* function. Gentle treatment results in better matrix preservation and thus alternative methods of valve preservation should focus on removal of cells from the tissue in the presence of inhibitors of hydrolytic enzymes such that matrix structure remains unchanged or changed in such a manner as to facilitate recellularization *in vitro* or *in vivo*. There is extensive literature indicating that changes in extracellular matrix proteoglycan correlate with *in vivo* mineralization of cartilaginous tissues.[15–18] Wolfinbarger and colleagues have suggested that mineralization of transplanted human aortic heart valves may

be due to processing-induced proteoglycan changes in a manner analogous to the "programmed" mineralization of cartilage in bone of infants.[13] Such changes in aggregate size of proteoglycans have been observed in the osteoid of mineralizing bone and may also occur post-transplantation of heart valves due to release of enzymes by dead and dying donor cells or invading recipient cells in a manner analogous to new bone formation. It is important that processing residuals, whether used in the cryopreservation or decellularization of cardiovascular tissues, not induce an apoptotic state in the infiltrating cells as these cells may contribute to subsequent calcification of these tissues as such dead and dying cells may contribute to calcification in cryopreserved tissues post transplantation.

Section 1

Harvesting and Transportation of the Donor Heart

The valve leaflets consist of a cellular component and an acellular component. The major acellular components are collagen types I and III, elastin and glycosaminoglycans. A network of tropocollagen molecules covalently cross-linked form the fibrous protein matrix of valve leaflet tissue. Heart valves also contain acid glycosaminoglycans (GAGs), which consist of polysaccharide (about 95%) and protein (about 5%). The main GAGs in heart valves are hyaluronic acid, dermatan sulfate and chondroitin sulfate. Small amounts of heparan sulfate and oversulfated dermatan sulfate are also present. These very large polyanions bind with water and cations, thereby forming the ground substance of the heart valve leaflet. That these molecules are primarily in the medial volume of conduit and leaflets of cardiovascular tissues probably have to do with the need for such molecules to "lubricate" the differential movements of the adventitial and ventricular aspects of these tissues. With advancing age, the proportions of hyaluronic acid and chondroitin 4-sulfate tend to increase, whereas those of chondroitin 6-sulfate, dermatan sulfate and heparan sulfate tend to decrease.[19] Overall these GAGs decrease in concentration with advancing age.[19] If changes in proteoglycan structure and content are indeed associated with a tendency of transplanted valves to calcify,[13] these observed changes in GAGs with advancing age may suggest a reason for avoiding valves obtained from older donors.

The cellular composition of heart valve leaflets includes fibroblasts and endothelial cells. The fibroblasts are responsible for maintenance of the extracellular matrix and are relatively insensitive to the pre-cryopreservation processing steps. The effects of prolonged post-procurement ischemia, in 4°C cell culture medium for up to 113 hours, upon heart valve leaflet fibroblast protein synthesis, ribonucleic acid synthesis, and glucose phosphorylation have been studied.[10] These studies indicated that there were no statistically significant changes in fibroblast functions during the first 42 hours of post-procurement cold ischemia.

Based upon these observations the total combined warm and cold ischemia tolerance time of human heart valve leaflet fibroblasts, prior to heart valve dissection, appears to be at least 48 hours. The American Association of Tissue Banks currently recommends that "Tissues obtained from living and non-living donors shall be retrieved and preserved within the time interval compatible with intended use of that tissue."[20] The European standards for cryopreserved heart valves currently permit a maximum of 48 hours for combined warm and cold ischemia providing that donor body refrigeration starts within 6 hours of death.[21] Analyses of subgroups of patients receiving aortic valve allografts suggested that valves treated with antibiotics and stored in fresh nutrient media provided improved durability when the period between harvesting and storage was short and when the storage times were also relatively brief, implying that cellular viability was an important feature.[1,22–25] Kadoba et al. demonstrated using a sheep model that a 48 hour delay at 4°C from donor death to harvesting did not have a significant effect on conduit function. This study suggests that it may be possible to expand the donor pool for allografts providing leaflet

durability and matrix structure are not compromised or that there are no increased risks of bacterial contamination with prolonged harvest times.

After heart valve dissection there is evidence from several groups indicating that the fibroblasts survive at least one week of refrigerated storage.[6,7] In contrast, the endothelial cells appear to be easily dislodged during processing—perhaps as early as at the time of procurement. Hearts are typically washed in cold saline or lactated Ringer's solution to remove blood products and cool the valve tissue prior to transport in tissue culture medium. In perfused human hearts[26] and rat livers,[27] the endothelium detaches after 3 to 8 hours at 4°C while in human kidneys,[28] dog saphenous veins,[29] rabbit aortas[30] and rat lungs,[31] it detaches after 1 to 4 days.

Various mechanisms explaining the chilling sensitivity of cells, which involves the cell membrane, have been proposed and include increased leakage of ions due to membrane ion pump shutdown,[32,33] membrane phase transition changes,[34,35] decreased cell energy charge,[36] increased cytosolic free calcium,[37,38] and phospholipase A_2 activation.[39,40] Reduction in temperature differentially affects the sodium-potassium pump[41] and cells typically swell because of the associated ionic imbalance. In classic experiments, Collins and associates[42] reported that perfusion of dog kidneys with solutions designed to protect cells from swelling during refrigeration storage, containing 115 mM potassium, 30 mM $MgSo_4$, 57.7 mM phosphate, and 140 mM glucose, resulted in functional kidneys. Acquatella and coworkers[43] suggested that such solutions tended to stabilize the water and ion content of tissues during hypothermic storage by mimicking the intracellular ion content and "protect cells from cell swelling at lower temperatures." The most popular organ procurement solution in use today is Viaspan™ (also known as UW solution).[44] This solution was designed to mimic the intracellular electrolyte composition resulting in a decrease in the gradient for sodium and potassium across cell membranes. Furthermore, the presence of lactobionate, raffinose and hydroxyethyl starch in Viaspan™ reduce transcapillary and osmotic fluid flow.

Washing freshly procured heart valves in lactated Ringer's or saline, rather than an organ preservation solution designed to mimic the intracellular environment, probably results in swelling of the endothelial cells enhancing their subsequent loss from the surface of the leaflet matrix during processing. Matrix fibroblasts may be expected to be somewhat protected by the matrix from this swelling phenomenon, thereby increasing their chance of survival. It has been shown that solutions rich in impermeant ions and potassium provide for retention of cellular viability after subzero storage in the presence of DMSO, so it is suggested that if retention of endothelial cells is desired then organ transport solutions should be used for both washing and transport of freshly procured heart valves. However, it should be noted that most processors advocate use of conditions which do not promote survival of endothelial cells due to concerns about tissue immunogenicity, which may be elevated by increasing the number of surviving endothelial cells.

Bilayer membranes are composed primarily of phospholipids, cholesterol and proteins (glycoproteins). As the temperature decreases, the lipids tend to preferentially associate with other lipids, excluding membrane proteins, in a process called "lateral phase separation." As a result of this process, regions of the membrane contain high densities of membrane proteins floating like islands in a homogeneous "sea" of lipids. Many of these membrane proteins span the bilayer membrane, being exposed to both the aqueous phase of the extracellular solvent and the cell cytoplasm. As the temperature continues to decrease, the lipid components undergo a "fluid-to-gel" transition where the vibrational energy (and lateral movement) of the lipids also decreases. The temperature at which this fluid-to-gel transition occurs depends on a number of factors, including but not restricted to: chain length of the fatty acids of the phospholipids (transition temperature increases with increasing chain length); degree of saturation/unsaturation of the fatty acids (unsaturated fatty acids decrease the tendency to form a "gel" at lower temperatures and thus lower the transition temperature); heterogeneity of fatty acid composition and charge distri-

bution of the phosphatide group (e.g., choline, serine, inositol); and the presence of cholesterol (cholesterol tends to lower the phase trasition temperature.[45] The depression of transmembrane ionic pump activities is a function of both direct temperature effects and membrane fluidity. The activities of all enzymes are modulated by solvent viscosity,[32,46–52] and the increased viscosity of membrane phospholipids is thought to contribute to the decrease in activity of membrane bound enzymes that is seen at low temperatures.[52] The membrane transition temperature of different cell types is inversely proportional to their sensitivity to hypothermia.[53]

Lipid modification, as a means of protecting bull spermatozoa during cryopreservation, has been studied with some success.[54] As an additional complication, in complex tissues, cell-to-cell contacts are made through membrane glycoproteins (gap junctions), and thus different cell populations within the tissue may experience different reactions to temperature changes; moreover, the transmembrane junctions between cells may also be variable in terms of permitting solute movement. For a more thorough discussion of this subject, refer to the articles by Quinn[55] and Morris and Clarke.[56]

The reduction of kinetic energy which occurs as temperature is lowered also has effects on the rates at which biochemical reactions occur. At 0°C biological materials metabolism is reduced to about 5% of normal physiologic temperature metabolism. Different biological reactions are reduced to varying degrees. The factor by which a metabolic reaction velocity is decreased for a reduction of 10°C is often described as a Q_{10} effect.[57] There is often a break temperature for the membrane bound enzymes below which the Q_{10} for the reaction is magnified, i.e. the Q_{10} for K+-stimulated Na+ turnover in rate aorta is 2.4 over the temperature range of 17–37°C, but is 8.8 over the range of 4–17°C. A consequence of this metabolic activity during hypothermia is tissue acidification due to intracellular hydrolysis of adenosine triphosphate and accumulation of lactic acid.

The role of free radicals in the production of damage to tissues during exposure to hypothermic conditions has been reviewed.[58,59] In nor-mothermic perfused conditions free radical production is balanced by production of perox-idases and other antioxidants. Displacement of the equilibrium between free radical produc-tion and removal included by hypothermia can have detrimental biological consequences. Radicals are chemical species with unpaired electrons in their orbital shells. In the process of restoring normal electron pairing, super-oxide, hydrogen peroxide, and hydroxyl rad-icals are created. These chemical species are extremely reactive with cellular components. Lipid peroxidation of the cell membranes renders the cells permeable to calcium. Extra-cellular calcium influx and redistribution of intracellular calcium can contribute to the development of irreversible cell injuries.

The combination of unbalanced metabolism, generation of free radicals and consequences of cell specific membrane phase changes of tis-sues exposed to hypothermia combine to give endothelial cells and fibroblasts in heart valve tissues very different survival periods. Endothe-lial cells persist several hours while the major-ity of fibroblasts can survive for at least a week. Longer periods of storage with retention of viable fibroblasts require the utilization of frozen storage techniques. From an immuno-logical perspective it is likely that the success of allograft heart valves is in part due to the loss of the highly immunogenic endothelial cells prior to transplantation. Efforts to increase endothelial cell viability by employing organ transport solutions might result in a higher probability of graft rejection by the valve recip-ient's immune system.

If heart valves are to be cryopreserved the duration of exposure to hypothermia should be minimized and the conditions of hypothermic exposure should be optimized.[60] It is likely that short ischemia times and minimal handling prior to cryopreservation result in better graft performance. Perhaps the least controlled vari-able in valve preparation is the first step of har-vesting. During harvesting, subcellular changes may alter the sensitivity of the cells to subse-quent processing steps.[60–62] Historically, strate-gies for minimizing injury have been derived from studies using relatively crude markers of

injury, and the experimental tissues were typi-cally exposed to minimal ischemia, unlike most clinical situations, and were unlikely to detect synergistic causes of injury.[63,64] More recent studies indicate that inhibition of adenosine deaminase and nucleoside transport in heart valves immediately after harvest or incubation of heart valves after hypothermic exposure, but prior to cryopreservation, at 37°C in nutrient media may prevent or correct reversible meta-bolic deficiencies.[65,66]

Section 2

Valve Preparation, pH Buffers and Antibiotic Sterilization

Valve Preparation

Valve dissection technique is discussed in Chapter 28. During valve dissection it is im-portant to both maintain sterility by dissection under appropriate conditions and to keep the tissues both moist and cool. This will prevent tissue dehydration and help in maintenance of fibroblast viability. An excellent means of keeping tissues cool during dissection is to employ a dissection tray with a cooling system built into the base.

Hearts for heart valve isolation are usually shipped on ice and exposed to antibiotics at 4°C. Cells that are metabolically depressed after tissue processing may not recover sufficiently to survive transplantation into a recipient. Simply incubating the heart valves at 37°C prior to cry-opreservation results in higher levels of meta-bolic activity following cryopreservation and thawing. This process known as revitalization results in increased 2-deoxyglucose phosphory-lation in allograft heart valve leaflets during the initial hours after thawing.[66,67] Alternatively, administration of the nucleoside transport inhibitor p-nitrobenzy-thionosine and the adenosine deaminase inhibitor erythro-9-(2-hydroxy-3-nonyl) adenine at procurement prevents loss of high energy phosphates during subsequent processing steps.[65] It would be interesting to learn what role induction of heat shock proteins due to fluctuations in temperature of such tissues have on subsequent cellular viability via some induced apoptosis event(s).

Low Temperature-Compatible pH Buffers

Biocompatible pH buffered solutions should consist of at least a basic salt solution, an energy source (i.e., glucose) and a buffer capable of maintaining a neutral pH at refrigerated temperatures. In the blood of mammals the pH rises in parallel with the neutral point of water during cooling in the range of 0°C to 40°C.[68] The rate of change of pH with temperature is −0.017 pH units/°C. This phenomenon is referred to as alpha-stat regulation in recognition of the fact that both the intracellular pH and the blood pH buffering is dominated by the degree of ionization of the imidazole moieties of proteins.[69] In contrast to the majority of mammals, hibernating animals maintain their arterial pH at 7.4 irrespective of systemic temperature (pH stat regulation). Many studies have shown that the electrical stability, contractility, and hemodynamics of the heart are better preserved during hypothermia when the α-stat scheme is followed in contrast to constraining pH to 7.4.[70–72] Most buffer anions (such as phosphate and bicarbonate) in common medical use have large temperature coefficients and acid dissociation constants which make them ineffective in maintaining normal pH as temperature is reduced. N-2-hydroxyethylpiperazine-N-2-ethanesulphonate (HEPES) is one of 12 buffers described by Good et al.[70] where buffer concentration, temperature, and ionic composition of the medium have a minimal influence on buffer dissociation. HEPES has been documented to be highly effective in combating the alterations in acid-base homeostasis of ischemic hearts.[73,74] Several of Good's buffers have been found to be effective in cryobiology applications.[75–78] However HEPES is the only member of this group of buffers that has been employed in heart valve cryopreservation protocols.

Antibiotic Sterilization

Early investigations of sterilization methods for heart valves included ethylene oxide,[79] irradiation, and β-propriolactone[80] in combination with a variety of storage techniques.[81] These methods killed the heart valve leaflet cells, damaged the leaflet material properties, and resulted in poor clinical performance. Kosek et al.[81a] recognized the damaging effects of the above sterilization methods and suggested that the use of fresh allografts would be clinically superior in patient outcome. Subsequently, it was shown that antibiotic treatment of allograft heart valves followed by short-term refrigerated storage[82–85] or long-term cryopreserved storage[86] produced the best clinical results.

A variety of antibiotic cocktails and conditions of treatment have been employed (Table 16.2). Generally, all the methods indicated in Table 16.2 are microbiologically effective, but the effects on cell viability have not, in most

Table 16.2. Antibiotic Treatment Methods.

Antibiotic Cocktail	Medium	Duration (h) and Temperature (°C)
Gentamycin, Methicillin, Erythromycin-lactobionate, Nystatin[4,166]	Hanks Soln., TC 199 w/10% FBS, Hams F-10	24h at 4°C
Penicillin, Streptomycin, Kanamycin, Amphotericin B[166,167]	Hanks Soln.	24–72h at 4°C
Gentamycin, Azlocillin, Flucloxacillin, Metronidazol, Amphotericin B[168]	RPMI 1640 w/20% FBS	Extended at 4°C
Cefoxitin, Lincomycin, Polymyxin B, Vancomycin, Amphotericin B[167,169,170]	TC 199 or RPME	24–48h at 4°C
Penicillin, Streptomycin, Amphotericin[170]	Eagles Minimum Essential Medium	24h at 37°C

cases, been clearly defined. The antibiotic concentrations should be non-toxic to valve cells, yet effectively sterilize the allografts.[87] Certain antibiotics (e.g. penicillin) may decrease cell viability.[87] Testing of new antibiotics must be performed because antibiotic resistant organisms are continually evolving. The effects of antibiotics(s) will be combination, concentration, time and temperature dependent. Antibiotic incubations will probably be more effective at 37°C, but there may be a risk of increased cell damage versus incubation at 4°C. Amphotericin B, in the form of Fungizone™, has traditionally been employed as an anti-fungal agent during treatment of allograft heart valves. Hu et al.[88] provided the first indication that amphotericin B was toxic for heart valve fibroblasts by demonstrating that cellular viability was zero in porcine heart valve leaflets after 12 h of incubation with amphotericin B at 4°C. Subsequently, Brockbank and Dawson reported that the cytotoxicity of amphotericin B for human valve leaflet fibroblasts is amplified by cryopreservation.[89] Autoradiographic assessment of human leaflets treated with 10 µg amphotericin B for 4 hours at 37°C demonstrated only an 11% loss in cell viability while leaflets treated and cryopreserved demonstrated a 53% decrease in cell viability. The mechanism of amphotericin B toxicity involves binding to cell membrane steroids. This association results in cytotoxicity by formation of transmembrane channels what cause cellular ionic and osmotic alterations.[90–92] The therapeutic effect of amphotericin B in treatment of fungal infections is due to stronger binding to ergosterol, the primary fungal sterol, than to cholesterol the mammalian counterpart.[93–95]

Section 3

Selection of Cryoprotectants, and Cooling Protocol

Cooling Protocol

An "average" adult heart valve to be cryopreserved is typically 6 cm in length from the annulus to the distal aspect of the aortic conduit. The valves are sized based on internal diameter and the average thickness of the aortic wall is approximately 1.6 mm. Valves are usually frozen in a total volume of 100 ml and the valve typically constitute 7–15% of the total volume to be frozen.

Several considerations must be taken into account in the cryogenic preservation of biological tissues. The rate of change from room temperature to 1–2°C below the freezing point of the solution may have a major effect on ultimate viability if the cells are sensitive to thermal shock; that is not the case with heart valve cells. Between −3.5 and −5°C, the sample is induced to freeze either by the introduction of an ice crystal, by touching the surface of the media with a cold probe, by mechanical vibration, or by rapidly lowering the temperature until ice nucleation occurs. The latter approach is usually employed for heart valves. Since freezing is an exothermic process, heat release (known as the heat of fusion or crystallization) during ice formation must be conducted away from the freezing material. In the case of heart valves this is usually done by maintaining the freezing chamber at a much lower temperature than the heart valves to provide a substantial heat sink or to place the valve package between heat conducting plates to improve heat transfer. The rate of cooling from the nucleation point of a sample to at least −40° is usually controlled using a programmable freezer.

Rapid cooling is generally regarded as harmful to the viability of cells. Rapid cooling may conveniently be defined as a freezing rate consistent with an absence of cell shrinkage due to osmotically driven dehydration. Consequently, the random formation of microscopic ice crystals during rapid freezing may occur either within the cellular cytoplasm or in the extracellular space. Because the volume of the extracellular solvent is greater, nucleation preferentially occurs there, and ice crystal growth spreads rapidly. The membrane barrier surrounding each cell restricts the spread of ice into the cell, and as ice formation continues, the concentration of solute outside the cells increases and the cells begin to lose water by osmotically induced shrinkage. Cells that are rapidly cooled during freezing generally appear unshrunken and contain intracellular ice. The damage to the cells caused by intracellular ice probably occurs during thawing rather during the actual freezing process. This is discussed in more detail later.

Slow cooling during freezing is also harmful to cells, albeit via mechanism(s) different from rapid cooling. Slow cooling may be defined as the rate of cooling during freezing that permits significant cell shrinkage (dehydration) without the formation of intracellular ice. As with rapid cooling, the preferential formation of extra-cellular ice during slow cooling increases the extracellular solute concentration. As water is osmotically drawn from the cells, they shrink until their osmolality reaches that of the external solution at each successively lower temperature. For example, the NaCl concentration in non-frozen iso-osmotic saline is 0.15 M, but the eutectic concentration (at $-21.6°C$) is 5.2 M. The importance of this observation lies in the solute-induced reduction of the temperature at which the cellular components actually solidify. As mentioned earlier, the eutectic point is that temperature at which the solvent and solute mixture solidifies; the formation of natural eutectic mixtures probably aids in cell survival following slow cooling by avoiding the formation of intracellular ice. However, with slow cooling during freezing, high intracellular and extracellular solute concentrations occur, and these conditions are the most probably cause of cell damage. High salt concentrations are generally regarded as being disruptive to cell membrane and protein structure, and certain ionic components are more harmful than others. For example, phosphates are stronger lyotropes than sulfates, the latter of which are routinely used in salt induced precipitation of proteins, i.e. ammonium sulfate. Thus, the use of phosphate buffers in the cryopreservation of cells and tissues should be avoided whenever possible, not only for their observed instability with respect to buffering activities but due to their strong tendency to precipitate proteins at elevated protein concentrations which may occur during the freezing process.

The work of van der Berg and associates[96,97] has provided phase diagrams of eutectic temperatures and associated pH changes in a variety of salt combinations. They reported that pH changes occur with eutectic changes and are relatively independent of temperature.

It is well known that calcium and potassium precipitate during the initial stages of freezing, and sodium ions cause considerable fluctuations in pH during freezing. Potassium ions, to the contrary, cause little change in pH during freezing. The temperature and concentration dependence of phosphate buffers, associated with the appropriate activity coefficient (0.98 at 0.001 M H_2PO_4 versus 0.74 at 0.1 M H_2PO_4) readily explains the dramatic pH changes observed.

The cell damage occurring during freezing correlates with solute concentration changes is supported by the work of Lovelock[98] in which hemolysis produced by freezing red blood cells could also be produced by exposing these same cells to salt concentrations equivalent to those experienced at successively lower temperatures.

Alternatively, Schneider and Mazur[99] suggested that eight-cell embryos were not affected by the high concentrations of salts produced by freezing. They suggested that cellular survival may be determined by that fraction of extracellular solute that remains unfrozen, and that cellular distortion may cause significant damage to cells.

Studies on the survival of various cell types frozen at a variety of cooling rates suggest that optimal survival occurs at a cooling rate somewhere between fast and slow. For most mammalian cells frozen either in glycerol or dimethylsulfoxide, the optimal cooling rate usually lies between 0.3 and 10°C per minute. This optimal rate varies with different cell types (i.e., different volume-to-surface areas and different solvent permeabilities of membranes) and appears to correspond to those rates at which intracellular ice just begins to form. Indeed, Leibo and associates[100] and Rall[101] reported that the cooling rate that produces a reduction in survival of mouse embryos was the same rate that produces intracellular ice crystals in about 20 percent of cells.

In general terms, each cell type has a freezing "window" in which the change in temperature with time provides for optimal cell survival

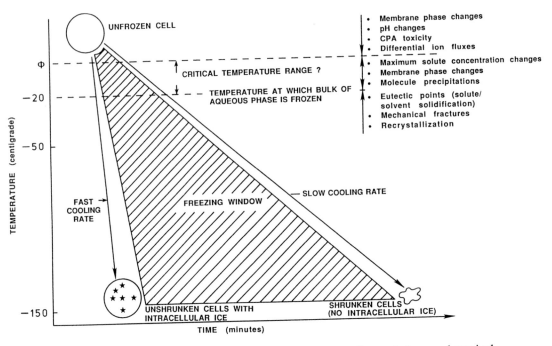

FIGURE 16.1. Effects of cooling rates during freezing on cell morphology and survival.

(Figure 16.1). This proposed "window" is narrow at high temperatures and becomes increasingly wider as the temperature decreases, suggesting that deviation from a given freezing rate at high temperatures may be more critical to cell survival than deviations at low temperatures. The survival of cells frozen by what is termed a two-step method, cells are frozen to a subzero temperature (usually $-20°C$, i.e., just above a critical eutectic point) and held at that temperature for a short period of time prior to resumption of cooling, which may now occur at a more rapid rate. Presumably, extracellular ice crystals forming during what is designated the freeze ($0°$ to $-20°C$) period cause a sufficiently large increase in external solute concentration to shrink the cells, reducing the probability of intracellular ice forming during rewarming.

During cryopreservation of human heart valves, a consistent phenomenon in the cooling rate occurs at $-18°C$ to $-19°C$. At this point, the temperature of the freezing chamber must be rapidly increased in order to prevent a dramatic increase in the cooling rate of the valve tissue

solvent (Figure 16.2). It is presumably at this temperature that the bulk of the extracellular water has frozen and the remaining solute-solvent mixture begins to solidify. Freezing programs presently in use by LifeNet maintain a constant $-1°C$/minute decrease down to $-40°$ and a more rapid cooling rate down to $-100°C$.

As illustrated in Figure 16.2, failure to properly control the freezing program during cryopreservation of a heart valve can lead to deviation from the desired freezing rate. By continually monitoring the process and by proper manipulation of the chambers temperature it is possible to control the sample freezing rate to match the theoretical (or desired) freezing rate. A problem with existing controlled-rate freezers, however, is a reliance on temperature probes inserted into a control (or reporter) pouch (which may or may not contain valve tissues) to assess sample temperature. It is not economical, or perhaps reasonable based on a potential for valve contamination, to insert a temperature probe into every valve that is being cryopreserved. In that the temperature probe represents an excellent heat sink, it is expected that heat dissipation from the control (reporter) pouch will be more rapid than heat dissipation from a sample pouch lacking the temperature probe. In the absence of non-invasive temperature assessment, the most appropriate approach to successfully controlling differential heat transfer, with respect to report and sample pouches, may involve the use of heat sinks such as those described by Prof. Dr. Nikolaus Mendler (Deutsches Herzzentrum Munchen, Personal Communication).

Cryoprotective Agents

Glycerol and DMSO are the most commonly employed cryoprotective agents used in heart valve cryopreservation. Fetal bovine serum (FBS) is commonly employed in cryopreservation solutions by heart valve processors, but it is not a cryoprotective agent and may be an unnecessary solution component.[102] Salts such as magnesium chloride have been reported to be cryoprotective agents;[103] Dextrans, glycols and starches as well as sucrose and polyvinyl pyrolidine appear to confer considerable cryoprotection to a variety of biologic systems.[104] Many chemicals with cryoprotective activity for one or more biological systems have been reported (Table 16.3). According to Mazur,[104] cryoprotectants protect slowly frozen cells by one or more of the following mechanisms: suppression of salt concentrations in the unfrozen fraction; reduction of cell shrinkage at a given temperature; and reduction in the fraction of the solution frozen at a given temperature.

The phase rule may apply to the major function of cryoprotective agents for protecting cells. This rule states that the total concentration of solutes is fixed at a given temperature. In short, a single solute system (i.e., NaCl), the required solute concentration must arise from that solute, whereas in a two-solute system, e.g.,

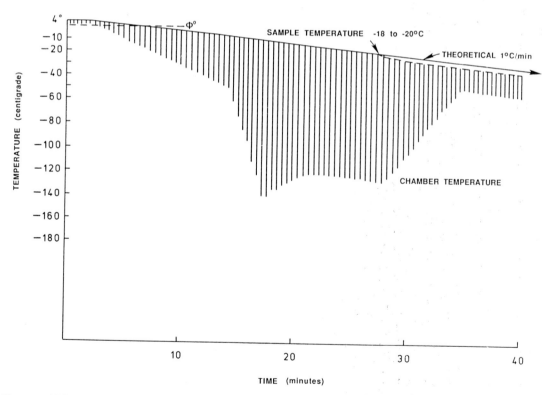

FIGURE 16.2. Portion of controlled-rate freezing curve. Note the deviation from the theoretical cooling rate, indicating the need to rapidly rewarm the freezing chamber when the sample temperature approaches −18° to −20°C.

TABLE 16.3. Chemicals with Demonstrated Cryoprotective Activity.

Acetamide	Ethylene glycol	Mannitol	Pyridine N-oxide
Agarose	Ethylene glycol	Mannose	Ribose
Alginate	Monomethyl ether	Methanol	Serine
Alanine	Formamide	Methoxy propanediol	Sodium bromide
Albumin	Glucose	Methyl acetamide	Sodium chloride
Ammonium acetate	Glycerol	Methyl formamide	Sodium iodide
Chondroitin sulfate	Glycerophosphate	Methyl ureas	Sodium nitrate
Chloroform	Glyceryl monoacetate	Methyl glucose	Sodium nitrite
Choline	Glycine	Methyl glycerol	Sodium sulfate
Dextrans**	Hydroxyethyl starch**	Phenol	Sorbitol
Diethylene glycol	Inositol	Pluronic polyols	Sucrose**
Dimethyl acetamide	Lactose	Polyethylene glycol	Triethylene glycol
Dimethyl formamide	Magnesium chloride	Polyvinylpyrrolidone**	Trimethylamine acetate
Dimethyl sulfoxide**	Magnesium sulfate	Proline	Urea
Erythritol	Maltose	Propylene glycol**	Valine
Ethanol			Xylose

** Chemicals that have conferred substantial cryoprotection in a wide variety of biological systems. (Modified from Shlafer.[107])

DMSO plus NaCl, the solute concentration obtained for a given temperature is the sum of the NaCl and DMSO concentrations. Inclusion of DMSO in the freezing solution effectively reduces the concentration of other solutes at each successive temperature in the freezing process.

Because the total solute concentration at any subzero temperature is fixed, the higher the cryoprotective agent/salt ratio present at the beginning of cooling, the lower is the concentration of salt, at a given subzero temperature. This reduction in non-cryoprotective agent solute concentration is presumably the basis for the reduced solute damage to cells that occurs during slow freezing. However, studies to evaluate this assumption have found that replacement of ionic agents with an osmotically equivalent amount of nonelectrolyte (mannitol) still results in cellular damage, presumably due to the cryoprotectant.[105]

Although cryoprotective agents also reduce the amount of extracellular ice at each subzero temperature with a resultant increase in the volume of the unfrozen fraction, it is not known if fewer ice crystals are responsible for any of the reduction in cell damage.[99] The latter function of cryoprotective agents may also relate to their role in reducing membrane fusion during cryopreservation.[45] Consider, for example, that a decrease in the volume of the aqueous (unfrozen) component during freezing increases the density of cells within it (cell suspensions) and thus increases the potential for cell-cell interactions. Solutions of low osmolality would be expected to have a smaller percentage of the unfrozen fraction at each subzero temperature than a solution of high osmolality (i.e., presence of cryoprotective agents) and cell-cell interactions would be more pronounced. Pegg[106] reported increased hemolysis of human erythrocytes when they were frozen at high densities. Cellular fusion at low temperatures is less of a problem during cryopreservation of dilute cell suspensions or of complex tissues, but may well be of considerable significance during cryopreservation of a concentrated cell suspension. For complex tissues, the relative volumes of crystalline ice and amorphous glass (solidified unfrozen fraction) surrounding and/or encompassing the tissue may contribute significantly to retention of structure and function of that tissue post-thawing and implantation. With cell suspensions, as ice crystal growth proceeds, the cells are progressively crowded into smaller and smaller volumes. With complex tissues such crowding cannot occur and the ice crystals must grow into the water volume space of the tissues. The pharmacologic effects of cryoprotective agents such as MDS and glycerol were reviewed by Shlafer.[107]

Combinations of cryoprotectants may result in additive or synergistic enhancement of tissue cell survival.[108,109] However, there have been no published studies on heart valves.

Comparison of chemicals with cryoprotectant properties reveals no common structural features. These chemicals are usually divided into two classes: 1) intracellular cryoprotectants with low molecular weights which penetrate cells, and 2) extracellular cryoprotectants with relatively high molecular weights (greater than or equal to sucrose [342 daltons]) which do not penetrate cells. Intracellular cryoprotectants, such as glycerol and dimethyl sulfoxide at concentrations from 0.5 to 3 molar, are effective in minimizing cell damage in many slowly frozen biological systems.

Extracellular cryoprotective agents such as polyvinylpyrrolidone or hydroxyethyl starch are more effective at protecting biological systems cooled at rapid rates. Such agents are often large macromolecules which affect the properties of the solution to a greater extent than would be expected from their osmotic pressure. Some of these non-permeating cryoprotective agents have direct protective effects on the cell membrane. However, the primary mechanisms of action appears to be the induction of vitrification (extracellular glass formation). When cryoprotectants are used in extremely high concentrations (at least 50% v/v), ice formation can be eliminated entirely, both intra- and extra-cellularly.[110] Vitrification techniques have not yet been applied to heart valves, but have been successfully applied to rabbit kidney slices, human Islets of Langerhans, monocytes, red blood cells, cultured liver cells, certain plants and plant tissues, and a variety of animal embryos and egg cells. It has been applied with partial success to human corneas. The subject of vitrification has been extensively reviewed[110] and is not discussed further in this chapter. Vitrification techniques will eventually be developed to solve the problems associated with ice formation by prevention of ice formation during heart valve preservation.

Another unexplored avenue for future research in heart valve preservation is control of ice formation. Through millions of years of evolution, nature has produced several families of proteins which help animals and plants survive in cold climates. These proteins are known collectively as antifreeze proteins (AFPs). AFPs have the ability to modify ice structure, the fluid properties of solutions, and the response of organisms to harsh environments. The antifreeze molecules are diverse in structure and, to date, four main types have been characterized. The first to be discovered were the antifreeze glycoproteins (AFGPs) found in Antarctic fish and northern cod species. Subsequently, additional types of AFPs were identified (Table 16.4). Similar proteins have also been found in a number of overwintering insects and plants. The fish-derived antifreeze molecules adsorb preferentially to the prism face of ice or to internal planes that also result in inhibition of ice crystal growth perpendicular to the prism face.

Conflicting results have been obtained by scientists following up on the proposal of Knight and Duman that many of the problems associated with ice formation during cryopreservation might be limited by the addition of naturally occurring AFP. Organ preservation experiments using AFGP at −3°C to 4°C have yielded contrasting results.[111,112] However, the studies of Hansen, Smith and Brockbank[113]

TABLE 16.4. Natural Antifreeze Molecules.

Characteristic	AFP Type I	AFP Type II	AFGP
Molecular Mass	3300–4500	6500	2600–33,000
Composition	Alanine-rich 11 Unit repeats	General	Ala-Ala-Thr repeats O-linked disaccharide
Secondary structure	α-helical	β-sandwich	Expanded
Tertiary structure	100% helical	Not determined	Not determined
Fish source	Winter flounder Sculpin	Ocean pout Wolf fish	Antarctic nototheniids Northern cod

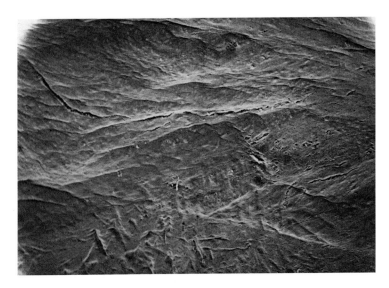

FIGURE 16.3. Fracture formation when human tissue is immersed directly in liquid nitrogen. Cryopreserved valves must remain in the vapor-phase of a liquid nitrogen valve storage system.

demonstrated that AFP Type I inhibited ice recrystallization in the extracellular milieu of cells, but increased ice crystal growth associated with the cells, and resulted in AFP concentration-dependent cell losses compared to untreated control cultures.

These AFP's are believed to absorb to ice by lattice matching or by dipolar interactions along certain axes. Fahy[110] suggested that "insight into the mechanism of AFP action opens the possibility of designing molecules which may be able to inhibit ice crystal growth in complementary ways, e.g., along different crystallographic planes."

Synthetic ice blockers (SIBs), which modify both ice crystal growth rates and form, are being developed. SIBs will be combined with naturally occurring AFPs and conventional cryoprotectants to develop improved preservation methods in which both the cells and the extracellular matrices are preserved.

Section 4

Tissue Storage and Transportation Conditions

It is well established that storage and shipping temperatures have a major impact on maintenance of product quality and can result in cell death via ice formation. If storage temperature is sufficiently low (below the glass transition point of the freezing solution [approximately −135°C]), little, if any, change occurs in biological materials.[3,4] Human heart valve leaflets demonstrate retention of protein synthetic capabilities for at least 2 years of storage below −135°C.[7] Degradative processes may occur at and above the solution's glass transition temperature. For example, it has been shown that cells in cryopreserved human heart valve leaflets are negatively affected by storage at temperatures warmer than −100°C.[7]

Immersion of cryopreserved human valves directly into liquid nitrogen for as little as 5 minutes may result in tissue fractures (Figure 16.3, illustration of fractures).[114] Therefore, it is important to avoid submersion in liquid nitrogen, where rapid and dramatic temperature changes can occur, either during storage or during transport from one storage facility to another. This problem came to light when a vapor-phase liquid nitrogen valve storage system in a hospital overfilled during an automatic refill cycle. Valves from this accident were discovered to have numerous full thickness fractures of the valve conduit, following normal thawing procedures in the operating room.[115] Kroener et al.[116] reproduced this phenomena experimentally demonstrating that sudden and dramatic changes in the temperature of a cryopreserved heart valve resulted in the formation of stress fractures in the ice/amorphous glass materials. The rationale for development of stress fractures in frozen matrices appears to relate to differential expansion/contraction of ice versus the amorphous glass phases in the solidified matrix and a presumptive "sliding" of one phase across the "face" of the second phase can lead to abrupt changes in the physical properties of the solidified tissue matrix-stress fractures. Kroener and Luyet[117] described abrupt temperature-dependent changes in aqueous glycerol solutions. Subsequently, they reported[117] that the formation and the disappearance of cracks depended on the interaction of several factors, in particular the mechanical properties of the material, the concentrate of solute, the temperature gradients, the overall temperature, and the rate of temperature change. Differential contraction and expansion coefficients for ice versus amorphous glass phases in a cryopreserved tissue can be expressed as stress in the solidified matrix and this stress is frequently relieved by a sudden and dramatic fracture along the stress plane.[114,115] Where this stress fracture cuts across tissues, a distinct cut or small abrasion will occur in the tissue post-thawing. Such events have been described as full thickness- or micro-fractures in cryopreserved heart valves

and other cardiovascular tissues.[114,115,118] Studies of frozen biological materials have also supported the presence of mechanical forces in cryopreserved tissues.[119,120]

Cryopreserved tissues are frequently stored in the vapor phase of liquid nitrogen in commercially available storage systems. Such systems are typically provided with a simple storage rack which sits above the liquid nitrogen on which items to be stored are placed. Such systems are to be avoided in that they provide a storage space which will be warmer than minus 130°C at heights greater than 12–14 inches above the liquid nitrogen. In addition, such systems experience sudden and dramatic changes in temperature during a refill cycle and it is possible that with improperly stored tissues, i.e., not in an insulated container, stress fractures can occur following repeated refill cycles. Liquid nitrogen storage freezers without a proper racking system for storage of the tissues can result in undesirable temperature gradients and fluctuations (Figure 16.4).[121,122] In an un-racked system the average temperatures were −72.40 ± −10.96°C near the top of the chamber, −115.46 ± −10.00°C near the mid-level of the chamber, and minus 158.75 ± −10.00°C just above the liquid nitrogen in the chamber.

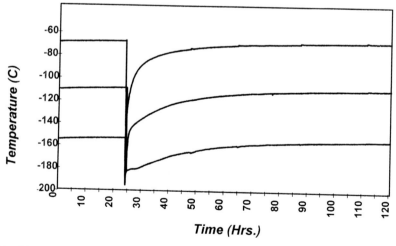

FIGURE 16.4. Liquid nitrogen storage freezers with proper racking result in undesirable temperature gradients from the top of the chamber (upper line) through the mid-level (middle line) and lowest (bottom line). Note the marked fluctuation associated with a refill cycle and the different rates of homeostasis for each of the different positions within the chamber.

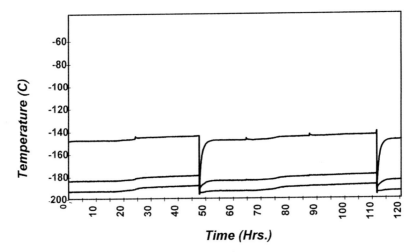

FIGURE 16.5. Racking system in which the lower portion of the rack is partially immersed in the liquid nitrogen results in minimal temperature gradients and more stable tissue temperatures. This system consistently maintains sample temperatures below −130°C.

Thus, the system presents a temperature gradient of 86.36°C over the approximately 20 inches from the top to bottom of the freezer storage compartment. Only the lower levels of the freezer consistently maintain temperatures below −130°C. In addition, the sudden and dramatic temperature fluctuations which can be experienced by tissues in the upper and middle levels of the freezer can be similar to plunging of vapor phase stored tissues into liquid nitrogen, the latter of which has been shown experimentally to produce tissue fractures.[114] Use of a racking system or employment of a mechanical freezer results in more stable storage conditions with consistent maintenance of tissues below −135°C (Figure 16.5). Use of a heat sink in the form of a racking system for tissues, such that the rack is partially immersed in the liquid nitrogen, results in minimal temperature gradients from top to bottom of the storage chamber and as a result of such minimal temperature gradients, tissues experience far less extremes of rapid and sudden changes in temperature during a routine filling cycle. Mechanical freezers are far superior to liquid nitrogen storage systems in maintenance of

a stable temperature. However, mechanical ultra-low freezers have been notoriously unreliable and can represent considerable expense during establishment of a cryopreservation storage facility. One of the authors, L. Wolfinbarger, has had excellent experience with the Cryostar® mechanical ultra-low freezer provided by Revco/Lindberg. As illustrated in Table 16.5 and Figure 16.6, this mechanical storage system provides extremely stable ultra-low temperatures.

TABLE 16.5. Temperature Related Data for Ultralow Temperature Storage Systems.

	Warmest	Coldest	Difference
Mechanical Freezer	−144	−153	9
Liquid Nitrogen (Racked)	−147	−191	44
Liquid Nitrogen (Un-racked)	−72	−159	87

Values in table expressed as °C. The value indicated as "difference" illustrates the average temperature from the bottom to the top of the storage chamber. (Data provided by Vicki Sutherland.)

Section 5

Processing Steps and Valve Handling Performed in the Surgical Suite

Thawing of Cryopreserved Tissues

It is generally accepted that rapid thawing of cells enhances survival. This observation is especially important for rapidly cooled cells and has been suggested to favor cell survival by suppressing the phenomenon known as re-crystallization (the thawing and re-freezing of water molecules which may occur during warming).

Recrystallization is a phenomenon common to solutions that have been frozen under non-equilibrium conditions. Slow cooling typically results in the formation of large crystals, whereas rapid cooling produces smaller crystals. Small ice crystals are unstable because of their high surface energy, and they tend to re-form into large crystals to improve their thermodynamic stability. Such transitions readily occur during the warming and may result in cell damage that was not present during the actual freezing event (although recrystallization could occur at the time of freezing). Cells frozen by a slow cooling process have fewer intracellular ice crystals and larger crystals, and thus are presumably less sensitive to the rate of thawing.

Rapid thawing is the preferred route for rewarming cryopreserved heart valves, as it restricts recrystallization. The process is normally accomplished by first warming the tissues to approximately −100°C, to restrict formation of stress fractures, followed by rapid immersion of the frozen valve in a large volume of water warmed to 42°C. Thawing is normally completed in less than 6 minutes; and so long as care is taken during packaging and when handling the valve during the thawing process, little mechanical damage occurs.

Slow thawing may better preserve the viability of certain cell types. Mammalian embryos and red blood cells appear to do better with a slow thawing rate.[123,124] This observation is probably explained by solute effects and solvent movements. Consider, for example, during freezing a cell that is slowly cooled has minimal intracellular ice and is considerably shrunken in volume. During rapid thawing, these cells experience considerable differences in solute concentrations and rapid rehydration by solvent (water).[84] Because red blood cells typically lack microvilli, the expandability of their surface area is limited, and they would be expected to be more sensitive to rapid osmotic changes (volume changes) than a typical mammalian cell. A slower thawing rate would tend to minimize osmotic imbalances by providing time for the rehydrating solvent to enter the cell. Conversely, rapidly cooled cells would be expected to contain intracellular ice and not be

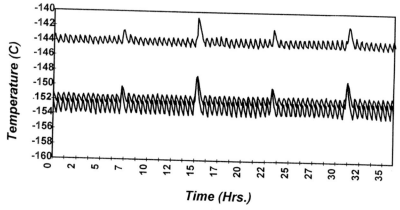

FIGURE 16.6. Mechanical freezer storage system is an alternative to the racked vapor phase system with maintenance of stable ultra-low temperatures.

shrunken in volume. During rapid or slow thawing, these cells would not be expected to experience dramatic osmotic imbalances or solute toxicity, and recrystallization would presumably be the major cause of cell damage. It is for this reason that it is best to always add (slowly) cryoprotectant solutions to cells or tissues than to add cells or tissues to cryoprotectant solutions.

The warming rate may also play a major role in the formation of tissue fractures or cracks. Traditionally, most valve processors have incorporated safeguards in their warming procedures to reduce the initial warming rate of their tissues, for instance the valve is removed from the storage freezer or shipper at some distance from the operating room and is wrapped in a towel and carried without additional cooling if the distance is short, shipped on dry ice, or placed on dry ice if the distance is more than a couple of rooms away. Alternatively, a set time before initiation of the rapid thaw can be determined such that the tissue reaches approximately $-100°C$ before placing the tissue in a water bath. Wassenaar et al.[125] demonstrated a correlation between the formation of cracks in cryopreserved aortic grafts and rapid initial thawing.

Cryoprotectant Removal

After thawing cryopreserved tissues, current opinion is that the cryoprotective agents must be removed. Although the mechanism for DMSO toxicity has not been determined, its ability to affect membrane fluidity,[126] induce cell differentiation[127] and modify cell structure by induction of changes in cytoplasmic microtubules has been well documented.[128,129] DMSO also forms stable coordination complexes with metals.[107] Cryoprotective agents are generally removed by a stepwise dilution procedure. Measurements of cell volume changes during this process clearly demonstrate that the cells undergo dramatic volume changes at each dilution step.[104,130,131]

Cells embedded within a tissue matrix may survive step changes more readily than cell suspensions because of the restricted movement of solutes through the ion-exchange action or viscosity of the macromolecular matrix or through a mechanism similar to that afforded by removal of the cryoprotectant in the presence of a non-permeating solute such as sucrose. Both conditions may restrict cell swelling, as the cryoprotectant diffuses out of the cells along its concentration gradient.

Until recently, following thawing, heart valves have been placed, in a stepwise manner, in serially diluted cryopreservation medium solutions prior to a final rinse in 300–320 mOsm/Kg medium without DMSO. Cryoprotectants have been removed gradually by changing the concentration (osmolality) of the extracellular solution in a stepwise fashion because DMSO enters and leaves cells at a slower rate than water. Therefore, there is a tendency for cells to swell as its environment returns to isotonicity. Even though the cell volumes will return to normal as the DMSO equilibrates, excessive volumetric excursions and the associated osmotic water fluxes can result in cell damage. However, the benefits of slow, stepwise cryoprotectant removal must be weighed against the increased exposure times to DMSO.

Modeling of cryoprotectant transport in tissues has been performed in several model systems. However, these studies usually follow cryoprotectant loading, not removal. Borel Rinkes et al.[132] assessed DMSO diffusion through a collagen matrix containing a hepatocyte monolayer. Using mathematical equations, which described the coupled diffusion of multiple chemical species through an interstitial matrix,[133] it was found that the DMSO concentration achieved by diffusion was 95% after 15 minutes of exposure at $22°C$.[133] Direct measurement of DMSO penetration of tissues has been measured using both nuclear magnetic resonance spectroscopy[134,135] and high pressure liquid chromatography.[88,136] Specific diffusion times may vary from minutes to hours depending upon the composition and geometry of the tissue, however Hu and Wolfinbarger[88] demonstrated that tissue DMSO approximated equilibrium conditions after as little as 80–100 minutes of incubation in medium made with 10% (v/v) DMSO. Mass transport limitations in tissues may create concentrations gradients.[136]

Obviously, these tissue conditions also exist during cryoprotectant removal. Thus, there may be large differences in DMSO concentration between the surface and interior of tissues even after prolonged incubation in DMSO removal medium.[88] In such cases cells in the interior of tissues may still be exposed to toxic concentrations of DMSO in spite of the ability to achieve non-toxic DMSO concentrations in the surface layers.

In addition, it has been reported[137,138] that many cell types tolerate cryoprotectant removal better at 37°C than at 0°C. Thus, the osmotic imbalances may be more quickly restored, and the cell(s) may more easily repair the damaging effects incurred by cryopreservation.

In 1992, Carpenter and Brockbank[139] introduced a one step method of cryoprotect removal from cryopreserved cardiovascular tissues. Cell viability results following cryoprotectant elution by one step methods in heart valves[139] and blood vessels[140] demonstrated that single step methods yielded essentially the same viability results as the historically employed multistep approach. An explanation for cell survival in heart valves thawed by the one step method is that cells embedded within a tissue matrix may survive large osmotic changes in environments into which a valve is placed more readily than cell suspensions or cells on the surface of a tissue because the movement of solutes may be restricted through the ion-exchange action of the macromolecular matrix. The addition of an impermeant solute may also help to reduce the risk of osmotic shock to heart valve cells during one step cryoprotectant removal protocols.[139] In contrast, studies in other tissue models, such as that of Taylor using a corneal model, have indicated that serial dilution of DMSO was preferred to one step removal.[141] Furthermore, the one step method was not found to be very effective at removing DMSO from cryopreserved heart valves. This formulation can be used in the one step dilution process over at least about a five to ten minute period to reduce a pre-dilution DMSO tissue concentration of about 10% (v/v) to a pre-transplant DMSO tissue concentration of about 5% (v/v) or

lower.[139] The major advantage of the one step method appears to be that it is easier for the operating room staff to perform than the multistep procedure in which the valve must be moved to the next step in the dilution process every few minutes. The major theoretical disadvantage of the one step method is that more residual DMSO will remain in the valve resulting in an increased risk of patient reactions to the DMSO and exhaled DMSO breakdown products and the patient may experience localized cell and tissue damage.

A method of cryoprotectant removal, AlloFlow™, recently developed for and used by LifeNet (US Patent ≠ **5,879,876**) combines positive features of both the multistep and the single step methods. From the perspective of tissue handling this method is simple since it involves only "one step." However, the method is essentially composed of many dilution steps performed in a continuous manner with the resulting reduction in risk of osmotic shock associated with both the single and multistep methods (Figure 16.7). Using the AlloFlow™ technology, a thawed valve is placed, with its freezing solution, into a Continuous Perfusion Chamber, and the continuously flowing dilution solution is perfused in a circular motion through and around the tissue before exiting the chamber to waste. The tissue DMSO gradient is thus maximized by the continuous clearance of the DMSO as it is eluted from the tissue. Like the single step process, the continuous process incorporates a non permeating solute in the wash solution and results in heart valve tissues containing approximately 2% (v:v) DMSO after as little as 7 to 10 minutes. An additional benefit of the continuous process is that wash-out is performed at room temperature to permit more rapid restoration of metabolic imbalances and the process proceeds without continual monitoring or handling. At completion of the process, the valve remains in a volume of washout solution and is ready for transplantation. Thus, in tissues treated by the continuous elution AlloFlow™ method, the osmotic imbalances may be quickly restored, and the cell(s) may more easily repair the damaging effects incurred by cryopreservation.

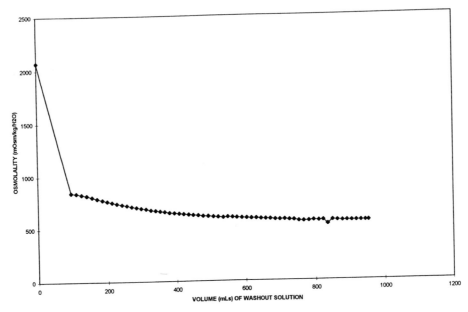

FIGURE 16.7. Continuous wash-out method for cryoprotectant removal reduces the risk of osmotic shock associated with single or even step-wise methods.

Conclusion

In this chapter we have reviewed the biology of heart valve preservation and indicated some of the pitfalls associated with cryopreservation and, where possible, the means to overcome them. Some of the more exciting areas of future research indicated were in tissue extracellular matrix preservation, decellularization of tissues, and in new preservation methods employing vitrification and molecules which modify the way ice forms by binding to ice nuclei. However, this review would not be complete without some discussion of the immune response to cryopreserved allogeneic heart valves.

Freedom from tissue failure for cryopreserved valves in adults is excellent and it averages about 80% at 10 years.[142,143] In contrast to adult valve recipients, young recipients have a significantly higher failure rate.[144–146] Freedom from allograft failure in patients less than three years of age at operation is only 45% at 6 years.[12] A marked diminution of the cellular component has been observed in explanted valves with progressively severe loss of normal layered structure and connective tissue cells.[147] Neither the structural basis of performance nor the pathophysiology of failure are understood.[148] Controversies are ongoing concerning the contribution of cryopreservation variables, immune responses, cellular viability, durability of the extracellular matrix and modes of failure.[146,147]

Allograft valves are usually used without HLA-ABO matching of donors and recipients. There is no direct evidence of a linear correlation between immunologic response and late valve failure.[147,149,150] Both HLA-specific antibody and T-cell activation have been demonstrated in patients, but the clinical performance of the viable allografts was not affected.[151–153] However, Clarke and colleagues[12,146] clearly believed that the cause of allograft failure in young children may have involved an immune response. The only non-calcified explant of six explants from children contained lymphocytes. Four children not requiring valve explantation received post operative treatment with anti-inflammatory agents and one child was receiving cyclosporin therapy with the original valve. There have been several reports with experimental allograft valves supporting the hypothesis that allograft valves retain their ability to stimulate an immune response following cryopreservation in animal models[154-156] and recent studies, stimulated by the observations of Clarke,[12,146] have demonstrated the development of donor specific HLA antibodies in pediatric recipients of cryopreserved heart valves.[157,158] Both human valve endothelium and fibroblasts have been shown to be immunogenic in vitro, however in contrast to endothelial cells, fibroblasts induced only a limited proliferation of peripheral blood mononuclear cells and CD4+T cells did not respond to MHC Class II bearing fibroblasts.[159] Even though it has not been demonstrated that the immune response causes allograft valve failure, HLA sensitization of allograft heart valve recipients has at least the potential of limiting the future opportunity for heart transplantation in these patients. A search of the literature on cryopreserved tissue transplantation reveals many suggestions that processing steps can be introduced in tissue preservation procedures which may reduce tissue immunogenicity including decellularization. Immunologic tolerance induction has been attempted by both graft treatment prior to implantation and by subsequent treatment of the graft recipient.[160,161] Both skin grafts and Islet of Langerhans grafts have been shown to have better survival as allografts when cryopreservation protocols designed to reduce dendritic cells are utilized.[162,163] Cryopreserved veins have reduced immunogenicity when compared with fresh allografts.[161,164] Mulligan et al.[165] reported decreased expression of leukocyte adhesion molecules by allogeneic rat aortic valves *in vivo*, suggesting that cryopreserved valves may have a diminished immunological response. It is clear, however, that there is a need for development of tissue preservation protocols which alleviate concerns regarding the immune response in young children.[166-170] At present, the most likely method of tissue preservation involves the removal of the cellular elements from tissues with either none or minimal changes in matrix structure.

Finally, this chapter would not be complete without a brief introduction of new technolo-gies under development by a number of heart valve providers. These new technologies almost universally involve the removal of the cellular components from the heart valves. They differ in the methods by which these cells are removed, but most involve some use of surfactants (detergents) in solubilization of the plasma membranes of cells and inhibitors of hydrolytic enzymes. Most methods are claimed not to alter the matrix structure of the valve and such acellular technologies may ultimately provide heart valves which can be repopulated by recipient cells either prior to or after transplantation, which are non-immunogenic (even in children), which may originate from animal sources other than human, and which may not require cryopreservation. As with most technologies, a primary ingredient to any decellularization technology lies in the appropriate choice of process and in not leaving residuals of processing reagents or a matrix structure that restricts recellularization or that induces an apoptotic response in the cells infiltrating the acellular matrix with subsequent probable calcification. Such acellularization technologies have been developed and are being applied to a variety of soft tissues (cardiovascular and musculoskeletal), but as this chapter is on cryopreservation, will not be discussed. As we enter into the next millennium, we should expect much from development of new technologies as we finally begin to understand existing technologies.

References

1. O'Brien MF, Stafford EG, Gardner MA, Pohlner PG, McGiffin DC. A comparison of aortic valve replacement with viable cryopreserved and fresh allograft valves, with a note on chromosomal studies. J Thorac Cardiovasc Surg 1987;94:812–823.

2. Polge C, Smith AY, Parkes AS. Revival of spermatozoa after vitrification and dehydration at low temperatures. Nature 1949;164.

3. Karow AM. Biophysical and chemical considerations in cryopreservation. In Karow JrAM, Pegg DE (eds). Organ Preservation for Transplantation. New York: Marcel Dekker 1981: 13–30.

4. Mazur P. Freezing of living cells: mechanisms and implications. Am J Physiol 1984;247:125.

5. Hu J, Gilmer L, Wolfinbarger L, Hopkins RA. Assessment of cellular viability in cardiovascular tissue as studied with 3 H-proline and 3 H-inulin. Cardiovasc Res 1990;24:528–531.

6. Mochtar B, Van der Kamp A, Roza-DeJong E, Nauta J. Cell Survival in canine aortic heart valves stored in nutrient medium. Cardiovasc Res 1974;18:497.

7. Brockbank KGM, Carpenter JF, Dawson PE. Effects of Storage Temperature on Viable Bioprosthetic Heart Valves. Cryobiology 1992;29:537–542.

8. Messier RH, Bass BL, Aly HM. Dual structural and functional phenotypes of the porcine aortic valve interstitial characteristics of the leaflet myofibroblast. J Surg Res 1994;57:1–21.

9. Watts LK, Duffy P, Field RB, Stafford EG, O'Brien MF. Establishment of a viable homograft cardiac valve bank: a rapid method of determining homograft viability. Ann Thorac Surg 1976;21:230–236.

10. Brockbank KG, Dawson PE. Influence of whole heart postprocurement cold ischemia time upon cryopreserved heart valve viability. Transplant Proc 1993;25:3188–3189.

11. VanDerKamp AWM, Nauta J. Fibroblast function and the maintenance of aortic valve matrix. J Cardiovasc Res 1979;13:167–172.

12. Clarke DR. Invited letter concerning: accelerated degeneration of aortic homograft in infants and young children. J Thorac Cardiovasc Surg 1994;107:1162–1164.

13. Shon YH, Wolfinbarger L. Proteoglycan content in fresh and cryopreserved porcine aortic tissue. Cryobiology 1994;31:121–132.

14. Allen MD, Shoji Y, Fujimura Y, Gordon D, Thomas R, Brockbank KGM, Disteche CM. Growth and Cell Viability of Aortic Versus Pulmonic Homografts in the Systemic Circulation. Circulation 1991;84(suppl III):III-94–III-99.

15. Hirschman A, Dziewiatkowski DD. Protein-polysaccharide loss during endochondral ossification: Immunological evidence. Science 1966;154:393–395.

16. Joseph AB. Proteoglycan structure in calcifying cartilage. Clin Orthop 1972;172:207–232.

17. Larsson R, Ray R, Keuttner K. Microchemical studies on acid glycosaminoglycans of epiphyseal zones during endochondral calcification. Calcif Tissue Res 1973;13:271–285.

18. Lohmander S, Hjerpe A. Proteoglycans of mineralized rib and epiphyseal cartilage. Biochim Biophys Acta 1975;404:93–109.

19. Murata K. Acidic glycosaminoglycans in human heart valves. J Mol Cell Cardiol 1981;13:281–292.

20. American Association of Tissue Banks. Standard for Tissue Banking. Page 12. 1989.

21. European Homograft Bank International. Yearly Report of the Medical Director. 1991. Brussels, Belgium.

22. Angell JD, Christopher BS, Hawtrey O, Angell WM. A fresh viable human heart valve bank-sterilization sterility testing and cryogenic preservation. Transplant Proc 1976;8(Suppl 1):127–141.

23. Danielson GD, McGoon DC, Wallace RB, et al. Pediatric cardiology. Edinburgh: Churchill Livingston 1978.

24. VanDerKamp AWM, Visser WJ, van Dongan JM, Nauta J, Galjaard H. Preservation of aortic heart valves with maintenance of cell viability. J Surg Res 1981;30:47.

25. Wain WH, Pearce HM, Riddell RW, Ross DN. A re-evaluation of the antibiotic sterilization of heart valve allografts. Thorax 1977;32:740–742.

26. Billingham ME, Baumgartner WA, Watson DC, et al. Distant heart procurement for human transplantation: Ultrastructural studies. Circulation 1980;62(Suppl 1):I11–I19.

27. McKeown CMB, Edwards V, Phillips MJ, et al. Sinusoidal lining cell damage. The critical injury in cold preservation of liver allografts in the rat. Transplantation 1988;46:178–191.

28. Gattone VH, Filo RS, Evan AP, et al. Time course of glomeral endothelial injury related to pulsatile perfusion preservation. Transplantation 1985;39:296–399.

29. Brockbank KGM, Bank HL, Schmehl MK. Ischemia and saphenous vein endothelial integrity. Transplant Proc 1989;21:1384–1388.

30. Torok J, Kristek F, Mokrasova M. Endothelium-dependant relaxation in rabbit aorta after cold storage. Eur J Pharmacol 1993;228:313–319.

31. Pickford MA, Gower JD, Dore C, et al. Lipid peroxidation and ultra-structure changes in rat lung isografts after single-passage organ flush and 48-hour cold storage with and without one-hour reperfusion in vivo. Transplantation 1990;144:210–218.

32. Kamm KE, Zatzman MOL, Jones AW, et al. Effects of temperature on ionic transport in

aortas from rat and ground squirrel. Am J Physiol 1979;237:23–30.

33. Kimzey SL, Willis JS. Temperature adaptation of active sodium-potassium transport and of passive permeability in erythrocytes of ground squirrels. Jour Gen Physiol 1971;58:634–649.

34. Morris GJ, Clarke A. Cells at low temperature. In Grout BWW, Morris GJ (eds). The Effects of Low Temperatures on Biological Systems. London: Edward Arnold 1987:72–119.

35. Klein RA. Thermodynamics and membrane processes. Quart Rev Biophys 1982;15:667–757.

36. Hochachka PW. Defense strategies against hypoxia and hypothermia. Science 1986;231:234–241.

37. Nicotera P, Orrenius S. Ca^{2+} and cell death. Ann N Y Acad Sci 1992;645:17–27.

38. Orrenius S, McConkey DJ, Bellomo G, et al. Role of Ca^{2+} in toxic cell killing. Trends in Pharm Sci 1989;10:281–285.

39. Kannagi R, Koizumi K. Effects of differential physical states of phospholipid substrates on partially purified platelet phospholipase A_2 activity. Biochim Biophys Acta 1979;556:423–433.

40. Op den Kamp JAF, de Gier J, van Deenen LLM. Hydrolysis of phosphatidylcholineliposomes by pancreatic phospholipase A^{2+} at the transition temperature. Biochim Biophys Acta 1974;345:253–256.

41. Elford BC. Temperature dependence of cation permeability of dog red blood cells. Nature 1974;248:522.

42. Rossi MA, Braile DM, Teixeira DR, Carillo SV. Calcific degeneration of pericardial valvular xenografts implanted subcutaneously in rats. Int J Cardiol 1986;12:331–339.

43. Acquatella H, Perez-Gonzalez M, Morales JM, Whittembury G. Ionic and histological changes in the kidney after perfusion and storage for transplantation. Transplantation 1972;14:480.

44. Ploeg RJ, Goossens D, Vreugdenhil P, McAnulty JF, Southard JH, Belzer FO. Successful 72-hour cold storage kidney preservation with UW solution. Transplant Proc 1988;20:935–938.

45. Ladbrooke BD, Williams RM, Chapman D. Studies on lecithin-cholesterol-water interactions by differential scanning calorimetry and x-ray diffraction. Biochim Biophys Acta 1968;150:333–340.

46. Willis JS. Membrane transport at low temperatures in hibernators and nonhibernators. In Heller HC, Muscchia XJ, Wang LCH (eds). Living in the Cold: Physiological and Biochemical Adaptations. New York: Elsevier 1986:27–34.

47. Lyons JM, Raison JK. Oxidation activity of mitochondria isolated from plant tissues and resistant to chilling injury. Plant Physiol 1970;45:386–389.

48. Raison JK, Lyons JM. Hibernation: alteration of mitochondrial membranes as a requisite for metabolism at low temperature. Proc Nat Acad Sci 1971;68:2092–2094.

49. Inesi G, Milman M, Eletr S. Temperature-induced transitions of function and structure in sarcoplastic reticulum membranes. Jour Mol Biol 1973;81:483–504.

50. Madeira VMC, Antunes-Madeira MC, Carvalho AP. Activation energies of the ATPase activity of sarcoplastic reticulum. Biochem Biophys Res Comm 1974;65:997–1003.

51. Gavish B, Werber MM. Viscosity-depentent structural fluctuations in enzyme catalysis. Biochem J 1979;18:1269–1275.

52. Cossins JR, Lee JAC, Lewis RN, Bowler K. The adaptation to the cold of membrane order and (Na+-K+)-ATPase properties. In Heller HC, Muscchia XJ, Wang LCH (eds). Living in the Cold: Physiological and Biochemical Adaptations. New York: Elsevier 1986:13–18.

53. Hansen TN. Correlation between chilling-induced injury in human cells and phospholipid membrane phase transition. Transplant Proc 1993;25:3179–3181.

54. Graham JD, Foote RH. Effect of several lipids, fatty acyl chain length, and degree of unsaturation on the motility of bull spermatozoa after cold shock and freezing. Cryobiology 1987;24:42–52.

55. Quinn PJ. A lipid-phase separation model of low-temperature damage to biological membranes. Cryobiology 1985;22:128–146.

56. Morris GJ, Clarke A. Effects of low temperatures on biological membranes. In New York: Academic Press 1981:241–377.

57. Prosser CL. Comparative Animal Physiology. Philadelphia: W.B. Saunders 1973.

58. Southard JH, Marsh DC, McAnulty JF, Belzer FO. Oxygen-derived free radical damage in organ preservation: Activity of superoxide dismutase and xanthine oxidase. Surgery 1987;101:566–570.

59. Fuller BJ, Gower JD, Green CJ. Free radical damage and organ preservation: Fact or fiction? Cryobiology 1988;25:377–393.

60. Messier R, Jr., Domkowski P, Hopkins RA, Aly H, Wallace R, et al. High energy phosphate depletion in leaflet matrix cells during processing of cryopreserved heart valves. J Surg Res 1992;52:483–488.

61. Messier RH, Jr., Domkowski PW, Abd-Elfattah AS, Aly HM, Crescenzo DG, Analouei AR, Hilbert SL, Wallace RB, Hopkins RA. Analysis of the total adenine nucleotide pool in 25 cryopreserved human cardiac valves. Circulation 84 (Suppl) II. 1991.

62. Crescenzo DG, Hilbert SL, Messier JrRH, Domkowski PW, Barrick MK, Lange PL, Ferrans V, Wallace RB, Hopkins RA. Human cryopreserved allografts: Electron microscopic analysis of cellular injury. Ann Thorac Surg 1993;55:25–31.

63. Yankah AC, Hetzer R. Procurement and viability of cardiac valve allografts. In Yankah AC, Hetzer R, Miller DC, Ross DN, Somerville J, Yacoub MH (eds). Cardiac Valve Allografts 1962–1987. New York: Springer-Verlag; 1988:23–34.

64. Heacox AE, McNally RT, Brockbank KGM. Factors affecting the viability of cryopreserved allograft heart valves. In Yankah AC, Hetzer R, Miller DC, Ross DN, Somerville J, Yacoub MH (eds). Cardiac valve allografts. New York: Springer-Verlag;1989:37–42.

65. Abd-Elfattah AS, Messier RH, Domkowski PW, Crescenzo DG, Wallace RB, Hopkins RA. Inhibition of adenosine deaminase and nucleoside transport: utility in a model of homograft cardiac valve preimplantation processing. J Thorac Cardiovasc Surg 1993;105:1095–1105.

66. Brockbank KGM, Dawson PE, Carpenter JF. Heart valve leaflet revitalization. Tissue and Cell Report 1993;1:18–19.

67. Carpenter JF, Brockbank KGM. Tissue Revitalization Method. [5,171,660]. 1992. United States.

68. Rosenthal TB. The effect of temperature on the pH of blood and plasma in vitro. J Biol Chem 1948;173:25–30.

69. Rahn H, Prakash O. Acid-Base Regulation and Body Temperature. Boston: Martinus Nijhoff Publishers 1985.

70. Good NE, Winget GD, Winter W, Connolly TN, Izawa S, Singh RMM. Hydrogen ion buffers for biological research. Biochem J 1996;184:547–554.

71. Swan H. The importance of acid-base management for cardiac and cerebral preservation during open heart surgery. Surg Gynecol Obstet 1984;158:391–414.

72. Vander Woude JC, Christlieb IY, Sicard GA, Clark RE. Imidazole-buffered cardioplegic solution. J Thorac Cardiovasc Surg 1985;90:225–234.

73. Swan H, Cowan M, Tornabene M, Owens L. Aminosulphonic acid buffer preserves myocardium during prolonged ischemia. Ann Thorac Surg 1994;57:1590–1596.

74. Garlick PB, Radda GK, Seeley PL. Studies of acidosis in the ischaemic heart by phosphorus nuclear magnetic resonance. Biochem J 1996;184:547–554.

75. Taylor MJ, Pignat Y. Practical acid dissociation constants, temperature coefficients and buffer capacities for some biological buffers in solutions containing dimethyl sulfoxide between 25 and −12°C. Cryobiology 1982;19:99–109.

76. Taylor MJ. The role of pH* and buffer capacity in the recovery of function of smooth muscle cooled to −13°C in unfrozen media. Cryobiology 1982;19:585–601.

77. Taylor MJ, Hunt CJ, Madden PW. Hypothermic preservation of corneas in a hyperkalaemic solution (CPTES): II.Extended storage in the presence of chondroitin sulphate. Br J Ophthalmol 1989;73:792–802.

78. Taylor MJ, Hunt CJ. A new preservation solution for storage of corneas at low temperature. Current Eye Research 1985;4:963–973.

79. Hudson RE. Pathology of the human aortic valve homograft. Br Heart J 1966;28:291–301.

80. Smith JC. The pathology of human aortic valve homografts. Thorax 1967;22:114–138.

81. Domkowski P, Messier R, Jr., Aly H, Abd-Elfattah A, Crescenzo D, Analouei A, Hilbert S, Wallace R, Hopkins R. Determination of adenine nucleotide pool metabolite levels in leaflet cells at each step between harvest and thawing of cryopreserved cardiac valves. Cryobiology 5. 1990.

81a. Kosek J, Iven A, Shumway N. Angell W. Morphology of fresh heart valve homografts. Surgery 1969;66:269–274.

82. Al-Janabi N, Ross DN. Enhanced viability of fresh aortic homografts stored in nutrient medium. Cardiovasc Res 1973;7:817–822.

83. Okita Y, Franciosi G, Matsuki O, Robles A, Ross DN. Early and late results of aortic root replacement with antibiotic-sterilized aortic homograft. J Thorac Cardiovasc Surg 1988;95:696–704.

84. Deck JD. Endothelial cell orientation on aortic valve leaflets. Cardiovasc Res 1986; 20:760–767.

85. Stark J. Do we really correct congenital heart defects? J Thorac Cardiovasc Surg 1989;97: 1–9.

86. Kirklin JW, Blackstone EH, Maehara T, Pacifico AD, Kirklin JK, Pollock S, Stewart RW. Intermediate-term fate of cryopreserved allograft and xenograft valved conduits. Ann Thorac Surg 1987;44:598–606.

87. Strickett MG, Barratt-Boyes BG, MacCulloch D. Disinfection of human heart valve allografts with antibiotics in low concentration. Pathology 1983;15:457–462.

88. Hu JF, Wolfinbarger L. Dimethyl sulfoxide concentration in fresh and cryopreserved porcine valve conduit tissues. Cryobiology 1994;31:461–467.

89. Brockbank KGM, Dawson PE. Cytotoxicity of amphotericin B for fibroblasts in human heart valve leaflets. Cryobiology 1993;30:19–24.

90. Gale EF. The release of potassium ions from Candida albicans in the presence of polyene antibiotics. J Gen Microbiol 1974;80:451–465.

91. Holz RW. Mechanism of action of anteukaryotic and antiviral compounds. In Gottlieb D, Shaw PD (eds). Antibiotics. New York: Springer-Verlag 1979:313–340.

92. Kerridge D. The polyene macrolide antibiotics. Postgrad Med J 1979;55:653–656.

93. Chen WC, Bittman R. Kinetics of association of amphotericin B with vesicles. Biochem J 1977;16:4145–4149.

94. Readio JD, Bittman R. Equilibrium binding of amphotericin B and its methyl ester and borate complex to sterols. Biochim Biophys Acta 1982;685:219–224.

95. Singer C, Kaplan MH, Armstrong D. Bacteremia and fungemia complicating neoplastic disease: a study of 364 cases. Am J Med 1971;62:731–742.

96. van der Berg L, Rose D. Effects of freezing on the pH and composition of sodium and potassium phosphate solutions: The reciprocal system $KH_2PO_4-NaHPO_4-H_2O$. Arch Biochem Biophys 1959;81:319.

97. van der Berg L, Soliman FS. Composition and pH changes during freezing of solutions containing calcium and magnesium phosphates. Cryobiology 1969;6:10–14.

98. Lovelock JE. The mechanism of the protective action of glycerol against haemolysis by freezing and thawing. Biochim Biophys Acta 1953; 11:28.

99. Schneider U, Mazur P. Relative influence of unfrozen fraction and salt concentration on the survival of slowly frozen eight-cell mouse embryos. Cryobiology 1987;24:17–41.

100. Leibo SP. Water permeability and its activation energy of fertilized and unfertilized mouse ova. J Membr Biol 1980;53:179–188.

101. Rall WF. Physical Chemical aspects of cryoprotection of human erythrocytes and mouse conbryoes. PhD dissertation, Univ. Tennessee, 1979.

102. Nakayama S, Ban T, Okamoto S. Fetal bovine serum is not necessary for the cryopreservation of aortic valve tissues. J Thorac Cardiovasc Surg 1994;108:583–586.

103. Karow AM, Carrier O, Jr. Effects of cryoprotectant compounds on mammalian heart muscle. Surg Gynecol Obstet 1969;128:51.

104. Mazur P. Fundamental cryobiology and the preservation of organs by freezing. In Karow AM, Jr., Pegg DE (eds). Organ Preservation for Transplantation. 2nd edition. New York: Marcel Dekker 1981:143–175.

105. Fahy GM, Karrow AM, Jr. Prosthypertonic osmotic shock and myocardial injury. Cryobiology 1975;12:577.

106. Pegg DE. The effect of cell concentration on the recovery of human erythrocytes after freezing and thawing in the presence of glycerol. Criobiology 1981;18:221–228.

107. Shlafer M. Pharmacological considerations in cryopreservation. In Karow AM (ed). Organ Preservation for Transplantation. 2nd edition. New York: Marcel Dekker 1981:177–212.

108. Brockbank KGM, Smith KM. Synergistic interaction of low-molecular-weight polyvinylpyrrolidones with mimethyl sulfoxide during cell preservation. Transplant Proc 1993; 25:3185.

109. Brockbank KGM. Method for cryopreserving blood vessels. [5,145,769 and 5,158,867]. 1992. United States.

110. Fahy GM. Vitrification. In McGrath JJ, Diller KR (eds). Low Temperature Biotechnology: Emerging applications and engineering contributions. New York: ASME 1988:118.

111. Wang T, Zhu Q, Yang X, Layne JR, DeVries AL. Antifreeze glycoproteins from Antarctic Notothenioid fishes fail to protect the rat cardiac explant during hypothermic and freezing preservation. Cryobiology 1994;31:185.

112. Rubinsky B, Arav A, Hong JS, Lee CY. Freezing of mammalian livers with glycerol and antifreeze proteins. Biochem Biophys Res Comm 1994;200:732.

113. Hansen TN, Smith KM, Brockbank KGM. Type I antifreeze protein attenuates cell recovery following cryopreservation. Transplant Proc 1993;25:3186.

114. Adam M, Hu JF, Lange P, Wolfinbarger L. The effect of liquid nitrogen submersion on cryopreserved human heart valves. Cryobiology 1990;27:605–614.

115. Wolfinbarger L, Adam M, Lange P, Hu JF. Microfractures in cryopreserved heart valves: valve submersin in liquid nitrogen revisited. Applications of Cryogenic Technology 1991; 10:227–233.

116. Kroener C, Luyet B. Formation of cracks during vitrification of glycerol solutions and disappearance of the cracks during rewarming. Biodynamica 1966;10:47–51.

117. Kroener C, Luyet B. Discontinuous change in expansion coefficient at the glass transition temperature in aqueous solutions of glycerol. Biodymanica 1966;10:41–45.

118. Hunt CJ, Pegg DE, Song YC. Fractures in cryopreserved arteries. Cryobiology 1994;31: 506–515.

119. Rubinsky B, Lee C, Bastacky J, Onik G. The process of freezing in the liver and the mechanisms of damage. Proceedings, CRYO 87–24th Meeting 1987.

120. Rajotte RV, Shnitka TK, Liburd EM, Dossetor JB, Voss WAG. Histological Studies on Cultured Canine Heart Valves Recovered from –196 C. Cryobiology 1977;14:15–22.

121. Asano M, Masuzawa-Ito K, Matsuda T. Charybdotoxin-sensitive K+ channels regulate the myogenic tone in the resting state of arteries from spontaneously hypertensive rats. Br J Pharmacol 1993;108:214–222.

122. Quast U. Potassium channel openers: pharmacological and clinical aspects. Fundam Clin Pharmacol 1992;6:279–293.

123. Miller RH, Mazur P. Survival of frozen-thawed human red cells as a function of cooling and warming velocities. Criobiology 1976;13:404.

124. Whittingham DG, Leibo SP, Mazur P. Survival of mouse embryos frozen to –196 degrees and –269 degrees C. Science 1972;178:411–414.

125. Wassenaar C, Wijsmuller EG, van Herverden LA, Aghai Z, van Tricht C, Bos E. Cracks in cryopreserved aortic allografts and rapid thawing. Ann Thorac Surg 1995;60 Suppl: S165–S167.

126. Barnett RE. The effects of dimethyulsulfoxide and glycerol on Na+, K+-ATPase and membrane structure. Cryobiology 1978;15:227.

127. Miranda AF, Nette G, Khan S, Brockbank KGM, Schonberg M. Alteration of myoblast phenotype by dimethylsulfoxide. Proc Natl Acad Sci USA 1978;75:3826–3830.

128. Katsuda S, Okada Y, Nakanishi I. Dimethyl sulfoxide induces microtubule formation in cultured arterial smooth muscle cells. Cell Biol Int Rep 1987;11:103–110.

129. Katsuda S, Okada Y, Nakanishi I, Tanaka J. The influence of dimethyl sulfoxide on cell growth and ultrastructural features of cultured smooth muscle cells. J Electron Micros 1984; 33:239–241.

130. Mazur P, Miller RH. The use of permeability coefficients in predicting the osmotic response of human red blood cells during the removal of intracellular glycerol. Cryobiology 1976;13: 126.

131. Jackowski S, Leibo SP, Mazur P. Glycerol permeabilities of fertilized and unfertilized mouse ova. J Exp Zool 1980;212:329.

132. Borel Rinkes IHM, Toner M, Ezzell RM, Tomkins RG, Yarmush ML. Effects of dimethly sulfoxide on cultured rat hepatocytes in sandwich configuration. Cryobiology 1992; 29:443–453.

133. Schreuders PD, Diller KR, Beaman JJ, Paynter HM. An analysis of coupled multicomponent diffusion in interstitial tissue. J Biomed Eng 1994;116:164–171.

134. Bateson EAJ, Busza AL, Pegg DE, Taylor MJ. Permeation of rabbit common carotid arteries with dimethyl sulfoxide. Cryobiology 1994;31: 393–397.

135. Fuller BJ, Busza AI, Proctor E. Studies on cyroprotectant equilibration in the intact rat liver using nuclear resonance spectroscopy: a noninvasive method to assess distribution of dimethylsulfoxide in tissues. Cryobiology 1989;26:112–118.

136. Carpenter JF, Dawson PE. Quantitation of dimethyl sulfoxide in solutins and tissues was performed by high-performance liquid chromatography. Cryobiology 1991;28:210–215.

137. Farrant J. General observations on cell preservation. In Ashwood-Smith MJ, Farrant J (eds). Low Temperature Preservation in Medicine and Biology. London: Pitman; 1980: 1–18.

138. Thorpe PE, Knight SC, Farrant J. Optimal conditions for the preservation of mouse lymph node cells in liquid nitrogen using cooling rate techniques. Cryobiology 1976;13: 126.

139. Carpenter JF, Brockbank KGM. Process for preparing tissue for transplantation. [5,160,313]. 1992. United States.

140. Muler-Schweinitzer E. Applications for cryopreserved blood vessels in pharmacological research. Cryobiology 1994;31:57–62.

141. Taylor MJ. Clinical cryobiology of tissues: Preservation of corneas. Cryobiology 1986;23:323–353.

142. O'Brien MF, McGiffen DC, Stafford EG. Allograft aortic valve replacement: long-term comparative clinical analysis of the viable cryopreserved and antibiotic 4 degree stored valves. J Card Surg 1991;6(suppl):534–543.

143. Kirklin JK, Smith D, Novick W, et al. Long-term function of cryopreserved aortic homografts: a ten year study. J Thorac Cardiovasc Surg 1993;106:154–166.

144. Hawkins JA, Bailey WW, Dillon T, Schwartz DC. Midterm results with cryopreserved allograft valved conduits from the right ventricle to the pulmonary arteries. J Thorac Cardiovasc Surg 1992;104:910–916.

145. Yankah AC, Alexi-Meskhishvili VA, Weng Y, Schorn K, Lange RE, Hetzer R. Accelerated degeneration of allografts in the first two years of life. Ann Thorac Surg 1995;60 Suppl:S71–S77.

146. Clarke D, Campbell D, Hayward A, et al. Degeneration of aortic valve allografts in young recipients. J Thorac Cardiovasc Surg 1993;105:934–942.

147. Mitchell RN, Jonas RA, Schoen F. Structure-function correlations in cryopreserved allograft cardiac valves. Ann Thorac Surg 1995;60:8108–8133.

148. Angell WW, Oury JH, Lamberti JJ, Koziol J. Durability of the viable aortic allograft. J Thorac Cardiovasc Surg 1989;98:48–55.

149. Hopkins RA. Cardiac reconstructions with allograft valves. New York: Springer-Verlag; 1989.

150. Bodnar E, Matsuki O, Parker R, Ross DN. Viable and nonviable aortic homografts in the subcoronary position: a comparative study. Ann Thorac Surg 1989;47:799–805.

151. Smith JD, Ogino H, Hunt D, et al. Humoral immune response to human aortic valve homografts. Ann Thorac Surg 1995;60:S127–S130.

152. Fischlein T, Schutz A, Haushofer M, Free R, Utilize A, Detter C, Reichart B. Immunologic reaction and viability of cryopreserved homografts. Ann Thorac Surg 1995;60 Suppl:S122–S126.

153. Brandl U, Schutz A, Breuer M, Engelhardt M, Reichart B, Kemkes BM. Acute Rejection in Heart Valves. The Journal of Heart and Lung Transplantation 1992;11.

154. Yankah AC, Wottge HU, Muller-Hermelink HK, Feller AC, Lange P, Wessel U, Dreyer H, Bernhard A, Müller-Ruchholtz W. Transplantation of aortic and pulmonary allografts, enhanced viability of endothelial cells by cryopreservation, importance of histocompatibility. J Card Surg 1987;2:209–220.

155. Cochran RP, Kunzelman KS. Cryopreservation does not alter antigenic expression of aortic allografts. J Surg Res 1989;46:597–599.

156. Lupinetti FM, Cobb S, Kioschos HC, Thompson SA, Walters KS, Moore KC. Effect of immunological differences on rat aortic valve allograft calcification. J Card Surg 1992;7:65–70.

157. Barratt-Boyes BG, Jaffe WM, Hong Ko P, Whitlock RML. The Zero Pressure Fixed Medtronic Intact Porcine Valve: An 8.5 Year Review. J Heart Valve Dis 1993;2:604–611.

158. Den Harner I, Hepkema J, Prop J, Eizenga N, Ebels T. HLA antibodies specific for cryopreserved heart valve "homografts" in children. J Thorac Cardiovasc Surg 1997;113:417–419.

159. Johnson DL, Rose ML, Yacoub MH. Immunogenicity of human heart valve endothelial cells and fibroblasts. Transplant Proc 1997;29:984–985.

160. Lafferty KJ, Babcock SK, Gill RG. Prevention of rejection by treatment of the graft: an overview. In Meryman HT (ed). Transplantation: Approaches to graft rejection. New York: Alan R. Liss 1986:87–117.

161. Brockbank KGM. The immune response to allogenic grafts. In Brockbank KGM (ed). Principles of Autologous, Allogenic, and Cryopreserved Venous Transplantation. Austin, New York: R.G. Landes, Co. and Springer-Verlag 1995:73–83.

162. Taylor MJ, Foreman J, Biwata Y, Tsukikawa S. Prolongation of islet allograft survival is facilitated by storage conditions using cryopreservation involving fast cooling and/or tissue culture. Transplant Proc 1992;24:2860–2862.

163. Ingham E, Matthews JB, Kearney JN, Gowland G. The effects of variation of cryopreservation protocols on the immunogenicity of allogeneic skin grafts. Cryobiology 1993;30:443–458.

164. Augelli NV, Lupinetti FM, Khatib H, Sanofsky SJ, Rossi NP. Allograft vein patency in a canine model. Additive effects of cryopreservation and cyclosporine. Transplantation 1991;52:466–470.

165. Mulligan MS, Tsai TT, Kneebone JM, et al. Effects of preservation techniques on in vivo expression of adhesion molecules by aortic valve allografts. J Thorac Cardiovasc Surg 1994;107:717–723.

166. Lockey E, Al-Janabi N, Gonzalez-Lavin L, Ross DNA. Method of sterilizing and preserving fresh allograft heart valves. Thorax 1972; 27:398.

167. Barratt-Boyes BG, Roche AH. A review of aortic valve homografts over a six and one-half year period. Ann Surg 1969;170:483–492.

168. Yankah AC, Sievers HH, Bürsch JH, Radtcke W, Lange PE, Heintzen PH, Bernhard A. Orthotopic transplantation of aortic valve allografts. Early hemodynamic results. Thorac Cardiovasc Surg 1984;32:92–95.

169. Armiger LC, Gavin JB, Barratt-Boyes BG. Histological assessment of orthotopic aortic valve leaflet allografts: its role in selecting graft pre-treatment. Pathology 1983;15:67–73.

170. McNally RT, Heacox A BK, Bank HL. Method for cryopreserving heart valves. [4,890,457]. 1990. United States.

17
Cell Viability and Problems with Its Quantification

Diane Hoffman-Kim and Richard A. Hopkins

A series of valid but limited observations shaped the initial thoughts about viability of homograft valve transplants. First, the resistance to hypoxic injury by fibroblasts and fibroblast-like cells was well appreciated. It was repeatedly demonstrated that viable fibroblast cells could be harvested from cardiac valve leaflets for days following death of the donor, particularly when cold storage of the cadaver had been accomplished relatively soon following demise.[1] Additional studies demonstrated that these cells could be harvested and grown in the laboratory as well as demonstrating metabolic activity.[2] Thus the clinical usage during these early days of cold/wet storage of harvested valves was supported by the concept that these cells were alive and were protected by the cold storage and tissue culture media as long as they did not become infected. And, to a great extent, these observations were true. In addition, since the very first implants in 1962, the fact that these transplants had such good performance characteristics and durability implied to the clinicians that there must be some element of viability. However, the explant studies ultimately failed to support that concept. While the 1986 paper by O'Brien purported to demonstrate at least one cell that was of donor origin (based on chromosomal studies of different sex, donor and recipient) the images published in the paper actually demonstrate a matrix fairly barren of cells.[3,4] There was also the concept of immune privilege in which clinicians felt that because the leaflet matrix cells were buried in a collagen matrix

that they weren't necessarily exposed to the blood stream and immune attack. However, clearly the base of the leaflets were revascularized and the wall of the conduits underwent immune rejection and foreign body-type reaction with ultimate fibrosis and calcification. The concept that the immune response did not routinely destroy the leaflets became well entrenched as a peculiar advantage of unmatched allograft valve transplants. In sum, the operating concepts of the 1980s incorporated the following thoughts:

1. When cardiac valves were harvested within a reasonable time after death and particularly with good cold storage of the cadaver, there were viable cells at the time of implantation.
2. Formal DMSO cryopreservation enhanced viability at the time of implantation.
3. Viability was a good thing in that it apparently (in most cases) did not engender an immune response, yet teleologically, seemed to be advantageous for valve durability.

The alternative theory was suggested that the valve leaflet viability at the time of implantation suggested excellent handling of the tissues with perhaps better retention of the cellular matrix components and that it was not the viability *per se* that confirmed medium term durability characteristics. Evidence for this was that no study suggested that increased quantitative viability had any kind of positive correlation with durability and the limited explant studies which were available did not seem to support long-term cell survival.[5–10] In addition, studies

TABLE 17.1. Tests for Cell Viability.

Test	Test Characteristics	Determinants of Test	Advantages of Test	Disadvantages of Test	References
Light Microscopy	Observe cells with light microscope	Cell volume changes can indicate death, cytocellular changes also indicate damage	Easy, cheap, can assess living cells, can observe state of each cell	Potentially transient nature of morphological changes, need dispersed cells	11–13
Electron Microscopy	Examine cell ultrastructure via transmission electron microscopy	Ultrastructural characteristics associated with reversible and irreversible injury, including mitochondrial flocculant densities, karyolysis, membrane disruption	Can observe state of each cell	Need to assess many cells, only for fixed cells, may not reflect subtle changes until late.	14
In Vitro Proliferation Studies	Observe cells in culture, count cells	Ability to reproduce in culture	Simple, sensitive, easy to quantify	Need single cells, sterile cultures. Need to wait days/weeks to assess	15–19
Dye Exclusion Test	Damaged membrane allows large charged molecules that cell normally excludes to access inside of cell	Exclude dyes (Trypan blue, Propidium iodide) = viable	Rapid evaluation, large numbers, good statistical accuracy	Membrane damage is not always the first sign of damage. Doesn't detect damage until overt membrane damage has occurred.	20–23
Dye Inclusion Test	Molecules quickly diffuse in; are cleaved to an impermeable, charged molecule	Undamaged cells retain labeled molecule (fluorescein diacetate)	Rapid evaluation, large numbers, good statistical accuracy	Membrane damage is not always the first sign of damage. Doesn't detect damage until overt membrane damage has occurred.	24
^{3}H Thymidine Incorporation	Autoradiography of liquid scintillation counting	Number of silver grains per cells reflect DNA synthesis	Can observe status of groups or individual cells	Can only measure in reproductively dividing populations	25
^{3}H Hypoxanthine Incorporation	Autoradiography of liquid scintillation counting	Number of silver grains per cells reflect RNA synthesis	Can observe status of groups or individual cells	Can only measure in reproductively dividing populations	26
Glucose Metabolism	Measure glucose incorporation or 2-Deoxy-D-Glucose	Viable cells utilize glucose	Rapid, no specialized equipment, non-destructive, quantifiable	Indirect assessment of one molecule used by the cell; cell may not synthesize all other necessary molecules	26,27
Amino Acid Incorporation	Protein synthesis	Cells that synthesize proteins (with proline) are deemed viable	Rapid, no specialized equipment, non-destructive, quantifiable, prolene is found in collagen	Indirect assessment of one molecule used by the cell; cell may not synthesize all other necessary molecules	2,17,19,25,26,28–30
Intermediate Metabolism	NMR, HPLC used to measure ATP, TAN	ATP, TAN levels compared to known healthy tissue	Can evaluate overall metabolic state of a group of cells in one experiment	Decreased levels do not necessarily mean dead cells. Cannot tell which cells are affected.	31–34

by a number of groups suggested that the cryopreservation process, while effective in maintaining significant population of seemingly "viable" cells, was not really innocuous and did exact a tremendous metabolic toll. Thus viability at the time of implantation would not necessarily correlate with prolonged donor cell viability.

During this era, many different tests of viability were used, each of which had its own advantages but none were perfect in terms of defining an ultimate or true viability. Tests which were used are listed in Table 17.1.

Each of the tests of viability had distinctive advantages and disadvantages and clearly, to obtain a coherent picture, multiple tests would be required. In addition, tests of viability at the time of implantation of a valve do not necessarily predict prolonged cell survival. This question can only be answered by chronic implant studies, both animal and human. The retention of the full phenotypic expression capacity of these cells, now known to be myofibroblasts, obviously requires multiple tests as a retention of fibroblasts capable only of scar formation (collagen type III). Secretory function, no matter how many cells are present, would not be retention of a native population with leaflet characteristics.

Ultimately, our own definition of viability includes the following components:

1. Morphologic cellular integrity retained.
2. Characteristic phenotypic expression of the cells appropriate to their location in the valve leaflet cell retained, including secretory and contractile components of the myofibroblasts.
3. Mitotic potential in individual cells.
4. Retained ability by the population of cells to regenerate an appropriate cell density, tissue morphology and functional capacity.
5. Ability of the cell population to accomplish growth of the tissue (size and density) and to remodel the tissue in response to appropriate stimuli (e.g. changing hemodynamics of hypertension resulting in thicker leaflets due to increased collagen synthesis).

References

1. Khan AA, Gonzalez-Lavin L. Viability assessment of allograft values by autoradiography. Yale J Biol Med 1976;49:347–350.
2. VanDerKamp AWM, Nauta J. Fibroblast function and the maintenance of aortic valve matrix. J Cardiovasc Res 1979;13:167–172.
3. O'Brien MF, Stafford EG, Gardner MA, Pohlner PG, McGiffin DC. A comparison of aortic valve replacement with viable cryopreserved and fresh allograft valves, with a note on chromoso-

mal studies. J Thorac Cardiovasc Surg 1987; 94:812–823.
4. O'Brien MF, Stafford G, Gardner M, Pohlner P, McGiffin D, Johnston N, Brosnan A, Duffy P. The viable cryopreserved allograft aortic valve. J Card Surg 1987;2:153–167.
5. Mitchell RN, Jonas RA, Schoen FJ. Pathology of explanted cryopreserved allograft heart valves: comparison with aortic valves from orthotopic heart transplants. J Thorac Cardiovasc Surg 1998;115:118–127.
6. Hilbert SL, Luna RE, Zhang J, et al. Allograft heart valves: assessment of cell viability by confocal microscopy. Circulation 1997;96(suppl): I508.
7. Mitchell RN, Jonas RA, Schoen F. Structure-function correlations in cryopreserved allograft cardiac valves. Ann Thorac Surg 1995;60:8108–8133.
8. Schoen FJ, Mitchell RN, Jonas RA. Pathological considerations in cryopreserved allograft heart valves. J Heart Valve Dis 1995;4:S72–S76.
9. Ferrans VJ, Arbustini E, Eidbo EE, et al. Anatomic changes in right ventricular-pulmonary artery conduits implanted in baboons. In Bodnar E, Yacoub M (eds). Biologic and Bioprosthetic Valves. New York, NY: Yorke 1986:316.
10. Gavin JB, Herdson PB, Monro JL, Barratt-Boyes BG. Pathology of antibiotic-treated human heart valve allografts. Thorax 1973;28:473–481.
11. Gavin JB, Barratt-Boyes BG, Hitchcock GC, Herdson PB. Histopathology of "fresh": human aortic valve allografts. Thorax 1973;28:482–487.
12. Van der Kamp A, Visser W, Van Dongen J, et al. Preservation of aortic heart valves with maintainence of cell viability. J Surg Res 1981;30:47–56.
13. Rajotte RV, Shnitka TK, Liburd EM, Dossetor JB, Voss WAG. Histological Studies on Cultured Canine Heart Valves Recovered from -196 C. Cryobiology 1977;14:15–22.
14. Crescenzo DG, Hilbert SL, Messier JrRH, Domkowski PW, Barrick MK, Lange PL, Ferrans V, Wallace RB, Hopkins RA. Human cryopreserved allografts: Electron microscopic analysis of cellular injury. Ann Thorac Surg 1993;55:25–31.
15. Messier RH, Bass BL, Aly HM. Dual structural and functional phenotypes of the porcine aortic valve interstitial characteristics of the leaflet myofibroblast. J Surg Res 1994;57:1–21.
16. Filip DA, Radu A, Simionescu M. Interstitial Cells of the Heart Valves Possess Characteristics

Similar to Smooth Muscle Cells. Circulation Research 1986;59:310–319.

17. Henney AM, Parker DJ, Devies MS. Estimation of protein and DNA synthesis in allograft organ cultures as a measure of cell viability. Cardiovascular Research 1980;14:154–160.

18. Reichenbach DD, Mohri H, Sands M, Merendino KA. Viability of connective tissue cells following storage of aortic valve leaflets. J Thorac Cardiovasc Surg 1971;62:690–693.

19. McGregor CGA, Bradley JF, McGee J, Wheatley DJ. Tissue culture protein and collagen synthesis in antibiotic sterilized canine heart valves. Cardiovasc Res 1976;10:389–397.

20. Evans HM, Schuleman W. The action of vital stains belonging to the benzodine group. Science 1914;35:443–454.

21. Pappenheimer AM. Experimental studies upon lymphocytes. Journal of Experimental Medicine 1917;25:633–640.

22. Pavlik EJ, Flanagan RC, Van Nigell JR, Hanson MB, Donaldson ES, Keaton KK, Doss B, Bartmas J, Denady DE. Esterase activity, exclusion of propidium iodide, and proliferation in tumor cells exposed to anticancer agents: phemomena relavent to chomosensitivity determination. Cancer Investigation 1985;3:413–420.

23. Funa K, Dawson N, Jewett BP, Agren H, Ruckdeschel JC, Bunn PA, Gazdar AS. Automated fluoroescent analysis for drug-induced cytotoxicity assays. Cancer Treatment Reports 1986;70:1147–1151.

24. Rotman B, Papermaster BW. Membrane properties of living mammalian cells as studied by enzymatic hydrolysis of fluorogenic esters. Proceedings of the National Academy of Sciences USA 1966;55:134–141.

25. Mochtar B, Van der Kamp A, Roza-DeJong E, Nauta J. Cell Survival in canine aortic heart valves stored in nutrient medium. Cardiovasc Res 1974;18:497.

26. Brockbank KG, Dawson PE. Influence of whole heart postprocurement cold ischemia time upon cryopreserved heart valve viability. Transplant Proc 1993;25:3188–3189.

27. Watts LK, Duffy P, Field RB, Stafford EG, O'Brien MF. Establishment of a viable homograft cardiac valve bank: a rapid method of determining homograft viability. Ann Thorac Surg 1976;21:230–236.

28. Hu J, Gilmer L, Wolfinbarger L, Hopkins RA. Assessment of cellular viability in cardiovascular tissue as studied with 3 H-proline and 3 H-inulin. Cardiovasc Res 1990;24:528–531.

29. Al-Janabi N, Gibson K, Rose J, Ross DN. Protein synthesis in fresh aortic and pulmonary value allografts as an additional test for viability. Cardiovasc Res 1973;7:247–250.

30. VanDerKamp AWM, Visser WJ, van Dongan JM, Nauta J, Galjaard H. Preservation of aortic heart valves with maintenance of cell viability. J Surg Res 1981;30:47.

31. Domkowski PW, Messier RH, Crescenzo DG, Aly HA, Abd-Elfattah AS, Hilbert SL, Wallace RB, Hopkins RA. Preimplantation Alteration of Adenine Nucleotides in Cryopreserved Heart Valves. Ann Thorac Surg 1993;55:1–7.

32. St. Louis J, Corcoran P, Rajan S, Conte J, Wolfinbarger L, Hu J, Lange PL, Wang YN, Hilbert SL, Analouei A. Effects of warm ischemia following harvesting of allograft cardiac valves. EJCTS 1991;5:458–64; discus.

33. Messier R, Jr., Domkowski P, Hopkins RA, Aly H, Wallace R, et al. High energy phosphate depletion in leaflet matrix cells during processing of cryopreserved heart valves. J Surg Res 1992;52:483–488.

34. Messier RH, Domkowski DW, Aly HM, Hilbert SL, Crescenzo DG, Hopkins RA, et al. Adenine nucleotide depletion in cryopreserved human cardiac valves: the "stunned" leaflet interstitial cell population. Cryobiology 1995;32:199–208.

18
Factors Affecting Cellular Viability During Preimplantation Processing

Richard A. Hopkins, Diane Hoffman-Kim, Robert H. Messier, Jr., and Patrick W. Domkowski

Extensive clinical durability of allograft valves has long been suggested to be linked to cellular viability and extracellular matrix integrity at the time of implantation.[1-3] Efforts to standardize processing procedures for valve transplantation and optimize the longevity of the valves provided the original impetus for researchers to examine the effects of each processing step. This chapter focuses on the series of studies that resulted from this work. As reviewed in the previous section, viability can be evaluated in a number of ways, depending on which parameters are of interest for the study. In this chapter, we summarize the results using various methodologies to assess the health of leaflet cells following preimplantation processing.

Porcine Cardiac Valve Leaflet Studies

Initial studies noted that clinical harvesting of allograft heart valves necessitates a time period of warm ischemia, corresponding to the time from cessation of donor heartbeat to the time of transport. Leaflet cell metabolic response to varying warm ischemic time intervals was characterized in porcine aortic valve leaflets by magnetic resonance spectroscopy (Figure 18.1).[4] Two hours following donor death, aerobic metabolism ceased, as evidenced by total depletion of adenosine triphosphate (ATP), no phosphorus production, and signifi-

cant lactate accumulation; these results suggest that oxidative phosphorylation stopped, high energy phosphate stores were depleted, and metabolism was converted to anaerobic processes. At 24 hours, proline incorporation ended, signifying that protein synthesis had ceased. Between 24 and 36 hours after death, lactate production ceased, showing that anaerobic metabolism had stopped, and most cells exhibited ultrastructural evidence of irreversible cellular injury.

Initial ischemia may be only one factor in the series of valve preparation steps that leads cumulatively to interstitial cell injury. After variable ischemic times, cardiac valves undergo two additional steps prior to transplantation: antibiotic disinfection and cryopreservation. Early metabolic markers of cellular injury were assessed biochemically via high performance liquid chromatography (HPLC) analysis of components of the adenine nucleotide pool.[5] This cascade of high-energy phosphates and purine byproducts is a dynamic metabolic pathway with elements that react quickly to metabolic changes and respond with substrate deprivation or enzymatic inhibition. The aims of this study were to define the reduction in energy reserves of leaflet cells during the initial phases of processing-associated injury, and to determine if such damage might be reversible. These changes in phosphate metabolism may ultimately lead to changes in energy-dependent cell functions including proliferation, protein transport, and synthesis (Figure 18.2). While variable periods of ischemia were examined,

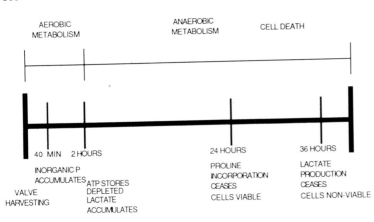

FIGURE 18.1. Progression of porcine aortic valve leaflet metabolic state in response to increasing ischemic time. Phosphorus accumulates significantly following 40 minutes post harvest warm ischemia. Metabolism becomes anaerobic after two hours, as shown by depletion of ATP reserves and accumulation of lactate. Viable cells persist with anaerobic metabolism, up to 24–36 hours.

the maximal 24-hour period of harvest ischemia did not fully deplete ATP or total adenine nucleotides (TAN). Subsequent pre-implantation processing steps of disinfection and cryopreservation decreased ATP and TAN following any ischemic interval, with the greatest damage following the longest ischemic time of 24 hours. However, even under the most stressful conditions, leaflet cells maintain significant metabolic capacity, as evidenced by residual high energy phosphate reserves.

A subsequent series of experiments was performed to separate out further the individual effects of the warm ischemic time, cold ischemic time, antibiotic treatment, and cryopreservation steps on cells' metabolic states (Table 18.1) (Figure 18.3).[6] As demonstrated in the previous study, warm ischemic times up to 24 hours did not appear to have significant detrimental effects on porcine aortic valve leaflet cells. Following an additional 24 hour cold ischemic time, there was a 17% reduction in ATP, and

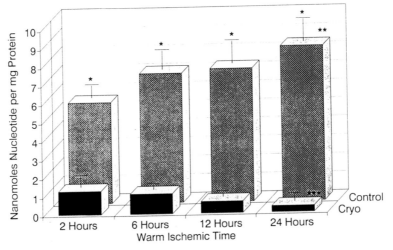

FIGURE 18.2. Total adenine nucleotides ([TAN] = [ATP] + [ADP] + [AMP]) of control leaflets (exposed to cadaveric ischemia only) and cryopreserved leaflets (cadaveric ischemia and cryopreservation processing). At each ischemic time, antibiotic treatment and cryopreservation lead to dramatic reduction in TAN. TAN of control leaflets are significantly higher after 24 hours; this accumulation may reflect ATP degradation or partial metabolic restoration through other salvage pathways. Leaflets undergoing 24 hrs ischemia and cryopreservation exhibit the largest reductions. (*P < 0.05 control versus corresponding ischemic time cryopreservation groups; **P < 0.05 control versus 2 hr controls; ***P < 0.05 in 24 hr cryopreserved versus 2 and 6 hr cryopreserved groups). CRYO, cryopreserved.

TABLE 18.1. Levels of Metabolites (nmol/mg Protein)[a] Following Each Leaflet Processing Phase.

	Group I (WIT only)	Group II (WIT + 24h 4°C Ischemia)	Group III (WIT + 24h 4°C Antibiotic Disinfection)	Group IV (WIT + 4°C Ischemia + Cryopreservation)	Group V (WIT + 4°C Disinfection + Cryopreservation)
ATP	1.78 ± 0.25	1.48 ± 0.12	0.91 ± 0.13[b]	0.46 ± 0.11[b]	0.25 ± 0.04[b]
ADP	0.59 ± 0.07	0.55 ± 0.05	0.33 ± 0.07	0.27 ± 0.05	0.25 ± 0.03
AMP	0.40 ± 0.10	0.78 ± 0.21	1.00 ± 0.40	0.14 ± 0.07	0.18 ± 0.07
Adenosine	0.18 ± 0.06	1.20 ± 0.29	6.10 ± 3.50	0.52 ± 0.10	3.10 ± 0.70
Inosine	1.50 ± 0.30	0.72 ± 0.20	0.87 ± 0.20	0.50 ± 0.50	0.71 ± 0.13
Hypoxanthine	1.70 ± 0.25	0.78 ± 0.16	0.73 ± 0.24	0.12 ± 0.06	0.07 ± 0.03
Xanthine	0.00 ± 0.00	1.10 ± 0.63	0.10 ± 0.08	0.09 ± 0.08	0.05 ± 0.04
NAD[+]	0.50 ± 0.04	0.33 ± 0.04	0.29 ± 0.12	0.07 ± 0.04	0.23 ± 0.04

[a] Adenine nucleotide metabolite concentrations (± standard error of the mean) existing at the completion of each step of preimplantation processing. [b] $p < 0.05$ vs. group I by analysis of variance. ADP = adenosine diphosphate; AMP = adenosine monophosphate; ATP = adenosine triphosphate; NAD[+] = nicotinamide adenine dinucleotide, oxidized form; WIT = warm ischemia.

evidence that ATP degraded only to ADP and AMP, perhaps because ATP was not broken down completely or was partly restored through other pathways. Cold antibiotic disinfection reduced the leaflets' ATP by almost 50%, while increasing purine byproducts 55%; thus, half of the ATP was broken down to ADP and AMP, and the TAN partly degraded to adenosine, inosine, hypoxanthine, and xanthine. These results suggest that most of the degraded ATP was broken down in a reversible way; this is important since maintaining total high energy phosphates (not just ATP) is crucial to a cell's basal functional capacity. Of all the processing steps, however, cryopreservation is responsible for the largest reduction in ATP (74%). The consequences of the cryopreservation step

augment the effects of cold ischemic and antibiotic disinfection. Therefore, in the effort to balance beneficial processing steps with detrimental ones, antibiotic treatment appears to be a useful step; it does not have a high relative metabolic cost in the overall cryopreservation process. All steps in the processing were synergistic in their reduction of the adenine nucleotide pool. However, even after the complete harvesting and cryopreservation processing, some leaflet cells maintained quantifiable high-energy phosphates. This correlated with the morphologic studies in suggesting that some cells were able to tolerate processing-related stresses.

Because leaflet cells appeared to retain some metabolic capacity following processing, treat-

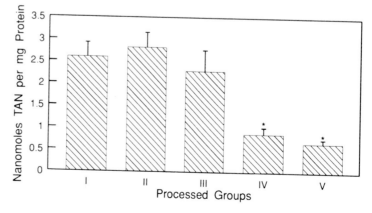

FIGURE 18.3. Total adenine nucleotides ([TAN] = [ATP] + [ADP] + [AMP]) measured after each step in leaflet processing; (I) warm ischemia, (II) cold transport, (III) antibiotic disinfection, (IV) cryopreservation, and (V) cryopreservation with antibiotics. (*P < versus groups I, II, III.)

ment with inhibitors of adenosine deaminase and nucleoside transport was explored in an attempt to salvage adenosine pools and as validation of the degradation observations (Figure 18.4 and 18.5).[7] HPLC showed that with minimal ischemic times (40 minutes) the processing steps of disinfection and cryopreservation independently disrupt the ATP-ADP cycle. However, treatment with restitution therapy maintained nucleotide levels at baseline harvest concentrations, and so such agents may be able to protect leaflet cells from catabolism, as is possible in myocardium. This study provided

further evidence that although injured, the entire valve leaflet cell population does not become metabolically inert following ischemia and processing, and in fact, cumulative metabolic damage may be minimized via adenine nucleotide protection.

The HPLC series of experiments served to demonstrate profound energy store depletion yet some potential for manipulation of the metabolic pathways. Without such protection and in fact by using the harvesting and processing protocols contemporary in the 1980s and 1990s, these experiments suggested that

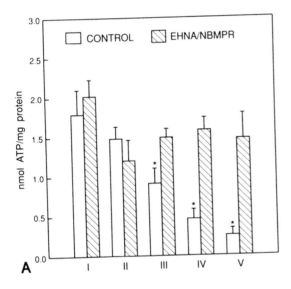

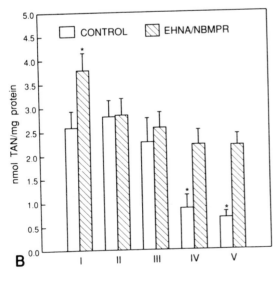

FIGURE 18.4. Adenine nucleotide levels in control valves and in valves treated with restitution therapy consisting of the nucleoside transport inhibitor p-nitrobenzy-thioinosine (NBMPR) and the adenosine deaminase inhibitor erythro-9 (2 hydroxy—3-nonyl) adenine (EHNA). (A) ATP levels. Significant reductions are seen following disinfection (control group III), cryopreservation after warm and cold ischemia only (control group IV), and cryopreservation after warm ischemia and cold disinfection (control group V). EHNA/NBMPR-treated groups showed prevention of ATP loss (*p < 0.05 versus control group I and corresponding EHNA/NBMPR-treated group). (B) Total adenine nucleotide levels ([TAN] = [ATP] + [ADP] + [AMP]). Disinfection processing (group III) did not result in significant depletion of TAN as it did with ATP. This likely reflects an early phase of processing-associated damage with respect to phosphorylated adenine nucleotides. Processing steps in groups IV and V did lead to significant losses in TAN, which were prevented by EHNA/NBMPR treatment (*p < 0.05 versus control group I).

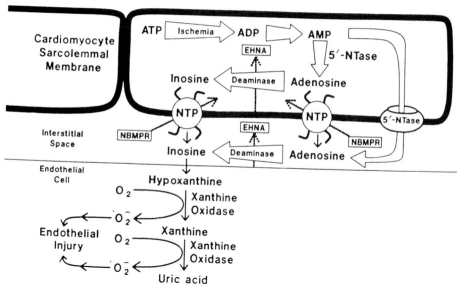

FIGURE 18.5. Diagram of biochemical pathways and active sites of EHNA/NBMPR. Nucleoside transport protein (NTP) facilitates adenosine and inosine export. NBMPR allows intracellular retention of adenosine. EHNA competes with adenosine deami-nase to inhibit it both within the cell and extracellularly. Adenosine hydrolysis to adenosine is almost completely prevented, leading to "restitution": increases in phosphorylated adenine nucleotides by reversal of the degradation pathway.

while many cells might be morphologically intact at the time of implantation, they were likely "doomed" to early death simply from metabolic depletion.

Human Cryopreserved Cardiac Valve Homografts

To determine if the response of human leaflet cells to clinical pre-implantation processing was similar to that observed in porcine valves, a series of human valves was subjected to the following: a warm ischemic interval in the donor of between 0 and 20 hours, followed by 24 hours of cold antibiotic disinfection, then cryopreservation. It is important to note that each human valve was originally intended for transplantation, and was included in the study only when it was deemed unsuitable, typically for anatomical reasons. Because of its initial designation, each valve in the study underwent the complete series of cryopreservation processing steps, in contrast to the processing in much of the com-parative work on porcine valves. The effects of these processing steps on cell metabolic state and ultrastructure were assessed with HPLC and electron microscopy (Figure 18.6).[8,9] Warm ischemic intervals of less than 2 hours resulted in virtually no evidence of damage at the ultrastructural level. Generally, the longer the ischemic time interval, the greater the extent of cellular injury. Ultrastructural changes providing evidence of damage gradually increased over time from endoplasmic reticulum dilatation, cytoplasmic edema, and mitochondrial swelling, to mitochondrial flocculent densities, karolysis, and plasma membrane disruption. Up to 12 hours of warm ischemia, cells exhibited morphology reflecting mostly reversible cellular injury, with minimal ultrastructural evidence of irreversible injury. However, after 12 hours, evidence of irreversible damage increased dramatically, and the amount of injury correlated with increased warm ischemic time. Following 20 hours of warm ischemia, 80% of the cells were injured. In contrast, in porcine valves subjected to warm ischemia but no other processing, ultrastructural evidence of irreversible

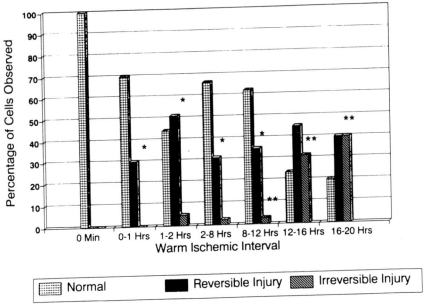

FIGURE 18.6. Percentage of human aortic valve leaflet cells exhibiting normal ultrastructure of evidence of reversible or irreversible cellular injury. Time intervals of warm ischemia for each group are noted on the x-axis. Cochran-Mantel-Haenszel trend analysis demonstrates a positive correlation (*p < 0.0001) for reversible injury during the first 12 hours of warm ischemic time and a positive correlation (**p < 0.001) between 12 and 20 hours of warm ischemia for irreversible cellular injury.

cellular injury manifested later than in this study's human valves—detectable only after 24 hours of warm ischemia. Taken together, these studies suggest that post-ischemia processing steps contribute substantially to cellular damage in human cryopreserved homografts.

The total adenine nucleotide depletion was substantial at harvest ischemic times greater than 2 hours (Table 18.2; Figure 18.7).[9] ATP depletion was similar to that observed in porcine experiments, and in 76% of the valves, ATP, ADP, and AMP were undetectable. Increased levels of catabolites confirmed that energy consumption was extremely high, and depletion occurred predominantly during pre-implantation processing rather than during harvest associated ischemic time.

Another assay of membrane integrity and metabolic activity, measurement of 3H-2deoxyglucose phosphorylation, has been used to evaluate human leaflets after cryopreservation.[10] Cryopreservation processing steps as described above resulted in a 30% decrease in phosphorylation as compared to fresh valves. This decrease could be partially reversed by incubating the valves at 37°C prior to transplantation.

These experiments supported the concept of a "stunned" leaflet cell population following processing, a population of cells devoid of energy reserves and thus at high risk for cell death, during the stress of transition following implantation. These findings possibly explained the potentially conflicting data that purported to show excellent cell "viability" as defined by morphology but contrasted with sparse cellularity at leaflet explants.[2,11]

Resuscitation of Leaflet Cells

Taken together, the work of other researchers and our own studies of porcine and human valves provided evidence that pre-implantation processing had significant detrimental effects on leaflet interstitial cell viability and functionality. The work also demonstrated consistently that a few robust cells remain following

TABLE 18.2. Metabolic Concentrations of the Adenine Nucleotide Pool (Individually Eluted, nmol Metabolite/ng Leaflet Protein) in Cryopreserved Human Valves.

Valve	WIT	Type	Donor Age/Sex	Cause of Donor Death	Reason Rejected	ATP	ADP	AMP	ADO	INO	HX	X	Urate	NAD$^+$
1	<1	Aortic	5/M	Suffocation	+Cx	0	0	0	1.870	0	0	0	0	0
2	<1	Aortic	46/F	Multiple trauma	+Cx	0.355	0.266	0	1.060	0.887	0	0	0	0.266
3	<1	Aortic	9/M	Multiple trauma	+Cx	0	0.442	0.737	2.500	1.470	0	0	0	0
4	1	Aortic	49/F	Multiple trauma	+Cx	0.404	0.101	0.908	1.410	1.110	0	0	0	0.303
5	1	Pulmonic	33/F	Multiple trauma	TE	0	0.327	0.762	0.544	0.436	0	0	0	0
6	1	Aortic	11/F	Multiple trauma	TE	0.663	0.663	1.330	0.663	0.442	0	0	0	0.221
7	3	Pulmonic	18/M	Multiple trauma	Ann.hem.	0	0	0	2.220	0.910	0	0	0	0
8	4	Pulmonic	2/M	Multiple trauma	TE	0	0	0	1.240	0.742	0	0	0	0
9	4	Aortic	14/M	Multiple trauma	+Cx	0	0	0	0.271	1.080	0.452	0	0	0.181
10	4	Aortic	44/F	Multiple trauma	TE	0	0	0	0	2.280	0	0	0	0
11	6	Aortic	8/M	CHI/MVA	SD	0	0	0	0	0	0	0	0	0
12	6	Aortic	3/F	CHI/MVA	TE	0.351	0	0	2.072	0.777	0	0	0	0.259
13	7	Aortic	40/F	MI	+Cx	0	0	0	1.520	0	0	0	0	0.234
14	8	Pulmonic	40/F	MI	+Cx	0	0	0	0.940	0.416	0	0	0	0.195
15	9	Aortic	33/F	MI	+Cx	0	0	0	0.584	0.973	0	0	0	0.173
16	9	Pulmonic	33/F	MI	+Cx	0.433	0	0	0.433	0	0	0	0	0.169
17	9	Aortic	7/M	CHI/MVA	+Cx	0	0.169	0	0.674	0.590	0	0	0	0
18	10	Pulmonic	7/M	CHI/MVA	+Cx	0	0	0	0.420	0.737	0	0	0	0
19	11	Pulmonic	47/M	Multiple trauma	+Cx	0.357	0	0	0.990	0.713	2.420	0	0	0.143
20	13	Aortic	23/M	Multiple trauma	+Cx	0	0	0	0.500	0	0	0	0	0
21	13	Aortic	35/M	Multiple trauma	+Cx	0	0	0	0.504	0.705	0	0	0	0.201
22	15	Aortic	16/F	Multiple trauma	+Cx	0	0	0	0.294	0	0	0	0	0
23	16	Pulmonic	19/M	Multiple trauma	+Cx	0	0	0	0.813	0	0	0	0	0
24	20	Aortic	27/M	Multiple trauma	+Cx	0	0	0	0.204	0.511	0	0	0	0
25	20	Aortic	19/F	CHI/MVA	+Cx	0	0.343	0	0.257	0.429	0	0	0	0

WIT = warm ischemic time; ATP = adenosine triphosphate; ADP = adenosine diphosphate; AMP = adenosine monophosphate; ADO = adenosine; INO = inosine; HX = hypoxanthine; X = xanthine; NAD$^+$ = nicotinamide adenine dinucleotide (oxidized form). Clinical characteristics of cryopreserved donor valves were assayed by HPLC. CHI = closed head injury; MVA = motor vehicle accident; CHF = congestive heart failure; MI = myocardial infarction; TE = technical error; +Cx = positive donor blood culture; Ann. Hem. = annular hematoma; age in years: M = male; F = female.

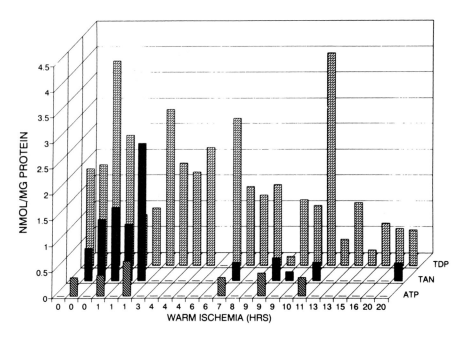

FIGURE 18.7. Depletion of adenine nucleotide pool in cryopreserved human valves. Major high energy phosphates and catabolites are only slightly retained at shorter ischemic time intervals (x-axis). This graft suggests that processing contributes more than ischemia to leaflet energy losses. Key: Σ[ATP] + [ADP] + [AMP]; TDP, Σ[adenosine] + [inosine] + [xanthine] + [hypozanthine]. Front bars, ATP; middle bars, TAN; rear bars, TDP.

ischemia, disinfection, and cryopreservation. Yet, the presence after processing of even a small number of live leaflet cells with metabolic reserves and intact healthy ultrastructure led investigators to hypothesize that perhaps leaflet cells could be resuscitated prior to implantation (for review see Chapter 14). In fact, incubation of cryopreserved porcine aortic valves in organ culture (37°C, media with 15% serum) for 8 days prior to implantation was able to restore the normal LIC population and matrix composition to the leaflets (Figure 18.8).[12]

Ovine Implant Model

The preceding body of work has provided a careful analysis of the effects of pre-implantation processing on various aspects of leaflet viability, and furthered our understanding of the state of the leaflet at the time of implantation. Of ultimate importance is the state of the valves, especially the state of the cells and matrix, while in the recipient. Another recent study has examined leaflet cellularity after implantation into a chronic ovine model, with a specific focus on the mechanisms responsible for cell loss.[13] This study has specifically addressed the hypothesis that apoptosis may be the mechanism underlying the acellularity seen in implanted aortic allograft valves. In an ovine model, fresh and cryopreserved aortic valves were examined following implantation times ranging between 2 days and 20 weeks. Leaflet interstitial cells exhibited losses in proliferating cell nuclear antigen (a marker of mitotic function) as well as positive nick end labeling, nuclear condensation, pyknosis, and formation of apoptotic bodies containing remnants of nuclear material. This evidence of mitotic cessation and apoptosis was detectable by 2 days following implantation. It reached a peak at 10–14 days, and by 20 weeks, grafts were completely acellular.

The cell state of human cryopreserved allograft valves and valves of transplanted hearts

FIGURE 18.8. Viable leaflet interstitial cells. Cells were released from leaflets by collagenase digestion, and viability was assessed via Trypan blue exclusion. Groups: Ischemia – warm ischemia only. Processing – ischemia + disinfection + cryopreservation. Restoration – processing + organ culture, M199 15% FBS, 37°C, 8 days. Processing significantly reduced cell numbers, but restoration treatment led to dramatic repopulation of the leaflets.

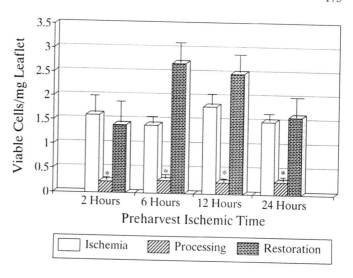

that did not undergo cryopreservation have recently been compared by Mitchell et al., 1998.[14] Explanted allograft valves displayed decreased cellularity, with morphological similarities to the valves of this study. In distinct contrast, aortic valves of orthotopically transplanted hearts maintained normal cellularity and morphology. Pre-implantation processing of allograft valves differs from that for heart allografts in that it contains periods of hypoxia, disinfection, and cryopreservation; this work gives further support to the idea that valve processing contributes to the loss of leaflet cellularity and the development of apoptosis, as well as possibly implicating an immune component.

Conclusion

The metabolic and morphological studies from the our laboratory have defined a severely stressed population of donor cells. Such metabolic "stunning" is by itself likely inconsistent with survival for a large fraction of the cell population unless some intervention is made prior, during, or after transplantation. The apoptosis findings suggest that this stress could result in limited long-term viability by two mechanisms. First, the early phase cell survival is likely low following transplantation due to the limited cellular energy reserves. Second, either the stress of pre-implantation processing or the abnormal environment in which the injured matrix cells

find themselves following transplantation (in particular, no native endothelium) triggers the apoptosis sequence. This could fit with some observations of moderate matrix and cellular viability early after implantation. Means by which to promote and augment valve viability in the recipient remain to be fully developed, and successful initial efforts at resuscitation through organ culture lend an optimistic note to these efforts. However, mere retention of donor cells may allow for preservation of synthetic function for a time following transplantation. These retained cells could restore matrix components and thus initially enhance physical leaflet characteristics and by this actually improve durability. This potential value of retained donor cells has to be balanced against the negative effects of provoking an immune response (*vida infra*). Cell loss by apoptosis may be preferable to necrosis as the former process is by definition non-inflammatory while necrotic cell debris are both extremely inflammatory and antigenic and could lead to accelerated degeneration, fibrosis and calcification of the transplanted allograft valve tissues.

References

1. Lockey E, Al-Janabi N, Gonzalez-Lavin L, Ross DNA. Method of sterilizing and preserving fresh allograft heart valves. Thorax 1972;27:398.
2. O'Brien MF, Stafford G, Gardner M, Pohlner P, McGiffin D, Johnston N, Brosnan A, Duffy P.

The viable cryopreserved allograft aortic valve. J Card Surg 1987;2:153–167.

3. VanDerKamp A.W.M., Nauta J. Fibroblast function and the maintenance of aortic valve matrix. J Cardiovasc Res 1979;13:167–172.

4. St. Louis J, Corcoran P, Rajan S, Conte J, Wolfinbarger L, Hu J, Lange PL, Wang YN, Hilbert SL, Analouei A. Effects of warm ischemia following harvesting of allograft cardiac valves. EJCTS 1991;5:458–64; discus.

5. Messier RH, Jr., Domkowski PW, Aly HM, Abd-Elfattah AS, Crescenzo DG, Wallace RB, Hopkins RA. High energy phosphate depletion in leaflet matrix cells during processing of cryopreserved cardiac valves. J Surg Res 1992; 52(No. 5):483–488.

6. Domkowski PW, Messier RH, Crescenzo DG, Aly HA, Abd-Elfattah AS, Hilbert SL, Wallace RB, Hopkins RA. Preimplantation Alteration of Adenine Nucleotides in Cryopreserved Heart Valves. Ann Thorac Surg 1993;55:1–7.

7. Abd-Elfattah AS, Messier RH, Domkowski PW, Crescenzo DG, Wallace RB, Hopkins RA. Inhibition of adenosine deaminase and nucleoside transport: utility in a model of homograft cardiac valve preimplantation processing. J Thorac Cardiovasc Surg 1993;105:1095–1105.

8. Crescenzo DG, Hilbert SL, Messier JrRH, Domkowski PW, Barrick MK, Lange PL, Ferrans V, Wallace RB, Hopkins RA. Human cryopreserved allografts: Electron microscopic analysis of cellular injury. Ann Thorac Surg 1993;55: 25–31.

9. Messier RH, Domkowski DW, Aly HM, Hilbert SL, Crescenzo DG, Hopkins RA, et al. Adenine nucleotide depletion in cryopreserved human cardiac valves: the "stunned" leaflet interstitial cell population. Cryobiology 1995;32:199–208.

10. Brockbank KGM, Dawson PE, Carpenter JF. Heart valve leaflet revitalization. Tissue and Cell Report 1993;1:18–19.

11. VanDerKamp AWM, Visser WJ, van Dongan JM, Nauta J, Galjaard H. Preservation of aortic heart valves with maintenance of cell viability. J Surg Res 1981;30:47.

12. Messier R, Bass BL, Domkowski PW, Hopkins RA. Interstitial Cellular Matrix Restoration of Cardiac Valves Following Cryopreservation. J Thorac Cardiovasc Surg 1999;118:36–49.

13. Hilbert SL, Luna RE, Zhang J, Wang Y, Hopkins RA, Yu ZX, Ferrans VJ. Allograft heart valves: the role of apoptosis-mediated cell loss. J Thorac Cardiovasc Surg 1999;117:454–462.

14. Mitchell RN, Jonas RA, Schoen FJ. Pathology of explanted cryopreserved allograft heart valves: comparison with aortic valves from orthotopic heart transplants. J Thorac Cardiovasc Surg 1998;115:118–127.

19
Cell Origins and Fates Following Transplantation of Cryopreserved Allografts

M.G. Hazekamp, D.R. Koolbergen, J. Braun, J.A. Bruin, C.J. Cornelisse, Y.A. Goffin, and J.A. Huysmans

Efforts in preservation of allograft heart valves aim at remaining cellular viability. Viability in this respect always means fibroblast viability as endothelial cells are almost completely lost in the sequence of dissection, sterilization, cryopreservation, thawing and implantation.[1,2] Cryopreservation is now considered to be the method of choice of allograft heart valve preservation and banking. Cellular viability after cryopreservation has been well documented.[3–5] The length of donor ischemia time is one of the factors that influence the quantity and quality of remaining viable donor cells.[6,7] Cytotoxicity of antibiotics and DMSO, and to a lesser degree cryopreservation itself also are of negative influence on cellular viability.[8–10]

The fate of the donor cells after allograft implantation has been object of discussion. It has been stated that the presence of viable donor cells after implantation is essential for graft function and longevity. Viable donor cells were believed to play a key role in maintaining the integrity of matrix and fiber structures in the valve leaflets.[3,11] The number of publications contradicting this theory is increasing. Explant studies commonly show little or no cellularity.[2,12,13] Furthermore, the presumed presence of viable donor cells increases antigenicity, which is thought to be detrimental to allograft function and longevity.[13–15]

Cellular elements presenting in explanting allografts may be of donor or recipient origin. Before questions concerning the role of surviving donor cells can be answered we must be able to distinguish between donor and recipients cells. The origin of fibroblasts and other cells in allograft explants can be determined if a sex difference between donor and recipient is present. Many techniques are dependent on tissue culture. Demonstration of Barr bodies in cultured fibroblasts is another sex-related technique that has been used to demonstrate the presence of remaining donor fibroblasts.[11] DNA fingerprinting is a third method to distinguish between donor and recipient cells. DNA fingerprinting can distinguish between cells without the need of a sex difference.[2] These three techniques (Barr body demonstration, chromosome banding and DNA fingerprinting) share one major disadvantage: They cannot be used to determine cell origin on location. Thus, the presence or absence of donor and recipient cells can be confirmed in allograft explants but morphology, number distribution and localization of these cells will remain unknown.

The above listed disadvantages can be overcome with the aid of *in situ* hybridization. If a sex mismatch between donor and recipient is present, DNA *in situ* hybridization for the Y chromosome can reliably distinguish between donor and recipient cells on location, that is in the tissue sections. Sensitivity and specificity of this technique are high. As this method can be applied on location, the morphology and distribution of donor and recipient cells can be established.

Semi-quantitative estimation of both donor and recipient cell populations can be obtained. Using a DNA probe for the porcine Y chromosome we were able to determine accurately the origin and localization of both donor and recipient porcine cells in explanted porcine cryopreserved aortic allograft valves.[16] Analysis of human allograft explants with the aid of *in situ* hybridization for the Y chromosome has started more recently in our department.

The technique of ISH in itself cannot determine whether a cell is viable or not. Hybridization requires an intact DNA, but the fact that hybridization occurs does not necessarily mean that the cells are capable of protein synthesis. In our studies, cellular morphology was used to support the probability of viable cells.

Technique of DNA *In Situ* Hybridization for the Y Chromosome

In situ hybridization, which has its roots in the field of pathology, allows the detection of specific nucleic acid sequences in histological sections.[17] All chromosomes contain nucleic acid sequences in histological sections.[17] All chromosomes contain nucleic acid sequences that are specific for that chromosome. Detection by ISH of such Y-chromosome specific sequences in a cell nucleus demonstrates the male origin of that specific cell.

The principles of ISH are schematically outlined in Figure 19.1. DNA consists of two complementary strands of nucleic acids. First, these strands have to be separated to expose the specific nucleic acids complementary to the target sequence. Given the right circumstances, the probe DNA will bind (hybridize) to the target DNA. After this hybridization step has taken place, actual demonstration of probe presence can be achieved in several ways; we have chosen a fluorescent technique for practical purposes. First, a detectable reporter molecule has to be incorporated into the probe before starting ISH. This reporter molecule carries a protein that can be detected using specific antibodies, which in turn are coupled to a fluorescent molecule. Finally, a dye that binds to all chromosomal DNA is applied to the tissue section thereby revealing all nuclei present in the section. In our experiments we have used a green fluorescent molecule to demonstrate the Y chromosome and a red dye for nuclear counterstaining. The tissue sections can then be analyzed using a fluorescence microscope. Presence of the fluorescent signal in a cell nucleus indicates the presence of the Y chromosome specific probe and consequently that of the Y chromosome, thereby affirming its male origin. When a cell does not contain the fluorescent signal, it should be considered as of female origin. Further technical details have been described by Braun and Hazekamp.[18]

Tissue sections can be subjected both to ISH as to normal HE staining. In this way, both origin and morphology of the cellular elements can be determined on location.

The technique has proven its reliability in terms of sensitivity and specificity, which theoretically may both reach 100%. In practice, for each application of ISH, optimal conditions have to be established empirically to obtain high values for both parameters.

Cell Origin in Porcine Cryopreserved Allograft Explants

Before examining human allograft explants, we studied the feasibility of establishing an ISH protocol to determine cell origin in allograft explants in a experimental setting, using a porcine model.[16] Previous experience convinced us of the usefulness of the growing young pig model for valve research purposes.[19] In a small series, three aortic grafts—one from a male pig donor, two from female pigs—were cryopreserved according to the standards for human allografts, and then implanted in the subcoronary mode in pigs of opposite sex. After five months, the animals were euthanized and the allografts were explanted, together with the native pulmonary valves that were used as a control. All valves were examined macroscopically and were then prepared for microscopic studies. The consecutive frozen sections that were made from each cusp were paired and alternately used for conventional haematoxylin-eosin staining and ISH.

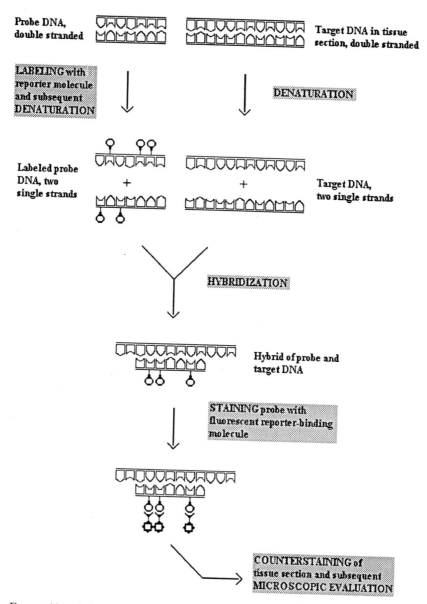

FIGURE 19.1. Schematic representation of the in situ hybridization technique.

Apart from a distinct thickening of the leaflet, which was more pronounced at the hinge area, the allograft explants in our series did not show macroscopic abnormalities.

Light microscopic evaluation of the explants revealed the presence of young, star-shaped fibroblasts located in the cuspal hinge area. In all cases, a fibrous sheathing had formed over the graft wall, extending onto the leaflets to a certain extent, being more prominent on the inflow side. Cellularity in the cusps had diminished when compared to the aspect of a native porcine aortic valve. All cusps contained several areas of varying sizes that were totally devoid of cellular components. Endothelial cells were not discovered on the leaflet surfaces.

After we had established the optimal conditions for ISH using a porcine Y chromosome specific probe, we were able to attain levels of sensitivity and specificity.

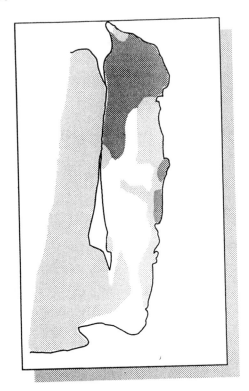

had decreased considerably. Most of these donor cells were found in distal parts of the leaflets; some leaflets also contained small isolated foci of donor cells located more proximally. When studying the same explants with HE staining techniques, we found that the donor cells all had the appearance of fibroblasts. There were no morphologic signs of cellular or nuclear lysis. In contrast to the observations made in the graft leaflets, we did not discover persisting donor cells in the graft walls.

Recipient cells were detected in all explants. They were observed to occupy the full thickness of the graft wall—apparently having replaced the donor cells—with large extensions

FIGURE 19.2. Schematic drawing of a longitudinal section through the non-coronary cusp of a porcine allograft explant (male donor, female recipient). Graft wall is shown on the right side, leaflet on the left. Dark shaded areas represent Y-positive (donor) cells, light shaded areas represent Y-negative (recipient) cells. White areas do not contain cellular elements. From Hazekamp et al.,[16] by permission of Mosby-Year Book, Inc.

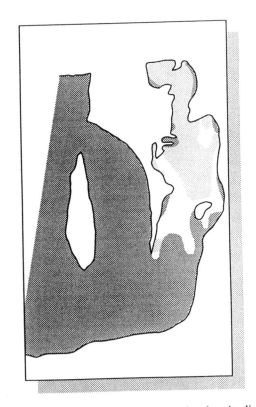

We then examined representative sections made from all aortic allograft explants, whereafter we were able to make a reliable distinction between cells that did or did not contain the Y chromosome. The presence of Y-positive and Y-negative cells was subsequently marked in schematic drawings, two of which are shown in Figures 19.2 and 19.3. Using these maps, we could establish the distribution of host and donor cells throughout the allografts. After we had studied the explants, some observations were found to be consistent as they occurred in all allografts in our series.

Five months after implantation, all cryopreserved porcine allograft explants still contained cells of donor origin, although their number

FIGURE 19.3. Schematic drawing of a longitudinal section through the left coronary cusp of a porcine allograft explant (female donor, male recipient). Graft wall is shown in the right side, leaflet on the left. Dark shaded areas represent Y-positive (recipient) cells, light shaded areas represent Y-negative (donor) cells. White areas do not contain cellular elements. From Hazekamp et al.,[16] by permission of Mosby-Year Book, Inc.

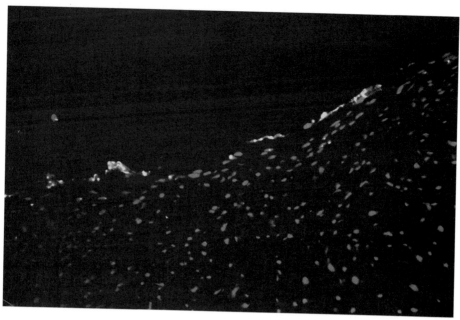

FIGURE 19.4. ISH photomicrograph of a longitudinal section through the right coronary cusp of a porcine allograft explant (female donor, male recipient). Detail from the leaflet surface, showing a sheath of green, Y-positive recipient cells growing red Y-negative remaining donor cells. Original magnifi- cation × 250. Reprinted from *Journal of Thoracic and Cardiovascular Surgery*, Vol 110, Hazenkamp et al, "In situ hybridization: a new technigue to determine the origin of fibroblasts in cryopreserved aortic homograft valve explants," 248–257. © 1995, with permission from Elsevier.

into the hinge area. In this area, we also found evidence of recipient originated neovasculariza- tion in some cases. Host cells were also seen in the fibrous sheathing; other cells were found to penetrate from these sheaths into deeper layers of the leaflet tissue, occasionally even reaching full thickness of the cusp (Figures 19.4 and 19.5; see color insert). We repeatedly observed the presence of superficially located foci of recipient cells that did not make contact with the afore- mentioned extensions, neither those extending from the graft wall nor those from the fibrous sheath. The location of these cells, which on routine light microscopy appeared to be a mixed population of fibroblasts and mononu- clear cells, suggests that they may have been blood-borne. Other host cells were fibroblasts in most cases. Mononuclears were also detected, but to a considerably lesser extent.

With this experimental study, we have estab- lished a new, reliable and reproducible method for determination of cell origin in allograft explants. Obviously, our next project focused on the adaptation of the ISH protocol to provide a comparable tool for the study of explanted human cryopreserved allografts.

Cell Origin in Human Cryopreserved Allograft Explants

The study of human allograft explants with the aid of the *in situ* hybridization technique for the Y chromosome is still under way. At the moment of writing the number of studied explants is too small to allow for definite conclusions.

To illustrate the value of DNA *in situ* hybridization (ISH) the preliminary results of ISH analysis of five human allograft explants will be discussed. Except for one, these cryop- reserved aortic and pulmonary allograft valves were explanted because of dysfunction. Mal- function was due to technical failure with para- valvular leakage in 2 explants (A and B) that were removed 6 months and 2 weeks after

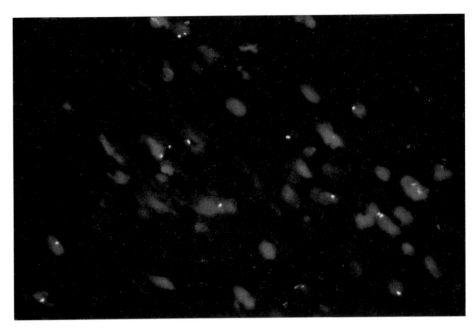

FIGURE 19.5. ISH photomicrograph of a longitudinal section through the left coronary cusp of a porcine allograft explant (female donor, male recipient). Detail from the cuspal hinge area, showing ingrowing Y-positive recipient cells amidst some Y-negative remaining donor cells. Original magnification × 640.

implantation. One pulmonary valve with important insufficiency was replaced 2 years and 4 months after first surgery (C). Noncardiac death led to explantation of an aortic allograft that had been *in situ* for 5 months (D). The fifth explant (E) was a stenotic and insufficient pulmonary allograft that had been implanted for 3 years and 10 months. In all cases a sex mismatch between donor and recipient existed. Radial tissue sections were made of allograft wall and leaflet. These sections alternately underwent HE staining for routine histologic examination and the ISH procedure.

Explant A

Explant A is an aortic allograft from a female adult (heart beating) donor. Cryopreservation was with DMSO 10% after antibiotic sterilization. The allograft was used for subcoronary aortic valve replacement in an adult male recipient with aortic valve stenosis. Six months later the allograft was explanted because of paravalvular leakage.

Macroscopy showed slightly thickened leaflets and an elastic aortic wall without calcifications. Routine HE histologic examination showed a variable but still prominent cellularity and a layer architecture that had almost disappeared. The cells appeared to be mainly myofibroblasts. Lymphocytic cellular infiltration was observed near the donor/host interface in the allograft aortic wall and leaflet base. Donor cells were strongly reduced in number and the majority of cells appeared to be of recipient origin. ISH demonstrated Y-positive (male, recipient) cells in a variable amount throughout the allograft aortic wall and in the proximal two thirds of the leaflet. On the leaflet surface and in the deeper layers areas with 80–90% of the cells showing Y-positive signals (male, recipient) could be observed. Some areas in leaflet and aortic wall, particularly those with poor cellularity, were completely Y-negative (female, donor).

Explant B

Explant B is an aortic allograft from a male adult (heart beating) donor. The allograft was DMSO cryopreserved after antibiotic sterilization. It was used for subcoronary replacement of the aortic valve in a female adult patient and had to be explanted after 2 weeks because of technical failure (paravalvular leakage).

The allograft appeared normal at macroscopic examination. Histology showed a slightly decreased cellularity with some acellular parts in the aortic wall. Trilaminar leaflet architecture has already started to blur. Some small areas on leaflet and aortic wall surface presented an increased cellularity with recipient inflammatory cells (mostly lymphocytes and macrophages). ISH showed clusters with reduced numbers of Y-positive (donor) cells in the leaflet and sporadically Y-positive cells in the aortic wall.

Explant C

Explant C is a pulmonary allograft from a male adolescent (heart beating) donor. It had been cryopreserved with DMSO 10% without previous antibiotic treatment. The allograft was used as a conduit from right ventricle to pulmonary artery in a 9 year old girl with Tetralogy of Fallot. The graft was explanted after 2 years and 4 months because of valvular insufficiency.

The arterial wall and leaflet appeared rather normal, pliable and without calcifications. The leaflets were slightly thickened and retracted, causing valvular insufficiency. The collagen was completely homogenized with disappearance of the normal layer structure. Cellularity in the atrial wall was strongly reduced. The leaflet was acellular, except for an endothelial-like monolayer of Y-negative recipient cells covering the leaflet surface. ISH showed no Y-positive (male, donor) cells. Remaining cells were of recipient origin.

Explant D

Aortic allograft explant D originated from a female adult (heart beating) donor. It was cryopreserved with DMSO 10% following antibiotic treatment and implanted in the aortic root of a male adult because of prosthetic valve endocarditis. It was explanted 5 months later, after the patient died in a car accident.

No allograft aortic wall tissue was available for study as only the leaflets were explanted. The leaflets were thickened but pliable with a smooth surface. Histology showed a slight increase in cellularity due to some inflammatory infiltration of the whole leaflet with lymphocytes and granulocytes. Fibroblasts in a layered architecture could still be recognized, although the interstitium showed homogenized collagen and was thickened due to some edema. Gram staining failed to show any bacteria. ISH demonstrated the inflammatory cells to be of male, recipient origin, with the majority of the fibroblasts also staining Y-positive (male, recipient-derived). The number of donor cells was strongly reduced.

Explant E

Pulmonary allograft E was derived from a male adult (heart beating) donor. Cryopreservation was with DSMO 10% without antibiotic treatment. This allograft had been implanted as a conduit in the right ventricular outflow tract of a 14 year old girl with Tetralogy of Fallot. After 3 years and 10 months, it was explanted because of stenosis and valvular insufficiency.

The arterial wall of the allograft was thickened but without macroscopic calcifications. The leaflets appeared thin, small and retracted. Histology showed a reduced cellularity in the arterial wall and an almost acellular leaflet. Layer structures had disappeared. No inflammatory cells were noticed. The allograft arterial wall showed some sclerotic alterations. ISH failed to demonstrate Y-positive (male, donor) cells. All cells were of recipient origin.

Comments

Despite the sometimes excellent harvest and cryopreservation techniques, most studies underline that before implantation there is at least some loss of cellular viability. This is consistent with the also common finding that cellularity in clinical allograft explants is highly variable but always less than before implantation. It is the consensus that there is always some loss of (viable) donor cells. Furthermore, substantial loss of endothelial cells pre- and post-implantation has been described in several studies.[1,2,6,8,12,20]

When inflammatory cells can be distinguished in allograft explants they are presumably of recipient origin although macrophages can be present in the normal, unimplanted valve.[2]

From remaining (myo)fibroblast populations it is difficult to say whether they are from donor or recipient origin, especially because in most cases trilaminar architecture of the valve tissue is disturbed or totally absent.[2,12] In some studies, DNA fingerprinting techniques showed that these remaining fibroblast populations can be of donor and/or recipient origin.[2]

Current techniques, first culturing cells from the valve tissue before testing, leave uncertainty about the quality of donor or recipient cells, and the finding of one population does not exclude the presence of the other. Furthermore, the current techniques give no insight into the question of where the remaining cell populations are localized in the valve.

The discussion about cell fate and origin is still open; first because of the proportionally few explants that have been examined on this issue and second because the examined valves were in great majority explanted because of dysfunction, leaving us uninformed about the valves that perform well.

The DNA in situ hybridization technique for the Y chromosome, as described previously, gives more insight into the quantity and distribution of donor and recipient cell populations in tissue sections of allograft explants. Applied on a series of explants, these data can be related to preimplantation condition, implantation time and clinical performance. It may enable us to draw conclusions about the significance of donor and recipient cell populations.

References

1. Lupinetti FM, Tsai T, Kneebone J, et al. Effect of cryopreservation on the presence of endothelial cells on human valve allografts. J Thorac Cardiovasc Surg 1993;106:912–7.
2. Goffin Y, Henriques de Gouveia R, Szombathelyi T. European Homograft Implants: a five year pathology study with reference to inimplanted valves. Proceedings of the 4th symposium of the European Homograft Bank, Brussells 1994;55–60.
3. VanDerKamp AWM, Visser WJ, van Dongan JM, Nauta J, Galjaard H. Preservation of aortic heart valves with maintenance of cell viability. J Surg Res 1981;30:47.
4. Brockbank K. Cell viability in fresh, refrigerated, and cryopreserved human heart valve leaflets [letter]. Ann Thorac Surg 1990;49:848–9.
5. Armiger LC, Thomson RW, Strickett MG, Barratt-Boyes EG. Morphology of heart valves preserved by liquid nitrogen freezing. Thorax 1985;40:778–86.
6. Crescenzo DG, Hilbert SL, Barrick MK, Corcoran PC, St. Louis JD, Messier RH, Ferrans VJ, Wallace RB, Hopkins RA. Donor heart valves: electron microscopic and morphometric assessment of cellular injury induced by warm ischemia. J Thorac Cardiovasc Surg 1992;103: 253–257.
7. St.Louis J, Corcoran P, Rajan S, Conte J, Wolfinbarger L, Hu J, Lange PL, Wang YN, Hilbert SL, Analouei A. Effects of warm ischemia following harvesting of allograft cardiac valves. EJCTS 1991;5:458–64; discus.
8. Abd-Elfattah AS, Messier RH, Domkowski PW, Crescenzo DG, Wallace RB, Hopkins RA. Inhibition of adenosine deaminase and nucleoside transport: utility in a model of homograft cardiac valve preimplantation processing. J Thorac Cardiovasc Surg 1993;105:1095–1105.
9. Crescenzo DG, Hilbert SL, Messier JrRH, Domkowski PW, Barrick MK, Lange PL, Ferrans V, Wallace RB, Hopkins RA. Human cryopreserved allografts: Electron microscopic analysis of cellular injury. Ann Thorac Surg 1993;55:25–31.
10. Hu J, Gilmer L, Hopkins R, Wolfinbarger L. Effects of antibiotics on cellular viability in

porcine heart valve tissue. Cardiovasc Res 1989; 23:960–964.

11. O'Brien MF, Stafford EG, Gardner MA, Pohlner PG, McGiffin DC. A comparison of aortic valve replacement with viable cryopreserved and fresh allograft valves, with a note on chromosomal studies. J Thorac Cardiovasc Surg 1987;94:812–823.

12. Schoen FJ. The first step to understanding valve failure: an overview of pathology. EJCTS 1992; 6(Suppl 1):50–3.

13. Clarke D, Campbell D, Hayward A, et al. Degeneration of aortic valve allografts in young recipients. J Thorac Cardiovasc Surg 1993;105:934–42.

14. Wheatley D, McGregor G. Influence of viability on canine allograft heart valve structure and function. Cardiovasc Res 1977;11:223–30.

15. Gonzales-Lavin L, Bianchi J, Graf D, Amini S, Gordon CL. Degenerative changes in fresh aortic root homografts in a canine model: evidence of an immunologic influence. Transplant Proc 1988;20:815–819.

16. Hazekamp M, Koolbergen D, Braun J, et al. In situ hybridization: a new technique to determine the origin of fibroblasts in cryopreserved aortic homograft valve explants. J Thorac Cardiovasc Surg 1995;110:248–57.

17. Cornelisse C, Devilee P, Raap A. In situ hybridization. In Bullock G, Van Velzen D, Warhol M (eds). Techniques in diagnostic pathology. London: Academic Press 1991:201–13.

18. Braun J, Hazekamp M, Koolbergen D, et al. Identification of host and donor cells in porcine aortic homograft heart valve explants by in situ hybridization. J Histochem Cytochem 1997; Submitted.

19. Hazekamp M, Goffin Y, Huysmans H. The value of the stentless biovalve prosthesis: an experimental study. EJCTS 1993;7:514–9.

20. Goffin Y. The stability and performance of bioprosthetic heart valves. In Williams D (ed). Current perspectives on implantable devices. London: JAI Press Ltd. 1990:65–120.

20
Resolution of the Conflicting Theories of Prolonged Cell Viability

Richard A. Hopkins

A large body of evidence has shown that following current methods of processing allograft heart valves, modest populations of viable cells persist within the leaflet tissue. However, the ability of cryopreservation to maintain a normal cellular state in processed valves for transplantation is a myth. Whether transplanted cryopreserved allograft valves are in fact normal and, indeed, how "normal" is defined, are important questions to resolve. Recent studies have examined these issues, following transplantation either into human patients or into juvenile sheep. Together, they suggest that cryopreserved allograft cardiac valves do not maintain the characteristics of native valves after processing and subsequent transplantation.

Review of Current Studies

The recent work of Mitchell et al.[1] augments the *in vitro* work demonstrating that few allograft valve cells are able to tolerate the processing steps involved in cryopreservation nor retain healthy metabolic status and ultrastructural characteristics. This study compared the post-transplantation states of allograft valves that were implanted either as cryopreserved valve replacements or within orthotopic heart replacements. Cryopreserved valves showed early cell ultrastructural degeneration with complete acellularity at later time points, and morphological alteration of matrix. In contrast, aortic valves of orthotopic heart transplants

retained near-normal cell and matrix morphology with no evidence of the injury exhibited by cryopreserved valves. None of the valves from either group showed evidence of immune-mediated injury, suggesting that this is not the underlying mechanism of cellular degeneration in these valves. Thus, these results point to preimplantation processing as a cause of the acellularity of valve tissue, since valves within the orthotopic heart transplants, that did not undergo cryopreservation processing, displayed healthy cellularity.

Examining how valve cells tolerate transplantation on a molecular and cellular mechanistic level, Hilbert et al. have recently investigated the fate of cells within cryopreserved allografts post-transplantation.[2] As early as 2 days after transplant into a juvenile sheep model, allograft cells began to develop evidence of cessation of mitosis, leading to apoptosis. These states were characterized by the loss of proliferating cell nuclear antigen, the presence of nuclear condensation, pyknosis, nick end labeling, and apoptotic bodies. Changes peaked at 2 weeks and no cells populated the allografts by 20 weeks, the longest time point observed. This work suggests that apoptosis contributes directly to the acellularity of allografts following transplantation.

The recipient reaction to implanted allograft valve tissue has included a distinct ensheathing response. Hilbert et al. have observed a layer of connective tissue ensheathing the allograft cusps of valves transplanted into a Hufnage sheep model.[3] This fibroelastic sheath was of host origin, and contained proteoglycans, collagens, interstitial myofibroblasts, and surface endothelial cells. The presence of sheathing tissue correlated with cuspal thickening and contraction. We have observed a similar phenomenon in our own 20 week sheep implants. Fibrous sheathing has also been seen in xenograft bioprosthetic valved conduits in young baboons.[4] Past reports of cryopreserved valves retrieved from human patients at the time of reoperation for valvular dysfunction did not show extensive sheath formation.[1,5–8] However, in recent studies of explanted antibiotic-treated human valve allografts, approximately half the cusp was covered by fibrous sheathing.[9]

After observing and beginning to understand the mechanisms of processing-associated damage, the obvious question arises of whether it can be prevented and/or reversed. Current studies indicate that valve leaflet interstitial cells of cryopreserved allografts can be "resuscitated" both in dissociated cell culture and in organ culture within intact leaflets (Chapter 4, this volume).[10] Incubation with 15% fetal bovine serum restores normal cell number, ultrastructure, and functional markers to valve leaflets.

Comprehensive Definition of Post-Transplantation Leaflet Cellular Viability

As discussed earlier in this section, a thorough definition of functional cell viability would include the following: the presence of cells whose morphologic integrity is intact and which express phenotypic markers appropriate to their location, including the specific dual secretory and contractile characteristics of myofibroblasts. Thus, theory proposes that viable cells would retain the capability of mitosis for regeneration of cells at densities appropriate for tissue function. Finally, these cells would be able to grow and remodel their tissue appropriately in response to stimuli generated by the body of the patient.

Current Theories: Stunning, Apoptosis and Prolonged Donor Cell Viability

The first great mythology of the cryopreservation era for allograft valve transplantation has been that donor leaflet cells remain viable and persist for years, replicating and functioning as typical matrix cells and providing a substrate for normal re-endothelialization. This has been shown by many studies to not be the natural history of these cells and that the mythology of prolonged viability is just that—a mythology. In fact, efforts to enhance viability of the matrix cells may actually have been counterproductive when it extended to the donor endothelial cells. It is likely that endothelial cells have greater antigenic potential, have more exposure to the blood stream and thus would provoke an enhanced immune response, whereas with deliberate stripping of the endothelium during preimplantation processing, the donor cells which definitely retain antigenic potential, would have a more limited exposure and perhaps some limited viability.

It is our belief that as currently practiced, cryopreservation of heart valves with subsequent unmatched allograft transplantation does not result in donor cells that survive in large numbers for a prolonged period of time (i.e. years). Studies reviewed in this book indicate that a significant loss of cellular morphologic integrity with irreversible cell death occurs during harvesting and processing. However, at the time of implantation, there are indeed a significant number of intact cells that are viable by morphologic criteria. The intermediate metabolism studies suggest that a large percentage of these are severely depleted metabolically and thus doomed to early death as a consequence of metabolic stunning. Further, the Hilbert paper[2] suggests that the stress inherent to the entire process initiates apoptosis and that, even if the transplanted cells survive and regain metabolic activity following implantation, they are unable to enter the regenerative cell cycle, and thus are not viable in the sense of our comprehensive definition. At best, these cells may provide some transitional secretory (and thus matrix sparing) function which could be very helpful in the short to medium term.

Immune Response

The other major myth of the cryopreservation era was that these homografts were essentially "immunologically privileged" in part because the myofibroblasts were buried within the matrix. This mythology led to commercial processing by some companies of human homografts with modifications in the technique to enhance viability, ultimately not only of fibroblasts, but also of endothelium. This enhanced viability was "marketed" without any evidence that this retained viability actually contributed to prolonged durability. In contrast, valves processed by the techniques of at least one not-for-profit tissue processor were intentionally exposed to solutions to remove endothelium, while the remainder of the processing steps were kinder to myofibroblasts. The decreased durability of cryopreserved allografts in younger children (especially in neonates) has been consistently attributed to an immune response-mediated accelerated valve failure. Both T cell and B cell infiltration has been demonstrated[11,12] as well as a persistence of human leukocyte antigen (HLA) antibodies in children receiving cryopreserved allografts.[13–16] Proliferative and inflammatory responses have also been demonstrated with intimal proliferation which may be the passive sheathing phenomenon we have noted (*vida infra*) or it has been attributed to a low grade immune response.[11,14,17] Shaddy and coworkers did not find ABO compatibility to be associated with shortened durability in their study of homografts in the pulmonary position,[12] but others have.[19] Work by Hoekstra,[20,21] Smith[22] and Shaddy[13,23] have demonstrated persistently positive panel reactive antibodies suggesting a significant HLA antibody response to implantation of allograft valves in both children and adults. The Geneva group reported a 91% durability at 5 years with ABO compatible homografts in RVOT reconstructions in chil-

dren versus 69% for incompatible transplants and concluded ABO immunogenicity plays a significant role in accelerated homograft fibrocalcification.[19]

Thus, the concept of immune privilege has been shown to be untrue. Any cells which might be spared metabolic, morphologic, or apoptotic doom are ultimately susceptible to immune attack. As a "foreign body," there is also risk of non-specific inflammation and scarring. Taken together, the variable "viability" status of the cells at the time of transplantation and the clearly demonstrated immune response suggests that few donor cells would persist for a prolonged period of time (i.e. years). This is consistent with the human explant studies as described in Section VII (Allograft Heart Valves: Morphologic, Biochemical, and Explant Pathology Studies).

Sheathing

The above review of the effects of stunning, apoptosis and immune responses must be correlated with the actual pretty good clinical results achieved with current cryopreservation technologies and classical implantation methods. It is our clinical hypothesis that patients in whom an immune response is avoided by the lack of retention of endothelium and the gradual death of matrix cells can achieve durable, functional benefit from allograft valves for many years based upon the passive performance characteristics of the retained collagen, elastin and matrix. The lack of physical failure of the leaflets during early and medium terms (three to fifteen years) may also be partially a consequence of the fibroblast proliferative sheathing response which may either be a normal low-level immune response or even a non-immune mediated inflammatory response to a foreign body in the circulation.

The studies and results from our own laboratory's chronic sheep implant and human explant studies suggest that the durability of homograft valve transplants likely depends on a passive retention of matrix physical and chemical properties.[1,2] This may be enhanced by a transition phase restoration of soluble proteins to the matrix and an absence of damage to the collagen substrate. In addition, the "sheathing" phenomenon which we have observed in both human explants and chronic animal models may influence durability. In this process, the recipient lines the donor valve leaflet (denuded of endothelium) with recipient fibroblast and pseudo-intima. While these fibroblasts appear to secrete primarily Type III collagen as opposed to Type I collagen (in the matrix of normal leaflets), it does provide splinting and living viscoelastic properties to the leaflets. It is our belief that this fibrous sheathing is important to the long-term durability of current generation cryopreserved human semilunar valves,[19] and when successfully accomplished correlates with prolonged valve function. If there is a heightened immune response due to the presence of endothelium or to the neonatal transplant setting, or for some other reason the protective sheath does not have time to develop, then durability of the ultimately acellular valve leaflet is likely adversely affected.

While these concepts do not invalidate the clinical practice of fresh or cryopreserved homograft transplantation, they do suggest that the original theories of prolonged donor cell viability are wrong, and that it might even be contraindicated to attempt to maximally enhance donor cell viability, unless the immune response is modified. If cell necrosis could be avoided and either immune tolerance enhanced or antigenicity reduced, then maximizing the cell population in the leaflets at the time of transplantation would be very attractive.[10] Alternatively, decellularization is likely preferable to donor cell retention especially if physical integrity of the valve matrix can be preserved and especially if recellularization with recipient cells can be accomplished either *in vivo* or with *in vitro* seeding.[24,25] There are certain caveats in regards to the attractiveness of decellularization: First, the processing treatment necessary must not weaken or degrade the physical material properties (i.e. strength and viscoelasticity) of the valve complex. Second, *all* cellular debris must be removed as

residual cell remnants can be pro-inflammatory, potentially initiating a non-specific inflammatory response that could then enhance an immune reaction, causing sensitization and/or more destruction, than the gradual ebbing of a cell population by apoptosis. Third, the processing must not alter or expose the structural and matrix proteins in such fashion as to be inflammatory or even antigenic (e.g. xenograft decellularized tissues). And finally, the decellularization process must result in a protein scaffold commodious to recellularization with phenotypically appropriate cells (i.e. myofibroblasts and endothelial cells) and not result in the typical fibroblastic scar response which simply mimics the optimal scenario for cryopreserved allografts (see sheathing *vida supra* and Chapter 65).

Current data suggest that cryopreservation methods which maximally enhance donor cell viability likely contribute to enhanced immune and inflammatory recipient responses which markedly shorten functional durability of homografts, especially when transplanted across ABO and HLA compatibility. Conversely, more aggressive cryopreservation, harvesting and storage methods which strip endothelium and reduce more superficially positioned interstitial cells while leaving deeply imbedded matrix myofibroblasts (for protein synthesis) may be the best expression of current cryopreservation methodologies. Such a theory could explain the recent reports of increasingly poor results (as measured by duration of valve durability) when "maximum viability" processing is used. Further complicating so-called gentle or optimal viability cryopreservation is the issue of "cell fate" following such processing. If "imbedded" myofibroblasts are lost by apoptosis rather than induced cell necrosis, then the inflammatory response should be muted. Conversely, cryopreservation methods that "enhance" early cell "viability" but which leave significant cell remnants (endothelial and/or myofibroblast) and especially when followed by matrix cell necrosis (stunned or doomed cells) could actually potentiate inflammation and immune rejection (that older methodologies likely, and perhaps inadvertently, muted).

References

1. Mitchell RN, Jonas RA, Schoen FJ. Pathology of explanted cryopreserved allograft heart valves: comparison with aortic valves from orthotopic heart transplants. J Thorac Cardiovasc Surg 1998;115:118–127.

2. Hilbert SL, Luna RE, Zhang J, Wang Y, Hopkins RA, Yu ZX, Ferrans VJ. Allograft heart valves: the role of apoptosis-mediated cell loss. J Thorac Cardiovasc Surg 1999;117:454–462.

3. Hufnagel CA, Gomes MN. Late follow-up of ball-valve prostheses in the descending aorta. J Thorac Cardiovasc Surg 1976;72:900–909.

4. Ferrans VJ, Arbustini E, Eidbo EE, et al. Anatomic changes in right ventricular-pulmonary artery conduits implanted in baboons. In Bodnar E, Yacoub M (eds). Biologic and Bioprosthetic Valves. New York, NY: Yorke 1986:316.

5. Hilbert SL, Luna RE, Zhang J, et al. Allograft heart valves: assessment of cell viability by confocal microscopy. Circulation 1997;96(suppl): I508.

6. Mitchell RN, Jonas RA, Schoen F. Structure-function correlations in cryopreserved allograft cardiac valves. Ann Thorac Surg 1995;60:8108–8133.

7. Schoen FJ, Mitchell RN, Jonas RA. Pathological considerations in cryopreserved allograft heart valves. J Heart Valve Dis 1995;4:S72–S76.

8. Goffin YA, de Gouveia H, Szombathelyi T, et al. Morphologic study of homograft valves before and after cryopreservation and after short term implantation in patients. Cardiovasc Pathol 1997; 6:35–42.

9. Gavin JB, Herdson PB, Monro JL, Barratt-Boyes BG. Pathology of antibiotic-treated human heart valve allografts. Thorax 1973;28: 473–481.

10. Messier R, Bass BL, Domkowski PW, Hopkins RA. Interstitial Cellular Matrix Restoration of Cardiac Valves Following Cryopreservation. J Thorac Cardiovasc Surg 1999;118:36–49.

11. Rajani B, Uree RB, Ratliff NB. Evidence for rejection of homograft valves in infants. J Thorac Cardiovasc Surg 1998;115:111–117.

12. Vogt P, Stallmach T, Niederhauser U, Schneider J, Zund G, Lachat M, Kunzli A, Turina M. Explanted cryopreserved allografts: a morphological and immunohistochemical comparison between arterial allografts and allograft heart valves from infants and adults. EJCTS 1999;15: 639–645.

13. Shaddy RE, Thompson DD, Osborne KA, Hawkins JAFT. Persistence of human leukocyte antigen (HLA) immunogenicity of crypreserved valve allografts used in pediatric heart surgery. American Journal of Cardiology 1997;80:358–359.

14. Motomura N, Imakita M, Yutani C, Kitoh Y, Kawashima Y, Oka T. Histological change in cryopreserved rat aortic allograft. Journal of Cardiovascular Pathology 1995;36:53–60.

15. Neves JP, Gulbenkian S, Ramos T, Martins AP, Caldas MC, Mascarenhas R, et al. Mechanisms underlying degeneration of cryopreserved vascular homografts. J Thorac Cardiovasc Surg 1997;113:1014–1021.

16. Neves J, Monteiro C, Santos R, et al. Histologic and genetic assessment of explanted allograft valves. Ann Thorac Surg 1995;60:141–145.

17. Hoekstra FM, Witvliet M, Knoeep CY, Wassenaar C, Boger JJC, Weimar W, Claas FHJ. Immunogenic human leukocyte antigen Class II antigens on human cardiac vlave induce specific alloantibodies. Ann Thorac Surg 1998;66:2022–2026.

18. Wagner E, Roy R, Marois Y, Douville Y, Guidoin R. Fresh venous allografts in peripheral arterial reconstruction in dogs: effects of histocompatibility and of short-term immunosuppression with cyclosporine A and mycophenolate mofetil. J Thorac Cardiovasc Surg 1995;110:1723–1744.

19. Christenson JT, Vala D, Dierra J, Beghetti M, Kalangos A. Blood group incompatibility and accelerated homograft fibrocalcifications. J Thorac Cardiovasc Surg 2003; In Press.

20. Hoekstra F, Knoop C, Jutte, et al. Effect of cryopreservation and HLA-DR matching on the cellular immunogenicity of human cardiac valve allografts. J Heart Lung Transplant 1994;13:1095–1098.

21. Hoekstra FM, Witvliet M, Knoop C. Donor-specific anti-human leukocyte antigen class I antibodies after implantation of cardiac valve allografts. Journal of Heart and Lung Transplantation 1997;16:570–572.

22. Smith JD, Ogino H, Hunt D, et al. Humoral immune response to human aortic valve homografts. Ann Thorac Surg 1995;60:S127–S130.

23. Shaddy RE, Hunter DD, Osborn KA. Prospective analysis of HLA immunogenicity of crypreserved valved allografts used in pediatric heart surgery. Circulation 1994;94:1063–1067.

24. Maish MS, Hoffman-Kim D, Krueger PM, Souza JM, Harper JJ, Hopkins RA. Tricuspid Valve

Biopsy—A potential source of cardiac myofibroblast cells for tissue engineered cardiac valves. J Heart Valve Dis 2002; In press.

25. Hong T, Maish MS, Cohen J, Fitzpatrick P, Bert A, Harper J, Hoffman-Kim D, Hopkins RA. Reproducible echocardiography in juvenile sheep and its application in the evaluation of a pulmonary valve allograft implant. Contemporary Topics in Laboratory Animal Science 2000; 39:15–21.

Section VII
Allograft Heart Valves: Morphologic, Biochemical, and Explant Pathology Studies

21
Overview: Allograft Heart Valves

Stephen L. Hilbert, Frederick J. Schöen, and Victor J. Ferrans

Pulmonary and aortic valves transplanted from one human to another (referred to as *homografts* or *allografts*) have been used for valvular replacement and ventricular outflow tract reconstruction for approximately 40 years.[1-5] Predominantly derived from cadaver donors, allograft valves may also be taken from hearts in which the aortic valve is explanted intact at cardiac transplantation.

The objective of this chapter is to review the morphological features, functional relationships and explant pathology findings in aortic and pulmonary allograft valves. This presentation will address heart valve anatomy and histology, biomechanics, the effects of preimplantation processing and storage on valvular tissue components, and valve-related pathology. Preclinical and clinical studies involving porcine, ovine and human valvular tissues will be discussed.

Allograft Valves and Other Replacement Heart Valves

The first clinical implantation of a mechanical replacement heart valve was performed in 1958 using a ball-in-cage valve inserted in the descending thoracic aorta.[6] The first orthotopic valve replacements were accomplished in 1960 (aortic position)[7] and 1961 (mitral position).[8] Mechanical heart valve designs continued to evolve, with the current prosthetic designs consisting of ball-in-cage, tilting disk and bileaflet

valves. The occurrence of thromboembolic events and of sudden, life-threatening modes of structural failure[9,10] have continued to stimulate interest in the use of biologic (allografts and autologous tissues) and bioprosthetic (glutaraldehyde-crosslinked porcine aortic valve and bovine pericardial tissues) heart valves.

Bioprosthetic and biologic heart valves became the prosthetic valves of choice during the 1970s, since they did not require long-term anticoagulation and demonstrated less restriction of central flow through the valve orifice. However, as long-term clinical experience increased, the durability of biologic and bioprosthetic valves became a limiting factor, principally because of primary tissue failure (e.g., tissue abrasion, cuspal dehiscence and calcification) and cuspal thickening (e.g., fibrous sheath formation) resulting in significant alterations in hemodynamic performance (i.e., stenosis; regurgitation). Leaflet tears and dehiscence have also occurred as a consequence of the technique used to attach pericardial and porcine valve tissue and allograft valves to polymeric and metallic stents (Figures 21.1 and 21.2).[11-16] The incidence of tissue failure secondary to cuspal calcification (Figures 21.1 and 21.3) was shown to be particularly high in porcine aortic valve bioprostheses implanted in children and adolescents.[17,18] Currently, allograft valves are used extensively for the reconstruction of the right ventricular outflow tract in children.[19,20] The clinical modes of failure of biologic and bioprosthetic valves are typically more gradual and less catastrophic than those

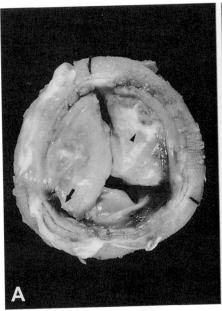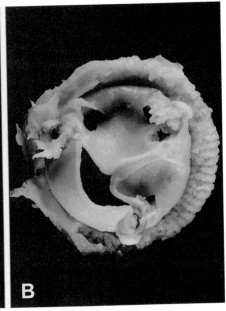

FIGURE 21.1. Gross photographs depicting bioprosthetic valve primary tissue failure. (A) Inflow surface of a porcine aortic valve showing cuspal dehiscence (arrow) and calcification (arrowhead). (B) Ionescu-Shiley bovine pericardial valve demonstrating leaflet tears located adjacent to the commissural stent posts.

of mechanical valves. However, the rate of reoperation after implantation of bioprosthetic valves has been reported to be approximately 40% following 8 to 10 years of use.[21] The current usage of cardiac replacement valves worldwide is estimated to be: approximately 70% mechanical valves (predominantly the St. Jude bileaflet valve); 28% bioprostheses (predominantly porcine aortic valves); and 2% cryopreserved allograft heart valves.[22]

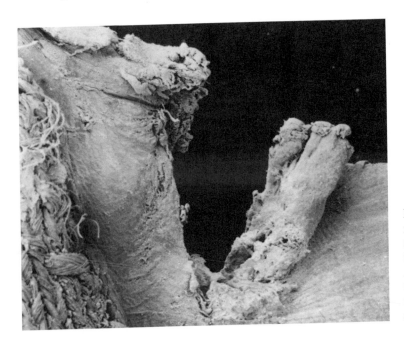

FIGURE 21.2. Scanning electron micrograph of the commissural region of an explanted Ionescu-Shiley bovine pericardial valve. A leaflet tear resulting from the use of an alignment suture to ensure leaflet coaptation is shown. X 15.

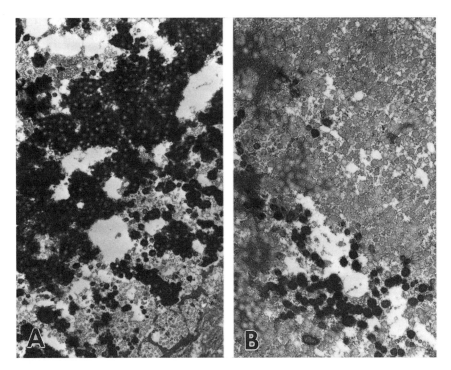

FIGURE 21.3. Transmission electron micrographs depicting intrinsic leaflet calcification localized to the surface of the collagen fibrils (A) and involving entire collagen fibrils (B). Uranyl acetate/lead citrate stain. A, X 14,000; B, X 10,000.

The development of replacement heart valves continues to progress with the use of a variety of biomaterials and tissues (e.g., pyrolytic carbon, polyurethane, parietal pericardium, dura mater, and aortic, mitral and pulmonary valvular tissues)[23–26] as well as with modifications in tissue processing (e.g., zero-pressure tissue fixation, anti-calcification treatments, non-aldehyde cross-linking agents),[27–37] the development of stentless bioprostheses,[36,37] and the application of tissue engineering concepts.[38,39] However, with the exception of the use of cryopreserved allograft valves and pulmonary autografts (i.e., Ross procedure), which have demonstrated a modest increase in long-term durability,[40–43] the clinical efficacy and actuarial freedom from primary tissue failure of the next generation of stentless bioprosthetic and autologous tissue valves remains to be demonstrated.

There has been a renewed interest in the use of allograft and heterograft mitral valves for the replacement of atrioventricular valves.[24,44–46] However, despite optimistic initial reports, the demonstration of long-term mitral valve allograft function remains to be established.[46] Preclinical studies of mitral valve allografts used as mitral valve replacements in juvenile sheep (surviving 12 to 24 weeks) have demonstrated two distinct mechanisms of allograft failure.[24] Characteristic morphologic changes occurred in the allografts depending on whether the mitral valves where glutaraldehyde-treated or stored in a cold antibiotic solution before implantation. Marked calcification and chordal rupture (secondary to calcific deposits) were observed in the glutaraldehyde-treated allografts, while leaflet perforations and ruptured chordae due to connective tissue deterioration were noted in the antibiotic stored valves (Figure 21.3). Cryopreserved mitral valve allografts have been used as either partial or total mitral valve replacements in conjunction with the use of an annuloplasty ring.[46] Clinical findings following fourteen months of implantation are encouraging with continued retention of valve function; however, long-term studies will be required to establish the effectiveness of this reconstructive mitral valve technique.

Allograft Valve Processing and Storage

Sterilization and Disinfection

The disinfection or sterilization of allografts have been accomplished by various methods, such as exposure to gaseous (ethylene oxide) or chemical (glutaraldehyde-formaldehyde mixtures, beta-propiolactone) sterilants, antibiotics (disinfection) and gamma or electron beam irradiation. Chemical sterilants, such as aldehydes, ethylene oxide and beta-propiolactone, are considered to be less than optimal, since these agents significantly alter the mechanical properties of the valvular tissue.[47] In contrast, exposure to low levels of radiation and antibiotic solutions does not markedly alter the valvular biomechanical properties or leaflet geometry and does not adversely affect performance.[48,49] However, allograft valves sterilized with ethylene oxide or beta-propiolactone prior to implantation have been reported to have an increased incidence of primary tissue failure (e.g., cuspal tears) as compared to valves stored in cold, antibiotic containing solutions. (759, 536, 318, 388) Treatment with beta-propiolactone has also been observed to result in cuspal thickening,[50] which is believed to be secondary to tissue shrinkage[47] and may induce regurgitation.

Storage Methods

Lyophilization (freeze-drying), storage in cold antibiotic solutions and cryopreservation (freezing and subsequent storage in liquid nitrogen vapor) have been traditionally used as a practical means of banking allograft valves.[50–55] The majority of the valves currently in clinical use are cryopreserved.[41,42,56–58]

Studies of short-term valve replacement in animals demonstrated that the performance of lyophilized allografts was comparable to that of fresh allograft valves; however, an increased incidence of cuspal tears was observed following the long-term clinical use of lyophilized allografts.[50,59,60] These cuspal tears were located either at the cusp-aortic wall junction or in the free edge of the leaflet, close to the commissure.[50] In addition to tissue failure secondary to alterations in mechanical properties, lyophilized valves also may be susceptible to calcification.[61]

Storage in cold antibiotic solutions has proven to be effective,[62] without inducing significant alterations of mechanical properties or morphologic changes in collagen and elastin (the principal fibrous connective tissue components). However, a significant reduction in the number of viable cells has been reported in leaflets following two to four weeks of storage in cold Hank's balanced salt solution or nutrient media, with complete loss of viable cells occurring after one month of storage.[63] Until recently, the majority of the allograft valves in clinical use had been stored in cold antibiotic or nutrient media before implantation.[52,56,62]

The loss of cell viability secondary to storage in cold antibiotics or nutrient media (referred to as "fresh" allografts) stimulated the use of cryogenic methods for the preservation of allograft valves. The objective of maintaining leaflet cell viability at the time of implantation has been facilitated by the use of cryopreservation and the development of improved tissue harvesting, disinfection and thawing protocols.[64] However, the influence of cell viability on the long-term durability of allograft valves is unknown, although an increase in the actuarial freedom from primary tissue failure and reoperation has been demonstrated with the use of cryopreserved allografts.

References

1. Ross DN. Replacement of the aortic and mitral valve with a pulmonary valve autograft. Lancet 1967;2:956–958.
2. Pillsbury RC, Shumway NE. Replacement of the aortic valve with the autologous pulmonic valve. Surg Forum 1966;17:176–177.
3. Barratt-Boyes BG. Homograft aortic valve replacement in aortic incompetence and stenosis. Thorax 1964;19:131–150.

4. Ross DN. Homograft replacement of the aortic valve. Lancet 1962;2:487.

5. Murray G. Homologous aortic valve segment transplants as surgical treatment for aortic and mitral insufficiency. Angiology 1956;7:466–471.

6. Hufnagel CA, Gomes MN. Late follow-up of ball-valve prostheses in the descending aorta. J Thorac Cardiovasc Surg 1976;72:900–909.

7. Harken DE, Soraff HS, Taylor WJ, Lefemine AA, Gupta SK, Lunter S. Partial and complete prostheses in aortic insufficiency. J Thorac Cardiovasc Surg 1960;40:744–762.

8. Starr A, Edwards ML. Mitral replacement: Clinical experience with a ball valve prosthesis. Ann Surg 1961;154:726–740.

9. Ericsson A, Lindblom D, Semb G, et al. Strut fracture with the Bjork-Shiley 70 convexo-concave valve: An international multi-institutional follow-up study. Eur J Cardiothorac Surg 1992;6:339–346.

10. Vongpatanasin W, Hillis LD, Lange RA. Prosthetic heart valves. New Eng Journ Med 1996;335:407–416.

11. Gallo I, Nistal F, Arbe E, Artinano E. Comparative study of primary tissue failure between porcine (Hancock and Carpentier-Edwards) and bovine pericardial (Ionescu-Shiley) bioprostheses in the aortic position at five- to nine-year follow-up. Am J Cardiol 1988;61:812–816.

12. Bortolotti U, Milan A, Thiene G, et al. Early mechanical failure of the Hancock pericardial xenograft. J Thorac Cardiovasc Surg 1987;94:200–207.

13. Schoen FJ, Fernandez J, Gonzalez-Lavin L, Cemaianu A. Causes of failure and pathologic findings in surgically-removed Ionescu-Shiley standard bovine pericardial heart valve bioprostheses: emphasis on progressive structural deterioration. Circulation 1987;76:618–627.

14. Hilbert SL, Ferrans VJ, McAllister HA, Cooley DA. Ionescu-Shiley bovine pericardial bioprostheses: histologic and ultrastructural studies. Am J Pathol 1992;140:1195–1204.

15. Christie GW, Gavin JB, Barratt-Boyes BG. Graft detachment, a cause of incompetence in stent-mounted aortic valve allografts. J Thorac Cardiovasc Surg 1985;90:901–906.

16. Allard MF, Thompson CR, Baldelli RJ, et al. Commissural region dehiscence from the stent post of Carpentier-Edwards bioprosthetic cardiac valves. Cardiovasc Pathol 1995;4:155–162.

17. Sanders SP, Levy RJ, Freed MD, Norwood WI, Castaneda AR. Use of Hancock porcine xeno-grafts in children and adolescents. Am J Cardiol 1980;40:429–438.

18. Silver MM, Pollock J, Silver MD, et al. Calcification in porcine xenograft valves in children. Am J Cardiol 1980;45:685–688.

19. Hopkins RA, Reyes A, Imperato DA, et al. Ventricular outflow tract reconstructions with cryopreserved cardiac valve homografts: a single surgeon's 10 year experience. Ann Surg 1996;223:544–553.

20. Stark J, Bull C, Stajevic M, Jothi M, Elliott M, De Leval MR. Fate of subpulmonary homograft conduits: determinants of late homograft failure. J Thorac Cardiovasc Surg . 1997.

21. Foster AH, Greenberg GJ, Underhill DJ, McIntosh CL, Jones M, Clark RE. Intrinsic failure of Hancock mitral bioprostheses: 10 to 15 year experience. Ann Thorac Surg 1987;44:568–577.

22. Schoen FJ. Approach to the analysis of cardiac valve prostheses as surgical pathology or autopsy specimens. Cardiovasc Pathol 1995;4:241–255.

23. Hilbert SL, Ferrans VJ, Tomita Y, Eidbo EE, Jones M. Evaluation of explanted pulyurethane trileaflet cardiac valve prostheses. J Thorac Cardiovasc Surg 1987;94:419–429.

24. Tamura K, Jones M, Yamada I, Ferrans VJ. A comparison of failure modes of glutaraldehyde-treated versus antibiotic-preserved mitral valve allografts implantedin sheep. J Thorac Cardiovasc Surg 1995;110:224–238.

25. Love JW, Schoen FJ, Breznock EM, Shermer SP, Love CS. Experimental evaluation of an autologous tissue heart valve. J Heart Valve Dis 1992;1:232–241.

26. Puig LB, Verginelli G, Iryia K, Kawabe L, Bellotti G, Sosa E, Pilleggi F, Zerbini EJ. Homologous dura mater cardiac valves. Study of 533 surgical cases. J Thorac Cardiovasc Surg 1975;69:722–728.

27. Moore MA, Bohachevsky IK, Cheung DT, et al. Stabilization of pericardial tissue by dye-mediated photo-oxidation. J Biomed Mater Res 1994;28:611–618.

28. Noishiki Y, Kodaira K, Furuse M, et al. Method of preparing antithrombogenic medical materials. [4,806,599]. 1989. United States.

29. Sung H, Cheng W, Chuiu I, Hsu H, Liu S. Studies of epoxy compound fixation. J Biomed Mater Res 1997;33:177–186.

30. Broom ND, Thomson FJ. Influence of fixation conditions on the performance of glutaraldehyde-treated porcine aortic valves: towards a more scientific basis. Thorax 1979;34:166–176.

31. Hilbert SL, Barrick MK, Ferrans VJ. Porcine aortic valve bioprosthesis: A morphologic comparison of the effects of fixation pressure. J Biomed Mat Res 1990;24:773–787.

32. Gott JP, Chih P, Dorsey L, Jay J, Jett GK, Schoen FJ, et al. Calcification of Porcine Valves: A Successful New Method of Antimineralization. Ann Thorac Surg 1992;53:207–216.

33. Vyavahare NR, Chen W, Joshi RR, et al. Current progress in anti-calcification for bioprosthetic and polymeric heart valves. Cardiovasc Pathol 1997;6:219–229.

34. Flomenbaum MA, Schoen FJ. Effects of fixation back pressure and antimineralization treatment on the morphology of porcine aortic bioprosthetic valves. J Thorac Cardiovasc Surg 1993; 105:154–164.

35. Vyavahare N, Hirsch D, Lerner E, et al. Prevention of bioprosthetic heart valve calcification by ethanol preincubation: efficacy and mechanisms. Circulation 1997;95:479–488.

36. David TE, Pollic C, Bos J. Aortic replacement with stentless porcine aortic bioprosthesis. J Thorac Cardiovasc Surg 1990;99:118.

37. Angell WW, Pupello DF, Hiro SP, Lopez-Cuenca E, Glatterer MSJ, Brock JC. Implantation of the unstented bioprosthetic aortic root: an improved method. Jour Card Surg 1993;8:466–471.

38. Shinoka T, Breuer CK, Tanel RE, et al. Tissue engineering heart valves: valve leaflet replacement study in a lamb model. Ann Thorac Surg 1995;S513–S516.

39. Schoen FJ, Levy RJ. Pathology of substitute heart valves: new concepts and developments. J Card Surg 1994;9(Suppl):222–227.

40. Ross D, Jackson M, Davies J. The pulmonary autograft—a permanent aortic valve. EJCTS 1992;6:113–116; discuss.

41. O'Brien MF, Stafford EG, Gardner MAH, Phaler PG, McGiffin DC, Kirklin JW. A comparison of aortic valve replacement with viable cryopreserved and fresh allograft valves with a note on chromosomal studies. J Thorac Cardiovasc Surg 1987;94:812–823.

42. Angell WW, Oury JH, Lamberti JJ, Koziol J. Durability of the viable aortic allograft. J Thorac Cardiovasc Surg 1989;98:48–55.

43. Messier RH, Bass BL, Aly HM. Dual structural and functional phenotypes of the porcine aortic valve interstitial characteristics of the leaflet myofibroblast. J Surg Res 1994;57:1–21.

44. Pomar JL, Mestres CA. Tricuspid valve replacement using a mitral homograft: surgical technique and initial results. J Heart Valve Dis 1993; 2:125–128.

45. Vrandecic M, Gontijo BF, Fantini FA, et al. Anatomically complete heterograft mitral valve substitute: surgical technique and immediate results. J Heart Valve Dis 1992;1:254–259.

46. Acar C, Tolan M, Berrebi A, et al. Homograft replacement of the mitral valve. Graft selection, technique of implantation, and results in forty-three patients. J Thorac Cardiovasc Surg 1996; 111:367–379.

47. Hilbert SL, Ferrans VJ, Jones M. Tissue-derived biomaterials and their use in cardiovascular prosthetic devices. Med Prog Technol 1988;14: 115–163.

48. Malm JR, Bowman FO, Jr., Harris PD, Kovalik AT. An evaluation of aortic valve homografts sterilized by electron beam energy. J Thorac Cardiovasc Surg 1967;54:471–477.

49. Harris PD, Kowalik AT, Malm JP. Factors modifying aortic homograft structure and function. Surgery 1968;63:45–59.

50. Ross D, Yacoub MH. Homograft replacement of the aortic valve. A critical review. Prog Cardiovasc Dis 1969;11:275–293.

51. Bodnar E, Wain WH, Martelli V, Ross DN. Long term performance of 580 homograft and autograft valves used for aortic valve replacement. Thorac Cardiovasc Surg 1979;27:31–38.

52. Barratt-Boyes BG, Roche AH, Subramanyan R, Pemberton JR, Whitlock RM. Long-term follow-up of patients with the antibiotic-sterilized aortic homograft valve inserted freehand in the aortic position. Circulation 1987;75:768–777.

53. Davies H, Missen GA, Blandford G, Roberts CI, Lessof MH, Ross DN. Homograft replacement of the aortic valve. A clinical and pathologic study. Am J Cardiol 1968;22:195–217.

54. Barratt-Boyes BG. Long-term follow-up of aortic valve grafts. Br Heart J 1971;33:Suppl:60–Suppl:65.

55. Ingegneri A, Wain WH, Martelli V, Bodnar E, Ross DN. An 11-year assessment of 93 flash-frozen homograft valves in the aortic position. Thorac Cardiovasc Surg 1979;27:304–307.

56. O'Brien MF, McGiffen DC, Stafford EG. Allograft aortic valve replacement: long-term comparative clinical analysis of the viable cryopreserved and antibiotic 4 degree stored valves. J Card Surg 1991;6(suppl):534–543.

57. Angell WW, Angell JD, Oury JH, Lamberti JJ, Grehl TM. Long-term follow-up of viable frozen aortic homografts: a viable homograft valve

bank. J Thorac Cardiovasc Surg 1987;93:815–822.

58. Kirklin JK, Smith D, Novick W, et al. Long-term function of cryopreserved aortic homografts: a ten year study. J Thorac Cardiovasc Surg 1993; 106:154–166.

59. Pate JW, Sawyer PN. Freeze dried aortic grafts: a preliminary report ot experimental evaluation. Am J Surg 1986;86:3–13.

60. Reichenbach DD, Mohri H, Merendino KA. Pathological changes in human aortic valve homografts. Circulation 1969;39:I-47–I-56.

61. Brock L. Long-term degenerative changes in aortic segment homografts, with particular reference to calcification. Thorax 1968;23:249–255.

62. Knaghani A, Dhalla N, Penta A, et al. Patient status 10 years or more after aortic valve replacement using antibiotic sterilized homografts. In Bodnar E, Yacoub M (eds). Biologic and Bioprosthetic Valves. New York: Yorke; 1986:38–46.

63. Angell WW, Shumway NE, Kosek JC. A five-year study of viable aortic valve homografts. J Thorac Cardiovasc Surg 1972;64:329–339.

64. Grunkemeier GL, Bodnar E. Comparison of structural valve failure among different "models" of homograft valves. J Heart Valve Dis 1994;3:556–560.

22
Morphology: Allograft Heart Valves

Stephen L. Hilbert, Frederick J. Schöen, and Victor J. Ferrans

Aortic and Pulmonary Valves

General Morphologic Features

Aortic and pulmonary valves are referred to collectively as semilunar valves. The normal aortic valve is non-obstructive when open, competent when closed, non-thrombogenic, non-injurious to blood cells, durable, resistant to infection and, capable of continuously remodeling its extracellular matrix and repairing itself when injured. The dilated pockets of aortic root behind the valve cusps bulge with each systolic ejection of blood and are called *sinuses of Valsalva*.[1] Normally, the three aortic valve cusps fold back into their respective sinuses of Valsalva when the left ventricular (LV) pressure exceeds that in the aortic root (in ventricular systole). When aortic root pressure exceeds that in the LV cavity, the cusps fall back across the outflow tract. Prolapse into the LV is prevented by their concave semilunar shape and coaptation of cuspal free edges (in ventricular diastole).

Aortic valve function normally relies on its 3 cusps, the annular fibrous tissue, and aortic root/sinuses of Valsalva. The aortic valve cusps attach to the aortic wall in a crescentic fashion, ascending to sites where adjacent cusps are separated by only a small distance (*commissures*) and descending to the trough of each cusp.[1] The three commissures are spaced circumferentially approximately 120° apart and occupy the three points of a triradiate crown. The aortic valve cusps are named for their rela-tionship to the coronary artery ostia; thus, a normal valve has right, left and non-coronary cusps. The structure of the pulmonary valve and surrounding tissues is similar to that of the aortic valve, except for a thinner structure, lack of well-developed sinuses behind the cusps and absence of coronary arterial orifices.

The three aortic cusps have a similar shape, resembling that of a half-moon (frequently referred to as semilunar cusps), but are usually unequal in size. The thin, crescentic region of each cusp between its free edge and closing edge, termed the *lunula*, defines the coaptive region of the cusps. During valve closure, the individual halves of the lunulas of one cusp contact the corresponding regions of both adjacent cusps, thereby effecting a competent seal. A fibrous mound, known as the *nodule of Arantius* (*nodulus Arantii*), is located on the ventricular surface, in the middle of the free edge of each cusp.[1] Visible semilunar ridges 2 to 3 mm from the cuspal free edge define the lower edge of the lunula and rise to meet the nodule of Arantius. Coaptation of the three nodules ensures complete central closure of the valve orifice during ventricular diastole. Since the cross-sectional area of the aortic root is smaller than the total surface area of the cusps, normal aortic valve cusps overlap as much as 40% of their area in the closed position.

Although it is common to have fenestrations (holes) near the free edges as a developmental or degenerative abnormality, this generally has no functional significance, since the lunular tissue does not contribute to separating aortic

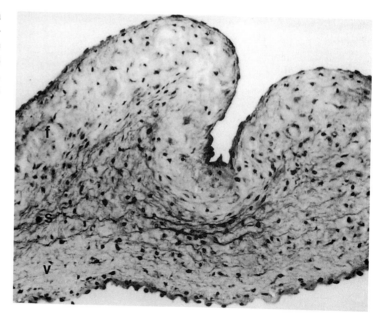

FIGURE 22.1. Light micrograph illustrating the characteristic histologic appearance of a porcine aortic valve. Three distinct regions are present: the ventricularis (v), the spongiosa (s), and the fibrosa (f). H&E stain. × 100.

from ventricular blood during diastole. In contrast, fenestrations below the lunula cause incompetence and they suggest a previous or active infection.

The aortic and pulmonary valves have a well defined histologic structure[1] and lack intrinsic blood vessels, since they are sufficiently thin to receive nutrients by diffusion from surrounding blood. The presence of nerve fibers and nerve terminals have recently been demonstrated in aortic valve cusps, although the functional significance of this finding is unknown.[2]

The cusps of the semilunar valves consist of three distinct histologic layers (from the inflow surface): the ventricularis, the spongiosa and the fibrosa (Figure 22.1). These layers are similar in distribution in all semilunar valves; however, the pulmonary valve is thinner and more delicate in appearance.[1] Ultrastructural studies of the pulmonary valve have been limited.[3] Thus, the description which follows is based primarily on studies of the aortic valve in humans and in various animal species.[4–13] Among the latter, porcine aortic valves have been extensively studied, due to their use as bioprosthetic heart valves. The only significant morphologic difference between the human and the porcine aortic valve involves the right coronary cusp, which in swine is larger than the

other two cusps and contains a "muscle shelf" located in the basal one-third to one-half of the cusp. The "muscle shelf" consists of cardiac myocytes and their vascular supply and represents an extension of the ventricular septal muscle into the basal region of the cusp. This muscle layer also may be present, but to a lesser extent, in the non-coronary cusp.[6] Thus, the hemodynamic implications of the presence of a "muscle shelf" (such as an asynchronous, delayed opening of the cusp), a reduced effective orifice area, and the propensity of this region to postimplantation degenerative calcification, are of no concern with the use of human allograft valves.

Cellular Components

Four major types of cells are present in cardiac valves: 1) endothelial cells; 2) interstitial connective cells; 3) mononuclear cells derived from the blood, and 4) interstitial dendritic cells. The endothelial cells form a continuous monolayer that completely lines the surfaces of the valves and is contiguous with the endothelial cell layer of adjacent regions of the endocardium and/or great vessels. These cells are flattened, have single, centrally located nuclei, contain actin-like and intermediate (10 nm) filaments and are connected by junctional complexes[9] that provide a permeability barrier to the diffusion of substances from the blood into the valvular tissue. The interstitial connective tissue cells are present throughout all layers of the valve. Cell counts have demonstrated a relatively uniform distribution of cells within specific histologic regions of porcine aortic valve cusps, (e.g., a mean +/− S.D. of 1760 +/− 312 nuclei/mm^2 of tissue section in the spongiosa and 1960″68 in the fibrosa).[14] These interstitial cells usually are referred to as "valvular fibroblasts", even though they actually show a spectrum of morphologic differentiation.[10–12] This spectrum includes: 1) clearly fibroblastic cells (with relatively extensively developed rough-surfaced endoplasmic reticulum); 2) intermediate forms, such as myofibroblasts (with less abundant endoplasmic reticulum, more developed actin-like filaments and peripherally located dense bodies that serve as attachment sites for the filaments) and 3) typical smooth muscle cells, with few cisterns of endoplasmic reticulum but very abundant actin-like filaments, peripherally located dense bodies and well developed basement membranes. These cells have been shown to form a network in which they are interconnected by gap junctions.[12] Small numbers of macrophages and lymphocytes (mostly T-lymphocytes) are also present throughout the various layers of the valves. In addition, interstitial dendritic cells also have been demonstrated to be present in heart valves. These cells are thin, uninucleated and have very slender, elongated cytoplasmic processes, but lack basement membranes and actin filaments. They are similar to cells of this type that are present throughout a variety of other tissues, including the heart.[13] By the use of immunohistochemical techniques, they can be identified specifically and distinguished from smooth muscle cells and other types of connective tissue cells.[15,15a] These cells are presumed to function, as they do in other tissues, in the presentation and processing of antigens.

The ventricularis is an extension of the ventricular endocardium. It is subjacent to the spongiosa and is in direct contact with the endothelial cell layer lining the inflow surface of the cusp. The ventricularis contains connective tissue cells (as described above), multidirectionally oriented collagen fibers and an extensive network of elastic fibers. The most prominent elastic fibers are oriented perpendicular to the free edge of the cusp (Figure 22.2). The ventricularis is thickened in the region of cuspal coaptation at the *nodulus Arantii* in the aortic valve (*nodulus Morgagni* in the pul-

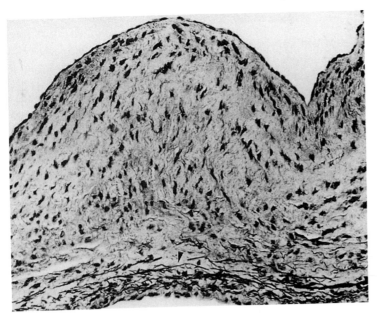

FIGURE 22.2. Histologic section of a porcine aortic valve demonstrating abundant, radially oriented elastic fibers (arrowhead) within the ventricularis. The inflow and outflow surfaces of the leaflet are lined by endothelial cells. Movat pentachrome stain. × 200.

FIGURE 22.3. Transmission electron micrograph of the outflow surface of a native porcine aortic valve. Note the presence of an intact endothelial cell layer, a cell-cell junctional complex (arrowhead) and reduplication of the basement membrane (arrow). Fibroblasts, collagen fibrils and elastic fibers (stained black) are seen in the fibrosa. Kajikawa stain. × 9,000.

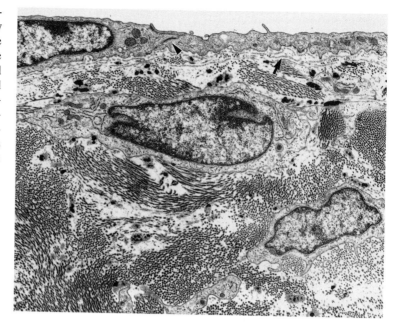

monary valve).[1] As a practical note, the ultrastructural study of cardiac valves involves a number of unusually difficult problems, particularly the proper identification of the inflow and outflow regions of the tissue specimen being examined. For this purpose, an elastic fiber stain (Kajikawa) (Figure 22.3) is preferable to routine electron microscopic stains, since it facilitates the identification of the ventricularis.[6]

The central layer of the cusp is referred to as the spongiosa. This layer is histologically similar in semilunar and in atrioventricular valves and is composed of loosely arranged collagen fibers, fibroblasts and other types of connective tissue cells embedded in an extracellular matrix rich in proteoglycans. The spongiosa is particularly prominent in the basal aspect of the cusp and does not extend to the free edge, which consists of only the fibrosa and the ventricularis.

The fibrosa is composed of fibroblasts, other types of connective tissue cells and dense collagen bundles, which serve as the major structural component of the outflow region of the cusp. The collagen bundles approaching the commissures are arranged into densely packed cords, which are integrated into the valvular

ring. A few connective tissue cells, including elongated fibroblasts and myofibroblasts,[10–12] and small numbers of elastic fibers are present in the fibrosa. Elastic fibers are prominently seen in the basal region of the cusp near the outflow surface and appear as a distinct histologic layer, referred to as the *arterialis*. A single layer of endothelial cells lines the outflow surface of the cusp. Reduplication of the endothelial basement membrane is a unique ultrastructural marker that serves to identify the outflow surface of the porcine aortic valve cusp (Figure 22.3).[6]

Morphologic studies of the aortic valve surface have provided insights into the effects of the physical forces (e.g., pressure, tension) applied to the valvular tissue at the time of histologic fixation.[4] The inflow surface is much smoother than the outflow surface, demonstrating radially oriented fine striations that correspond to the elastic fibers present in the ventricularis. The outflow surface has a corrugated appearance, due to the presence of coarse, circumferentially arranged collagen bundles in the fibrosa (Figure 22.4). These bundles consist of densely packed collagen fibrils, which appear wavy or crimped when in the relaxed state. As increasing pressure is

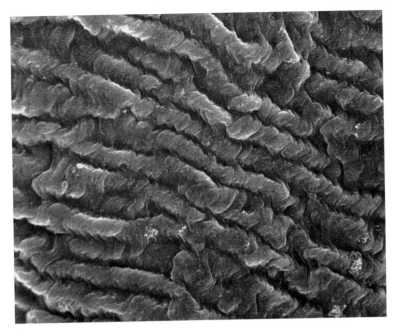

FIGURE 22.4. Scanning electron micrograph of the surface of a cryopreserved pulmonary valve allograft, demonstrating the corrugated appearance produced by the underlying collagen bundles and the marked retention of collagen crimp. × 750.

applied to the valvular tissue, the collagen fibrils become elongated or straightened, with consequent loss of crimp (Figure 22.5). Polarized light microscopy is particularly well suited for the assessment of the extent of collagen crimp (Figure 22.6). It is noteworthy that pressure gradients as small as 2 mm Hg are sufficient to significantly alter the magnitude of collagen crimp (Figure 22.7).[16,17]

Extracellular Matrix

Cardiac valves are primarily composed of extracellular matrix components of connective

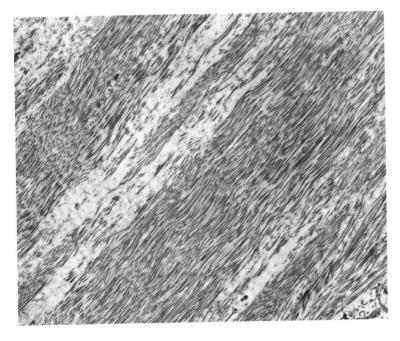

FIGURE 22.5. Transmission electron micrograph demonstrating the loss of collagen crimp, as shown by collagen fibril elongation or straightening. High pressure-fixed porcine aortic valve. × 2,900.

FIGURE 22.6. Polarized light micrographs depicting the morphologic appearance of the collagen bundles and collagen cords of a porcine aortic valve. (A) Characteristic birefringent banding pattern of collagen bundles in which crimp is retained. (B) Loss of collagen crimp (straightening) resulting from tissue elongation by the application of a 100 gram load to the leaflet. × 100.

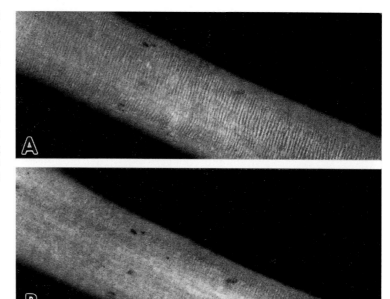

tissue. Maintained by the interstitial cells, these components consist mainly of collagen fibrils, elastic fibers and proteoglycans, which represent the bulk of the physical mass of the cusp. As described above, the histologic organization of these components into three distinct layers determines the unique biomechanical properties and resultant functional characteristics of cardiac valves.[9,18–22] Type I and Type III collagen are the most abundant extracellular proteins in cardiac valves; however, Type V collagen is also present as a minor component.[23] Recent studies

FIGURE 22.7. Histologic section illustrating the effects of pressure fixation on the morphologic appearance of a porcine aortic valve. Note the presence of three distinct histologic regions (ventricularis, spongiosa, fibrosa); however, due to the loss of collagen crimp, the collagen bundles have become elongated, resulting in the overall linear appearance of the valvular tissue. Compare with Figure 6.4. Toluidine blue stain. × 200.

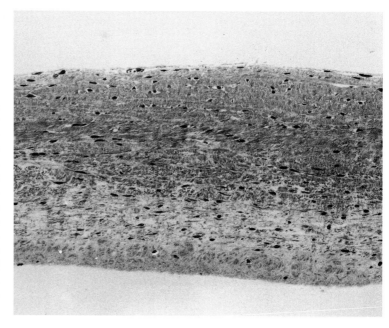

characterizing the types of collagen in cartilage have demonstrated that collagens may be present as either homogeneous fibrils or as mixed fibrils.[24] Similar studies of cardiac valve collagens have not been made.

The functional effects of proteoglycan-collagen interactions may involve the regulation of extracellular polymerization of collagen fibrils.[25,26] Domains of high positive charge density are located within the collagen fibril at sites of overlap of adjacent collagen molecules (i.e., carboxyl- and amino-terminal end of the polypeptide chain; staggered overlap region). These sites are involved in the formation of intermolecular cross-links in the collagen fibril. The extent of the cross-linking of the collagen fibrils may be regulated by the presence of proteoglycan glucosaminoglycan side chains and at these cationic sites.[25,26] These concepts are of theoretical and practical significance concerning the direction of future research on the viability of cells in cryopreserved allografts and on the mechanisms of renewal of the extracellular matrix of allograft valves.

In addition to the various morphologic characteristics of allograft valves, a variety of gender and age-related anatomic and histologic changes occur in human aortic valves. The following changes are most frequently observed in valves harvested from male donors: 1) degeneration of collagen fibers; 2) a fibroelastic "spur" along the coaptation surface; 3) a decrease in the number of cuspal fibroblasts and in the amount of proteoglycans; 4) accumulation of extracellular lipid (Figure 22.8) and 5) calcific deposits (Figure 22.9).[27–29] Because of the prevalence of these changes, current donor criteria for allograft heart valves include an age restriction and a negative medical history of previous cardiac surgery, uncontrolled hypertension, functional cardiac murmurs, rheumatic fever and malignant, autoimmune or vascular diseases.[29]

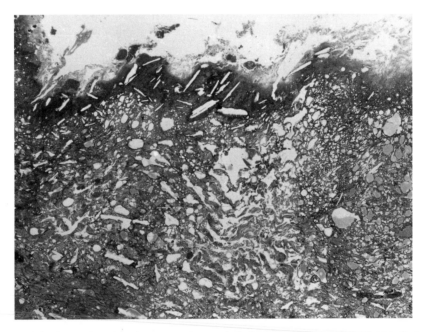

FIGURE 22.8. Explanted aortic valve demonstrating lipid accumulation, collagen fiber degeneration and the loss of typical valvular histologic features. The cleft-shaped inclusions indicate that cholesterol esters were present in the valvular tissue. H&E stain. × 200.

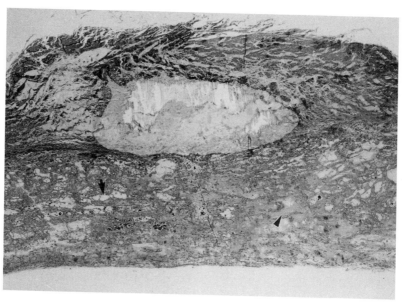

FIGURE 22.9. Histologic section of a calcific nodule within the spongiosa of a porcine aortic valvular bioprothesis. This nodule has resulted in deformation and disorganization of the collagen bundles in the fibrosa. Note the loss of the histologic layering of the valve and the insudation of plasma proteins (arrow) and lipids (arrowhead). Toluidine blue stain. Glycol methacrylate. × 100.

Mitral Valve

General Morphologic Features

The anterior mitral valve leaflet is significantly larger than the posterior leaflet; in addition, there are a few histologic differences.[1] The histologic appearance of the mitral valve leaflet is similar to that previously described for the semilunar valve cusps.

The *auricularis* of the mitral valve consists of an elastic lamina with interspersed collagen fibers and smooth muscle cells lying beneath a continuous layer of endothelial cells. The auricularis may comprise as much as 20% of the leaflet structure and represents a continuation of the atrial endocardium, extending over approximately 60% of the leaflet surface. At the free edge of the leaflet, all the histologic regions merge, and the elastic lamellae are less superficial and are covered by a layer of connective tissue containing collagen fibers and few cells.

The spongiosa is histologically similar to that of aortic and pulmonary valves. In contrast to semilunar valves, this layer dips into the insertion sites of the chordae tendineae.

The fibrosa contains fibroblasts and other types of connective tissue cells, as well as a continuous layer of crimped collagen bundles that are oriented parallel (circumferential) to the ventricular surface and continue into the chordae tendineae. The latter structures consist of an outer layer lined by endothelial cells and an inner core. The outer layer has a subendothelial region containing a few collagen and elastic fibers. As mentioned above, the inner core is a continuation of the valvular fibrosa and consists of longitudinally oriented, crimped collagen bundles. Fibroblasts and myofibroblasts are interspersed between the collagen bundles in these areas.

The ventricularis represents a continuation of the ventricular endocardium. It is covered by an endothelial cell layer with a subendothelial region rich in proteoglycans and elastic fibers. The elastic fibers in the ventricularis of the posterior cusp are shorter than those in the auricularis. The ventricularis of the anterior cusp, in contrast to that of the posterior cusp, is a continuation of the subaortic endocardium and can be readily identified by the presence of dense elastic fibers, which may be more prominent than those in the auricularis.

References

1. Gross L, Kugel MA. Topographic anatomy and histology of the valves in the human heart. Am J Pathol 1931;7:445–473.

2. Marron K, Yacoub MH, Polak JM, et al. Innervation of human atrioventricular and arterial valves. Circulation 1996;94:368–375.

3. Kolb R, Pischinger A, Stockinger L. Ultrastuktur der Pulmonalisklappe des meerschweinchens. Beitrag zum Studium der egetative-nervosen Pripheris. Z Mikrosk Anat Forsch 1967;76:184–211.

4. Clark RE, Finke EH. The morphology of stressed and relaxed human aortic leaflets. Trans Am Soc Artif Intern Organs 1974;20B:437–448.

5. Missirlis YF, Armeniades CD. Ultrastructure of the human aortic valve. Acta Anat (Basel) 1977; 98:199–205.

6. Ferrans VJ, Spray TL, Billingham ME, Roberts WC. Structural changes in glutarraldehyde-treated porcine heterografts used as substitute cardiac valves. Transmission and scanning electron microscopic observations in 12 patients. Am J Cardiol 1978;41:1159–1184.

7. Wheeler EE, Gavin JB, Herdson PB. A scanning electron microscopy study of human heart valve allografts. Pathology 1972;4:185–192.

8. Hammon JW, Jr., O'Sullivan MJ, Oury J, Fosburg RG. Allograft cardiac valves. A view through the scanning electron microscope. J Thorac Cardiovasc Surg 1974;68:352–360.

9. Swanson WM, Clarke RE. Dimensions and geometric relationships of the human aortic valve as a function of pressure. Circ Res 1974; 35:871–882.

10. Messier RH, Bass BL, Aly HM. Dual structural and functional phenotypes of the porcine aortic valve interstitial characteristics of the leaflet myofibroblast. J Surg Res 1994;57:1–21.

11. Mulholland DL, Gotlieb AI. Cell biology of valvular interstilial cells. Canadian Journal of Cardiology 1996;12:231–236.

12. Filip DA, Radu A, Simionescu M. Interstitial Cells of the Heart Valves Possess Characteristics Similar to Smooth Muscle Cells. Circulation Research 1986;59:310–319.

13. Gavriel Y, Sherman Y, Ben-Sasson SA. Identification of programmed cell death in situ via specific labeling of nuclear DNA fragmentation. J Cell Biol 1992;119:493–501.

14. Schoen FJ, Levy RJ, Nelson AC, et al. Onset and progression of experimental bioprosthetic heart valve calcification. Lab Invest 1985;52:523–532.

15. Zhang J, Yu ZX, Fuijita S, et al. Interstitial dendritic cells of the rat heart. Quantitative and ultrastructureal changes in experimental myocardial infarction. Circulation 1993;87:909–920.

15a. Maish M. Hoffman-Kim D, Krueger PM, Harper JJ, Hopkins RA. Tricuspid valve biopsy: A potential source of cardiac myofibroblast cells for tissue engineered cardiac valves. J Heart Valve Dis 2003;12:264–269.

16. Hilbert SL, Barrick MK, Ferrans VJ. Porcine aortic valve bioprosthesis: A morphologic comparison of the effects of fixation pressure. J Biomed Mat Res 1990;24:773–787.

17. Flomenbaum MA, Schoen FJ. Effects of fixation back pressure and antimineralization treatment on the morphology of porcine aortic bioprosthetic valves. J Thorac Cardiovasc Surg 1993;105:154–164.

18. Broom ND, Christie GW. The structure/function relationship of fresh and glutaraldehyde-fixed aortic valve leaflets. In Cohn LH, Gallucci V (eds). Cardiac Bioprostheses. New York: Yorke 1982:476–491.

19. Missirlis MF, Chong M. Aortic valve mechanics. I. Material properties of native porcine aortic valves. J Bioeng 1978;12:287–300.

20. Williams BT, Bellhouse BJ, Ashton T. Autologous superior vena cava as a material for heart valve replacement. J Thorac Cardiovasc Surg 1973;66:952–958.

21. Brewer RJ, Deck JD, Capati B, Nolan SP. The dynamic aortic root. Its role in aortic valve function. J Thorac Cardiovasc Surg 1976;72:413–417.

22. Thubrikar MJ, Aouad J, Nolan SP. Comparison of the in vivo and in vitro mechanical properties of aortic valve leaflets. J Thorac Cardiovasc Surg 1986;92:29–36.

23. Bashey RI, Jimenez SA. Collagen in Heart Valves. In Nimni ME (ed). Collagen. Boca Raton, FL: CRC Press 1988:257–273.

24. Scotten LN, Walker DK, Brownlee RT. The in vitro function of 19mm bioprosthetic heart valves in the aortic position. Life Support Systems 1986;5:145–153.

25. Ruggerri A, Benazza F. Collagen-proteoglycan interactions. In Ruggerri A, Motta PM (eds). Ultrastructure of the Connective Tissue Matrix. Boston: Nijhoff 1984:113–125.

26. Thyberg CJO. Electron microscopy of proteoglycans. In Ruggerri A, Motta PM (eds). Ultrastructure of the Connective Tissue Matrix. Boston: Nijhoff 1984:95–112.

27. Smith JC. The pathology of human aortic valve homografts. Thorax 1967;22:114–138.

28. Ross D, Yacoub MH. Homograft replacement of the aortic valve. A critical review. Prog Cardiovasc Dis 1969;11:275–293.

29. Lange PL, Hopkins RA, Brockbank K. Allograft valve banking: Techniques and technology. In Hopkins RA (ed). Cardiac reconstructions with allograft valves. New York: Springer-Verlag 1989:37–64.

23
Biomechanics: Allograft Heart Valves

Stephen L. Hilbert, Frederick J. Schöen, and Victor J. Ferrans

Aortic and Pulmonary Valves

The hemodynamic performance of the aortic valve is determined by the dynamics of the aortic root, the pattern of cuspal closure in response to small changes in pressure, and the sharing of mechanical and dynamic stresses between the cusps and the sinuses of Valsalva. Stresses within the valvular tissue result from the presence of a pressure gradient across the cusps when the valve is closed and from the reversal of the cuspal curvature as the valve responds to changes in pressure and flow during the cardiac cycle. Studies of the effects of increasing pressure applied across a closed aortic valve, as occurs during diastole, demonstrated that neither the commissural height nor the length of the free edge change with increasing pressure, although distension of the aortic annulus (rarely exceeding 10%) was noted between zero and 120 mm Hg.[1] However, the diameter of the sinuses of Valsalva and the elastic modulus increase (compliance decreases) with increasing pressure, while a corresponding decrease in coaptive surface area and cuspal thickness occurs. A progressive increase in radial (perpendicular to the free edge) stresses is observed from the base to the free edge, particularly near the *nodulus Arantii*. The dimensional changes that occur in response to increasing pressure serve to distribute circumferential (parallel to the free edge), uniform stresses along the coaptive surface. Circumferential stresses are negligible when

the peak diastolic pressure is reached. Increasing pressure also results in decreases in cuspal thickness and in bending stresses within the coaptive region. The bending stresses generated during cuspal opening and closure are lower in magnitude than the circumferentially distributed static stresses present in the tissue when the valve is closed.[1–7]

The biomechanical properties of the aortic valve correlate with and are dependent on the unique histologic organization of the valvular extracellular components.[3] The nonlinear viscoelastic properties of aortic valve tissue have been demonstrated by stress/strain studies. In addition, the elastic modulus is greatest in the circumferential direction, while the extensibility is greatest in the radial direction. The anisotropic properties of aortic valve tissue result from the circumferential orientation of the collagen bundles in the fibrosa and the radial orientation of the elastic fibers (primarily in the ventricularis). The circumferential compliance is determined by the extent of crimping present in the collagen bundles of the fibrosa. Changes in collagen crimp influence the biomechanical properties, such as circumferential compliance, of valvular tissue. The progressive loss of collagen crimp results in a gradual reduction in compliance. Complete elimination of collagen crimp (i.e., straightening of collagen fibers) significantly alters the fatigue behavior of valvular tissue, culminating in collagen bundle "kinking" (Figure 23.1) and ultimately fracture of the collagen fibers.[3,8] The integration of the cuspal extracellular connective tissue

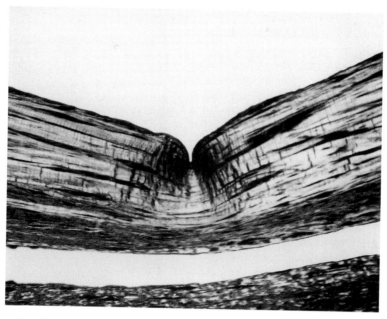

FIGURE 23.1. Glycol methacrylate section of a commissural cord illustrating a "kink" in the collagen bundles present in the fibrosa. High pressure fixed porcine aortic valve bioprosthesis. Toluidine blue stain. × 100.

components into the structure of the sinuses of Valsalva allows for the transfer of stresses from the cusp to the sinus wall. The basal region of the cusp at the junction with the sinus wall undergoes extensive bending stresses during systole. The stresses in this region are accommodated by an expanded wedge-shaped spongiosa that is rich in proteoglycans.[9] The marked expansion of the spongiosa and its increased proteoglycan content at this site serve to reduce the shear and bending stresses generated by the opposing motions of the fibrosa and the ventricularis. The fibrosa continues into the sinus wall, where the collagen bundles merge into the extracellular matrix of the aortic wall.[9]

It is notable that biaxial stress/strain studies have demonstrated an age-dependent change in the radial extensibility (referred to as radial stretch). A 40% decrease in radial stretch occurs between 15 and 25 years of age; however, aortic valve radial extensibility remains constant until 40 years of age and then decreases at a rate of approximately 1% per year. The impact of this observation on the selection of valve donors based on age is unknown.[10]

Mitral Valve

In contrast to that of semilunar valves, the function of atrioventricular valves depends not only on hemodynamic and leaflet biomechanics, but also on the active contraction of the annulus and the mitral valve apparatus (papillary muscles and chordae tendineae). As a result of papillary muscle contraction, the chordae tendineae elongate (with loss of collagen crimp), restricting leaflet movement and maintaining coaptation as the ventricular pressure rises.

The principal components of the extracellular matrix and their relative proportions (reported as a percentage of leaflet weight) are as follows: type I collagen, 60%; elastic fibers, 10%, and proteoglycans, 20%.[11,12] As previously discussed, the majority of the collagen fibrils are arranged in dense bundles running parallel to the free edge of the leaflet in the fibrosa. Collagen has the highest elastic modulus (stiffness) of the various extracellular matrix components. The predominance of circumferentially oriented collagen is responsible for the tensile strength of mitral valvular tissue. The anterior leaflet, which has a greater thickness and cross-sectional area, supports a greater tensile load than does the posterior leaflet. The unique histologic structure of valvular tissue and the proteoglycan-rich spongiosa greatly reduce the bending stresses within both the anterior and the posterior cusps. The auricularis and the spongiosa are quite prominent in the coaptive region of the valve and may be responsible for the observed reduction in cuspal stresses in this area during leaflet closure.

Finite element analysis has demonstrated that the principal stresses within the leaflet are oriented circumferentially, corresponding to the principal orientation of the collagen bundles in the fibrosa. In addition, this modeling technique has predicted that the combination of annular contraction and increasing tensile stress within the chordae tendineae (secondary to papillary muscle contraction) facilitates the optimal distribution of stresses in the mitral valve leaflet.[12]

Nonlinear stress/strain biomechanical properties have been described for both mitral valve leaflets, as tested in the circumferential and radial direction.[13,14] The anterior and posterior leaflets demonstrate anisotropic properties, since the elastic modulus is greater in the circumferential than in the radial direction. A significantly greater change in circumferential versus radial elastic modulus was observed in the anterior leaflet.

The posterior leaflet is more extensible than the anterior leaflet, although the post-transitional elastic moduli of the two leaflets are comparable. A comparison of uniaxial and biaxial stress/strain studies indicates that increasing the circumferential load markedly influences the radial extensibility and elastic modulus. It has been postulated that this finding may reflect the interaction between collagen fibers or bundles; however, additional factors, such as the number of chordae tendineae insertion sites, also may contribute to this observation.[14]

References

1. Swanson WM, Clarke RE. Dimensions and geometric relationships of the human aortic valve as a function of pressure. Circ Res 1974; 35:871–882.
2. Schoen FJ, Levy RJ, Nelson AC, et al. Onset and progression of experimental bioprosthetic heart valve calcification. Lab Invest 1985;52:523–532.
3. Broom ND, Christie GW. The structure/function relationship of fresh and glutaraldehyde-fixed aortic valve leaflets. In Cohn LH, Gallucci V (eds). Cardiac Bioprostheses. New York: Yorke 1982:476–491.
4. Missirlis MF, Chong M. Aortic valve mechanics. I. Material properties of native porcine aortic valves. J Bioeng 1978;12:287–300.
5. Thubrikar MJ, Aouad J, Nolan SP. Comparison of the in vivo and in vitro mechanical properties of aortic valve leaflets. J Thorac Cardiovasc Surg 1986;92:29–36.
6. Deck JD, Thubrikar MJ, Schneider PJ, Nolan SP. Structure, stress, and tissue repair in aortic valve leaflets. Cardiovascular Research 1988;22:7–16.
7. Van Steehoven AA, Veenstra PC, Reneman RS. The effect of some hemodynamic factors on the behavior of the aortic valve. J Biomech 1982; 15:941–950.
8. Broom ND. The stress/strain and fatigue behavior of gllutaraldehyde processed heart valve tissue. J Bioeng 1977;10:707–724.
9. Gross L, Kugel MA. Topographic anatomy and histology of the valves in the human heart. Am J Pathol 1931;7:445–473.
10. Christie GW. Age dependent changes in the radial stretch of human aortic valve leaflets determined by bi-axial testing. Ann Thorac Surg 1995;60: S156–S158.
11. Lis Y, Buarleigh MC, Parker DJ, Child AH, Hogg J, Davies MJ. Biochemical characterization of individual normal, floppy and rheumatic human mitral valves. Biochem J 1987;244:597–603.
12. Kunzelman KS, Cochran RP, Murphree SS, Ring WS, Verrier ED, Eberhart RC. Differential collagen distribution in the mitral valve and its influence on biomechanical behaviour. J Heart Valve Dis 1993;2:236–244.
13. Kunzelman KS, Cochran RP. Stress/Strain Characteristics of Porcine Mitral Valve Tissue: Parallel Versus Perpendicular Collagen Orientation. J Card Surg 1992;7:71–78.
14. May-Newman K, Yin FC. Biaxial mechanical behavior of excised porcine mitral valve leaflets. Am J Physiol 1995;269:H1319–H1327.

24
Effects of Preimplantation Processing on Allograft Valves

Stephen L. Hilbert, Frederick J. Schöen, and Victor J. Ferrans

Cellular Components

An increase in the actuarial freedom from primary tissue failure and reoperation has been reported following the use of cryopreserved allograft heart valves.[1-3] It has been hypothesized that the increased durability of cryopreserved heart valves is related to the retention of viable cuspal cells; however, other investigators have suggested that this observation is the consequence of tissue processing methods which do not necessarily preserve cell viability but minimally damage the valvular extracellular matrix.[4-9] If the retention of viable donor cuspal fibroblasts is responsible for the noted increase in allograft valve durability, then every effort should be made to optimally harvest and process allograft heart valve tissue in a manner that ensures minimal loss of viable cuspal cells.

Currently, in most clinical centers, allograft heart valves are harvested, disinfected and cryopreserved in the following manner: 1) warm ischemic time (see discussion to follow) is generally restricted to 24 hours or less; 2) cold temperatures (4°C) are used for dissection to procure the allograft and for subsequent transportation; 3) disinfection typically involves the immersion of the allograft for 24 hours (4°C) in solutions containing antibiotics (e.g., cefoxitin, lincomycin, polymyxin B, vancomycin); 4) the use of dimethylsulfoxide (10%) as a cryoprotectant, and 5) controlled-rate freezing (1 degree per minute to −70°C) of the allograft valve and subsequent storage in liquid nitrogen vapor (−170°C).

Independent of the processing method selected, there is an obligatory interval of time, referred to as the warm ischemic time, which elapses from the cessation of the donor's heartbeat to the initial cooling of the allograft in transport media. The duration of warm ischemia represents a period of potential cellular injury and cell death, which significantly alters the number of viable cells present in the cusp at the time of implantation. Detailed ultrastructural studies evaluating the extent of cellular injury induced by increasing the duration of the warm ischemic intervals have been conducted on porcine, and human aortic and pulmonary valves.[6,7,10] Morphologic indicators of reversible cellular injury (dilatation of endoplasmic reticulum, cytoplasmic edema, mitochondrial swelling) are observed early (e.g., 40 minutes) after the death of the donor and gradually progress to irreversible injury (mitochondrial flocculent densities, karyolysis, cell disruption) through 12 hours of warm ischemia. A significant increase (i.e., 10% to 25%) in the number of irreversibly injured cells occurs between 12 and 24 hours of warm ischemia.

Approximately 40% of the cuspal cells in human cryopreserved allograft valves demonstrate ultrastructural evidence of irreversible injury following 16 to 20 hours of warm ischemia.[6] As the warm ischemic time increases, a progressive loss of endothelial cells, fibroblasts and myofibroblasts occurs. Endothelial cell loss was most notable initially, while the morphology of leaflet interstitial cells began to significantly deteriorate after approximately 12 hours of warm ischemia. Similar observations have been made in aortic allograft conduits harvested 24 and 48 hours after death.[11] Extensive morphologic changes (i.e., pyknotic nuclei, cytoplasmic eosinophilia) were reported in smooth muscle cells in these grafts.[11] Flow cytometry studies utilizing fluorescent indicators of cell viability (e.g., FDA-PI) have demonstrated a significant negative correlation between warm ischemic time and cell viability.[5] A good correlation has been observed between estimates of the percentage of viable cells (as assessed by flow cytometry), and ultrastructural changes in cell integrity after 6 hours of warm ischemia.[5,7] Furthermore, the absolute number of cuspal cells may be expected to be further reduced as a consequence of additional processing (e.g., disinfection, cryopreservation, freezing and storage).

The effects of pre-harvesting warm ischemia, disinfection, cryopreservation and thawing on adenine nucleotide metabolism have been recently reported.[12–14] These studies indicate that both the duration of harvest-related warm ischemia and preimplantation processing (disinfection, cryopreservation, thawing) induce marked alterations in allograft valve metabo-lism, as shown by a decrease in adenine nucleotides and an increase in lactate production. An inverse relationship was also noted between the duration of warm ischemia and the levels of metabolites of high-energy phosphates. These findings indicate that a shift from aerobic to anaerobic metabolism occurred secondary to tissue hypoxia in an attempt to maintain adequate intracellular adenine nucleotide levels.

Extracellular Matrix

Increasing the duration of the warm ischemia or of the preimplantation processing results in a progressive loss of proteoglycans; however, the morphologic characteristics of the elastic fibers and collagen fibrils are retained (Figure 24.1). Collagen crimp (as demonstrated by polarized light microscopy) and the extent of collagen crosslinking were unaltered by extended periods of warm ischemia (i.e., 72 hours) and allograft processing (DG Crescenzo and SL Hilbert [unpublished results]).

It has been suggested that the clinical performance of allografts may be influenced by the duration of the warm ischemic interval and the method of preimplantation processing.[12,13,15] It

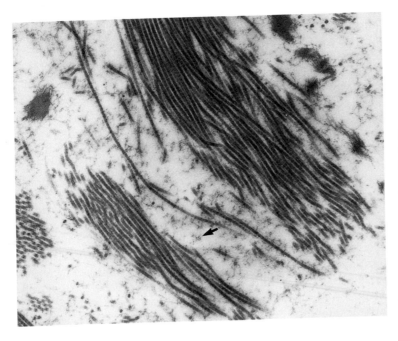

FIGURE 24.1. Transmission electron micrograph demonstrating the ultrastructural appearance of a porcine aortic valve exposed to 24 hours of warm ischemia before processing. A moderate loss of proteoglycans (arrow) is observed. Collagen fibrils and elastic fibers have retained their characteristic morphology. Uranyl acetate and lead citrate stain. × 14,000.

remains to be demonstrated whether or not there is any retention of a significant number of fibroblasts that remain viable, and whether or not the viability of such cells can have subsequent effects on the long-term durability of allograft valves. The presence of morphologically intact cellular and extracellular components may simply be an indicator of the adequacy of allograft valve harvesting, disinfection and cryopreservation protocols.

References

1. O'Brien MF, Stafford EG, Gardner MAH, Phaler PG, McGiffin DC, Kirklin JW. A comparison of aortic valve replacement with viable cryopreserved and fresh allograft valves with a note on chromosomal studies. J Thorac Cardiovasc Surg 1987;94:812–823.
2. O'Brien MF, McGiffen DC, Stafford EG. Allograft aortic valve replacement: long-term comparative clinical analysis of the viable cryopreserved and antibiotic 4 degree stored valves. J Card Surg 1991;6(suppl):534–543.
3. O'Brien MF, Stafford EG, Gardner AH, et al. Allograft aortic valve replacement: long-term follow-up. Ann Thorac Surg 1995;60:S65–S70.
4. Hilbert S, Jones M, Ferrans VJ. Flexible Leaflet Replacement Heart Valves. In Wise DJ, Trantolo DJ, Altobelli DE, Yaszemski MJ, Gresser JD, Schwartz ER (eds). Encyclopedic Handbook of Biomaterials and Bioengineering Part B: Applications. New York: Dekker 1995:1111–1152.
5. Niwaya K, Sakaguchi J, Kawachi K, Kitamura S. Effect of warm ischemia and cryopreservation on cell viability of human allograft valves. Ann Thorac Surg 1995;60:S114–S117.
6. Crescenzo DG, Hilbert SL, Messier JrRH, Domkowski PW, Barrick MK, Lange PL, Ferrans V, Wallace RB, Hopkins RA. Human cryopreserved allografts: Electron microscopic analysis of cellular injury. Ann Thorac Surg 1993;55: 25–31.
7. Crescenzo DG, Hilbert SL, Barrick MK, Corcoran PC, St.Louis JD, Messier RH, Ferrans VJ, Wallace RB, Hopkins RA. Donor heart valves: electron microscopic and morphometric assessment of cellular injury induced by warm ischemia. J Thorac Cardiovasc Surg 1992;103: 253–257.
8. Mitchell RN, Jonas RA, Schoen FJ. Pathology of explanted cryopreserved allograft heart valves: comparison with aortic valves from orthotopic heart transplants. J Thorac Cardiovasc Surg 1998;115:118–127.
9. Hilbert SL, Luna RE, Zhang J, Wang Y, Hopkins RA, Yu ZX, Ferrans VJ. Allograft heart valves: the role of apoptosis-mediated cell loss. J Thorac Cardiovasc Surg 1999;117:454–462.
10. Armiger L, Thomson R, Strickett M, et al. Morphology of heart valves preserved by liquid nitrogen freezing. Thorax 1985;40:778–786.
11. Kadoba K, Armiger L, Sawatari K, Jonas RA. Influence of time from donor death to graft harvest on conduit function of cryopreserved aortic allografts in lambs. Circulation 1991;84: III100–III111.
12. St.Louis J, Corcoran P, Rajan S, Conte J, Wolfinbarger L, Hu J, Lange PL, Wang YN, Hilbert SL, Analouei A. Effects of warm ischemia following harvesting of allograft cardiac valves. EJCTS 1991;5:458–464; discus.
13. Domkowski PW, Messier RH, Crescenzo DG, Aly HA, Abd-Elfattah AS, Hilbert SL, Wallace RB, Hopkins RA. Preimplantation Alteration of Adenine Nucleotides in Cryopreserved Heart Valves. Ann Thorac Surg 1993;55:1–7.
14. Messier RH, Domkowski DW, Aly HM, Hilbert SL, Crescenzo DG, Hopkins RA, et al. Adenine nucleotide depletion in cryopreserved human cardiac valves: the "stunned" leaflet interstitial cell population. Cryobiology 1995;32:199–208.
15. Angell WW, Shumway NE, Kosek JC. A five-year study of viable aortic valve homografts. J Thorac Cardiovasc Surg 1972;64:329–339.

25
Explant Pathology Studies

Stephen L. Hilbert, Frederick J. Schöen, and Victor J. Ferrans

Despite the wide clinical use of allograft heart valves, studies of the pathological features of explanted cryopreserved allografts have been reported only recently. Further analysis of explanted allograft valves is needed to clarify the following important issues: 1) whether and to what extent viable cells are retained in optimally cryopreserved allografts; 2) what mechanisms of cell death (e.g., necrosis, apoptosis) underlie their attrition; 3) whether and to what extent allograft cells are replenished or the graft repopulated by cells from the recipient; 4) whether allograft cell viability at the time of implantation is an important determinant of long-term function; 5) the extent to which the integrity of the extracellular matrix, independent of cell viability, contributes to the long-term function of the allograft and 6) whether immune-mediated inflammatory responses play a role in the loss of valvular function.

Preclinical Studies

Preclinical animal studies involving allograft heart valves have been conducted predominantly in non-orthotopic models in which an allograft valved-conduit (also referred to as an aortic root) has been implanted in the systemic circulation thus avoiding the need for cardiopulmonary bypass.[1,2] Reconstruction of the right ventricular outflow tract has been accomplished in lambs using cryopreserved and antibiotic-disinfected aortic valve allografts.[3]

To the best of our knowledge, orthotopic aortic valve replacement in animals has been limited by significant animal model-related adverse events (e.g., supravalvular stenosis secondary to aortotomy healing). However, mitral valve allografts and stentless porcine aortic valve bioprostheses have been evaluated in their respective orthotopic sites.[4-6]

One of us (SLH) has been involved in the development of a non-orthotopic allograft model in juvenile sheep. This model is suitable for the evaluation of aortic valve allograft hemodynamics and morphology.[1] Fresh and cryopreserved sheep aortic valve allografts were implanted in the mid-thoracic aorta (left thoracotomy, 4th intercostal space) by means of proximal and distal end-to-end anastomoses following the temporary placement of a bypass shunt (to prevent spinal cord ischemia/paraplegia). A 5 mm ePTFE vascular graft served as a shunt between the distal aortic arch (approximately 2 cm proximal to the allograft anastomosis) and the left atrium. The use of this shunt raised the left atrial pressure to approximately 12–14 mm Hg, but did not result in the subsequent development of congestive heart failure in chronic (20 weeks) animals. The shunt served to increase the aortic pulse pressure by decreasing the diastolic pressure (e.g., 10–15 mm Hg). The placement of this shunt provided the appropriate hemodynamic conditions necessary to ensure the full range of leaflet motion and coaptation, as confirmed by Doppler echocardiography. The leaflets were observed to simply flutter throughout the cardiac cycle when the

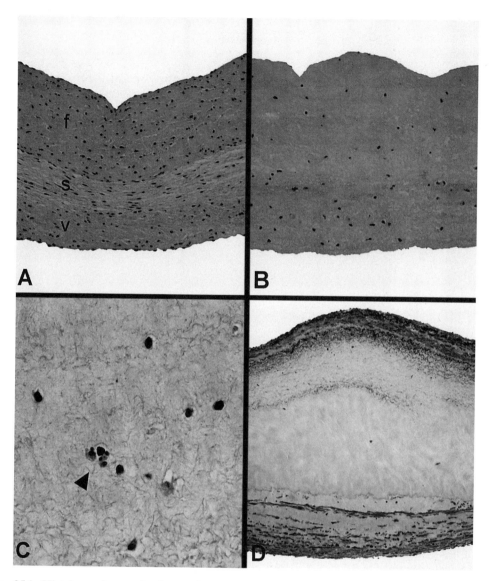

FIGURE 25.1. Histology of normal ovine aortic valve and implanted ovine aortic valve allografts. (A) Three distinct regions are present: the ventricularis (v), the spongiosa (s) and the fibrosa (f). H&E stain, × 100. (B) Cryopreserved ovine aortic valve allograft demonstrating the loss of the trilaminar histologic appearance of the cusp after 30 days of implantation. Note the loss of endothelial cells and a marked reduction in cuspal cellularity. H&E stain. × 100. (C) Cryopreserved ovine aortic valve allograft 30 days after implantaion. Pyknotic nuclei and apoptotic bodies in cells with increased cytoplasmic eosinophilia are depicted. Note the marked reduction in cuspal cellularity. H&E stain. × 100. (D) Low magnification view of section of a fresh ovine aortic valve allograft implanted for 20 weeks. The cusp is essentially acellular and encased by a thick fibrous sheath. Movat pentachrome stain. × 100.

aortic-left atrial shunt was cross-clamped or occluded.

The following histologic findings were similar in explanted fresh and cryopreserved allograft valves: 1) a marked reduction in leaflet cellu-larity occurred within the first 30 days of implantation (Figure 25.1A, B and C; see color insert); 2) an increase in cuspal thickness, primarily due to the formation of a layer of fibroelastic connective tissue (fibrous sheath) of recipient origin

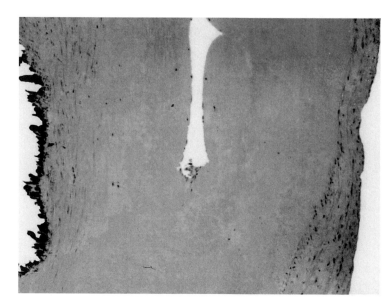

FIGURE 25.2. Histologic section of a fresh ovine aortic valve allograft 20 weeks after implantation. No cuspal calcification is apparent; however, extensive calcification (stained black) is present in the aortic wall. Note the fibrous sheath on the inflow aspect of the cusp. Von Kossa stain, × 100.

typically encased the allograft cusp by twenty weeks (Figure 25.1D); 3) macrophages were diffusely distributed in the extracellular matrix in long-term explants (i.e., 30 days or longer); 4) lymphocytes and plasma cells were rarely observed; 5) loss of an intact endothelial cell layer was consistently observed (see Figure 25.1B); 6) the characteristic trilaminar appearance of the aortic valve was significantly altered following 30 weeks of implantation, due to the loss of distinct boundaries between the ventricularis and spongiosa (Figure 25.1B); 7) cuspal calcification was not observed following 20 weeks of implantation, although the aortic wall was extensively mineralized (Figure 25.2) and 8) collagen crimp was typically present in short-term explants (i.e., less than 30 days) (Figure 25.3A), while prominent regions of collagen straightening (elongation) were present in long-term explants (e.g., 20 weeks) (Figure 25.3B). Collagen fibrils were not fractured.[1] In contrast to glutaraldehyde crosslinked bioprosthetic heart valves, extensive calcification was not observed in allograft valve leaflets.

We have recently studied the pathologic mechanisms responsible for the marked reduction in leaflet cellularity noted in allografts following 30 days or longer of implantation in the systemic circulation. Laser scanning confocal fluorescence microscopy methods were devel-oped for the simultaneous detection of Factor VIII, mitotic activity, cell density and apoptosis in allograft valves. Mitotic activity was assessed by an immunostaining method for the demonstration of proliferating cell nuclear antigen (PCNA). Leaflet cellularity was evaluated using 4′,6-diamidino-2-phenylindole, (DAPI), a fluorescent nuclear stain.

Apoptosis, also referred to as programmed cell death, is a selective nuclear process (e.g., cleavage of double stranded nuclear DNA; formation of nucleosomes) responsible for cell deletion during embryogenesis, normal cell turnover in various organ systems as well as in a variety of pathologic conditions.[7] Apoptosis was demonstrated by the nuclear incorporation of fluorescein-conjugated or biotinylated deoxynucleotides by terminal deoxynucleotydyl transferase (TUNEL).[1] In addition, transmission electron microscopic studies were conducted on selected tissue specimens to determine whether or not they contained apoptotic bodies derived from the nuclear fragmentation of cells undergoing apoptosis.

The results of this investigation demonstrated that a marked reduction in the mitotic activity of leaflet cells occurred within two days of implantation, as assessed by the loss of PCNA reactivity (Figure 25.4; see color insert). Endothelial cells are progressively lost from the leaflet surfaces after implantation, as demonstrated by Factor VIII immunostaining and by light and electron microscopy. Endothelial cells are focally present on the leaflet surface through 10 days of implantation, but are rarely seen after 30 days. Apoptosis occurred in leaflet connective tissue cells of allografts at two days after implantation as valved conduits in the systemic circulation (Figure 25.5A; see color insert). Apoptosis reached a peak between 10–14 days (Figure 25.5B) and resulted in the formation of numerous apoptotic bodies (Figure 25.5C and D; Figure 25.6), pyknotic nuclei (Figure 25.7) and in the progressive loss of leaflet cellularity following 30 days of implantation.

After twenty weeks of implantation, the following findings were observed: 1) the leaflets were essentially acellular, with the exception of rare myofibroblasts and macrophages (thought to be of donor origin); 2) no apoptotic bodies or PCNA-positive cells were observed; and 3)

the cusps were markedly thickened and contracted, due to extensive fibrous sheathing of host origin. The fibrous sheath consisted of a proteoglycan-rich extracellular matrix, interstitial myofibroblasts and a layer of Factor VIII-positive endothelial cells. The reaction for PCNA was negative in most of these cells, indicating that both the endothelial cell and the myofibroblast populations stabilize after a rapid, initial increase in number. Significant cuspal thickening and contraction resulted in either valvular insufficiency or complete immobilization of the leaflet against the aortic wall.

The results of this study suggest that apoptosis plays a major role in the loss of allograft cell viability and the subsequent decrease in leaflet cellularity observed in explanted allograft valves. Taken together, the histologic and metabolic preclinical studies reviewed in this chapter suggest that the improved long-term clinical performance of cryopreserved allograft

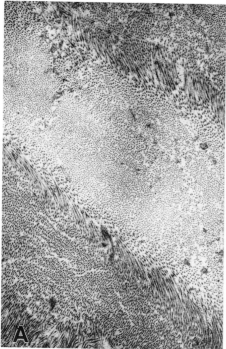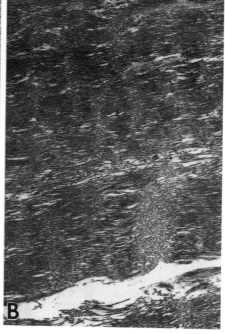

FIGURE 25.3. Transmission electron micrographs of collagen in ovine aortic valve allografts. (A) Collagen crimp is retained in this region of cryopreserved allograft implanted for 30 days. × 3,500. (B) Regions of straightening of the collagen crimp in the fibrosa of a fresh ovine aortic valve allograft after 20 weeks of implantation as a valved-conduit in the systemic circulation. × 2,900.

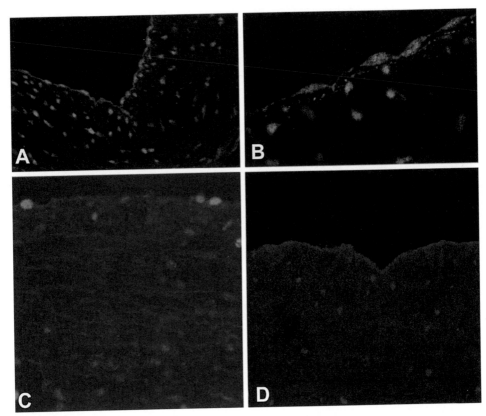

FIGURE 25.4. Confocal images demonstrating reactivity for PCNA and Factor VIII in native ovine aortic valve (A and B) and implanted ovine aortic valve allografts (C and D). (A) Native ovine aortic valve showing PCNA-positive nuclei (green fluorescence) in myofibroblasts and endothelial cells. × 400. (B) High magnification view demonstrating the presence of Factor VIII in the cytoplasm of endothelial cells (red fluorescence) lining the outflow surface of the fibrosa. PCNA-positive nuclei (green fluorescence) are also present. × 1,000. (C) The number of PCNA-positive nuclei is markedly reduced in the spongiosa and ventricularis of a cryopreserved ovine aortic valve allograft following 2 days of implantation. × 1,000. (D) Cryopreserved aortic valve allograft implanted for 30 days, demonstrating loss of endothelial cells from the surfaces and absence of reactivity for PCNA in cuspal tissue. Note the low level of autofluorescence in the extracellular matrix of the cusp. × 400.

valves may be related to the retention of critical components of the extracellular matrix rather than to the preservation of viable leaflet cells capable of remodeling valvular tissue.

The histologic findings noted in cryopreserved valves retrieved from patients at the time of reoperation for valvular dysfunction are similar to those observed in non-orthotopic animal models, with the exception of extensive fibrous sheath formation. The latter has been previously reported in bioprosthetic valved conduits implanted in young animals. One of us (SLH) has observed extensive fibrous sheathing in a single allograft used to reconstruct the right ventricular outflow tract in a patient with pulmonary atresia. The patient underwent reoperation because of calcific stenosis of the conduit at 5 years 9 months after implantation. Significant cuspal thickening, leaflet contraction and marked calcification of the aortic wall were present; however, calcific nodules were not seen in the leaflet tissue. Histologically, the leaflets were predominantly acellular, with diffusely distributed macrophages. Extensive fibrous sheathing was observed, with only the free edge of the cusp devoid of fibrous tissue. The trilaminar structure of the aortic valve cusp was lost, becoming homogeneous throughout. The incidence of fibrous sheath formation and the characteristics of the patient populations that may be at risk as the consequence of exuberant fibrous tissue response remains to be determined. In previous studies of human explanted antibiotic-treated human valve allografts approximately one-half of the cusp was covered by fibrous sheath.[8]

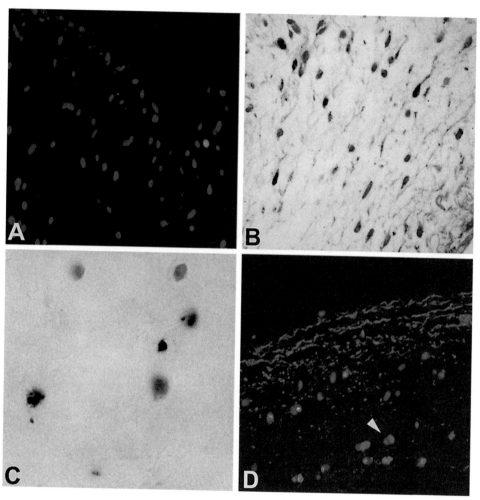

FIGURE 25.5. Apoptosis in ovine aortic valve allografts. (A) Cyropreserved allograft 2 days after implantation. Confocal image showing a single apoptotic nucleus (nick end labeling; green fluorescence). The leaflet cellularity is not reduced, and nonapoptotic nuclei are demonstrated by staining with DAPI (blue fluorescence). × 400. (B) Nick end labeling technique demonstrating apoptotic nuclei (black; peroxidase method) in the spongiosa of a fresh allograft implanted for 14 days. Nonapoptotic nuclei are counterstained with hematoxylin. × 630. (C) Cyropreserved allograft implanted for 30 days. Apoptotic nuclei and apoptotic bodies are demonstrated (black) by the peroxidase method for nick end labeling. × 1,000. (D) Apoptotic, pyknotic nuclei (nick end labeling; green fluorescence) and intracellular apoptotic bodies (arrowhead) are present in the ventricularis. Cusp cellularity is decreased as illustrated by nuclear counterstaining with DAPI (blue fluorescence). Elastic fibers in the ventricularis show moderate green autofluorescence. × 400.

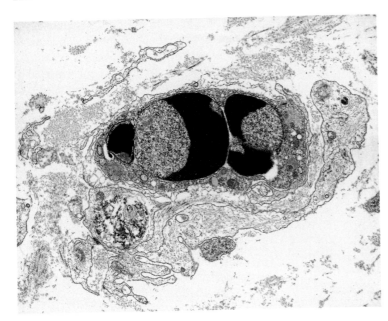

FIGURE 25.6. Transmission electron micrograph depicting the ultrastructural appearance of an apoptotic body. Note the presence of discrete nuclear fragments and crescent-shaped condensed nuclear chromatin. Cyropreserved aortic valve allograft implanted for 30 days. Uranyl acetate/lead citrate stain. × 6,000.

Clinical Studies

The pathologic changes that develop after implantation in non-cryopreserved allograft valves differ according to the method of preimplantation processing to which they are subjected.[8-13] Tissue processing, such as chemical sterilization, lyophilization and irradiation has been associated with cuspal rupture and calcification. As mentioned previously, less harsh methods of allograft processing, such as disinfection with antibiotics, storage at 4°C and cryopreservation, have resulted in a reduced incidence of primary tissue failure and calcification.[8,14] Cryopreserved allografts stored in liquid nitrogen vapor can also develop macroscopic or microscopic cracks which appear after

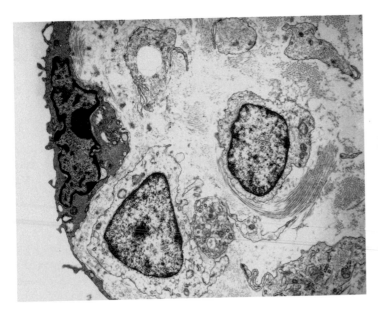

FIGURE 25.7. Ultrastructural features of a pyknotic endothelial cell present on the surface of the fibrosa are illustrated in this micrograph. Note marked condensation of the nuclear chromatin and contraction (darker staining) of the cytoplasm. Compare with normal chromatin and cytoplasm in adjacent fibroblasts. Uranyl acetate/lead citrate stain. × 4,800.

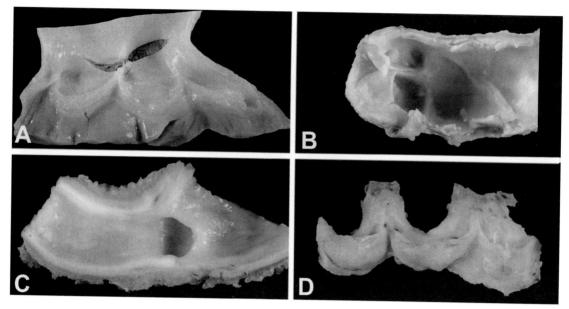

FIGURE 25.8. Failure modes of human cryopreserved allograft valves. (A) Macroscopic transmural crack in the aortic wall portion of a human aortic valve thawed after storage in liquid nitrogen vapor. (B) Gross photograph of an allograft valve implanted as a right-heart valved conduit in a child and explanted 7 months later because of stenosis. The valve cusps are thin; however the aortic wall is extensively calci-fied. (C) Allograft valve used for right ventricular outflow tract reconstruction and explanted 16 months later. Marked cuspal contraction and thickening are shown (compare to Figure 25.8). (D) Aortic valve allograft explanted 3 years after implantation because of central regurgitation secondary to cuspal elongation and prolapse.

rapid thawing (Figure 25.8A; see color insert).[15] The conditions which predispose to such defects have not been completely elucidated.

A recent study done in the laboratory of one of us (FJS) examined 33 explanted human cryopreserved allografts implanted from several hours to 9 years, serves to illustrate the pathological characteristics of these valves.[14] Of the explanted allografts, 20 had been used for aortic root replacements and 13 for right ventricle to pulmonary artery conduits. The latter were removed primarily because of structural deterioration (Figure 25.8B, C and D) of the valve, infection or growth-related stenosis of the valve or conduit. Also studied for comparison were 14 thawed cryopreserved human valves intended for implantation, but not used at surgery and 16 aortic valves from orthotopic allograft heart transplants removed at either autopsy or retransplantation. The orthotopic allograft heart transplant series had postopera-

tive intervals ranging from 2 days to >4 years, and included cases with fatal myocardial rejection and graft coronary arteriosclerosis. These valves were evaluated grossly and by light and electron microscopy and by methods for the immunohistochemical identification of endothelial cells, T- and B-lymphocyte subsets and macrophages.

Histologically, unimplanted cryopreserved and thawed human aortic and pulmonic valves retained their normal architecture (e.g., outflow surface corrugations formed by collagen bundle crimp within the fibrosa) and the trilaminar histologic characteristics of the native aortic valve. However, relative to normal valves the following morphologic features were observed: 1) mild autolysis with slight loss of the discrete collagen substructure and amorphous extracellular matrix; 2) variable nuclear pyknosis of the cuspal connective tissue cells; 3) loss of an intact endothelial cell layer lining the leaflet surfaces; 4) a minimal number of diffusely scattered mononuclear cells and 5) the absence of necrosis, cuspal hematoma, thrombosis and calcification (Figure 25.9A; see color insert). Moreover, normal human valves prepared as allografts have a low level, diffuse population of macrophages and T-lymphocytes present, perhaps as normal cellular constituents.

Cryopreserved allograft valve leaflets implanted for up to 18 days demonstrated progressive autolysis and structural deterioration, such as loss of distinct histologic layering, flattening of the normal outflow surface corrugations, and a variable, but occasionally marked, reduction in the number of connective tissue cells (Figure 25.9B and C). Endothelial cells were rarely seen on the leaflet surfaces. T-lymphocytes were the predominant type of inflammatory cells; however, these cells were not focally or diffusely increased in number. Cuspal hematomas[16] and superficial mural thrombi were frequently present. Further loss of leaflet histologic structure, fragmentation and reduced staining of elastic fibers, and flattening (thinning) of the cusps occurred in valves implanted for 2–11 months. Stainable residual connective tissue cells are rare. A mixed inflammatory cellular infiltrate, including T-lymphocytes, was prominent in those cases in which infective endocarditis necessitated explantation. A marked but unexplained lymphocyte infiltrate was noted in a single valve (Figure 25.10A; see color insert).

The cusps of allograft valves implanted for 1–9 years were uniformly flattened and thin, with loss of the corrugations in the outflow surface and an indistinct, non-layered histologic appearance (Figure 25.11D). Nevertheless, remnants of the normal trilaminar architecture, such as a residual elastin network in the ventricularis, could be demonstrated in most valves. Stainable cuspal cells or endothelial cells were rare. The progressive loss of cuspal cells noted above is consistent with the results of other recent studies, indicating that the endothelial cells and the interstitial cells in cryopreserved allograft valves implanted for relatively short periods of time (e.g., 1 to 2 months) are nonviable. Cuspal hematomas and mural thrombi (Figure 25.9D) were variably noted.

Focal cuspal calcification was found in some long-term implants. In stenotic valves present in right ventricular to pulmonary artery conduits explanted from children, arterial wall calcification was often extensive, but the cusps were generally not calcified (Figure 25.10B).

Morphologic studies of explanted cryopreserved allograft conduits demonstrated that the pulmonary and aortic arterial walls were acellular. Extensive medial autolysis and necrosis were observed as early as 3 days after implantation. In the walls of the great vessels, calcification appeared to be initiated in nucleation sites associated with nonviable cells and their remnants and, to a lesser extent, elastic fibers (Figure 25.10C) and collagen. In some cases, calcification of elastic fibers was prominent in conduits. These findings are consistent with the morphologic description of calcification observed in native and bioprosthetic valves and other cardiovascular tissues, including the aorta and atherosclerotic plaques.[17,18] Cuspal calcification (Figure 25.10D) was less frequent than arterial wall calcification, and is primarily associated with cuspal cells rather than with extracellular matrix.

The reason for the higher resistance to calcification in the cusps of cryopreserved allograft valves as compared to that of glutaraldehyde-fixed porcine bioprosthetic valves is unknown. We hypothesize that the extensive autolysis that occurs during harvesting, preimplantation processing, and even postimplantation, sufficiently alters the chemical composition of the residual cellular debris, reducing the numbers of nucleation sites for calcification. In addition, previous studies have indicated that the exposure of valvular tissue to glutaraldehyde, as occurs during the fabrication of bioprosthetic valves, further alters both the cellular and extracellular leaflet components and results in an increased potential for cuspal calcification.[19]

Transmission electron microscopy of long-term explants in our study (Figure 25.11) demonstrated abundant degenerated and fragmented cuspal cells, with focal microcalcifications (largely associated with cell membranes and organelles). Collagen bundles were preserved; however, a marked loss of collagen crimping was noted. Calcification of cuspal extracellular matrix

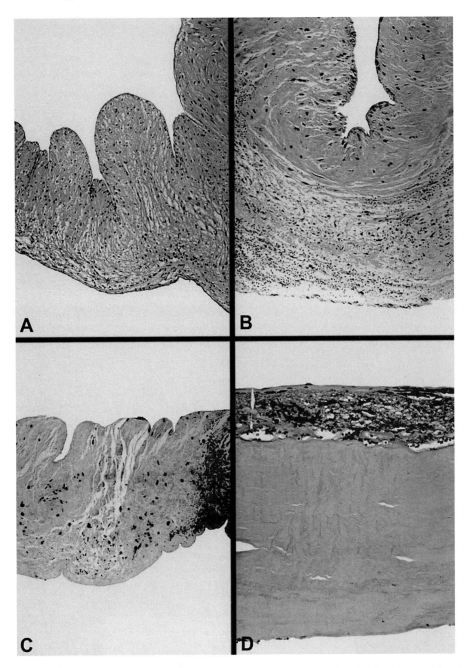

FIGURE 25.9. Histology of unimplanted and implanted human aortic valve allografts. (A) Unimplanted cryopreserved and thawed aortic valve allograft. Note the infolding (corrugations) of the fibrosa, the distinct histologic regions and the extent of cuspal cellularity. H&E stain. × 33. (B) Cryopreserved human aortic valve allograft implanted for eight days. The trilaminar histologic structure is retained; however, red blood cells are seen within the spongiosa and ventricularis. H&E stain. × 33. (C) Cryorpreserved human aortic valve allograft implanted for 18 days shows loss of distinct histologic layers and the lack of stainable cuspal cells. Sparse macrophages are present. An intracuspal hematoma is also present (right edge). Note the reduced eosinophilia of the extracellular matrix. Compare to Figure 6.22A&B. H&E stain. × 33. (D) Low magnification view of an allograft implanted for 7 years as a right-heart valved conduit. The cusp is essentially acellular, with pale staining of the extracellular matrix and loss of discrete trilaminar structure. Note the absence of endothelial cells. A mural thrombus is present on the outflow surface (top). H&E stain. × 33.

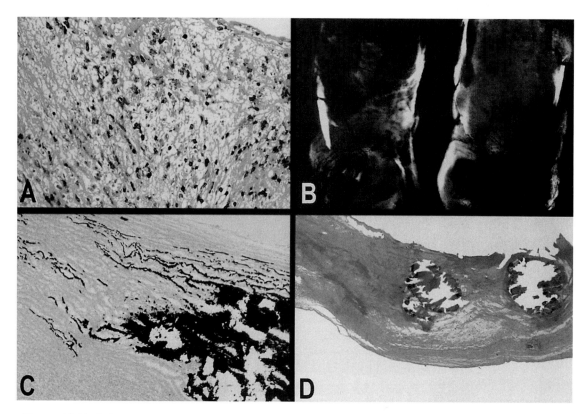

FIGURE 25.10. Inflammation and calcification in allograft valves. (A) Atypical histologic findings, demonstrating a marked inflammatory infiltrate (consisting predominantly of T-lymphocytes) are found in an explanted human aortic valve allograft. No histologic evidence (eg, bacteria; PMNs) consistent with endocarditis was noted. Immunohistochemical staining for T-lymphocytes (UCHL-1 antibody). Hematoxylin counterstain. × 50. (B) Radiograph demonstrating extensive calcification within the aortic wall of an allograft that was used to reconstruct the right ventricular outflow tract in a child and was explanted after 7 months because of conduit stenosis. The cal-

cification does not involve the aortic valve cusps. (C) Micrograph showing a calcific nodule and extensive calcification of the elastic lamellae in the aortic media of the wall of an explanted human aortic valve allograft that was implanted for 6 months as a pulmonary valved conduit. The media is essentially acellular. Von Kossa stain. × 33. (D) Low magnification view of two calcific nodules present within the cusp of a cryopreserved aortic valve allograft implanted for 5 years. Note the loss of the distinct histologic layers typical of an aortic valve cusp and the complete loss of cellularity. H&E stain. × 33.

components, such as collagen and elastic fibers was not observed.

The mode of late failure and its associated gross findings differed among valves implanted in the right and the left ventricular outflow tracts of the heart. Right ventricle-to-pulmonary artery conduits explanted from children typically demonstrated heavy calcification within the arterial walls (Figure 25.10B) and were stenotic; however, cuspal calcification was rarely observed. In contrast, flattened and

thinned noncalcified cusps were noted in regurgitant allograft valves explanted from the left side of the heart in adults. Fibrous sheathing was prominent only in a few of these valves. As in valves explanted from the right side of the heart, gross calcification of the cusps was rarely observed.

The postimplantation changes noted above, including loss of cellularity and cell viability, occur in the absence of significant mononuclear inflammatory cell infiltrates, even though patients are generally not immunosuppressed and the valves are implanted without regard to HLA or blood group status. The fact that inflammatory cells are rarely observed in explanted allograft valves suggests that immune-mediated mechanisms are not generally responsible for the loss of cell viability and marked reduction in cellularity. The paucity of inflammatory cells observed in our study does not support the concept presented by other investigators, who have hypothesized that the failure of cryopreserved allografts may have an immunologic (generally considered to be humoral) basis.[20,20–24]

In contrast to the significantly altered morphology of explanted cryopreserved allograft valves, aortic valves from long-term orthotopic cardiac transplants were essentially normal (Figure 25.12A and B; see color insert). Neither cuspal hematomas, mural thrombi or valvular calcification were noted in our study. Similar findings have been reported by other investigators in valves from transplanted hearts.[20] The morphologic findings in the valves of transplanted hearts failing due to severe rejection (Figure 25.12C) and transplantation-associated coronary arteriosclerosis (i.e., conditions in which a substantial mononuclear infiltrate is present)

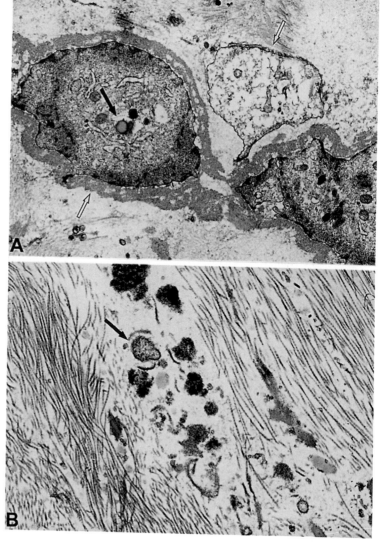

FIGURE 25.11. Transmission electron micrographs depicting cellular remnants and focal microcalcification in a long-term explanted aortic valve allograft cusp. Light microscopic study of this cusp did not demonstrate either cuspal cells or mineralization. (A) Cellular remnants (open arrow) and microcalcfication (solid arrow). (B) Collagen fibrils and cellular remnants (arrow). Note the loss of collagen crimp and the straightening of the collagen fibrils. Uranyl acetate/lead citrate stain. × 10,000. Reprinted from *Journal of Thoracic and Cardiovascular Surgery*, Vol 115, "Pathology of explanted cryopreserved allograft heart valves: comparison with aortic valves from orthotopic heart transplants," 118–127. © 1998, with permission from Elsevier.

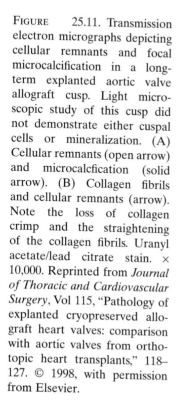

were not different from those in valves explanted from patients in whom immunological processes did not contribute to their demise. These findings further support the hypothesis that immune-mediated inflammatory mechanisms are not typically responsible for the loss of allograft valve cellularity following their use in patients or animals. The comparative histologic characteristics of cryopreserved allograft valves and aortic valves in orthotopic heart transplants are summarized in Table 25.1.

We also have examined three pulmonic-to-aortic autografts (Ross procedure) explanted after 18 days, 2 years (Figure 25.12D) and 6 years of function, respectively. The normal histologic structure of the cusps was retained in all three autografts. The pulmonary valve autograft that was explanted 6 years after implantation demonstrated a mild decrease in interstitial cellularity with an intact endothelial cell layer; focal intimal thickening of the pulmonary artery, without calcification, was also observed. In contrast to these findings, the cryopreserved allografts explanted 18 days and 2 years after use as a replacement for the auto-transplanted pulmonary valve were acellular,

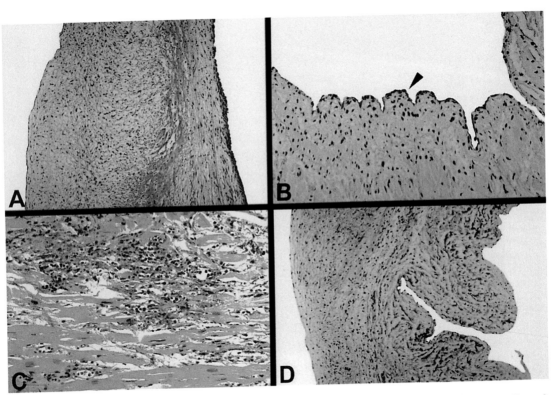

FIGURE 25.12. Histologic findings in valves (A and B) and myocardium (C) from human orthotopic cardiac allografts and after autotransplantation of aortic and pulmonary valves (Ross procedure) (D). (A) Micrograph demonstrating essentially normal aortic valve histology. Note the extent of cellularity and the presence of endothelial cells lining the surface of the cusp. H&E stain. × 25. (B) Higher magnification view demonstrating preservation of the endothelium on the surface of the fibrosa. Immunohistochemical staining for endothelial cells (CD31). Hematoxylin counterstain. × 50. (C) Histologic section of myocardium from an orthotopic cardiac allograft demonstrating dense infiltration of T-lymphocytes, consistent with myocardial rejection. Compare with Figure 25.10 A&B, noting that an inflammatory infiltrate is not present in the cuspal tissue in this transplanted heart. Immunohistochemical stain for T-lymphocytes (UCHL-1 antibody). Hematoxylin counterstain. × 50. (D) Pulmonary valve that was used in a Ross procedure and was explanted after 2 years. The histologic findings are essentially normal. H&E stain. × 25.

TABLE 25.1. Pathologic Features of Aortic/Pulmonic Cryopreserved Allograft Heart Valves and Aortic Valves from Orthotopic Heart Transplants.

	Cryopreserved Unimplanted	0–8 d	2–11 mo	1–9 y
Number of specimens	14	15	6	12
Trilaminar architecture	++	++	–	–
Stainable connective tissue cells	++	+/++	–	– to +[c]
Lymphocytic infiltrate (T-cells)	– to +	–/+	– to +++[b]	– to +
Intact endothelium	–/+	–/+	–	–
Intimal hyperplasia/pannus	–	–	–	+/–
Cuspal hematoma/thrombus	–	–/+	+/++	– to ++
Calcification				
cusps	–	–	–	– to +
walls	–	–	–	– to +++

[a] Cellularity and other morphologic measures of the valves semi-quantified as: – = not present, + = mild/minimal, ++ = moderate, and +++ = severe/marked.
[b] Substantial only in those valves with endocarditis.
[c] Predominantly associated with pannus.
Reprinted from *Journal of Thoracic and Cardiovascular Surgery*, Vol 115, "Pathology of explanted cryopreserved allograft heart valves: comparison with aortic valves from orthotopic heart transplants," 118–127. © 1998, with permission from Elsevier.

hyalinized and showed moderate loss of its trilaminar structure.

References

1. Hilbert SL, Luna RE, Zhang J, Wang Y, Hopkins RA, Yu ZX, Ferrans VJ. Allograft heart valves: the role of apoptosis-mediated cell loss. J Thorac Cardiovasc Surg 1999;117:454–462.
2. Allen MD, Shogi Y, Fujimura Y. Growth and cell viablility of aortic versus pulmonic homografts in the systemic circulation. Circulation 1991;84: III94–III99.
3. Jonas RA, Ziemer G, Britton L, Armiger LC. Cryopreserved and fresh antibiotic-sterilized valved aortic homograft conduits in a long-term sheep model. J Thorac Cardiovasc Surg 1988;96: 746–755.
4. Tamura K, Jones M, Yamada I, Ferrans VJ. A comparison of failure modes of glutaraldehyde-treated versus antibiotic-preserved mitral valve allografts implanted in sheep. J Thorac Cardiovasc Surg 1995;110:224–238.
5. Acar C, Tolan M, Berrebi A, et al. Homograft replacement of the mitral valve. Graft selection, technique of implantation, and results in forty-three patients. J Thorac Cardiovasc Surg 1996; 111:367–379.
6. Brown WMI, Jay JL, Gott JP, et al. Placement of aortic valve bioprostheses in sheep via a left thoracotomy. Implantation of stentless porcine heterograft. Trans Am Soc Artif Intern Organs 1991;37:M445–M446.
7. Gavriel Y, Sherman Y, Ben-Sasson SA. Identification of programmed cell death in situ via specific labeling of nuclear DNA fragmentation. J Cell Biol 1992;119:493–501.
8. Gavin JB, Herdson PB, Monro JL, Barratt-Boyes BG. Pathology of antibiotic-treated human heart valve allografts. Thorax 1973;28:473–481.
9. Hudson RE. Pathology of the human aortic valve homograft. Br Heart J 1966;28:291–301.
10. Smith JC. The pathology of human aortic valve homografts. Thorax 1967;22:114–138.
11. Ross D, Yacoub MH. Homograft replacement of the aortic valve. A critical review. Prog Cardiovasc Dis 1969;11:275–293.
12. Davies H, Missen GA, Blandford G, Roberts CI, Lessof MH, Ross DN. Homograft replacement of the aortic valve. A clinical and pathologic study. Am J Cardiol 1968;22:195–217.
13. Kosek JC, Iben AB, Shumway NE, et al. Morphology of fresh heart valve homografts. Surgery 1969;66:269–277.
14. Mitchell RN, Jonas RA, Schoen FJ. Pathology of explanted cryopreserved allograft heart valves: comparison with aortic valves from orthotopic heart transplants. J Thorac Cardiovasc Surg 1998;115:118–127.
15. Wassenaar C, Wijsmuller EG, van Herverden LA, Aghai Z, van Tricht C, Bos E. Cracks in cryo-

preserved aortic allografts and rapid thawing. Ann Thorac Surg 1995;60 Suppl:S165–S167.

16. Ichihara T, Ferrans VJ, Barnhart GR, Jones M, McIntosh CL, Roberts WC. Intracuspal hematomas in implanted porcine valvular bioprostheses, clinical and experimental studies. J Thorac Cardiovasc Surg 1982;83:399–407.

17. Ferrans VJ, Boyce SW, Billingham ME, et al. Calcific deposits in porcine bioprostheses: structure and pathogenesis. Am J Cardiol 1980;46:721–734.

18. Thubrikar MJ, Nolan SP, Aouad J, Deck JD. Stress sharing between the sinus and leaflets of canine aortic valve. Ann Thorac Surg 1986;42:434–440.

19. Golomb G, Schoen FJ, Smith MS, Linden J, Dixon M, Levy RJ. The role of glutaraldehyde-induced cross-links in calcification of bovine pericardium used in cardiac valve bioprostheses. Am J Pathol 1987;127:122–130.

20. Fishlein T, Schultz H, Haushofer M, et al. Immunologic reaction and viability of cryopreserved homografts. Ann Thorac Surg 1995;60:S122–S126.

21. Baskett RJ, Ross DB, Nanton MA, Murphy DA. Factors in the early failure of cryopreserved homograft pulmonary valves in children: preserved immunogenicity? J Thorac Cardiovasc Surg 1996;112:1170–1179.

22. Hogan P, Duplock L, Green M, Smith S, Gall KL, Frazer IH, O'Brien MF. Human aortic valve allografts elicit a donor-specific immune response. J Thorac Cardiovasc Surg 1996;112:1260–1267.

23. Smith JD, Ogino H, Hunt D, et al. Humoral immune response to human aortic valve homografts. Ann Thorac Surg 1995;60:S127–S130.

24. Batten P, McCormack AM, Rose ML, Yacoub MH. Valve interstitial cells induce donor-specific T-cell anergy. J Thorac Cardiovasc Surg 2001;122:129–135.

COLOR PLATE I

FIGURE 19.4. See page 179 for figure legend.

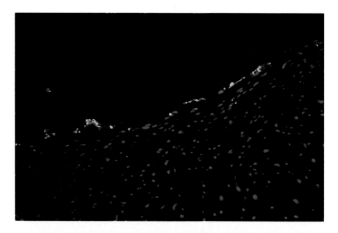

FIGURE 19.5. See page 180 for figure legend.

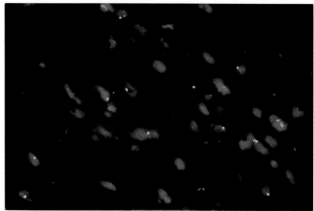

FIGURE 25.1. See page 217 for figure legend.

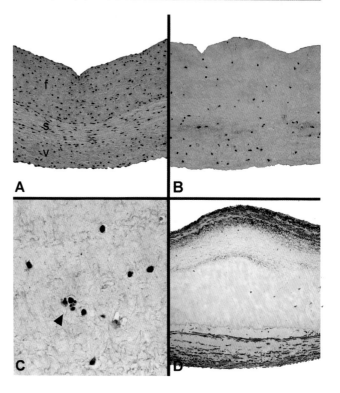

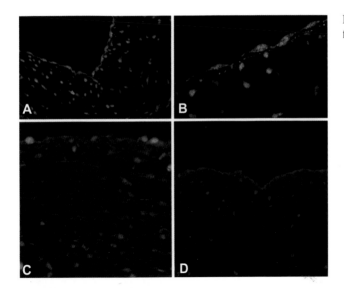

FIGURE 25.4. See page 220 for figure legend.

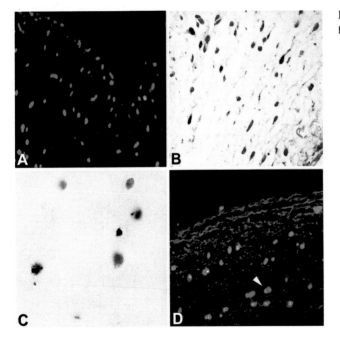

FIGURE 25.5. See page 221 for figure legend.

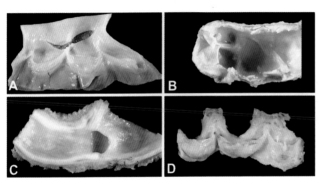

FIGURE 25.8. See page 223 for figure legend.

FIGURE 25.9.   See page 225 for figure legend.

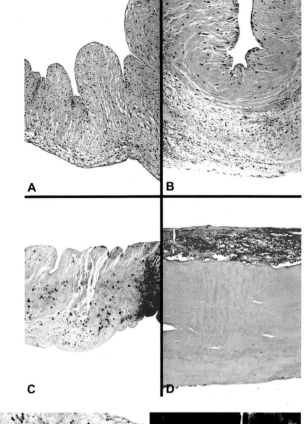

FIGURE 25.10.   See page 226 for figure legend.

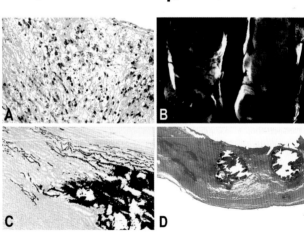

FIGURE 25.12.   See page 228 for figure legend.

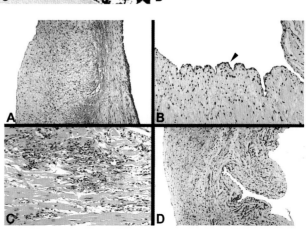

COLOR PLATE IV

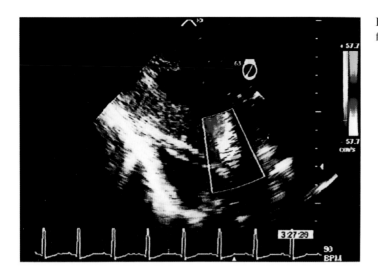

FIGURE 42.3. See page 400 for figure legend.

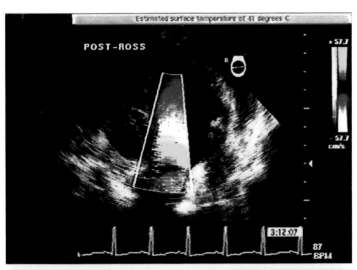

FIGURE 42.4. See page 400 for figure legend.

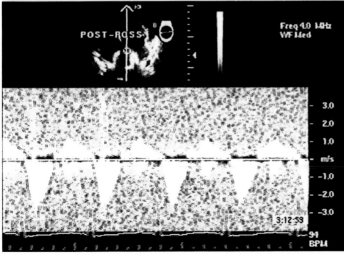

26
Implications of Explant Pathology Studies

Stephen L. Hilbert, Frederick J. Schöen, and Victor J. Ferrans

As described above, our collective preclinical and clinical experience has served to identify clearly the pathologic changes that occur following the implantation of fresh and allograft heart valves in the systemic circulation in juvenile sheep and in human patients. The morphologic findings in this series of investigations demonstrate that a marked reduction in mitotic activity occurs in both the endothelial cells and connective tissue cells of the allografts within a few days of implantation. The allograft valve cusps become acellular within one to two weeks of implantation. We have provided evidence, based on animal studies, that apoptosis is a major cause of the loss of cell viability in allografts during the first 30 days after implantation. We have shown that these changes occur in optimally harvested and processed fresh and cryopreserved allograft valves. The documentation of apoptosis by histochemical staining and by the ultrastructural demonstration of apoptotic bodies within allograft leaflets will have to be confirmed in clinically explanted allograft valves. These findings are in conflict with the expectation that viable cells are retained and are capable of replicating and participating in the remodeling of the allograft cusp.

The temporal evolution of the microscopic appearance of explanted cryopreserved allografts following implantation suggests that changes related to harvesting, handling, ischemic time, freezing and thawing are the factors which are most responsible for the loss of donor cell viability. Moreover, excessive neutrophilic and/or mononuclear inflammatory cell infiltrates are absent in most explanted cryopreserved valves at all time points, including those concurrent with histologic deterioration and loss of cellular staining. This leads to the conclusion that immunologic phenomena cannot be causally implicated in the processes involved in allograft degeneration. Moreover, evidence of immunologic injury to the valves is not seen (i.e., no valvular scarring or loss of cellularity) even in heart transplant patients in whom immunologic phenomena caused cardiac allograft failure, or in patients who sustained multiple episodes of parenchymal rejection.

Collectively, these results suggest that despite the demonstrable ability of allograft valves to induce a detectable humoral and/or cellular allogeneic response, some valves, depending on yet defined processing or innate variables, may be relatively resistant to immune injury, perhaps due to some combination of high flow, lack of valvular microvasculature, or low alloantigen expression, and/or lower expression of relevant adhesion or co-stimulator molecules. However, a recent study showed that all the aortic valve allografts explanted from infants had failed due to aortic insufficiency.[1] Intimal hyperplasia, extensive fibrous sheath formation and focal infiltrates of B-lymphocytes (CD20-positive) and T-lymphocytes (CD43-positive) were observed in the allografts retrieved from the infants. We are not aware of any investigations which have clearly demonstrated immunologically mediated allograft dysfunction, although many studies do indicate that transplanted allograft valves are immunogenic (e.g.—endothelial cells express HLA, MHC I and II antigens). Marked fibrous sheath formation is routinely observed in explanted xenograft bioprosthetic valves and conduits which are immunogenic but do not elicit an immune-mediated response resulting in valvular dysfunction.[2] Further investigations will be required to determine whether the early failure (i.e., aortic insufficiency with cuspal thickening and contraction) of some allografts explanted from infants is immunologically mediated or caused by a fibroelastic tissue response (i.e. fibrous sheath formation) secondary to flow conditions in the allograft (which may be exacerbated in infants and children).

It is also interesting to note that the mode of failure of allograft valves seems to be related to their placement in either the right versus left ventricular outflow tract (stenosis vs. insufficiency, respectively) or humans versus juvenile sheep (extensive fibrous sheathing develops in the latter). Extensive fibrous sheathing has been consistently observed in bioprosthetic valved conduits or allograft valves implanted in the systemic circulation of juvenile sheep and baboons. Further studies involving larger number of pediatric patients will have to be conducted to confirm this preclinical observation and to identify patient populations that may be at an increased risk for this failure mode (leaflet thickening and contraction).

Despite the loss of connective tissue cells and endothelial cells, calcification of the cusps of allografts does not result in significant primary tissue failure. This is in contrast to glutaraldehyde-fixed bioprosthetic valves in which this complication frequently occurs. The integrity of extracellular matrix components, primarily collagen and elastic fibers, is retained in long-term clinical explants, although collagen crimp and the characteristic trilaminar histologic structure of the valvular tissue are progressively lost. In spite of these changes, these valves show a satisfactory actuarial freedom from dysfunction and structural deterioration. The ultrastructural appearance of the cusps of explanted allograft valves is strikingly similar to that of glutaraldehyde-treated porcine bioprosthetic heart valves.[3]

The acellularity and the intact extracellular matrix of the leaflets suggest that the retention of the collagen and elastic fibers of cryopreserved allografts serves as the major structural basis for their long-term performance. These observations suggest that maintenance of long-term cell viability is not necessary for the proper function of allografts. Therefore, the number of potential allograft valve donors may be increased by less restrictive tissue harvesting and processing time constraints, which have been designed to maintain cell viability.

Conclusions

In conclusion, this section provides a review of allograft heart valve histology, biomechanics, tissue processing and the pathological changes that develop in these valves, particularly in cryopreserved allografts, after implantation in animal models and in patients. Although cryopreserved allograft valves have gained increased clinical acceptance, particularly for reconstruction of the right ventricular outflow tract, many fundamental scientific issues concerning these valves remain to be addressed, including: 1) the mechanisms responsible for the initiation of apoptosis of the valvular cells; 2) the development of approaches capable of mitigating this apoptosis; 3) the development of tissue processing and sterilization methods intended to enhance the long-term stability of the extracellular matrix components and the retention of their biomechanical properties; 4) the identification of unique failure modes that may be dependent on the age of the patient and the site of implantation; and 5) the possible liberalization of allograft harvesting criteria resulting in more allografts being available for transplantation, since the long-term viability of the cuspal cells are not maintained by current processing methods.

References

1. Rajani B, Uree RB, Ratliff NB. Evidence for rejection of homograft valves in infants. J Thorac Cardiovasc Surg 1998;115:111–117.

2. Ferrans VJ, Arbustini E, Eidbo EE, et al. Anatomic changes in right ventricular-pulmonary artery conduites implanted in baboons. In Bodnar E, Yacoub M (eds). Biologic and Bioprosthetic Valves. New York, NY: Yorke 1986:316.

3. Ferrans VJ, Spray TL, Billingham ME, Roberts WC. Structural changes in glutarraldehyde-treated porcine heterografts used as substitute cardiac valves. Transmission and scanning electron microscopic observations in 12 patients. Am J Cardiol 1978;41:1159–1184.

Section VIII
Allograft Valve Banking: Harvesting and Cryopreservation Techniques

27
Cryopreservation and Tissue Banking

Perry L. Lange and Richard A. Hopkins

The use of human allograft heart valves for replacement of congenitally defective or diseased heart valves has become normal practice in cardiothoracic surgery. From the early days of using wet-stored "nonviable" homografts to current methods of transplanting cryopreserved "viable" allografts, the superiority of human heart valve implants has been well documented.[1–7] Clinical demand for allograft heart valves is still growing. However, supply of this valuable human resource has become a limiting factor.

Donor selection and qualification is within the statutory purview of the FDA. The allograft tissue community has established its own overseeing body, the American Association of Tissue Banks (AATB). However, this is a voluntary accrediting organization so it is not mandatory. The AATB has established *"Standards for Tissue Banking"* ("Standards") reflecting the collective expertise and conscientious efforts of tissue bank professionals to provide a comprehensive foundation for the guidance of tissue banking activities.[8] These Standards address all aspects of tissue banking, from donor suitability to valve distribution, and assure allograft tissue recipients of receiving safe allograft cardiac tissue implants.

The United States Food and Drug Administration (FDA) began regulating allograft (human) heart valves as a Class III medical device in December of 1990 under a previous law aimed primarily at replacement heart valve manufacturers (mechanical, porcine, and bioprosthetic valves). The U.S. allograft processors

were instructed to file for pre-market approval (PMA) and enter into investigational device exemption (IDE) studies to prove their safety and effectiveness. This enforcement was withdrawn on October 14, 1994 (see Strong vs. FDA) and procedures were initiated to classify the allograft heart valve as a class II medical device. Since that time the FDA has issued notice that the classification for allograft heart valves will fall within the rules governing all human tissue (proposed 21 CFR 1271). Chapter 11 covers this unique series of regulatory events in more detail.

This review is based on the AATB Standards and the methods and procedures of LifeNet's cardiovascular tissue banking services. As a not-for-profit organization, LifeNet's goal is to provide the highest quality allograft heart valve at the lowest possible cost to the recipient. Recipient safety must be ensured through strict heart donor screening criteria and stringent quality control measures encompassing the entire heart valve preparation protocol.

Heart valve preparation protocols are divided into multiple areas: (A) donor suitability; (B) heart procurement; (C) heart valve dissection; (D) heart valve evaluation; (E) allograft sterilization/disinfection; (F) cryopreservation; (G) storage; (H) transportation and distribution; (I) thawing and dilution prior to surgical preparation of the allograft; and (J) quality review systems. Each of these areas is vital to the performance of the implanted allograft, and strict standards must be adhered to such that optimal replacement heart valves are provided for the recipient patient population.

References

1. Khanna SK, Ross JK, Monro JL. Homograft aortic valve replacement: seven years' experience with antibiotic-treated valves. Thorax 1981;36(5): 330–337.
2. Wain WH, Greco R, Ignegeri A, Bodnar E, Ross DN. 15 years experience with 615 homograft and autograft aortic valve replacements. Int J Artif Organs 1980;3:169–172.
3. Angell WW, Angell JD, Oury JH, Lamberti JJ, Grehl TM. Long-term follow-up of viable frozen aortic homografts: a viable homograft valve bank. J Thorac Cardiovasc Surg 1987;93:815–822.
4. O'Brien MF, Stafford EG, Gardner MA, Pohlner PG, McGiffin DC. A comparison of aortic valve replacement with viable cryopreserved and fresh allograft valves, with a note on chromosomal studies. J Thorac Cardiovasc Surg 1987;94:812–823.
5. Kirklin JW, Blackstone EH, Maehara T, Pacifico AD, Kirklin JK, Pollock S, Stewart RW. Intermediate-term fate of cryopreserved allograft and xenograft valved conduits. Ann Thorac Surg 1987; 44:598–606.
6. Barratt-Boyes BG, Roche AH, Subramanyan R, Pemberton JR, Whitlock RM. Long-term follow-up of patients with the antibiotic-sterilized aortic homograft valve inserted freehand in the aortic position. Circulation 1987;75:768–777.
7. Karp RB. The use of free-hand unstented aortic valve allografts for replacement of the aortic valve. J Card Surg 1986;1:23–32.
8. American Association of Tissue Banks. Standards for Tissue Banking. 1998.

28
Donor Suitability and Heart Procurement

Scott A. Brubaker

Donor Suitability

Permission for heart donation is usually obtained in writing or via a taped, documented telephone conversation with the donor's legal next of kin, even if a potential donor carries an organ donor card. Alternatively, a self-signed donor document can be accepted as long as it is in accordance with the Uniform Anatomical Gift Act and applicable state and local regulations. Once permission is obtained, the donor must be adequately screened to minimize any potential transfer of an infectious disease.

The 1998 edition of AATB Standards incorporated all FDA tissue donor screening criteria which was published in a Final Rule and Guidance Document for the Screening and Testing of Donors of Human Tissue Intended for Transplantation, that became effective on January 29, 1998 (21 CFR 1270). It was so mandated that each potential donor should be evaluated individually by obtaining and reviewing the following information: relevant medical records including those describing past medical history and current clinical course; an interview by trained personnel with the donor's next of kin or other knowledgeable historian to reveal possible behavioral risk factors the donor possessed that could be associated with HIV, hepatitis or other transmissible disease; physical evidence by examination that could reveal a possible risk associated with HIV or hepatitis; and a hemodilution (plasma dilution) assessment of the donor's blood sample(s) used

for serological screening. In the case of pediatric tissue donors who have been breast fed within the past 12 months and/or are 18 months of age or less, the natural mother's risk for transmission of disease must also be evaluated. Screening also includes investigation for evidence of malignancies, risk factors for prion-associated disease, and systemic bacterial/viral infection (sepsis). Additional AATB Standards require that if an autopsy was performed, the final report or a summary of the final report shall be evaluated by a physician Medical Director prior to tissue release for clinical distribution.

The AATB Standards for cardiovascular tissues (CV) also stipulate that heart valve donors shall meet the following criteria:

1. There shall be no history of bacterial endocarditis, rheumatic fever, or semilunar valvular disease, or a cardiomyopathy of viral or idiopathic etiology.

2. Any history of previous cardiac surgery, closed chest massage, penetrating cardiac injury, or other potentially deleterious cardiac intervention shall be evaluated on a case-by-case basis.

3. Recovery of valves from anencephalic infants shall begin only after asystole.

4. In the case of suspected Sudden Infant Death Syndrome (SIDS), an autopsy should be performed and results reviewed to confirm the cause of death.

The donor suitability criteria must be in accordance with the AATB Standards, however it is

239

possible for the Tissue Bank Medical Director to establish more stringent criteria. Note the following differences between AATB Standards and LifeNet policy:

- Age and size limits:
  (a) Lower size limit: AATB = generally 4 pounds; LifeNet = 8 pounds.
  (b) Lower age limit AATB = newborn; LifeNet = full-term newborn (36 weeks gestational age)
  (c) Upper age limit: AATB = 60 years; LifeNet = 55 years.

As discussed by several authors,[1,2] increasing heart donor age may yield a corresponding increase in calcification rates of transplanted allograft heart valves. Various age criteria of other programs[2–4] extend up to 65 years of age with good results, but LifeNet has set a conservative upper age limit of 55, as suggested by several studies.[1,2,5] Because the largest possible allograft should be implanted that will not be distorted within the recipient's native annulus, the lower age and size limits were established with actual implantable allograft sizes in mind.

LifeNet also maintains screening criteria that constitute the review of the donor's risk for cardiovascular disease. Histories which include the following risk factors are individually and collectively evaluated for acceptability: hypertension, long-term smoking, hypercholesterolemia, hyperlipidemia, gout, morbid obesity, diagnosed coronary artery disease, and advanced diabetes. If a donor presents with multiple risk factors and the cause of death is directly related to the risk for CV disease, those potential donors are ruled out.

The possibility of cardiac trauma is also considered. Many deaths are due to extensive traumatic injuries and it is important to consider that irreversible damage may have occurred to the heart valves and/or their outflow tracts. These traumas may be grossly visible or may only be detectable by microscopic evaluation. Crushing injuries and obvious blunt force trauma to the thoracic cavity should be scrutinized. Sternal trauma, rib fractures, flail chest, prolonged CPR, and traumatic recovery each can cause rupture of cardiac blood vessels. The release of heme from red cell destruction can adversely stain cuspal tissue resulting in localized areas of damage through autolytic processes. This release of heme may also cause moderate to severe staining of the aortic and pulmonic outflow tracts (conduits) which may render compromised tissue that is clinically suboptimal.

Heart Procurement

The time period from cessation of heartbeat until cardiac procurement as the "warm ischemic time" and the time interval from placement of tissue in cold transport solution to the beginning of disinfection as the "cold ischemic time." The AATB Standards permit cardiovascular tissue recovery to be established by each individual bank; however the following upper time limits for completion of retrieval and processing of cardiovascular tissues may not be exceeded:

1. Warm ischemic time shall not exceed 24 hours from asystole (or cross-clamp) if the body was cooled or refrigerated within 12 hours of asystole. The time limit shall not exceed 15 hours if the body was not cooled or refrigerated. Warm ischemia for cardiovascular tissue ends when the heart is rinsed or placed into a cold, sterile, isotonic solution.
2. Cold ischemic time should not exceed 24 hours.
3. Total ischemic time shall not exceed 48 hours.

LifeNet follows AATB Standards for cold and warm ischemia with the exception that warm ischemia time limit if the body is not cooled or refrigerated is only 12 hours. A consideration related to warm ischemia time is that the time of death that is determined to be accurate may actually be closest to the last time the donor was seen alive, versus the "official" pronouncement of death.

Studies have shown that valve leaflets recovered past the 8–12 hour ischemic specification may exhibit substantially decreased fibroblast viability; however, these "non-viable" heart valve allografts do have clinical applicability because they may still outperform other available prosthetic devices.[4-11] As discussed in Chapters 4, 5 and 6, retention of normal intact leaflet matrix structures may be a more important factor in long-term allograft valve function. It has been shown that extended warm ischemic times may have an even greater damaging effect on the non-cellular components of the valve leaflets vs. the effect on cellular viability. Since long-term durability may be the only compromised factor, recipients with a shortened life expectancy (where the allograft would outlive the recipient) or recipients who can be anticipated to outgrow their valve may still profit from the other inherent advantages of an allograft.

Donor hearts for allograft heart valve transplantation should ideally be obtained aseptically in an operating room setting but may also be recovered in less optimal arenas of recovery such as in a medical examiner suite, a morgue setting, or in a funeral home. Procurement techniques for the recovery of hearts in an autopsy setting have been published elsewhere.[12]

When the heart is to be recovered immediately following vascular organ donation, the original surgical preparation should be extended to anticipate a median sternotomy. As shown by Hopkins, et al., heart valve leaflets are relatively resistant to anoxia, but removal of the heart within the first two hours after cessation of heartbeat may be ideal. If the cardiectomy is to be performed as a separate tissue donor procedure, the heart should be recovered first and as soon after death as possible.

The key aspects of the procurement of hearts for heart valves are aseptic technique, proper length of the aorta and pulmonary artery (for future conduit usage in ventriculopulmonary artery reconstruction), and the avoidance of valve leaflet injury.

Detailed steps for sterile cardiectomy are as follows:

1. The general site of retrieval must be documented and area access restricted. Aseptic technique must be followed using sterile surgical packs, instrumentation and technique. All work surfaces to be used during the retrieval should be cleansed using a bactericidal agent or properly draped sterilely.

2. Shave and prepare the donor from chin to umbilicus to bilateral nipple line.

3. Cleansing, preparing, and draping the skin and surrounding area (steri-drape coverage is recommended). Persons performing the surgical retrieval shall perform a surgical scrub of their hands and forearms prior to retrieval. A head cover and mask shall be worn at the time of scrub, and a sterile gown and gloves shall be donned after the scrub with the same diligence used routinely for operative procedures.

4. The initial incision should be a median incision over the sternum. During the initial incision all areas of skin with abrasions or puncture wounds should be avoided.

5. Divide the subcutaneous tissue to expose the anterior surface of the sternum, xiphoid process to sternal notch.

6. Free the pericardium from the posterior sternum by blunt and sharp dissection. This procedure may need to be done intermittently during the sternotomy.

7. Perform median sternotomy with the Lebsche knife and mallet or sternal saw. Install chest spreaders/rib retractors. Weitlanders can be used for pediatric donors (position with handle towards umbilicus). Note: For a "Y-incision" approach, use heavy Mayo scissors or an automated saw to transversely cut the ribs at their midlength, then pull the remaining breastplate up and over the donor's head superiorly.

8. Incise pericardium to expose the heart and remove pericardial fluid. Using 3–0 silk sutures or towel clips, tack the pericardium back to the skin, to the breast plate, or to the spreader for full exposure. This will isolate the lungs from the sterile field desired for the cardiectomy.

9. Circumferentially dissect the ascending aorta to expose one cm of the brachiocephalic artery.

10. Circumferentially dissect the aortic arch to expose one cm of the left carotid and left subclavian arteries.

11. Expose and ligate the superior and inferior vena cava.

12. Expose the right and left pulmonary arteries.

13. Continue to dissect the pulmonary arteries to their first segment branch arteries, which requires dissection outside the pericardial cavity. Begin to cut major vessels only after adequate exposure is accomplished.

14. Transect the pulmonary arteries at their first segmental branches.

15. Transect the superior and inferior vena cava proximal to the ligatures.

16. Evert the heart and transect the pulmonary veins. While incising the posterior pericardium, avoid entering the esophagus or trachea, as it would grossly contaminate the operative field.

17. Ligate the aorta beyond the left subclavian artery. *Do not* cross-clamp the aorta anywhere proximal to this ligature, as intimal damage may result that can render the aortic valve unusable.

18. Transect the brachiocephalic, left carotid, and left subclavian arteries. Transect the aortic arch distal to its ligature.

19. Safely divide any remaining connective tissue and remove the heart.

20. Place the heart in a large basin containing approximately 1 liter of any cold isotonic solution (i.e. Normal saline, lactated Ringer's solution, PlasmaLyte, organ transplant perfusates, or tissue culture media)

21. The heart should immediately be rinsed free of blood, gently massaging the ventricles to remove as much blood as possible, and packaged in cold isotonic, sterile, solution using any acceptable organ recovery system that utilizes double sterile bags or containers. The volume of transport solution should be adequate to cover the entire heart, including vessels and valves, so that no surface area will become dry (damaged).

22. After packaging, the heart is handed off the sterile field, bagged, labeled, and placed in a fluid-tight shipping container designed to prevent contamination of the contents, and allow for aseptic delivery of the heart at the time of processing.

23. The heart transportation container is transported at wet-ice temperatures and is appropriately labeled as "Quarantined, Not Intended For Human Use In Current Form").

24. All available donor information, heartbeat cessation time, and cardiectomy time should be included with the heart shipment to facilitate the valve dissection procedures and to properly identify the quarantined tissue.

25. Following cardiectomy, the surgical site should be surgically closed and the body prepared for the retrieval of other tissues or for transportation to an appropriate facility (i.e., morgue, medical examiner's office, funeral home).

References

1. Khanna SK, Ross JK, Monro JL. Homograft aortic valve replacement: seven years' experience with antibiotic-treated valves. Thorax 1981; 36(5):330–337.

2. Armiger LC, Thomson RW, Strickett MG, Barratt-Boyes EG. Morphology of heart valves preserved by liquid nitrogen freezing. Thorax 1985;40:778–786.

3. Wain WH, Greco R, Ignegeri A, Bodnar E, Ross DN. 15 years experience with 615 homograft and autograft aortic valve replacements. Int J Artif Organs 1980;3:169–172.

4. O'Brien MF, Stafford EG, Gardner MA, Pohlner PG, McGiffin DC. A comparison of aortic valve replacement with viable cryopreserved and fresh allograft valves, with a note on chromosomal studies. J Thorac Cardiovasc Surg 1987;94:812–823.

5. Barratt-Boyes BG, Roche AH, Subramanyan R, Pemberton JR, Whitlock RM. Long-term follow-up of patients with the antibiotic-sterilized aortic homograft valve inserted freehand in the aortic position. Circulation 1987;75:768–777.

6. Kirklin JW, Blackstone EH, Maehara T, Pacifico AD, Kirklin JK, Pollock S, Stewart RW. Intermediate-term fate of cryopreserved allograft and xenograft valved conduits. Ann Thorac Surg 1987;44:598–606.

7. Angell JD, Christopher BS, Hawtrey O, Angell WM. A fresh viable human heart valve bank-sterilization sterility testing and cryogenic preservation. Transplant Proc 1976;8(Suppl 1):127–141.

8. Kay PH, Ross DN. Fifteen years' experience with the aortic homograft: the conduit of choice for right ventricular outflow tract reconstruction. Ann Thorac Surg 1985;40:360–364.

9. Allwork SP, Pucci JJ, Cleland WP, Bentall HH. The longevity of sterilized aortic valve homo-

grafts 1966–1972. J Cardiovasc Surg (Torino) 1986;27:213–216.

10. Fontan F, Choussat A, DeVille C, et al. Aortic valve homografts in the surgical treatment of complex cardiac malformations. J Thorac Cardiovasc Surg 1984;87:649–657.

11. Barratt-Boyes BG, Roche AHG, Whitlock RML. Six year review of the results of freehand aortic valve replacement using an antibiotic sterilized homograft valve. Circulation 1977;55:353–361.

12. Kirklin JW, Barratt-Boyes GB. Cardiac Surgery. New York: Wiley 1986.

29
Techniques and Technology: Dissection, Examination, Sterilization, and Cryopreservation

Mark VanAllman and Kelvin G.M. Brockbank

Heart Valve Dissection

Hearts must be received at the processing facility in time to allow for completion of dissection, evaluation and the initiation of antibiotic treatment within the established ischemic time limits.

Dissection of the allograft is performed in an aseptic "cleanroom" environment under laminar flow conditions. The working area should be sterile and draped according to normal surgical protocol. As well as using sterile instruments, ligatures, and grafts sizers, LifeNet utilizes a specifically designed "cold pan" to help keep the heart cool during dissection. This apparatus is a closed, double boiler type of system that externally circulates 4°C liquid that transfers and maintains cold temperatures within the basin. The internal basin is filled with 1 liter of cold normal saline, lactated ringer's solution, organ transport solution, or tissue culture medium; and most of the heart dissection is performed in the 4°C bath. Maintaining the cardiac tissue in the cold state maximizes cellular viability and matrix integrity. The AATB Standards state that methods and equipment shall be qualified to maintain temperatures within the range of 1 to 10°C during heart dissection.

AATB Standards also dictate that the dissection and processing of cardiovascular tissue shall be performed as stated above in a certified air quality environment found to be cleaner than or equal to a Class 1000 environment, such as a laminar flow or cleanroom facility. Tissues shall be processed in an aseptic fashion using sterile drapes, packs, solutions, and instruments.

The heart is removed from its sterile transport solution and placed onto the operative field within the cold pan. Dissection is begun with the heart apex directed away from the person performing the procedure, with the anterior surface of the heart projected superiorly. The steps involved in the dissection procedures are as follows:

- The anterior aspect of the aortic conduit is inspected and any gross peri-adventitial connective tissue removed until an even coverage remains over the entire length of the conduit, from the aorta to the aortic root. Arterial hemostats can be affixed to the most distal aspect of the conduit to provide counter traction. Note: Beware of the right and left coronary arteries and do not damage the ostia.
- Once the anterior aspect of the aorta has been grossly cleaned, turn to the posterior aspect of the heart. Repeat this procedure until the entire conduit is circumferentially cleaned from the aorta to the aortic root. Return to the anterior aspect of the heart.
- Incise the atrial adipose tissue covering the right coronary artery. Do not cut the artery. Dissect free the right coronary artery until 1 cm of artery is exposed. Ligate the artery with 3-0 silk ligature. Check this area of the aorta and the coronary artery itself for any nicks, holes or abrasions and make note of

such. Also look for any anatomical abnormalities such as coronary displacement.

- The left coronary artery is now dissected in a similar manner. The dissection is carried out just distal to the origin of the circumflex and left descending (LAD) arteries. The left coronary artery is ligated with a single 3-0 silk ligature at the circumflex LAD bifurcation and divided. Again, make note of any problem area.
- The entire base of the aorta can now be fully exposed to the aortic root-myocardial junction.
- Divide the pulmonary artery from the aortic arch, freeing both conduits.
- Open the right ventricle just below the right coronary artery with a full-thickness incision. Holding the pulmonary artery in one hand, remove the pulmonary artery with a full thickness cut in a circumferential manner. Leave a minimum of 1 cm of myocardium below the pulmonary valve leaflets. Note: Care must be taken when separating the base of the pulmonary artery from the aorta. The conus ligament/tendon, or the infundibulum, is often minute, and the aortic and/or pulmonary conduits can easily be damaged during this step.
- With the pulmonary artery dissected free, grossly remove the epicardial adipose tissue and maintain the pulmonary allograft in the cold pan solution until further dissection.
- With a full thickness cut, divide the aorta from the myocardium beginning at the previous right ventricular incision. Continue posteriorly through the right atrium until the atrial septum is reached.
- Return to the anterior aspect of the heart and transversely incise the ventricular septum. This full-thickness incision through the septum should be approximately midway down the septum, below the left ventricular mitral chordae tendineae attachments.
- Expose the entire left ventricle by making an incision to the heart apex. Care should be taken to stay well beyond the origins of the aortic valve leaflets in the Valsalva sinuses.
- In the opened left ventricle, transect the chordae tendineae of the anterior mitral valve leaflets.

- Make longitudinal incisions at both junctions of the anterior and posterior mitral valve leaflets. This maneuver divides the mitral valve.
- Remove the entire left atrial myocardium and posterior mitral valve leaflet from the aortic base, leaving the anterior mitral valve leaflet attached to the aortic root.
- Transversely, divide the ventricular septum 1 cm below the aortic valve leaflets. Remove any remaining myocardium from the aorta and free the allograft from the heart with the anterior mitral leaflet still attached to the aortic conduit.
- Trim excess myocardium, adipose, and connective tissue from the aortic base, leaving a uniform thickness of 2–3 mm of myocardium. Beware of the membranous portion of the septum near the aortic base and tricuspid valve junction. Avoid damaging any of the tissue in this area and leave at least 2 mm of myocardium attached.
- Return to the pulmonary valve conduit and remove excess tissue. Avoid any unnecessary contact with the allograft leaflets.
- The tissue shall be kept cold and moist at all times throughout the entire dissection procedure to prevent drying and possible cellular, tissue, and matrix deterioration.

Heart Valve Evaluation and Examination

The AATB Standards mandate a standardized evaluation and classification system for allograft heart valves. This evaluation should include sizing and a qualitative graft assessment. A system must be in place to notify the implanting surgeon of any graft's condition if requested prior to final dispensing.

Sizing the allograft is a vital aspect of the processing procedures; consistency and accuracy are of the utmost importance. Incorrect sizing of the allograft aortic root diameter could require tailoring of the recipient's annulus and prolong the patient's aortic cross-clamp time. Adequate conduit length is also mandatory in ventriculopulmonary artery reconstructions

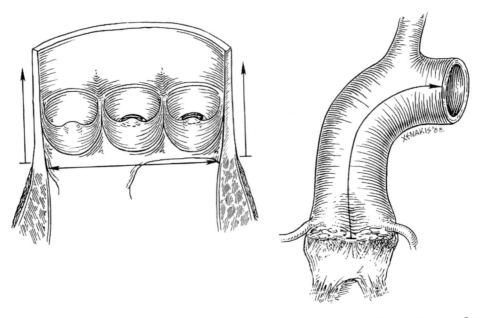

FIGURE 29.1. Valve diameter is measured as the internal diameter at the base of the aortic root. Length of conduit is as shown.

and aortic root replacement procedures. Proper communication between the implanting surgeon and the processing team is essential. All parties should be in agreement on the mechanics of sizing and know the parameters involved (Figures 29.1 and 29.2).

The internal diameter of the allograft root is determined and recorded. To obtain accurate sizing, the annulus must not be stretched or distorted. LifeNet uses specially designed sizing obturators made of high-grade stainless steel. Each obturator measures a specific size, from 15 mm to greater than 30 mm, and can be used to obtain the annular diameter measurement in a minimally invasive manner. For smaller pediatric valves, Hegar cervical dilators are utilized. Repeated obturator sizing of the valve has been found to damage the leaflets through the continued physical contact and should be avoided.[1] For this reason, each obturator or Hegar dilator measurement is confirmed using calipers. This sizing double

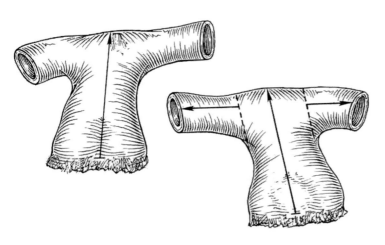

FIGURE 29.2. Pulmonary allograft dimensions: length of allograft and left and right pulmonary arteries.

check helps to ensure the accuracy of the measurement.

It is important that the implanting surgical team know that valve sizes are determined by internal root diameters. Most allograft internal roots average 3 mm less than the recipient's annulus, as determined by preoperative echocardiogram. This 3 mm differentiation must be kept in mind when requesting a specific allograft. LifeNet has found the pulmonary valve root to consistently be 2–4 mm larger than the aortic root, the differential increasing with the size of the heart.

The lengths of the aortic conduit and main pulmonary artery are recorded along with the size of the right and left pulmonary artery remnants. These sizes are recorded in centimeters. During the sizing period, the allograft should be kept cold and moist, and the leaflets should be carefully examined for any degenerative, traumatic, or congenital abnormalities.

At LifeNet, every allograft is assigned a quantifiable "categorical" rating to assess its overall condition. The following is a list of the qualifications and conditions observed for each specific numerical rating:

Category 2: Perfect valve

- Valve, conduit and attachments free of any problem area such as tears, lacerations, fenestrations, contusions, atheroma or calcific deposits

Category 1: Implantable valve with some imperfections

- Atheroma noted on intimal surface of conduit or on leaflets
- Calcific deposits not associated with leaflets, commissure or leaflet attachments
- Contusions of myocardium near valve root
- Leaflet fenestrations noted not affecting valve competency
- Leaflet hemoglobin staining
- Uneven collagen distribution changes on leaflet
- Conduit damaged or lacerated not affecting valve function

Category 0: Valve unacceptable for clinical use

- Bicuspid valve or other congenital defect
- Severe leaflet fenestrations affecting valve competency
- Leaflets torn or abraded
- Intimal peel throughout the entire conduit length
- Calcific deposits on the leaflet, commissures or leaflet attachments
- Conduit cut short or lacerated affecting valve function or commissural posts
- Severely damaged
- Severe leaflet hemoglobin staining
- Valve incompetent

When assessing graft quality, it is important to assess the valve and associated conduit as a single unit in regard to the graft's intended use. A perfect valve may have associated conduit tissue with a qualitative assessment that may render the graft as a whole unacceptable. Conversely, an incompetent valve with numerous fenestrations, may have associated conduit tissue which is in "perfect" condition. The processing technician must consider these issues when making decisions regarding acceptability and graft production. Due to the variety of congenital reconstructive applications for cardiac allografts, production options are not limited to just aortic and pulmonary valves. Non-valved "conduit grafts" provide the processing technician with a range of options intended to maximize this very precious resource.

Once the allograft condition is noted, all ratings, sizes, and comments are recorded in the donor chart along with the date and time of dissection. The manufacturers and lot numbers for all antibiotics and solutions used during the processing should be recorded. Each allograft should be assigned a separate identification number and all records maintained in a permanent donor chart.

Sterilization and Disinfection

In order to provide a disinfected allograft for transplantation, identification and elimination of any potential contaminants are required. AATB Standards dictate that processing shall include an antibiotic disinfection period followed by rinsing, packaging, and cryopreservation, and that "disinfection of cardiovascular tissue shall be accomplished via a validated, time specific antibiotic incubation". Disinfection involving incubation of the allograft in low-concentration, broad-spectrum antibiotics is well documented.[2,3] Many antibiotics mixtures have been utilized with varying degrees of effect on cellular viability, host ingrowth rate, disinfection efficiency, and valve survival rates.[1,4–10]

Just prior to exposure of the tissue to any disinfecting media, LifeNet performs a filter culture of solutions used in processing and obtains a representative tissue sample. These cultures are aimed at identifying any potential procurement or process-related microorganisms that may remain with the processed grafts as they enter the disinfection solution. It is important to identify this "pre-disinfection" bioburden to determine whether microorganisms that may be isolated at this time meet established acceptability criteria. If organisms are isolated that are known to exhibit a high degree of pathogenicity, or are not considered part of the normal respiratory flora, grafts may be discarded regardless of the results of post-disinfection cultures.

It has been suggested that hearts recovered from multi-organ donors are microbiologically sterile and may be immediately transplanted or cryopreserved.[11] However, Gonzalez-Lavin reports that 53% of his multi-organ donors' hearts yielded positive cultures (ibid.). At LifeNet, we found that approximately 32% of our hearts received were contaminated. LifeNet's primary contaminating bacteria historically have been Streptococcus viridans, Staphylococcus sp., and anaerobic diphtheroids. It is therefore suggested that all allograft heart valves enter into a disinfection program.

Varying antibiotic formulas using penicillin, gentamicin, kanamycin, axlocillin, metronidazol, flucloxacillin, streptomycin, ticarcillin, methicillin, chloramphenicol, colistimethate, neomycin, erythromycin, and nystatin have been tried by several authors. These solutions have proven unsatisfactory for a variety of reasons including: a decrease in cellular viability[12–14] and molecular cross-linkages with colla-

gen and mucopolysaccharides inhibiting host ingrowth into the disinfected valve leaflets.[9,15] LifeNet uses a modified version of the antibiotic treatment regimen recommended by Barrat-Boyes.[3] The following antibiotics are added to a sterile-filtered nutrient

Cefoxitin	240 µg/ml medium
Lincomycin	120 µg/ml medium
Polymyxin B	100 µg/ml medium
Vancomycin	50 µg/ml medium

Several nutrient media have been used, including modified Hank's solution, TCM 199, MEM Eagle's, and RPMI 1640.[3,4,16,17] LifeNet utilizes sterile filtered RPMI 1640 as a base medium for the disinfection solution, as recommended by others.[16,18]

The sterilization stage begins once the allograft is fully dissected. All antibiotics are reconstituted with sterile water and pre-mixed with the appropriate nutrient medium. This antibiotic solution has a shelf life of 72 hours when stored at 4°C. Buffer may need to be added to maintain the pH between 6.8 and 7.0. The allograft is placed in a suitable sterile container, and approximately 125 ml of the antibiotic solution is added. It is important that the solution completely covers the tissue.

The container should be large enough that the entire allograft be freely movable within the interior and not contorted in any way. It has been found that distorting the tissue to fit a small container may result in allograft conduit cracking after the freezing and thawing process.

The allograft tissue is stored at 4°C for 24 hours immersed in the antibiotic medium. The heart valve is then removed from cold storage, rinsed with tissue culture medium, and aseptically packaged for cryopreservation employing controlled-rate cooling.

Nearly all allograft heart valve programs advocate the use of antibiotics (Table 29.1). Many different antibiotics in various tissue culture media are being employed, but all are in relative low-doses, and with varying incubation times and temperatures.[19]

O'Brien initially reported incubating allografts in a solution containing penicillin, streptomycin and Amphotericin B for 24 hours at 37°C.[20] More recently, however, he has changed

TABLE 29.1. Allograft Heart Valve Programs.

Program	Antibiotics	Nutriment Medium
Yankah (et al., 1987):[39] German Heart Center Berlin	Gentamycin, Axlocillin, Flucloxacillan, Metronidazole Amphotericin B	RPMI 1640 & human serum
Kirklin (et al., 1987):[40] University of Alabama	Streptomycin, Penicillin, Amphotericin B	RPMI 1640
Gonzalez-Lavin (et al., 1987): [41] Deborah Heart & Lung Center, New Jersey	Cefoxitin, Ticarcillin Neomycin, Polymyxin Mycostatin	RPMI 1640 & Fetal calf serum
Angell (et al., 1987):[4] Scripp's Clinic San Diego	Colistimethate, Gentamicin, Kanamycin, Lincomycin	TC199
Barratt-Boyes (et al., 1987):[20] Green Lane Hospital Auckland	Cefoxitin, Lyncomycin Polymyxin B, Vancomycin, Amphotericin B	TC199
Almeida (1988):[42] American Red Cross Los Angeles	Cefoxitin, Lincomycin Vancomycin, Polymyxin B, Amphotericin	TCI199
O'Brien (et al., 1987, 1988):[43] Charles Hospital Brisbane	Streptomycin, Penicillin	Eagle's MEM
Ross (Khanna, et al., 1981):[44] Hospital London	Gentamycin, Methicillin, Nystatin, Erythromycin, Streptomycin	Modified Hank's: National Heart

to a sterilizing protocol of the gentler antibiotics with the complete avoidance of Amphotericin B in the disinfecting solution. He now incubates the heart valve allografts for only 6 hours at 37°C, with these changes aimed at maximizing leaflet cell viability (M.F. O'Brien, personal communication, 7 March 1988.) In 1988, LifeNet removed Amphotericin B from the antibiotic incubation.

Elimination of Amphotericin B from the antibiotics regimen used to sterilize the grafts highlights the importance of thorough donor screening. Permission for autopsy and obtaining pertinent medical history, including detection of symptoms related to those associated with systemic mycoses or infective endocarditis, is paramount to exclusion of fungal organisms originating from the donor graft. Strict sterile technique during recovery, transport at 4°C, and cold, sterile processing are additional measures to prevent fungal proliferation. Approximately 15% of all cases of infective endocarditis are due primarily to two fungal agents, Candida sp. and Aspergillus sp.[21] Histoplasma sp. has been implicated in rare numbers. Actinomyces sp. and Nocardia sp. have also

been implicated in myocarditis and endocarditis.[22] The coexistence of a bacterial agent and an undetected yeast infection occurs in human endocarditis,[23] so any donor history of endocarditis should be scrutinized. Fungal endocarditis is characterized by development of mycotic vegetation commonly attached to the aortic or mitral leaflets.[23] It is apparent that the fungal organisms have a tendency to accumulate on leaflets of the left heart due to the increased oxygen tension found here. It has also been reported that the right heart offers a more effective host response to defend against infection.[23] Most mycotic infections are acquired via airborne spores and ultimately manifest in the lungs, making the left heart most susceptible to vegetation, especially on the surface of the leaflets. For these reasons, the optimal tissue specimen for fungal cultures is obtained from the posterior mitral leaflet. A specimen that is void of bacterial contamination is preferred, as the presence of fungus would not be inhibited by overgrowth of competitive bacteria. Tissue contaminated with bacteria and sent for fungal culture may prove unsuitable for diagnostic procedures due to autolytic processes.[24] This supports the practice of obtaining the tissue (post, mitral cusp) for fungal cultures after antibiotic treatment, just prior to packaging and cryopreservation of the allograft, and discarding tissue when surveillance cultures are positive before or after antibiotics.

As noted by Wain and colleagues,[8] antibiotics cannot be expected to unfailingly disinfect every allograft. Originally, LifeNet tried touch-culturing and tissue remnant sampling (aorta and mitral valve sections) as the mode of testing for sterility. Of the initial 300 hearts tested using these techniques, only one allograft yielded a positive culture result following the antibiotic incubation period. However, it was determined that the touch culture and tissue sampling techniques could yield a high incidence of false-negative reports. Approximately 0.14 ml of antibiotic solution was carried with the tissue sample or transported within the culture swab to the thioglycollate broth. This small amount of disinfecting solution transported during the sampling procedure was enough to restrict the growth of low concentrations of microorganisms during incubation at 37°C in the thioglycollate broth. Carry-over of antibiotics would thus mask the presence of the low-concentration microbial contaminants present on the allograft tissue, resulting in the reporting of false-negative cultures. The carry-over effect of the antibiotic solution has been substantiated by Waterworth and associates.[7]

LifeNet currently utilizes a post-disinfection sterility control procedure. Following 24 hour incubation, heart valves are removed from the antibiotic solution. The solution is divided into two aliquots and each aliquot is filtered through a 0.22 µm Pall Gelman Laboratory filtration device (47 mm filter holder; Pall Gelman Laboratory, Ann Arbor, Michigan 48103). The filters (and all trapped microorganisms) are rinsed of residual antibiotics and placed directly onto trypticase soy agar with 5% sheep blood (Remel Microbiology, Lenexa, KS 66215) and CDC anaerobic blood agar (Remel Microbiology, Lenexa, KS 66215), respectively. Culture plates are incubated at 35°C +/−1° and then examined daily for three days. In addition, representative tissue samples are collected pre- and post-processing. In the past, these samples have been cultured using sterility test methods recommended in USP 23. More recently, LifeNet has validated the use of the BacTAlert™ automated microbial detection system (Organon Teknika Corp., Durham, NC) for culturing these samples.

Cryopreservation

Immediately following the antibiotic incubation period, packaging and subsequent cryopreservation of the grafts is begun. All packaging should be performed under strict aseptic conditions within a certified and qualified Class 100 (or cleaner) laminar flow environment. The allograft is removed from the antibiotic medium, rinsed in fresh antibiotic-free medium, and packaged with enough cryoprotectant solution to produce a total volume of 100 ml. At the time of packaging, cultures of all solutions, media, and representative samples are obtained.

The allograft and the appropriate amount of freezing solution are placed in a sterile pouch large enough to prevent distortions of the allograft. All air is removed from within the pouch, and it is heat-sealed. The allograft package is inserted into a slightly larger sterile pouch and again heat-sealed. This doubly packaged allograft is then taken to the freezing chamber for control-rate freezing. It is important to ensure that the pouches used in packaging the allografts are able to maintain their integrity at liquid nitrogen temperatures (−196°C). LifeNet currently utilizes a clear silicon oxide bag as the internal pouch (RollPrint Packaging Products, Inc., Addison, IL 60101) and a Kapton/Teflon bilaminate as the external pouch (American Flouroseal, Gaithersburg, MD 20877).

The freezing medium employed by LifeNet is similar to the solution utilized by Kirklin and coworkers.[16] RPMI 1640 tissue culture medium is amended with dimethyl sulfoxide (DMSO) to a 10% DMSO concentration and with a 10% fetal calf serum (FCS). The RPMI 1640 and the FCS may be pre-mixed and maintained at 4°C for up to 14 days (recommendation by Gibco Laboratories, Technical Service Department, Grand Island, New York 14072) or purchased directly from the manufacturer in a premixed condition (Bio Whittaker, Walkersville, MD 21793).

The DMSO is added to the cooled (4°C) solution, premixed at the time of allograft packaging. The DMSO cryoprotectant may be added at either room temperature or 4°C. Although DMSO may take longer to reach osmotic equilibration at 4°C, it results in less cytotoxicity to leaflet fibroblasts and therefore yields higher cell viability than addition of the cryoprotectant at 37°C.[25,26] Our studies have shown that the added DMSO comes to equilibrium in the freezing medium within approximately 15 minutes.

The use of FCS in the freezing medium is still the subject of debate. Most programs employ the use of 10–20% concentrations of FCS in the medium. The use of FCS or a high-molecular weight colloid substitute, e.g., albumin or pasteurized plasma protein fraction (PPF), is well documented.[27] These large macromolecules affect the properties of the freezing solution to a greater extent than would be expected from their osmotic pressure and act directly on the cell membrane.[25] The colloid is thought to provide a necessary balance of oncotic pressure, thereby regulating the activity of the unfrozen water in the freezing solution and its movement into the tissue.[27]

The same authors have also postulated that the addition of FCS or a high-molecular weight colloid to the cryopreservation solution may help protect the cell from the damaging effect of high concentrations of salts/solutes as they build up within the unfrozen fraction of the cryomedia.[25–27] FCS is also believed to minimize the dilution shock to the allograft tissue during thawing by restricting cell swelling.[25] It is well established that serum is a valuable additive to nutrient media during cell culture growth, and the addition of serum to the freezing solution may also assist in cell preservation during the DMSO equilibration period just prior to cell freezing.

However, questions have been posed regarding the potential heterologous antigenicity induced in heart valve allografts by the FCS. Bodnar and colleagues have suggested that the calf serum content of the nutrient medium infiltrates the aortic wall during allograft preservation and that it may induce a second-set immune reaction following transplantation.[28] They believe that FCS is not necessary during cryopreservation and have discontinued its use. Yankah also believes that the potential antigenicity of FCS may play a role in the rejection of allograft heart valves, and he is now using human-derived serum.[29] Some serum substitutes and plasma extenders are on the market, and the use of these agents may be warranted (Serum Plus; Hazleton Biologics, Inc., Lenexa, Kansas 66215). Nakamaya et al.[30] have presented data demonstrating excellent porcine valve cell viability in the absence of serum proteins.

Once the freezing medium is assembled and the allograft is packaged, the tissue should be cooled under defined conditions in a manner that allows the tissue to freeze at a predetermined rate with compensation for the heat of crystallization. Surrogate packs may be used to monitor the freezing program by insertion of a temperature probe within the pack. The use of surrogate packs should be validated and the use of a tissue sample within the surrogate pack should be considered, as this most closely represents the environment within the graft pouches destined for clinical use. If tissue is not used in the surrogate pack, the validation must ensure that the rate of cooling documented by monitoring the surrogate closely mimics the cooling rate of the grafts destined for clinical use. If freezing surrogates are used for monitoring the freezing program, the AATB Standards impose regular packing inspections and solution and tissue changes per the tissue bank's SOPs. In the cooling devices employed by LifeNet, the freezing chamber of the cooling device functions by monitoring such a surrogate placed in the chamber with the allograft(s). Monitoring for deterioration in freezing curve profiles is also mandated by the AATB Standards. Some general considerations of the freezing profile employed by LifeNet are that cardiovascular tissues should be cryopreserved to −100°C unless problems arise during the freezing cycle and acquisition of an accurate freezing profile is in jeopardy. In these instances, terminating the freeze cycle at −40°C

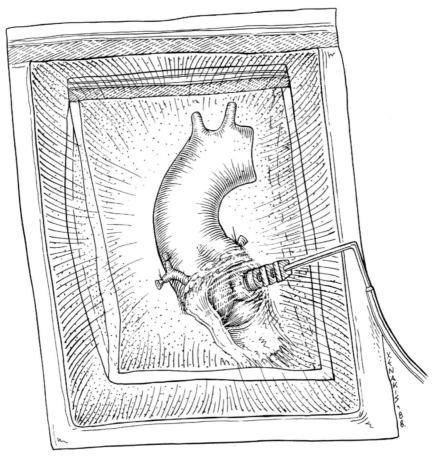

FIGURE 29.3. Control freezing pouch with temperature probe through a watertight portal.

or colder is acceptable. The cycle is not allowed to end before the sample temperature has reached −40°C. No more than 5 minutes of "flat time" is allowed at any time during the freezing cycle. The average rate for any one minute period between +4°C and −40°C is not allowed to exceed −5°C/min. Furthermore, other than during release if the latent heat of fusion, the sample temperature is not allowed to rise for a period exceeding one minute.

At the end of the procedure, the freezing profile should be reviewed to make sure that tolerance limits have been met.

The surrogate package must be assembled using the same type of pouch materials as the grafts intended for clinical use. This will help ensure that the heat transfer across the surrogate pack and the clinical grafts is similar. The freezing medium (RPMI + 10% FCS + 10%

DMSO) is added to yield 100 ml total volume. The control pouch must be constructed with an absolutely watertight portal that allows a temperature probe to be inserted. This can be accomplished by utilizing a double O-ring heparin-lock system as the portal (Figure 29.3). The system is capped with a latex injectable IV-bag port; the temperature probe may be inserted through this port, and freezing solution can be injected or withdrawn while maintaining the watertight integrity.

In our experience the control valve cryopreservation solution should be changed every time a new allograft batch is cryopreserved.

As stated by Arminger and associates,[31] acid mucopolysaccharides are known to readily diffuse out of tissues held in aqueous solutions. LifeNet has found consistent pH and osmolality changes within the control valve freezing medium with repeated freezing. Small-molecular weight solutes continually leach from the sample tissue contained within the surrogate pack, altering the makeup of the freezing medium and thus changing the freezing program. It should be noted however that there is no significant alteration in the content, molecular size, or distribution of mucopolysaccharides in allografts cryopreserved (frozen a single time) for transplantation.[32] It is not recommended that previously cryofrozen and thawed allografts be re-cryopreserved a second/multiple times.

If a heart valve is used in the surrogate pack, it should be stored in the frozen state at liquid nitrogen vapor temperatures ($-190°$ to $-150°C$) between allograft freeze runs. The control valve is thawed just prior to its use, and freezing solution is exchanged through the latex portal prior to its placement into the freezing chamber with the allograft tissue. Since every effort should be made to keep the physical makeup of the control sample as close as possible to the actual heart valve being cryopreserved, the freezing media of the control valve should be changed with each allograft freeze.

LifeNet allografts are cryopreserved in a freezing chamber (CryoMed Freezing Chamber 2600C, CryoMed, Mount Clemens, Michigan 48045) at the controlled cooling rate of $-1°C$ per minute utilizing a programmable controller (CryoMed Micro Controller 1010). Temperatures are continually monitored and recorded with a temperature chart recorder (CryoMed Recorder 500). AATB Standards indicate that "the tissue shall be frozen at a specific rate to a pre-determined specific endpoint (a temperature of $-40°C$ or cooler). The allograft is then transferred to permanent storage in vapor-phase liquid nitrogen. The allograft valve may be stored indefinitely at these temperatures.[2,27]

Upon completion of the freezing program employing controlled rate cooling methods, a record of the freezing profile must be evaluated, approved, and incorporated as a permanent part of the processing records. Typical freezing curves are shown in Figures 29.4, 29.5 and 29.6. Early in the freezing program, the valves are brought slowly to freezing temperatures. From the time the allograft heart valves are placed in cryopreservation media during packaging, until the solution and tissues begin to freeze, 30 to 45 minutes have elapsed. During this period, the allograft should not be allowed to warm as it has been suggested that subjecting human fibroblasts to warm temperatures may adversely affect their post-thawing viability.[33]

Once the allograft medium begins to freeze, adjustments in the freezing program must be made to compensate for the heat release that occurs as the freezing solution begins to crystallize. To compensate for this heat of fusion, the freezing chamber must quickly be cooled to temperatures below $-100°C$. Such supercooling allows the temperature of the allograft to decline at a steady $-1°C/minute$ rate, avoiding the cell damaging effects of inconsistent temperature fluctuations.

Significant changes in the freezing program can be made if a CryoSink® (Organ Recovery Systems, Inc., Charleston, SC 29403) is employed (Figure 29.6). LifeNet has found that the freezing process can be shortened and liquid nitrogen requirements reduced by placing the packaged allografts between two plates of snuggly fitted finned aluminum. Transfer and dissipation of the heat of fusion is optimized during ice nucleation. The inventor of this device, Professor Mendler of the Deutsches Herzzenentrum München, has processed more than 500 heart valves employing the CryoSink® (personal communication).

As the allograft temperature approaches $-20°C$, most of the extracellular water has frozen and the release of heat associated with water crystallization rapidly diminishes. To maintain a consistent $-1°C/minute$ freezing rate, the chamber must be rewarmed to temperatures just below the allograft's. From this point, temperature declines within the chamber are directly reflected in parallel temperature declines of the allograft tissue.

Different controlled cooling rates have also been investigated. Mermet and associates found $-1°C$ per minute to yield a superior viability rate versus $-0.1°C$ per minute or $-5°C$ per minute.[34] VanDerKamp and colleagues also reported that $-1°C$ per minute as the best

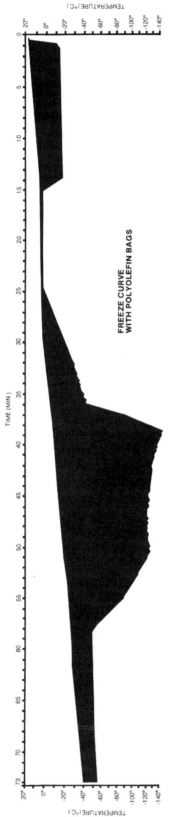

FIGURE 29.4. Computer controlled freezing curve. Time is from right to left. This curve is for a valve inside two polyolefin bags. The upper straight line is the 1°C/minute drop in tissue temperature. The lower curve described by the vertical lines is the chamber temperature.

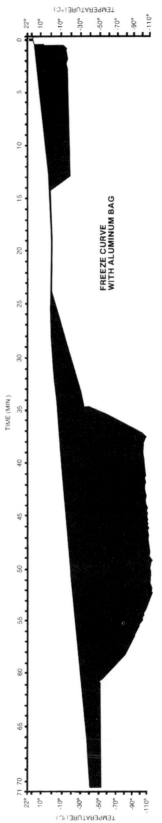

FIGURE 29.5. Freezing curve for a heart valve in an aluminum bag. Note the different chamber temperatures required to maintain the steady 1°C/minute linear freeze compared to Figure 29.4 and 29.6.

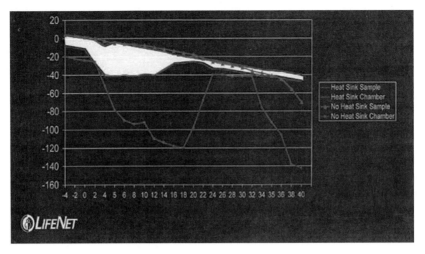

FIGURE 29.6. Freezing curve for a heart valve using Kapton packaging with the CryoSink® device. Reproduced, with permission, from LifeNet Tissue Services.

cooling rate to maximize fibroblast viability.[35] LifeNet, University of Alabama, and Prince Charles Hospital[36] are currently using −1°C per minute as their controlled cooling rate. However, Bodnar and Ross (E. Bodnar at The First Workshop on Homologous and Autologous Heart Valves, Chicago: Deborah Heart and Lung Center, 5 April 1987) and Armiger and Colleagues[31] used a −1.5°C per minute cooling rate.

Although most facilities utilize a microcomputer and freezing chamber[37] to control the freezing rate, Barratt-Boyes cryopreserved allografts using insulated heat sink boxes (B.G. Barratt-Boyes, personal communication, 5 April 1987). The heat sink method of cryopreservation has been shown to produce a cooling rate which varies between −1° and −2°C per minute.[38] However, control-rate freezing using heat sink boxes does not compensate for the latent heat released as ice crystals nucleate within the freezing solution.

The constituents of the freezing medium have a profound effect on cell and tissue freezing. Glycerol, DMSO, and ethylene glycol have all been tried as cryoprotective agents for allograft heart valves. Comparing DMSO, glycerol, and ethylene glycol, VanDerKamp and associates found that 10% DMSO yielded the highest number of viable fibroblasts.[35] They investigated varying concentrations of DMSO (5–20%) and found that 10% yielded superior cell survival. Kirklin and associates,[16] Karp,[18] and O'Brien and coworkers[36] use a 10% DMSO freezing medium, whereas Angell's group[4] employs a 7.5% concentration. Most programs now utilize DMSO as the cryoprotectant, with the possible exception of Bodnar and Ross who use a 15% glycerol formulation.

Another element in cryopreservation freezing solution is the variability of nutrient media into which the DMSO is added. Angell and associates use TC199 with HEPES amended with a 20% concentration of FCS.[4] Kirklin and colleagues,[16] Karp,[18] and LifeNet utilize RPMI 1640 tissue culture medium with 10% FCS. Whereas Bodnar, Ross, and Yankah use human serum to guard against the potential antigenicity of the calf sera (presented at The First Workshop on Homologous and Autologous Heart Valves. Chicago: Deborah Heart and Lung Center, 5 April 1987).

A number of other technical variables may affect the freezing rate of a heart valve allograft.

- There are several probes on the market that indicate the temperature of the control valve as it freezes. Blunt-tip probes (CryoMed Temperature Probes) can be inserted through the control package portal and situated with the tip of the probe either in the supraleaflet area of the control valve aorta or in the subleaflet area by entering through the proximal aortic root. A needle probe (Brymill Temperature Probe; Brymill Corporation—Cryosurgical Equipment, Vernon, Connecticut 06066) may be embedded in the aortic wall of the control valve or through one of the control leaflets. Altering probe placements affects temperature readings.

- Pouches used in packaging can be of several varieties, each of which may exhibit different heat transfer properties that may affect the freezing curve if changes are not made to the freezing program. This can be seen by comparing Figures 29.4, 29.5, and 4.6. Approximately 30% less chamber temperature was required to overcome the heat release of crystallization as the allograft was freezing when an aluminum foil outer pouch was used. An outer polyolefin bag required the chamber to drop to about −140°C, whereas the aluminum foil bag required a maximal low temperature of only −105°C. The metallic content of the foil pouch serves as a superior temperature conductor and insulator. The Kapton pouches currently used by LifeNet act as an insulator and thus require greater amounts of liquid nitrogen. External transfer devices such as the CryoSink® can offset this need and reduce liquid nitrogen requirements.

- The total volume of the control valve should be maintained at 100 ml. When replenishing freezing medium, a calibrated syringe should be used to exactly measure the amount of medium withdrawn. Alterations in the freezing curve have been observed when volume changes of as little at 5% are made.

- The number of allograft packages placed in the freezing chamber can also affect the control valve freezing curve. A pulmonary and an aortic allograft can be frozen simultaneously, but more than two allograft packages liberate too much heat into the freezing chamber. The heat release of three or more allograft packages causes a rise in the control valve package temperature, altering the freezing curve. A completely different freeze program must be developed when multiple allografts are frozen simultaneously unless a technician is available to constantly monitor and manually adjust the cooling rate.

- It was also found that freezing programs were altered by using different freezing chambers. Slight variations in door sealant moldings, liquid nitrogen fan speeds, and other chamber components yielded varying freezing results; the program should be recalibrated when equipment changes are made.

- Package placement within the freezing chamber is also important. The control valve and the allograft package should be placed equidistant from the liquid nitrogen source. Both packages should be situated at the same angle with equal package surface area exposed to the liquid nitrogen vapor. Allowing different freezing conditions to exist between the control and allograft package does not alter the control valve freezing rate, but the actual freezing curve of the allograft may not parallel that of the monitored control valve.

- The ratio of tissue versus medium within the allograft package is also a variable that affects the overall freezing program. It has been found that the smaller pediatric-size allografts (less tissue mass) freeze at a slightly slower rate than adult allografts (more tissue mass) using the same freeze program. The pediatric valve has a larger proportion of fluid within the total 100 ml volume, thus liberating more latent heat of crystallization as the larger amount of fluid freezes. It is suggested that different freeze programs and control valves be used for pediatric and adult allografts owing to differing amounts of tissue mass. LifeNet has validated the use of the CryoSink® device to overcome these differences.

- Altering the volume/surface ratio of the allograft package also affects the freezing rate. By increasing the total volume of the allograft package, more heat is liberated, thereby increasing the amount of liquid nitrogen that must be injected into the freezing chamber to compensate.

Once an allograft is determined to be acceptable for transplant, all donor and processing records are examined and approved by the Medical Director of the program, who should be a physician knowledgeable in allograft tissue banking.

References

1. Yacoub M, Kittle CF. Sterilization of valve homografts by antibiotic solutions. Circulation 1970;41 Suppl:29–31.
2. Ross DN, Martelli V, Wain WH. Allograft and autograft valves used for aortic valve replacement. In Ionescu MI (ed). Tissue Heart Valves. Boston: Butterworth 1979:127–172.
3. Strickett MG, Barratt-Boyes BG, MacCulloch D. Disinfection of human heart valve allografts with antibiotics in low concentration. Pathology 1983; 15:457–462.
4. Angell WW, Angell JD, Oury JH, Lamberti JJ, Grehl TM. Long-term follow-up of viable frozen aortic homografts: a viable homograft valve bank. J Thorac Cardiovasc Surg 1987;93:815–822.
5. Barratt-Boyes BG, Roche AHG, Whitlock RML. Six year review of the results of freehand aortic valve replacement using an antibiotic sterilized homograft valve. Circulation 1977;55:353–361.
6. Lockey E, Al-Janabi N, Gonzalez-Lavin L, Ross DNA. Method of sterilizing and preserving fresh allograft heart valves. Thorax 1972;27:398.
7. Waterworth PM, Lockey E, Berry EM, Pearce HM. A critical investigation into the antibiotic sterilization of heart valve homografts. Thorax 1974;29:432–436.
8. Wain WH, Pearce HM, Riddell RW, Ross DN. A re-evaluation of the antibiotic sterilization of heart valve allografts. Thorax 1977;32:740–742.
9. Gavin JB, Herdson PB, Monro JL, Barratt-Boyes BG. Pathology of antibiotic-treated human heart valve allografts. Thorax 1973;28:473–481.
10. Gavin JB, Barratt-Boyes BG, Hitchcock GC, Herdson PB. Histopathology of "fresh": human aortic valve allografts. Thorax 1973;28:482–487.
11. Gonzales-Lavin L, McGrath L, Alvarez M, Graf D. Antibiotic sterilization in the preparation of homovital homograft valves: Is it necessary? In

12. Cardiac Valve Allografts 1962–1987. New York: Springer-Verlag 1987:17–21.
12. Angell JD, Christopher BS, Hawtrey O, Angell WM. A fresh viable human heart valve bank-sterilization sterility testing and cryogenic preservation. Transplant Proc 1976;8 (Suppl 1): 127–141.
13. Girinath MR, Gavin JB, Strickett MG, Barratt-Boyes BG. The effects of antibiotics and storage on the viability and ultrastructure of fibroblasts in canine heart valves prepared for grafting. Aust N Z J Surg 1974;44:170–172.
14. Armiger LC, Gavin JB, Barratt-Boyes BG. Histological assessment of orthotopic aortic valve leaflet allografts: its role in selecting graft pre-treatment. Pathology 1983;15:67–73.
15. Gavin JB, Monro JL. The pathology of pulmonary and aortic valve allografts used as mitral valve replacements in dogs. Pathology 1974;6: 119–127.
16. Kirklin JW, Blackstone EH, Maehara T, Pacifico AD, Kirklin JK, Pollock S, Stewart RW. Intermediate-term fate of cryopreserved allograft and xenograft valved conduits. Ann Thorac Surg 1987;44:598–606.
17. Watts LK, Duffy P, Field RB, Stafford EG, O'Brien MF. Establishment of a viable homograft cardiac valve bank: a rapid method of determining homograft viability. Ann Thorac Surg 1976;21:230–236.
18. Karp RB. The use of free-hand unstented aortic valve allografts for replacement of the aortic valve. J Card Surg 1986;1:23–32.
19. Yankah AC. Cardiac valve allografts 1962–1987. New York: Springer Verlag 1988.
20. Barratt-Boyes BG, Roche AH, Subramanyan R, Pemberton JR, Whitlock RM. Long-term follow-up of patients with the antibiotic-sterilized aortic homograft valve inserted freehand in the aortic position. Circulation 1987;75:768–777.
21. Robbins SL. Pathologic Basis of Disease. Philadelphia: WB Saunders 1984.
22. Morehead RP. Human Pathology. New York: McGraw-Hill 1965.
23. McGinnis MR. Chapter 3. In McGinnis MR (ed). Current Topics in Medical Mycology. New York: Springer-Verlag 1985.
24. Sommerwith AC, Jarett L. Gradwohl's Clinical Laboratory Methods and Diagnosis. St. Louis: CV Mosby Co. 1980.
25. Bank HL, Brockbank K. Basic principles of cryobiology. Jour Card Surg 1987;2 suppl:137–143.

26. Ashwood-Smith MJ, Farrant J. Low Temperature Preservation in Medicine and Biology. London: Pitman 1980.

27. Karow AM, Pegg DE. Organ Preservation for Transplantation. New York: Marcel Dekker 1981.

28. Bodnar E, Olsen WGJ, Florio R, et al. Heterologous antigenicity induced to human aortic homografts during preservation. Eur J Cardiothorac Surg 1988;2:43–47.

29. Yankah AC. First Workshop on Homologous and Autologous Heart Valves. 1987. Chicago, IL, Deborah Heart and Lung Center. Ref Type: Conference Proceeding

30. Nakayama S, Ban T, Okamoto S. Fetal bovine serum is not necessary for the cryopreservation of aortic valve tissues. J Thorac Cardiovasc Surg 1994;108:583–586.

31. Armiger LC, Thomson RW, Strickett MG, Barratt-Boyes EG. Morphology of heart valves preserved by liquid nitrogen freezing. Thorax 1985;40:778–86.

32. Shon YH, Wolfinbarger L. Proteoglycan content in fresh and cryopreserved porcine aortic tissue. Cryobiology 1994;31:121–132.

33. Cryolife I. Clinical Program 101—Homgraft Heart Valves. 17. 1985. Marietta, GA, Cryolife, Inc. Ref Type: Conference Proceeding

34. Mermet B, Buch W, Angell W. Viable heart valve graft—preservation in the frozen state. Surgical Forum 1970;21:156.

35. VanDerKamp AWM, Visser WJ, van Dongan JM, Nauta J, Galjaard H. Preservation of aortic heart valves with maintenance of cell viability. J Surg Res 1981;30:47.

36. O'Brien MF, Stafford G, Gardner M, Pohlner P, McGiffin D, Johnston N, Brosnan A, Duffy P. The viable cryopreserved allograft aortic valve. J Card Surg 1987;2:153–167.

37. Kirklin JW., Barratt-Boyes GB. Cardiac Surgery. New York: Wiley 1986.

38. May SR, Guttman RM, Wainwright JF. Cryopreservation of skin using an insulated heat sink box stored at −70 degrees C. Cryobiology 1985; 22:205–214.

39. Yankah AC, Hetzer R. Procurement and viability of cardiac valve allografts. In Yankah AC, Hetzer R, Miller DC, Ross DN, Somerville J, Yacoub MH (eds). Cardiac Valve Allografts 1962–1987. New York: Springer-Verlag 1988:23–34.

40. Kirklin JK, Kirklin JW, Pacifico JAD, Phillips S. Cryopreservation of aortic valve homografts. In Yankah AC, Hetzer R, Miller DC, Ross DN, Somerville J, Yacoub M (eds). Cardiac Valve Allografts 1962–1987. New York: Springer-Verlag 1987:35–36.

41. Gonzalez-Lavin L, Bianchi J, Graf D, Amini S, Gordon CI. Homograft valve calcification: Evidence for an immunological influence. In Ross, Somerville J, Yacoub MH (eds). Proceedings of the Symposium on Cardiac Valve Allografts 1962–1987: Current Concepts on the Use of Aortic and Pulmonary Allografts for Heart Valve Substitutes. Berlin: Springer-Verlag 1987:69–74.

42. Almeida M. American Red Cross, Heart Valve Program, Los Angeles. Lange PE. 1988. Ref Type: Personal Communication.

43. O'Brien MF, Stafford EG, Gardner MA, Pohlner PG, McGiffin DC. A comparison of aortic valve replacement with viable cryopreserved and fresh allograft valves, with a note on chromosomal studies. J Thorac Cardiovasc Surg 1987;94:812–823.

44. Khanna SK, Ross JK, Monro JL. Homograft aortic valve replacement: seven years' experience with antibiotic-treated valves. Thorax 1981;36(5): 330–337.

30
Techniques and Technology: Storage, Transportation and Distribution, Thawing, Dilution, and Quality Systems

Perry L. Lange and Kelvin G.M. Brockbank

Storage

Upon termination of the freezing program at −40°C (or cooler), the allograft may be immediately removed from the freezing chamber. Cooling below −40°C causes no harm to the tissue. An identifying label should be stapled to the external pouch, affixed superior to the heat seal line such that pouch sterility is uncompromised. The label should include the individual allograft identification number and the valve size. The allograft package is then placed in a pre-cooled, pre-labeled, specifically designed cardboard storage box (Heart Valve Box; Dillard Paper Company, Greensboro North Carolina 27407). The storage box is placed in liquid nitrogen vapor-phase temperature (−150° to −190°C) storage. The time interval of allograft removal from the freezing chamber to liquid nitrogen vapor storage should be kept to a minimum in order to avoid thermal fluctuations of the tissue.

The key to long-term allograft storage is maintenance of the frozen tissue below the glass transition point of the freezing solution, approximately −130°C. At temperatures above −130°C, several changes in frozen tissue structure may occur that can affect cellular viability. Cells frozen at the relatively rapid rate of −1°C per minute yield small ice crystals. As the unstable small ice crystals coalesce to form larger ones, any tissue caught between the merging ice is damaged, and cellular viability is compromised. As the frozen allograft tissue tempera-

ture rises above −130°C, the rate of ice recrystallization accelerates.[1]

Macrocrystallization is the general phenomenon of small ice crystals coalescing to form larger crystals. Thermodynamically, small crystals are less stable than large ones because of their higher surface energy.[1] The small crystals naturally fuse in an effort to minimize their surface energies. Macrorecrystallization is of three types.[2]

1. Irruptive recrystallization: the method by which ice crystals rapidly resume their growth within a specific temperature range during slow rewarming and change from transparent to opaque under normal light conditions.
2. Migratory recrystallization: the growth of large ice crystals at the expense of small ones during gradual rewarming until the melting point is reached.
3. Spontaneous recrystallization: occurs during rapid cooling as the latent heat released during freezing is not dissipated enough to prevent a localized rise in temperature, thus giving rise to recrystallization within the local affected area.

It has also been postulated that any intracellular ice may recrystallize with existing extracellular ice through pores in the cell membrane,[3] thereby compromising cellular viability. Intracellular ice recrystallization has been detected at temperatures as low as −130°C,[4] so temperature fluctuations above this level are to be avoided.

259

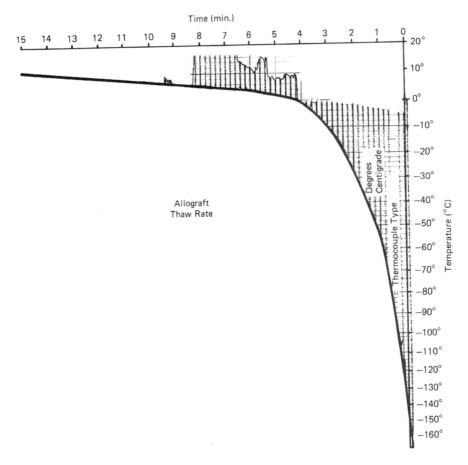

FIGURE 30.1. Freeze curve utilizing a CryoSink.

Below the glass transitional temperature of approximately −130°C, molecules still vibrate but do not move from one position to another, thus preventing chemical reactions.[5] Storage times of 10 years [6] to 32,000[5] years have been speculated. Even though some physical[7] and chemical[8] changes have been reported in cultures cells at −130°C, maintenance of the allograft below −130°C should ensure long-term allograft cell viability. Brockbank et al.[9] have demonstrated maintenance of cell viability in human heart valve leaflets for up to two years below −135°C.

Allowing the temperature of the frozen allograft to warm to temperatures of −100°C during storage or transportation can affect the long-term storage potential. At −100°C many cell types have been observed to age appreciably owing to enzymatic activity[10] and physical reactions,[6] thereby reducing viability.

Damage to the cryopreserved allograft has also been seen when the frozen tissue was allowed to become immersed within the liquid nitrogen pool. In the early days of the University of Alabama's program, the frozen tissue was routinely stored in liquid nitrogen.[11] Upon thawing, tissue fractures of the allograft were discovered, primarily affecting the aortic conduit. This same phenomena has been seen by us and others following accidental immersion of aortic allografts in liquid nitrogen. Cracking can generally be avoided by storage in vapor-phase nitrogen and by slowly warming the tissue to approximately −100°C. This warming is performed in the LifeNet thawing instructions by holding the graft pouch at room temperature for seven minutes before placement in a warm bath.

Several models of liquid nitrogen vapor-phase storage units are available (CryoMed, Mount Clemens, Michigan 48045; Minnesota Valley Engineering Inc., New Prague, Minnesota 56071; Taylor Wharton, Indianapolis, Indiana 46224). Regardless of the size unit employed, temperature gradients exist within the storage area dependent on the distance above the liquid nitrogen pool of −196°C.

In an in-house report published by Minnesota Valley Engineering (MVE),[12] it was determined that a maximum temperature of −150°C is attained at 15 inches above the liquid nitrogen level. This study utilized an MVE VPS-80 storage unit (current model XLC-440) with a storage cavity of 27 inches depth and 18 inches diameter and a reservoir of 4 inches of liquid nitrogen at the bottom. In a LifeNet study using the CryoMed CMS-328 freezer, a maximum temperature of −142°C was obtained at 12 inches above the liquid nitrogen level. The storage unit measured 27 inches depth and 31 inches diameter, and it contained 6 inches of liquid nitrogen. Thus, tissue temperatures under −130°C can easily be maintained using several types and sizes of liquid nitrogen storage freezers.

To increase the allograft storage capacity of the freezer unit, the liquid nitrogen vapor temperatures (−190° to −150°C) in the lower levels of the storage cavity must also be maintained in the upper cavity. For holding limited quantities of a heart valve inventory, single-layer storage on the freezer platform just above the liquid nitrogen level is recommended. Approximately 50 heart valves fit into a single storage layer of a freezer unit with a 30-inch diameter, and about 16 allografts can be held in an 18-inch diameter freezer unit.

Aluminum bars (0.25″ × 1.25″ × 24″) can be affixed to the storage platform, with the proximal 4 inches immersed in the liquid nitrogen pool and the distal 20 inches rising to the top of the storage cavity. Aluminum is an excellent thermal conductor. A LifeNet study found a decrease of 8°C in temperatures at the top of the storage cavity with the use of these rods.

However, for larger inventories, commercial inventory-control systems are available. Most of these systems utilize vertical aluminum racks to hold the cryopreserved allografts in their storage boxes. Three or four allografts can be held per individual rack and a standard liquid nitrogen freezer can hold up to 44 of these separate racks. It has been validated that a standard liquid nitrogen freezer can store up to 132 single allografts, with temperatures at the top of the unit held below −150°C.

Also, various thicknesses of styrofoam sublids are available. These inserts fit tightly within the diameter of the freezer unit and can be designed to rest within the storage cavity on top of the added aluminum bars or inventory racks. With a combination of these items, temperatures within the upper region of the liquid nitrogen storage freezer can be lowered an additional 10–20°C.

Transportation and Distribution

The goal of any cryogenic transport system is to provide the cryopreserved tissue without shipping damage and without subjecting the frozen allograft to injurious thermal fluctuations. Maintaining the biologic tissue below −130°C is imperative. Several systems of cryogenic transportation have been devised, dependent on the distance of travel and the length of time the tissue is subject to transfer.

In situations where the allograft processing and storage facility is in the same complex as the surgical suite, several options are available. The tissue can be thawed in warm saline while it is in transit to the surgical suite and then aseptically delivered to the sterile field for successive rinsing and further warming.[13] The allograft can also be transported to the operating room in insulated containers containing liquid nitrogen (FreezSaf Insulated Container; Polyfoam Packers Corporated, Wheeling, Illinois 60090). The frozen tissue is placed on retaining racks situated just above 4 inches of liquid nitrogen. At room temperature transport (20°–25°C), the entire pool of liquid nitrogen vaporizes in approximately 30 minutes but maintains temperatures below −130°C for only 10 minutes (in-house report: LifeNet, Virginia Beach, Virginia 23455). Thus the allowable distance from the liquid nitrogen storage unit to the surgical suite is limited.

In 1995 as presented at the 19th Annual AATB Meeting in Atlanta, Georgia, LifeNet developed a method of cryogenic transport which would allow up to approximately 10 hours of transport at temperatures well below −130°C. Modifying an existing 10-liter dewar flask with a loose-fitting lid, an additional internal cavity was constructed utilizing a calcium-based absorbent material (Kaylo™ silicate). The finished product, called a "cross-shipper," can be quickly pre-charged with liquid nitrogen and weighs only 17 pounds, yielding a safe, nonspillable "dry-shipper." This new method of lightweight cryogenic transportation can be used for all types of cryopreserved allograft tissue as well as human bone marrow. The "cross-shipper" is not approved for commercial air transport, but can safely be driven to local areas within the 10 hour static hold time limit.

Most commercial airlines do not accept containers containing spillable liquid nitrogen or closed pressurized systems of liquid nitrogen. To address the issue of transporting cryopreserved tissues over long distances, new methods of maintaining liquid nitrogen vapor temperatures (below −130°C) were developed. Several options of long distance cryogenic transport are available. A patented design[14] utilizing solid carbon dioxide impregnated with liquid nitrogen has been used to transport cryopreserved tissues. This system maintains temperatures of −120°C for up to 12 hours.[15] However, this design leaves room for potential thermal damage to the tissue as the temperature warms above −130°C or if the transportation is delayed longer than the 12-hour limit.

To guard against possible thermal damage to the frozen allografts, LifeNet in conjunction with MVE and CryoMed, has developed a cryogenic dry-shipper that maintains temperatures below −130°C for up to 14 days. A large 40-liter bulk cryoflask was developed as a dry-shipping unit and can carry up to five allografts per shipment. A calcium-based porous material was added to the flask cavity, and liquid nitrogen is poured directly into the material. With several fillings, the porous material becomes saturated with liquid nitrogen. The excess liquid nitrogen is poured off, and the absorbed liquid nitrogen is held in a non-spillable fashion by the calcium-based material. A loose-fitting, well-ventilated lid is attached, yielding a non-pressurized cryogenic shipper that optimizes transportation of cryopreserved tissues. This bulk dry-shipper, is available from CryoMed as model CMD-20.

When shipping the allografts, care must be taken to avoid damaging the tissue. The allograft packages are brittle at liquid nitrogen vapor temperatures, and damage to these packages has been seen. Packing cotton balls, surgical sponges, or other shock-absorbent materials around the packages within the retaining cardboard storage boxes provides some measure of protection. Also, packing the internal cavity of the shipper container with soft towels or other such material offers further resistance to shipping damage.

Most allograft heart valve programs in the United States now use packaging materials validated to withstand liquid nitrogen vapor temperatures. Since LifeNet began utilizing the previously noted silicon oxide/Kapton-Teflon pouches, very little (if any) packaging damage has been noted. This may also in part be due to the use of several pouch-suspension systems. Originally trademarked as the "CryoTainer System," a method of cushioning and supporting the frozen pouches within the allograft containing box was developed. The original design utilized custom-made Styrofoam box inserts, but LifeNet has recently validated an internal pouch support system which uses form-fitting foam rubber to cradle and support the fragile cryopreserved tissue pouches.

The AATB has published the *"Standards for Tissue Banking"* for labels and labeling of allogeneic tissues distributed for implantation (please refer to the AATB *Standards* for all details). The most recent edition of AATB *Standards* (August, 1998) is patterned after the FDA's Current Good Manufacturing Practices for Medical Devices (cGMPs) and covers such issues as:

- nomenclature and general requirements
- relabeling methods

- label inspection
- labeling control and storage
- container visual inspections
- package insert requirements
- label content
- external shipping box requirements and shipments

As a general rule, each allograft intended for transplantation should include a unique and traceable tissue identification number. The following information should also be included on the allograft container label or an accompanying package insert:

— Descriptive name of the tissue;
— Name(s) and address(es) of tissue bank(s) responsible for determining donor suitability, processing and distribution;
— Expiration date, if applicable, including the month and year;
— Disinfection or sterilization procedure utilized (if applicable);
— Preservative (if utilized) and/or method of preservation (if applicable);
— Quantity of tissue expressed as volume, weight, dimensions, or combinations of such units of measure, if applicable;
— Potential residues of processing agents/solutions (e.g., antibiotics, ethanol, ethylene oxide, dimethyl sulfoxide); and
— The statement "See package insert."

Additional information often required by AATB or requested by implanting surgeons include:

— Statement limiting use to specific health professionals (e.g., physicians);
— Statement that the tissue is intended for use in one patient, on a single occasion only;
— Known contraindications (if any) to the use of the tissue;
— Warnings and list of known possible significant adverse reactions;
— Statement that the tissue was prepared from a donor whose blood was negative or acceptable when tested using all the tests required by the AATB Standards;
— Statement that indicates that the tissue may transmit infectious agents;

— Statement that the tissue may not be sterilized;
— Donor age (and blood type, if available);
— Date of dissection or cryopreservation;
— Donor heart warm ischemic time;
— Donor heart cold ischemic time;
— Heart valve/conduit sizes (i.e., diameter and length);
— Heart valve/conduit physical descriptions and evaluations, including description of imperfections and evaluation criteria;
— Statement that it is the responsibility of the Tissue Dispensing Service and end-user clinician to maintain tissue intended for transplantation in appropriate storage conditions prior to transplant and that recipient records must be maintained for the purpose of tracing tissue post-transplantation.
— Statement that adverse outcomes potentially attributable to the tissue must be reported promptly to the tissue supplier;
— Type of antibiotics present;
— Concentration of preservatives;
— Presence of known sensitizing agents;
— The type of cryoprotectant and clear statement regarding the possibility of residuals;
— A description of the temperature-sensitive nature of the grafts, recommended storage conditions and tolerance limits;
— Instructions for opening the package and container;
— Warning against using a graft if there is evidence that the container has broken or the contents have thawed;
— Instructions for thawing contents, dilution of the cryoprotectant, and restoration of the ionic balance within the tissue;
— Expiration time following thawing; and
— Date of issue or revision of the package insert.

AATB also requires that agencies distributing allograft heart valves have in place procedures for the recall of an individual or group of allografts. Also, a mechanism should be in place for the distributing agency to receive adverse reactions, implant complications, and unexpected patient outcomes, as well as basic patient recipient implant information.

The need for expedient transport of allogeneic cardiovascular tissues is obvious. Several overnight carriers and courier services handle non-spillable liquid nitrogen containers. However, a prearranged service agreement and some preplanning is recommended in order to avoid possible delays in allograft delivery to the transplanting facility.

Thawing and Dilution Prior to Surgical Preparation of the Allograft

Preparing the frozen allograft for transplantation involves thawing the tissue at a specific rate, diluting the cryoprotective agents, and restoring the cryopreserved tissue to osmotic isotonicity. Careful handling of the allograft and strict adherence to protocols are imperative. To maximize cellular viability and matrix structure, heart valve leaflet manipulation should be kept to a minimum. After thawing and dilution, the "recovering" heart valve should be kept moist and bathed in a physiologic solution at all times during implantation.

Heart valve allografts frozen at a rate of $-1°C$ per minute are considered to be slowly cooled and should be thawed at a more rapid rate to enhance cell survival.[2,5] As discussed in Chapter 3, rapid warming serves to protect the cells that may have any intracellular ice formation by limiting the amount of migratory recrystallization. Farrant and Woolgar suggested that the injury to biologic tissue associated with intracellular ice formation occurs primarily during the rewarming phase and not during the initial crystallization of cooling.[7] Not only is cell damage seen during rewarming (as a function of ice recrystallization), but it has also been suggested that the melting of intracellular ice and the resultant restoration of osmotic gradients may also cause cellular injury.[7]

As published by Pegg and associates in 1997 (*Cryobiology*, 34, 183–192), fractures in arterial tissue are routinely seen if the initial thawing of the cryopreserved tissue is done too rapidly. It was found that the fractures occurred as a result of thermal events below $-100°C$. Pegg found the glass transition temperature of a standard

cryopreservation solution to be about $-123°C$. Reducing/slowing the initial warming rate to less than $50°C$/minute prevented such thermal damage, up to $-100°C$. Thus, LifeNet recommends that the cryopreserved tissue be removed from the vapor-phase storage and sit at room air for approximately seven minutes, followed by pouch placement into the warm bath. It has been validated that this initial "room air thaw" allows the frozen tissue to slowly come to about $-105°C$, thus inhibiting the potential for thermal thaw damage.

It is generally accepted that thawing the frozen allograft in a $37–42°C$ bath produces a warming rate rapid enough to inhibit migratory recrystallization and enhance cell survival.[5,13,16] When an allograft is thawed in a constantly maintained $40°C$ bath, the heart valve rapidly warms to approximately $-50°C$ after 1 minute from the initial prethaw temperature of $-100°C$. The frozen tissue then warms to $-30°C$ after 2 minutes ($30°C$ per minute), to $-14°C$ after 3 minutes ($16°C$ per minute), and is completely thawed in approximately 4 minutes. Allowing the bath to cool may expose the tissue to the recrystallization effects of a slow rewarming process (Figure 30.1).

LifeNet has investigated the thawing of nontransplantable heart valve allografts in heated baths in the range of $60°–80°C$. Though the thawing rate was much faster, several problems were noted: The extra allograft freezing medium warmed to temperatures above $10°C$ while intraconduit ice was still present; and a small percentage of the conduits developed full-thickness cracks during the thawing process. Therefore, thawing the allograft in a bath above $42°C$ is not recommended.

The allograft should be thawed within the surgical suite under aseptic conditions just prior to its use in surgery. An alternative method was presented by Kirklin and Barratt-Boyes[13] in which the frozen tissue is thawed during its transport from the off-site storage freezer to the operating room. Once the allograft external pouch is fully thawed under these nonsterile conditions, the heart valve is aseptically removed from its sterile inner pouch and the freezing medium dilution process is performed under sterile conditions within the operating suite.

Several protocols for thawing the allograft and diluting the cryoprotectant have been developed by Karp,[17] Angell and associates,[18] Kirklin and associates,[19] and others. These techniques involve immersion of the frozen allograft (or the entire allograft pouch) in a 37–42°C bath and then step-wise re-equilibration of the allograft to isotonicity over a 10- to 15-minute period. The gradual step-wise rinses employ an isotonic physiologic solution that gradually allows the dehydrated cryopreserved cells to establish osmotic equilibrium and to rehydrate. This step-by-step protocol also increasingly dilutes the cryoprotectant (DMSO) employed in the freezing solution.

The procedure followed for the preparation of LifeNet allograft heart valves is performed entirely within the operating room and is as follows:

Upon arrival at the operating room, assemble all recommended sterile equipment on a sterile back table (this should include a thermometer, a 5-liter basin, an AlloFlow™ basin, scissors, a clamp, and an IV tubing set). The recommended LifeNet procedure for thawing and dilution of cryopreserved cardiac allografts is essentially as follows:

1) Using insulated gloves, the circulator retrieves the boxed graft from the liquid nitrogen freezer or cryoshipper. Remove the graft from the box. Check for package integrity. Return the graft pouch to the fiberboard box and let the box sit at room temperature for 7 minutes (this step is crucial—see above explanation).

2) Place the thermometer in the large basin and add 2 liters of warm saline. Add room temperature saline to bring the temperature to 37–42°C. Caution: exceeding 42°C may damage the tissue.

3) After the initial seven minutes of "room temperature" thaw, remove the graft from the box and dry off any condensation thoroughly.

4) The circulating nurse opens the outer pouch by grasping the angled edge between thumb and forefinger and peels apart until the inner pouch is retrievable. Be careful not to contaminate or damage the inner sterile pouch. Note: Make sure to initiate the peeling sequence at the corner labeled "peel."

5) Present contents to the scrub nurse who will retrieve the inner sterile pouch with the clamp. The scrub nurse shall be double-gloved. Note: Do not puncture inner pouch.

6) Place the inner pouch in the large basin and gently agitate the pouch for 5–7 minutes.

7) Continue to add warmed saline to the large basin as needed to maintain the temperature at 37–42°C. Do not pour the warm saline directly on the pouch.

8) While the graft is thawing, attach the wash solution in-flow IV line to the lower port of the AlloFlow™ basin and place the AlloFlow™ basin in to the second large basin. The AlloFlow™ procedure is a continuous gradient cryoprotectant removal process described in more detail in Chapter 3. Make sure that the stopcock is fully closed and positioned on the IV line near the point of attachment to the AlloFlow™ basin.

9) After 5–7 minutes, when the ice has melted and the graft is freely movable, remove the pouch from the saline bath and dry the outside thoroughly. Do not palpate the graft to see if the ice has melted.

10) Open the pouch with sterile scissors and pour the entire contents in to the AlloFlow™ basin. Discard the outer gloves. A loose-fitting lid may be placed on to the basin.

11) Pass the inflow line to the circulator.

12) Circulator will attach the spiked inflow IV line to a one liter bag of LRD5 wash solution.

13) The scrub nurse will open the stopcock to allow the wash solution to run wide open in to the AlloFlow™ basin. The stopcock should be allowed to remain open once the LRD5 begins to flow.

14) Once the entire liter of LRD5 has emptied the graft is ready for implantation. The stopcock can now be closed and the IV line cut away if desired.

15) Keep the graft completely immersed in LRD5 solution until needed for implantation. Heparinized blood from CPE line can be added to bowl after 15 minutes.

The dilution process may be carried out at either 4° or 37°C.[16] Several cryobiologists believe dilution at 37°C enables cells to tolerate osmotic stress better than dilution at the colder temperatures.[5] However, prolonged exposure of the heart valve to the cryoprotectant at the warmer temperatures may prove to be toxic. It has been suggested that cellular preservation can be maximized by diluting the freezing medium at 4°C.[16] This may be performed in either one step, multiple dilution steps or as a continuous gradient using the AlloFlow™ process.[20]

Some heart valve preservation programs advocate avoidance of FCS in the dilution medium because of its potential antigenicity.[21] However, the presence of some type of serum or extracellular colloid has been advocated by Bank and Brockbank[22] and Ashwood-Smith and Farrant.[5] The serum helps reduce the trauma to the rehydrating cell and minimizes the dilution shock. The use of human serum,[23] a serum substitute, or no serum components at all[24] warrants further investigation.

During the thawing and dilution aspects of allograft heart valve preparation, several safety precautions are suggested to avoid damaging the tissue:

1. Do not allow the allograft package to become immersed in liquid nitrogen. Not only may it crack the cryopreservation pouches, but these extremely low temperatures may cause cracking in the allograft conduit if thawed too quickly.

2. Do not allow the frozen allograft to be removed from liquid nitrogen vapor storage until it is to be thawed for surgery. LifeNet in-house studies have demonstrated that a frozen allograft warms from −180°C to −130°C in approximately 3–4 minutes upon exposure to room air. Allowing the graft to warm for seven minutes in air prior to thawing in a warm bath prevents cracking of the graft due to rapid warming and minimizes the risks of recrystallization which may occur if the tissue was warmed in air to temperatures much warmer than −100°C.

3. If the most external sterile pouch cracks or sterility is compromised, the allograft can still be thawed under sterile conditions and used for transplantation. However, thawing should be done on a table separate from the one used for the dilution steps. All gowns and gloves should also be changed to avoid possible contamination of the sterile inner pouch.

4. Do not allow the freezing medium to warm much above 10°C when thawing. As discussed, DMSO may be toxic to human cells at warm temperatures. Remove the thawing allograft and solution from the warming bath once the medium has turned to slush but is not completely thawed.

5. Keep the allograft fully immersed at all times. Allograft exposure to air at the time of surgical implantation has been suspected to damage endothelial cells.[25] Allowing the entire tissue graft to dry out during its 45 minutes of surgical implantation greatly reduces cellular viability and may cause matrix structural damage. Judicious, constant wetting of the heart valve during insertion is strongly suggested.

6. Careful handling of the allograft is paramount: Avoid any contact with the leaflet structures, and handle the heart valve from the most distal aspect of the conduit only. It has been suggested that a major percentage of a cryopreserved heart valve's damage occurs during rough handling by the transplanting surgical team.[26]

Quality Systems

Today in the United States, multiple agencies are involved in the oversight of allograft heart valves. As discussed in Chapter 11, the FDA currently has government regulatory jurisdiction in areas regarding donor acceptability and allograft recipient safety. As previously discussed, the AATB has established voluntary *Standards* which cover all aspects of tissue banking, from donor screening to record keeping to tissue production and distribution. And finally, several banks (CryoLife, Inc. and LifeNet) have achieved ISO (International Standards Organization) 9000/1 registration. The overriding theme behind all these agencies is one of ongoing Quality Systems/Quality Assurance/Quality Control. General organizational issues such as training, administrative oversight, vendor qualification, contracts, supply/materials tracking, systems monitoring, internal audits, complaints/errors and accidents documentation and follow-up, etc. are all part of a complete organizational quality systems program. Though the general topic of "Quality Systems" is well beyond the scope of this chapter, prior to the release of an allograft heart valve, each donor and the associated valves should go through a thorough documented review process.

- Donor Acceptability: As previously discussed, the donor's medical, social, and behavioral history is reviewed and shall fall within all established criteria. This documented review includes the consent process, all pre-screening forms and next-of-kin interviews, physical assessment, time and age limit verifications, heart procurement-related items, infusion/transfusion data, and autopsy. It is important that this documented review be done by a physician Medical Director as required by AATB *Standards*.
- Laboratory Tests: All donor serology tests, microbiology tests, and blood work analysis are also reviewed by the Medical Director.
- Production/Processing: All technical work is reviewed by multiple parties involving both front-line technicians and cardiovascular managers. As discussed previously in this chapter, all dissection, sizing, schematics, valve evaluation, disinfecting parameters, packaging criteria, cryofreezing tolerances and cryopreservation procedures, supply lot number/expiration dates, graft and time limit specifications, and computer and manual entry data is reviewed and such review is documented.
- Storage/Distribution: As noted above, all labels and labeling items are approved for use. Other items such as storage and inventory control parameters; printed brochures, manuals, use instructions, and other publications; shipping containers, temperatures, and expiration dates; accompanying printed material and implant return cards; and allograft orders and transportation information are also reviewed prior to shipment.

All of the above and other QA/QC items are double-checked by multiple approved staff and documentation of their review is maintained.

It is important for everyone involved in the review process to keep in mind that allograft heart valves must meet all pre-established criteria/specifications and that the end result of our work and the donor family's generosity is the ultimate transplantation of the tissue into a recipient.

References

1. Karow AM, Pegg DE. Organ Preservation for Transplantation. New York: Marcel Dekker 1981.
2. Grout BWW, Morris GJ. The Effects of Low Temperatures on Biological Systems. London: Edward Arnold 1987.
3. Mazur P. The role of cell membranes in the freezing of yeast and other single cells. Annals of the New York Academy of Sciences 1965;125: 658.
4. Dowell LG, Rinfret AP. Low temperature forms of ice as studied by x-ray diffraction. Nature 1960;188:1144.
5. Ashwood-Smith MJ, Farrant J. Low Temperature Preservation in Medicine and Biology. London: Pitman 1980.
6. Luyet BJ. On various phase transitions occurring in aqueous solutions at low temperatures. Annals of the New York Academy of Sciences 1960;85: 549.
7. Farrant J, Woolgar AE. Possible relationships in between the physical properties of solutions and cell damage during freezing. In Farrant J, Woolgar AE (eds). The Frozen Cell. London: Churchill 1979.
8. Peterson WD, Stulbert CS. Freeze preservation of cultured animal cells. Cryobiology 1984; 1:80.
9. Brockbank KGM, Carpenter JF, Dawson PE. Effects of Storage Temperature on Viable Bioprosthetic Heart Valves. Cryobiology 1992; 29:537–542.
10. Josylyn MA. The action of enzymes in the dried state and in concentrated solutions. Proceedings of the Eighth International Congress of Refrigeration 1952;331.
11. Watkins C. University of Chicago Hospital Heart Valve Program. Lange PE. 1988. Personal Communication.
12. MVE Engineering. Temperature Profile. Test Report 212. 1985. New Prague, MN.
13. Kirklin JW, Barratt-Boyes GB. Cardiac Surgery. New York: Wiley 1986.

14. Cryolife I. Freezing agent and container. [4,597,266]. 1986. United States.
15. Cryolife I. Thermal cycling during transport of homograft tissue may compromise cell viability. CryoLife Technology Memorandum 1987;2.
16. Bank HL, Brockbank K. Basic principles of cryobiology. Jour Card Surg 1987;2 suppl:137–143.
17. Karp RB. The use of free-hand unstented aortic valve allografts for replacement of the aortic valve. J Card Surg 1986;1:23–32.
18. Angell JD, Christopher BS, Hawtrey O, Angell WM. A fresh viable human heart valve bank-sterilization sterility testing and cryogenic preservation. Transplant Proc 1976;8 (Suppl 1): 127–141.
19. Kirklin JW, Blackstone EH, Maehara T, Pacifico AD, Kirklin JK, Pollock S, Stewart RW. Intermediate-term fate of cryopreserved allograft and xenograft valved conduits. Ann Thorac Surg 1987;44:598–606.
20. Linthurst A, Braendle L, Burkart M, Brockbank KGM. A comparative study of cryopretectant removal methods. 1998. Pittsburgh, PA, International Society for Cryobiology.
21. Bodnar E, Olsen WGJ, Florio R, et al. Heterologous antigenicity induced to human aortic homografts during preservation. Eur J Cardiothorac Surg 1988;2:43–47.
22. Kirklin JK, Kirklin JW, Pacifico JAD, Phillips S. Cryopreservation of aortic valve homografts. In Yankah AC, Hetzer R, Miller DC, Ross DN, Somerville J, Yacoub M (eds). Cardiac Valve Allografts 1962–1987. New York: Springer-Verlag 1987:35–36.
23. Yankah AC. First Workshop on Homologous and Autologous Heart Valves. 1987. Chicago, IL, Deborah Heart and Lung Center.
24. Nakayama S, Ban T, Okamoto S. Fetal bovine serum is not necessary for the cryopreservation of aortic valve tissues. J Thorac Cardiovasc Surg 1994;108:583–586.
25. O'Brien MF. Cardiac Valve Allografts. Cardiac Surgery 1987;2 Suppl:169.
26. O'Brien MF, Stafford EG, Gardner AH, Pohlner P, McGiffin DC, Johnston N, Tesar P, Brosnan A, Duffy P. Cryopreserved viable allograft valves. In Yonkah AC, Hetzer R, Miller DCea (eds). Cardiac valve allografts 1962–1987. New York: Springer Verlag 1988:311–321.

Section IX
Surgical Techniques: Valve and Root Methods for Left Ventricular Outflow Tract Reconstructions

31
Indications and Contraindications: Valve and Root Methods

Richard A. Hopkins

The developing role for allograft transplants is reviewed in Sections I, II and III. The major controversies reside in the issues of durability, viability, and use of homografts versus the alternative of autotransplants and unstented heterografts in various patient subgroups. The hemodynamic performance of a properly placed allograft is clearly superior to stented xenograft or mechanical valve and the advantages concerning resistance to infection and the avoidance of anticoagulation are becoming more evident and attractive. Good long-term performance is dependent on an excellent technical surgical result. The surgeon must view the use of allograft tissue as a tool for the reconstruction of the left ventricular outflow tract rather than as an implant of a device. This requires mastering both the analysis of the outflow tract as well as multiple methods for its reconstruction.

The early allograft aortic valve replacements were referred to as "freehand" in the sense that the valve was sewn directly into the aortic root without stents. This "freehand" approach encompasses a range of techniques which must account for variations in annulus, aortic root, and coronary anatomy as well as ensuring the continued perfect function of the allograft semilunar aortic valve mechanism.

Although some authors have recommended that the allograft valve is the prosthesis of choice for all aortic valve replacements, limitation of availability and the requisite increase in aortic cross-clamp time requires selection.[1] In addition, there are anatomic situations that may increase the difficulty of inserting an allograft valve. In general, allograft valve transplant is considered for the following indications: (1) all aortic valve replacements and left ventricular outflow tract reconstructions in patients with more than a 10-year life expectancy in whom anticoagulation is undesirable (e.g., children, young women of childbearing age, and young active adults); (2) aortic root replacement: (3) aortoventriculoplasty; (4) small aortic annulus; (5) bacterial endocarditis;[2] and (6) reoperation for failure of an aortic valve prosthesis, particularly in patients with accelerated degeneration of a porcine bioprosthesis. Older patients may be well suited for unstented xenografts whereas younger patients with life expectancy exceeding 20 years should be considered for Ross autotransplant.

Relative contraindications to insertion of an allograft valve include the following: (1) severe asymmetric annular calcification precluding uniform, smooth "seating" or extensive calcification extending into the septum, mitral valve, and fibrous trigones; (2) lack of availability; (3) active immune complex or rheumatoid-like diseases (e.g., lupus, rheumatoid arthritis, collagen vascular disease, etc); (4) aortic root ectasia exceeding a diameter of 30mm;[3] aortic valve replacement being a small component of the total amount of cardiac surgery necessary in which cross-clamp times would be expected to 120 minutes; (6) severe left ventricular dysfunction; and (7) connective tissue disorders such as Marfan's syndrome or cystic medial necrosis.

Sizing of Aortic Root for Allograft Insertion

Careful matching of allograft size to aortic annulus is important for optimal performance. It requires a slightly different set of assumptions for the surgeon accustomed to using rigid stented prostheses, as the measured diameter of the allograft is the internal diameter (in contrast to the external diameter for standard prostheses) and thus allowance must be made for wall thickness. In addition, the hemodynamic performance of the smaller allograft aortic valves is markedly superior to mechanical or bioprosthesis such that a 19 to 20 mm (internal diameter, ID) allograft valve is usually adequate for most adults and hemodynamically analogous to a much larger prosthesis (See Appendix: Valve Diameters). A 16 to 17 mm or larger valve can usually be placed in patients who weigh more than 20 kg.

Preoperative estimation of the allograft size required for a given patient has been approached angiographically and echocardiographically. Yankah, from Germany, recommended angiographic measurement of the aortic "annulus" for preoperative determination of size. This technique involves an angiogram obtained in the lateral position during both systole and diastole, with the measurements being performed 1 mm above the sinuses.[4] However, others have thought that aortography gives unreliable estimates of aortic annulus size and, to be useful, the left ventriculography requires precise methodology.[5]

We have found a simple echocardiographic technique most helpful. A parasternal long axis view is obtained of the left ventricular outflow tract. The internal diameter of the outflow tract is measured at the point of the continuity of the anterior leaflet of the mitral valve and the aortic annulus just beneath the valve leaflet attachment and across to the septum (Figure 31.1). Multiple measurements are made, but the most important is during early systolic ejection, as a useful correlation within 1–2 mm is possible with this measurement (Figure 31.2). The

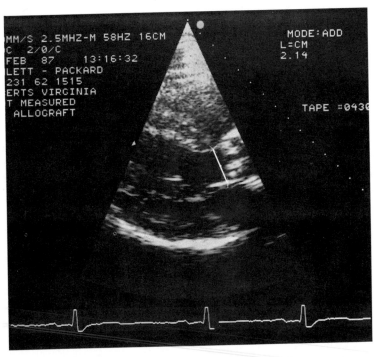

FIGURE 31.1. Parasternal, long axis two-dimensional echocardiographic view for allograft sizing. The white bar shows the plane in which the left ventricular outflow tract diameter is measured during the initial portion of systole for sizing for freehand aortic valve replacement.

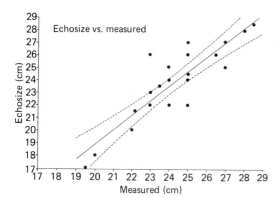

FIGURE 31.2. Correlation between internal diameter measurement of aortic "annulus" at surgery with the echocardiographic preoperative measurement. Dotted line represents ± 1SD. $n = 21$. Best fit: $y = 1.15x + (-4.12)$. Analysis of variance: $r^2 = 0.7769$.

ultimate internal diameter measurement is made during surgery. The measured estimated diameter of the base of the aortic outflow minus 3–4mm provides a "target size" so that a span of allograft sizes can be readily available.

Some authors have recommended external aortic root diameter measurement at the time of surgery as a guide to the internal diameter. The formula is approximately 8mm less than the external diameter measurement as measured by forceps at the base of the aortic root. This technique has been unreliable in our hands.

Direct internal measurements are made at operation after opening the aorta and excising the native valve. After adequate debridement, the size of the aortic outflow is measured with the Hegar dilators. Hegar dilators are preferred, as commercial prosthesis sizers vary significantly from their nominal measurements owing to purposely introduced manufacturers' "prosthetic specific factors,"[6] which accommodate for specific sizing issues for each prosthesis. This measurement can be made prior to the final meticulous debridement of the annulus but at such time that the actual size of the outflow is readily apparent. This measurement is then used to calculate the size of the aortic valve allograft selected. Because the wall thickness of an allograft is approximately 2mm, it is necessary to subtract 4mm from the measured internal diameter to obtain the size of the allo-

graft to implant. If there is not a large amount of calcium, in general one can increase the size of the allograft by 1–2mm such that only 2–3mm are subtracted from the internal diameter size. For example, if the internal measurement is 24mm, we would use a 21mm aortic allograft; but if there is much calcium, a 20mm allograft would be selected. If the measurement is 21.5mm, we would select an 18 or 19mm allograft. The more calcium in the annulus, the more one avoids a large allograft.

Preparation of Allograft for Insertion

The allograft is thawed. On obtaining the allograft, the surgeon inspects the aorta for cracks and the valve itself for fenestrations or congenital abnormalities. The aortic allograft is then filled with saline to test for aortic valve insufficiency, and the muscle at the base of the valve on the septal side is trimmed meticulously. As much of this tissue as can be removed safely is debrided. This step is easily accomplished by gently placing the wet gloved finger through the valve and using the carved portion of the scissors to gently pare away the muscle (Figure 31.3). Sufficient muscle must be removed that the fibrous skeleton can be visualized for accurate placement of the sutures. In addition, reducing the muscle bulk allows placement of a slightly larger prosthesis and reduces the need to rotate the valve. When the muscle has been meticulously removed, the aortic valve can be placed orthotopically without rotation in virtually all aortic roots. For the standard freehand aortic valve insertion, the anterior leaflet of the mitral valve is excised, leaving a 2mm remnant.

Cannulation

Cannulate the ascending aorta as high as possible, close to the innominate artery. If the proximal aortic root is short, we recommend cannulating the femoral artery or the aortic arch.

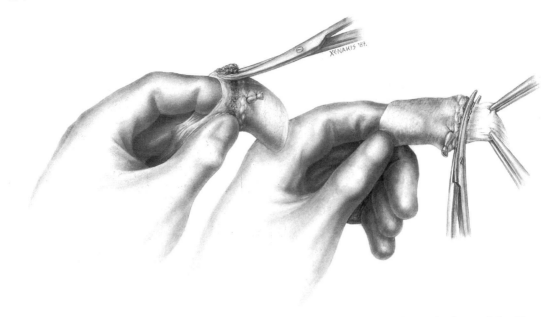

FIGURE 31.3. Trimming of the thawed allograft is begun by removing muscle at the base of the fibrous skeleton. The allograft is kept moist with saline during all manipulations.

Cardiopulmonary Bypass Management

A single atrial return cannula and left ventricular venting via the right superior pulmonary vein are used for aortic valve replacement, as is moderate total body hypothermia with cardioplegic arrest supplemented by topical cooling. Multiple doses of cardioplegia are delivered via direct coronary cannulas at 20 minute intervals; or after antegrade induction, maintenance cardioplegia is given via retrograde coronary sinus delivery.

References

1. Karp RB. The future of homografts. J Card Surg 1987;2:205–208.
2. Barratt-Boyes BG. The timing of operation in valvular insufficiency. (Review). Jour Card Surg 1987;2:435–452.
3. Barratt-Boyes BG, Roche AH, Subramanyan R, Pemberton JR, Whitlock RM. Long-term follow-up of patients with the antibiotic-sterilized aortic homograft valve inserted freehand in the aortic position. Circulation 1987;75:768–777.
4. Yankah AC, Hetzer R. Procurement and viability of cardiac valve allografts. In Yankah AC, Hetzer R, Miller DC, Ross DN, Somerville J, Yacoub MH (eds). Cardiac Valve Allografts 1962–1987. New York: Springer-Verlag 1988:23–34.
5. Imamura E, Tomizawa Y, Hashimoto A, et al. A comparative analysis of left ventriculography and root aortography for estimating aortic annular size. J Thorac Cardiovasc Surg 1987;93:592–596.
6. Bonchek LI, Burlingame MW, Vazales BE. Accuracy of sizers for aortic valve prostheses. J Thorac Cardiovasc Surg 1987;94:632–634.

32

"Freehand" Aortic Valve Replacement with Aortic Allograft Valve Transplant Aortotomy

Richard A. Hopkins

The aortotomy for aortic valve replacement should be different when using an allograft from that used when implanting other prostheses. A reverse "lazy S" incision is begun 4–5 cm vertically above the right coronary artery and is brought down to a level that is well above a point at which the allograft commissural pillars are estimated to reach; it is then deviated virtually transversely until reaching the midpoint above the non-coronary cusp (Figure 32.1). The incision is then completed by aiming down toward the anterior leaflet of the mitral valve; unless an extensive aortoplasty or annuloplasty is definitely planned, however, the incision is stopped well above the annulus, approximately at or just below the level of the aortic sinus ridge, to the right of the pillar between the left and non-coronary cusps. The exposure of this aortotomy is greatly facilitated by placement of the three stay sutures, two on the left "flap" and one on the surgeon's side of the aortotomy (Figure 32.2). This incision gives good exposure, leaves adequate native aortic wall for placement of the commissural posts, provides the option of extending the incision for annuloplastic maneuvers and allows aortoplastic augmentation or reduction. Other incisions have been suggested, including oblique standard incisions and transverse incisions. The transverse incision, although adequate if nothing needs to be done to the aortic root, is limiting if enlargement procedures or alterations in aortic root geometry are necessary. A standard oblique incision, as is usually performed for mechanical prostheses, can make placement of the allograft commissural pillar between the right and non-coronary sinuses more difficult because it is usually lower and would encroach on this region.

Surgical Technique for Standard Aortic Valve Replacement with Freehand Insertion of an Allograft Aortic Valve

Proximal Suture Line

After preparation of the allograft and resection of the native valve, three sutures of 4-0 monofilament polypropylene on a taper-point half-circle needle are placed as simple sutures, relating the middle of each recipient sinus to the donor coronary ostia (Figure 32.3). They are placed as simple sutures beginning with the base of the left sinus of the allograft lined up to a position directly underneath the left coronary of the recipient (Figure 32.4). Similarly, a simple suture is placed between the midportion of the right coronary sinus of the transplant and a point just underneath the right coronary ostia (presuming both coronary ostia are in the middle of their respective sinuses). The valve is thus placed orthotopically without rotation.

When the second suture is placed, an "adjustment" may be necessary. If either of the native coronary ostia are off center from their coronary sinuses (which they often are), the allograft left coronary sinus is centered to the left

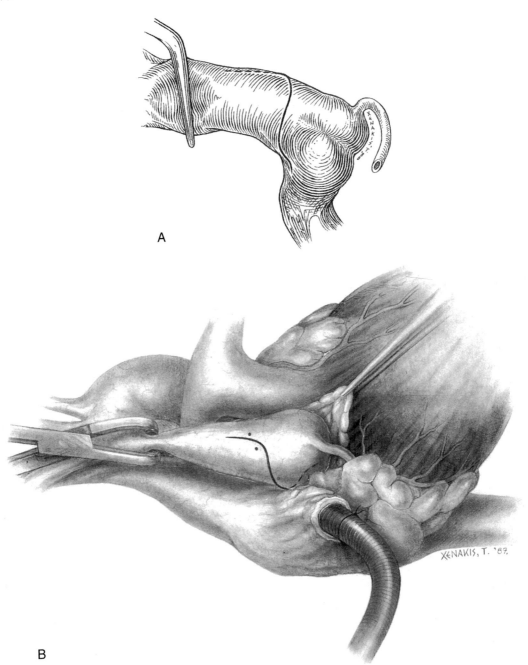

FIGURE 32.1. (A) Reverse S aortotomy for freehand aortic valve replacement with allograft aortic valve. Transverse portion of the incision is kept well above the commissural pillar between the right and non-coronary cusps. (B) Nonsurgical view demonstrates the deviation of the incision above the level of the commissural pillar and into the non-coronary cusp. Ending the incision just below the level of the sinus ridge in this position allows extension for annulus enlargement if necessary.

FIGURE 32.2. Positioning of stay sutures for exposure of the aortic root.

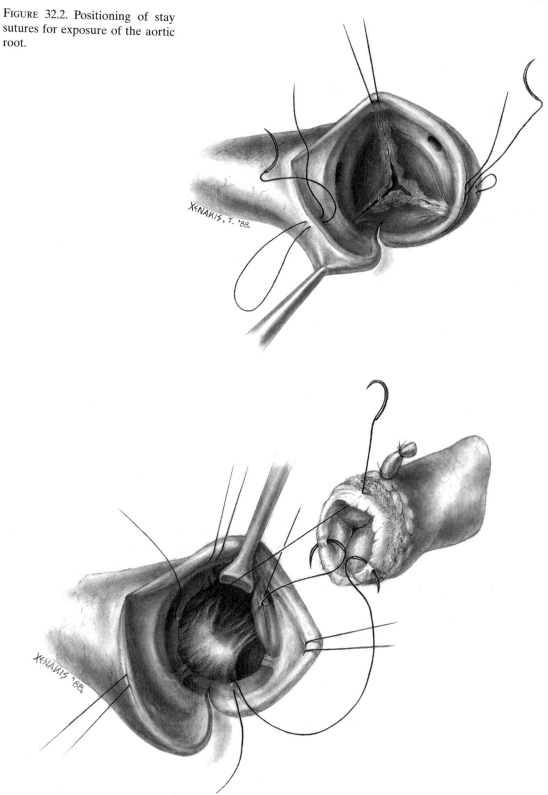

FIGURE 32.3. Three monofilament 4-0 half-circle needle sutures are placed for the proximal suture line so as to "line up" the allograft coronary sinuses to the recipient coronary ostia.

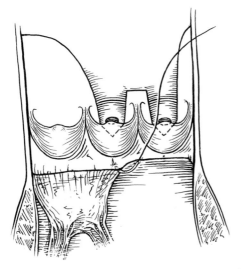

FIGURE 32.4. The first suture is placed at a point underneath the left coronary ostia of the recipient and line up to the midpoint of the coronary sinus of the allograft. When the sinus geometry between recipient and transplant are symmetric, the second suture relates the midpoint of the recipient right sinus below the right coronary ostia of the donor mid-sinus point.

coronary ostia. A rotational adjustment is then needed for positioning the midportion of the right coronary sinus to a point relevant to the recipient right coronary ostia (see the section on mini rotation below). This adjustment makes placement of the distal suture line possible without deviating the line of the commissural post to avoid the right coronary ostium, which would cause semilunar dysfunction. The third suture starts in the midportion of the non-coronary sinus through the fibrous skeleton of the base of the transplant valve and is then placed at a point equidistant from each of the other two sutures (midway on both recipient and transplant). These three sutures fix the rotation of the valve.

The valve is inverted into the left ventricular cavity (Figure 32.5). Beginning with the left suture, a running suture line is constructed with four or five simple sutures being taken with each limb such that the sutures meet at a midpoint between the starting points (usually underneath the commissures) (Figure 32.6). This measure allows a continuous suture line

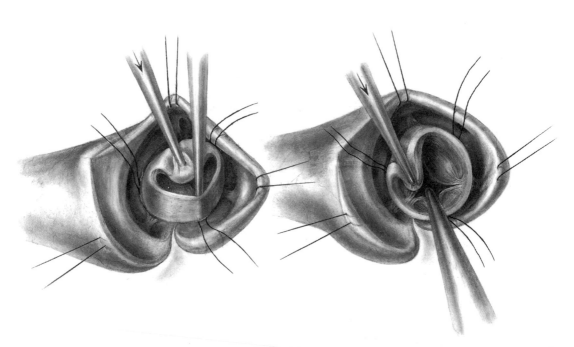

FIGURE 32.5. The valve is carefully inverted into the left ventricular cavity. Forceps are used to push the valve leaflets aside and not to grasp the delicate tissues. Three sutures of the proximal anastomosis are kept on light tension with rubber-shod clamps.

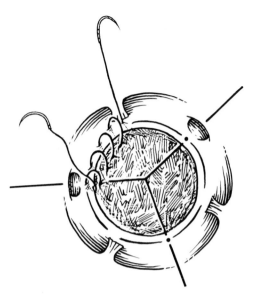

FIGURE 32.6. The three sutures are begun at the points indicated by the dots, and the six hemisutures are each run to a midpoint between their starting places, taking approximately four bites apiece.

but on which tension needs to be placed for only four or five suture "bites" to allow tightening without drag or cutting into the delicate allograft tissue; once all six hemisutures have been run to the midportions, they are snugged and tied (Figure 32.7). This point is a good time to repeat the cardioplegia with direct coronary cannulae (Spencer's). The valve is reverted (Figure 32.8).

Distal Suture Line

Guide traction sutures of 4-0 monofilament are placed at the apex of each commissural post (Figure 32.9) and the allograft coronary sinuses excised with scissors to provide an opening sufficient to suture around the native coronary ostia (Figure 32.10). We defer this step until now because it is at this time that the position of the coronary ostia relative to the transplanted coronary sinus can be best ascertained, thereby avoiding unnecessary dissection. 4-0 Soft braided sutures are then placed behind the commissural posts to the native aortic wall as nontransmural simple sutures to accomplish obliteration of that space (Figure 32.11) (analogous to the vertical mattress through-and-

through suture of Barratt-Boyes and Roche[1]). Then, with modest tension on the commissural posts by the assistant, 4-0 monofilament sutures on half-circle needles are started at the bottom of each coronary sinus (usually starting with the left) and the suture line run to the tops of each commissural post where the suture is brought outside the native aorta (Figure 32.12). Sutures are used to run from the bottom of each sinus, taking care to keep the lower portion of the distal suture line "flat" and to maintain commissural suspension for enhancement of semilunar function (Figure 32.13). These sutures are tied over pledgets outside the aorta (Figure 32.14).

There are basically three methods for handling the non-coronary sinus (Figure 32.15).

1. *Flange Technique.* In our practice, the "flange" technique of preparing the allograft is the most routine, as it leaves ample allograft tissue for sculpturing of the aortic root to ensure uniform commissural post architecture.

The allograft is trimmed as demonstrated (Figure 32.16). Care is taken to leave the length of the aorta in the region of the non-coronary sinus long—longer than one would think necessary. The three bottom sutures are placed as

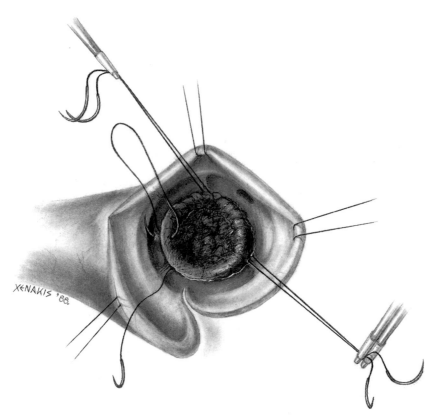

FIGURE 32.7. The loops of monofilament suture are not securely tightened until all have been run to allow displacement of the allograft in and out of the ventricular cavity, permitting accurate placement of the needle into both the recipient fibrous tissue and the fibrous skeleton of the allograft. Once all of the suture limbs have been run to each other, they are snugged securely and tied.

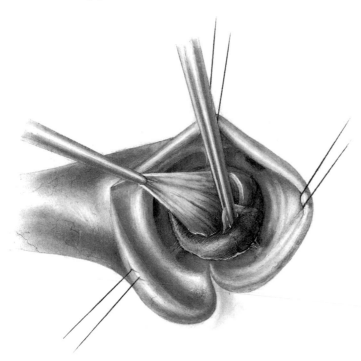

FIGURE 32.8. The valve is carefully reverted.

FIGURE 32.9. Monofilament guide sutures are placed at the apex of each allograft commissure pillar. They are then controlled by the assistant, which gives exposure of the sinuses and allows some stretch to be placed on the pillars during excision of sinus walls and the creation of the distal suture line.

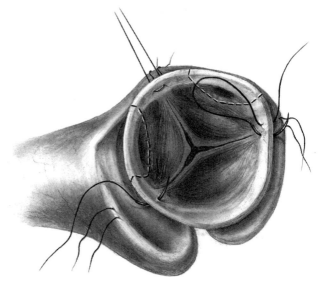

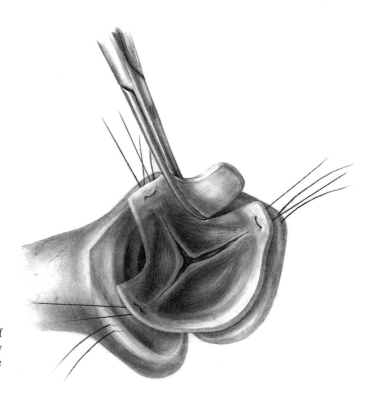

FIGURE 32.10. The coronary sinuses of the allograft are now excised as deeply as necessary to allow exposure of the native coronary ostia.

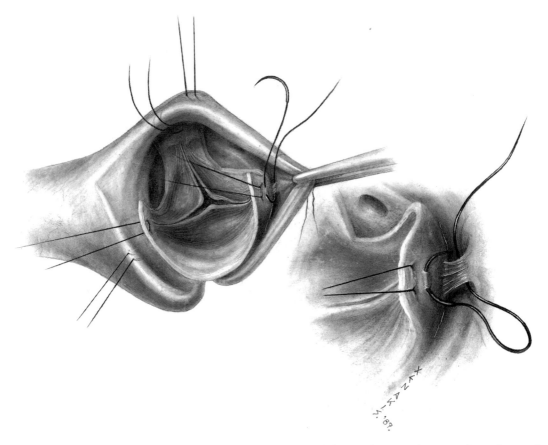

FIGURE 32.11. A nontransmural, soft-braided suture is used to obliterate the space between the native aortic wall and the commissural posts, and then it is tied.

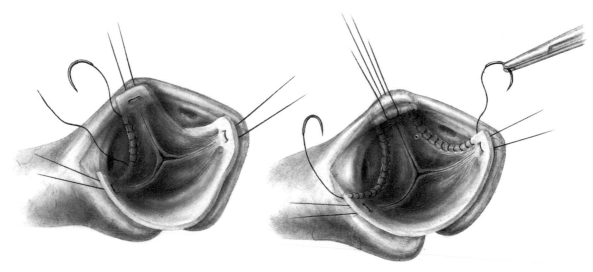

FIGURE 32.12. Creation of the distal suture line with running monofilament sutures beginning at the base of each coronary sinus.

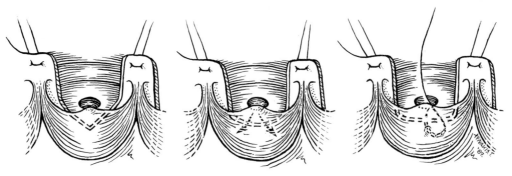

FIGURE 32.13. The base of the suture line underneath the coronary ostia is kept "flat" to avoid encroachment.

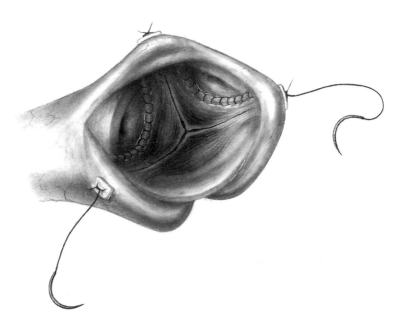

FIGURE 32.14. All three commissural pillars are suspended and their positions fixed. The next step is management of the non-coronary sinus.

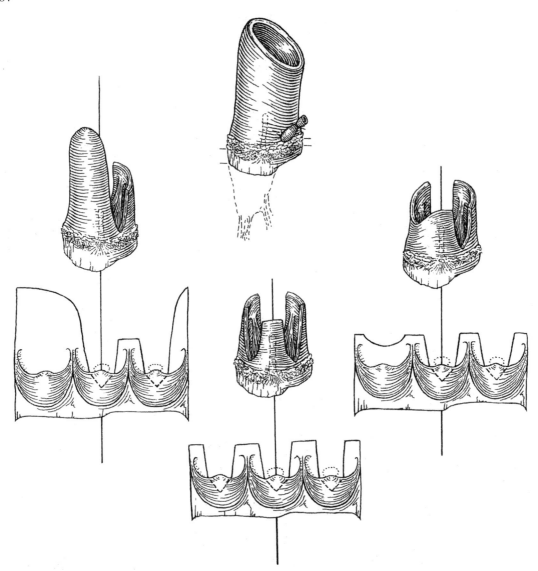

FIGURE 32.15. Representation of the three basic techniques for managing the non-coronary sinus, particularly the distal suture line. *Flange technique* (on the left) allows allograft augmentation of the non-coronary sinus, which when accomplished with annulus enlargement can enlarge the entire aortic root for placement of a larger valve. In the *classic technique* (middle) the sinuses of the allograft are excised and the suture lines run around each pillar, taking care to suspend the pillars for semilunar valvular function. It is the best technique when "rotation" of the allograft is planned within the recipient aortic root (i.e., aligning the allograft left sinus to the recipient right sinus). In the *scallop technique* (on the right) only a shallow scallop is removed from the non-coronary sinus. The maneuver allows primary closure of the aortotomy with deviation of the suture line of that sinus below the aortotomy site, but it does not remove much allograft tissue in that sinus, which helps preserve the alignment of the pillars.

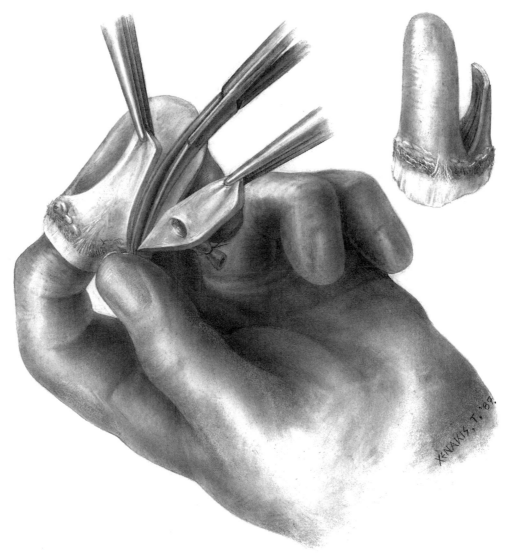

FIGURE 32.16. Trimming of the allograft for the flange technique of handling the distal suture line. It can be accomplished prior to the proximal suture line construction when aortic augmentation aortoplasty is definitely required or after reversion, if preferred.

previously described and the proximal suture line accomplished in the usual fashion (Figure 32.17). The valve is reverted, and the right and left coronary ostia are excised, leaving the commissural pillar between the right and left sinuses isolated but the non-coronary sinus and its flange of aorta intact (Figure 32.18). Stay sutures are placed at the top of each pillar. The distal suture line is then begun with a running 4-0 polypropylene suture on a half-circle taper-point needle. The suturing is begun at the base of the left coronary sinus (Figure 32.19). Care is taken to keep the suture line flat underneath the left coronary ostia. The suture line is run to the top of the pillar between the left and right coronary ostia, where it is brought outside the aorta. The right coronary sinus is handled similarly. The suture line is brought to the top of the other two pillars and outside the aorta. The stay sutures at the top of these two pillars are brought to the outside of the aorta, through a pledget, and tied (Figure 32.20). This measure

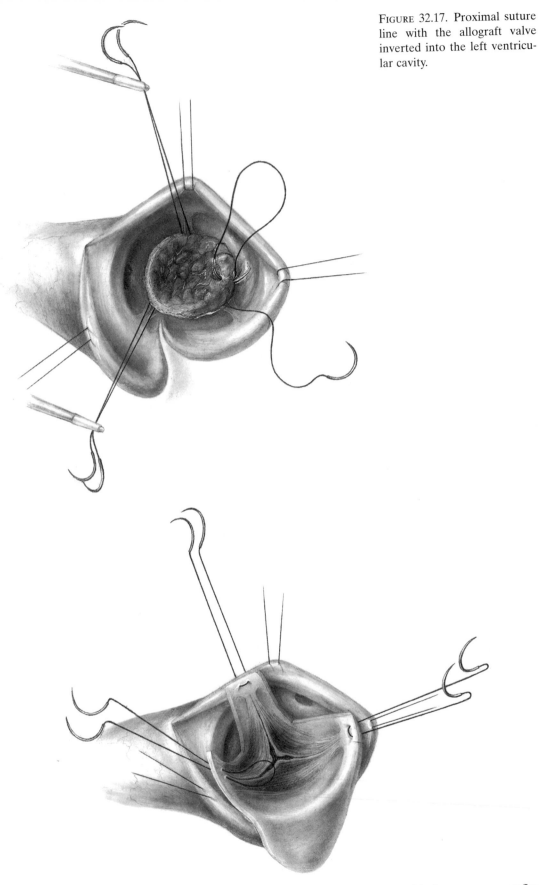

FIGURE 32.17. Proximal suture line with the allograft valve inverted into the left ventricular cavity.

FIGURE 32.18. Reverted allograft valve after excision of the coronary sinuses, with the non-coronary flange left intact and stay sutures placed at the top of each commissural pillar.

FIGURE 32.19. The distal suture line of the flange technique is begun in the left sinus below the left coronary ostia.

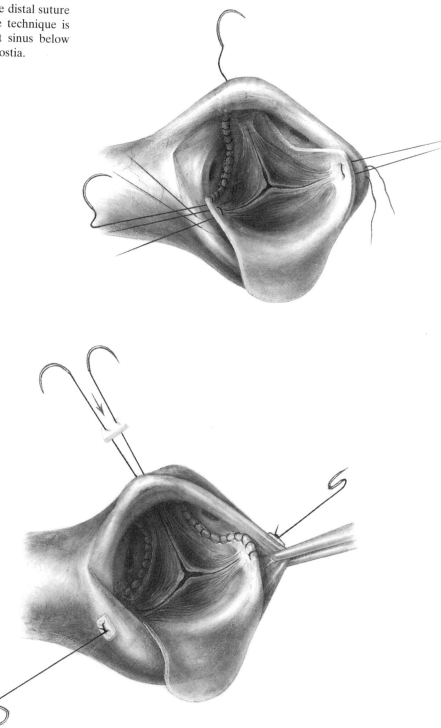

FIGURE 32.20. All three pillars' positions are fixed normal to the aortic long axis. The stay suture at the top of the pillars on either side of the non-coronary sinus are used for support so the continuous suture can be fixed at that point, and they are then continued to their meeting points with the aortotomy closure. (The aortotomy stay sutures have been left out for clarity.)

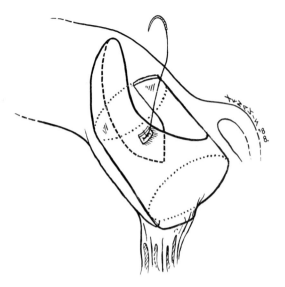

FIGURE 32.21. The flange of the allograft allows reconstruction of the aortic root to a symmetrical cylinder with the amount of augmentation necessary to allow maintain alignment of the pillars and also to allow a slight waist to be constructed at the level of the sinus ridge.

fixes the commissural posts but leaves the aortic wall of the allograft to fill however much is necessary of the non-coronary sinus to maintain the aortic root geometry (Figure 32.21). The sinus ridge (ie. top of the pillars) circumference should never be larger than the aortic annulus diameter of the transplanted valve and preferably should be reduced slightly but no less than a reduction of 20% below the value of the aortic annulus diameter.[2]

The aortotomy closure is begun at the base of the non-coronary sinus with a pledgetted suture (Figure 32.22). The suture is advanced superiorly along the aortic closure with transmural suturing through the native aorta to the wall of the allograft aortic wall. This suture line is run to the point where the distal line meets the aortotomy, then converted to a running edge-to-edge closure of the allograft aortic wall flange and the native aorta (Figure 32.23). The flange (trimmed as necessary) fills the aortotomy up into its transverse portion (Figure 32.24), providing controlled expansion of the non-coronary sinus.

If only a small amount of expansion of the non-coronary sinus is required, the suture line

can be deviated away from the native aortic edge. Sutures are transmural through the native aorta and nontransmural through the allograft until the top of the pillar is reached. At this point, the edge of the allograft is sutured to the inside of the aorta until the triangulation point is reached (Figure 32.25). The operation is completed by simply suturing the remainder of the aortotomy with a pledgetted technique, de-airing and removing the cross-clamp.

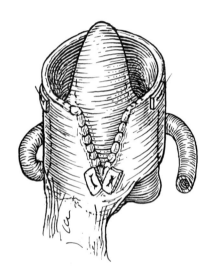

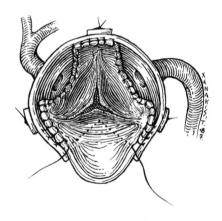

FIGURE 32.22. The distal suture line is continued to the points where the aortotomy closure sutures meet them, and they are then tied together. If no augmentation aortoplasty is necessary, the sutures are run to the top of the truncated flange and tied together outside the native aorta.

Figure 32.23. The inner distal suture line
is continued to the edge of the aortotomy
closure.

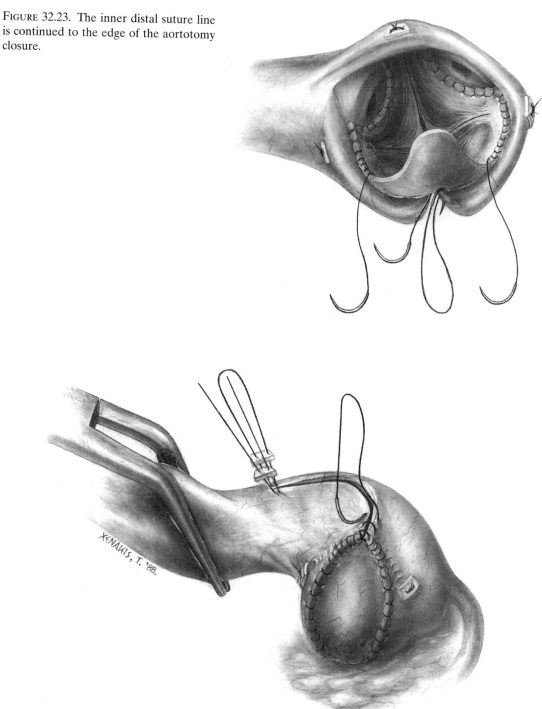

Figure 32.24. The inner distal suture line is tied to the outer sutures and the aortotomy closure continued in a standard fashion.

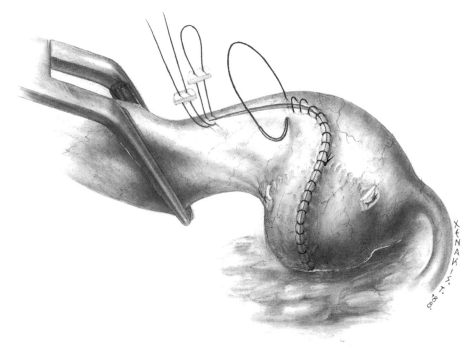

FIGURE 32.25. The amount of allograft aorta exposed relates to the amount of expansion of the sinus necessary. If no expansion is necessary, the aortotomy closure completely overlaps the allograft flange.

Classic Technique

With the classic subcoronary fully scalloped technique (similar to that originally developed by Barratt-Boyes, Ross, Karp and others) minimal allograft aorta is retained, and the allograft is dissected prior to beginning the proximal suture line (Figure 32.26).[3–5] All three sinuses are excised, leaving the commissural pillars as three posts, as in a crown (Figure 32.16). This technique is selected for an aortic root in which commissural post placement can be accomplished in such a manner that primary closure of the aortotomy incision results in appropriate architecture without splaying or narrowing of the posts or if rotation of the sinuses is desired. The distal suture line is constructed with three 4-0 polypropylene sutures, each begun at the bottom of a sinus and run to meet each other at the top of the pillars (Figures 32.27 and 32.28).

Although appearing to be the simplest technique conceptually, the classic technique limits later options for sculpturing the aortic root. The spacial geometry of the non-coronary sinus must be reassessed after suturing the allograft commissural posts. If the non-coronary sinus of the native aorta cannot be closed without deforming the commissures on either side, a patch of prosthetic material must be inserted (Figure 32.29). Air removal maneuvers are performed and the aortotomy closed with a running monofilament suture technique. The "classic" method of aortic valve replacement is best used when there is sufficient dilatation of aortic root to allow "sacrifice" of enough aorta at the aortotomy for adequate closure without distorting the non-coronary sinus and causing inward deflection of the commissural posts at the aortic sinus ridge. If the implants cannot be made in this way, attention to aortic root geometry mandates some minor changes in this method (*vida infra*).

FIGURE 32.26. Classic technique. All three allograft sinuses are excised, leaving minimal tissue for the distal suture line.

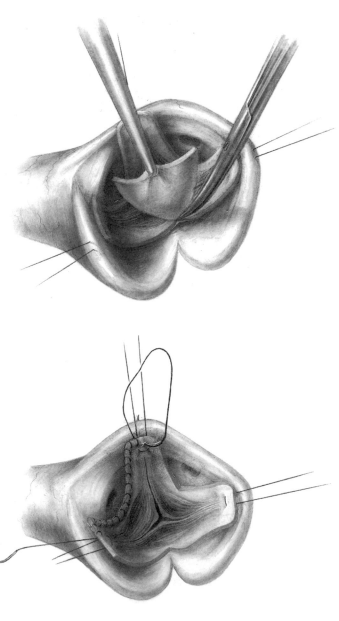

FIGURE 32.27. Suturing of the semilunar allograft valve pillars: distal suture line.

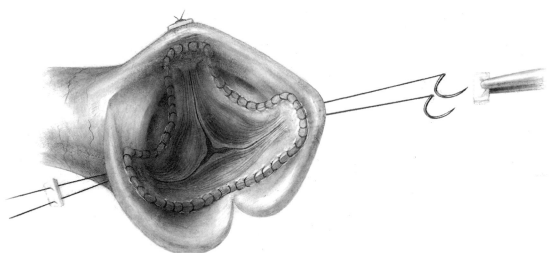

FIGURE 32.28. Supports to the native aorta. Pillars are secured to the outside pledgets.

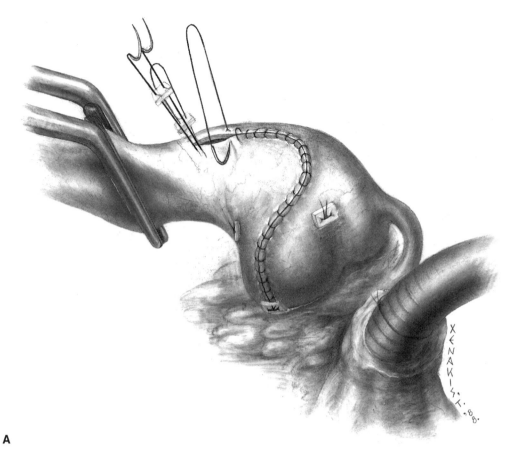

A

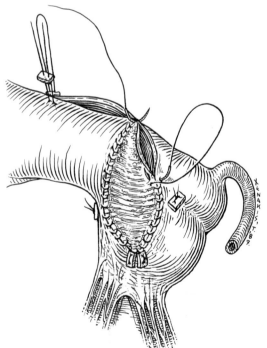

B

FIGURE 32.29. Aortotomy closure in the classic "pillars only" technique without (A) and with (B) a prosthetic patch.

Modified Scallop Technique (Minimal Scallop of Non-Coronary Sinus)

The modified scallop technique is similar to the later method of Ross,[6] as it leaves the non-coronary sinus relatively intact to buttress, or fill, the base of the aortotomy incision and allows deferral of the decision on what to do with the aortic root geometry until after the proximal suture line has been completed (Figure 32.16). To use this technique, the native aortic root must not need annulus enlargement or an augmentation aortoplasty at the level of the sinus ridge. The non-coronary sinus is only minimally "scalloped" (Figure 32.30). The usual aortotomy incision is performed but can be stopped at the top of the native commissures (the sinus ridge). The proximal suture line is the same as for all the other methods (Figure 32.31). The distal suture line is constructed in a fashion similar to that for the classic technique except the non-coronary sinus scallop is shallow (Figure 32.32). A suture is begun at the base of this scallop, run to the top of each commissural post, and tied over a pledget outside the native aorta. The spaces behind the pillars on either side of this non-coronary sinus have been obliterated with nontransmural 4-0 braided suture. The noncoronary sinus is only minimally scalloped so as to place the distal suture line of this portion of the allograft below the level of the aortotomy (Figure 32.33). Closure is accomplished with pledgetted simple technique (Figure 32.34).

Hints

Mistakes to avoid in "freehand" aortic valve replacement include stretching the commissural posts over dilated aortic sinuses and deviation of commissural post suspensions. The latter can be minimized by sighting the line of the new commissural post relative to the old commissures in native trileaflet valves. In the ideally simple implant, they are orthotopic to the native commissures. Most often, one or two allograft commissural posts are shifted parallel to the native commissural line (while being kept straight axially) so as to account for aortic root geometry and positioning of coronary ostia. If suspension of pillars is not maintained, sagging of semilunar cusps result in regurgitation; thus the tops of the allograft pillars are usually brought to a point superior to the native pillars (Figures 32.33, 32.35 and 32.36). Severe calcification that extends heavily into the anterior leaflet of the mitral valve and the trigones causes some risk for "cracking" and bleeding with a continuous proximal suture line. In these cases either an allograft should not be used or consideration is given to a pledgetted interrupted technique.

Variations in Technique

The preceding techniques are clearly derived from those described by the pioneers of allograft valve transplantation. Variations have been suggested by many authorities.

Placement of the initial three sutures can be underneath the commissural post rather than at the base of each sinus. A 120° counterclockwise rotation can be used as originally described by Barratt-Boyes.[5] We have found it easier to align the native coronary ostia to the analogous portions of the allograft coronary sinuses and allow the commissural posts to assume their necessary positions within the aortic root rather than the reverse. Doty recommended Teflon pledgets at the top of each commissural post on the inside of the aorta, whereas we prefer to place the pledgets outside in order to reduce thrombotic potential.[7,8] Ross did not recommend rotation of the allograft non-coronary within the aortic root and left the allograft non-coronary sinus, forming a backing to the aortotomy.[6] When using this method (Scallop technique), the aortotomy should be stopped above the level of this minimally scalloped sinus unless aortoplasty of the non-coronary aortic sinus is necessary. Similar to Ross, we find it easier not to rotate the allograft except in special situations, e.g. extreme left ventricular hypertrophy with a bulging septum. In this situation, it is advantageous to place the allograft with the least amount of annular bulk (i.e., aortic/mitral continuity) over the septum. Similarly, routine use of the orthotopic position lends itself to variations in annulus enlargement, as described below. Obviously, for

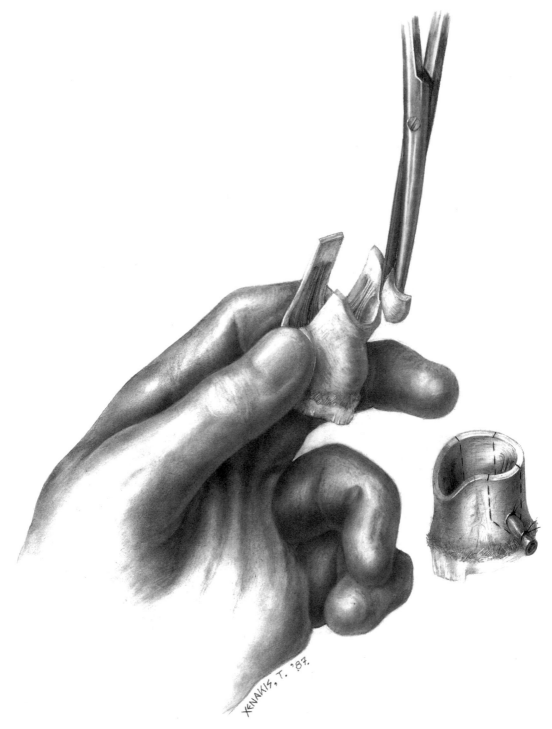

FIGURE 32.30. Sinus excision for the scallop technique.

FIGURE 32.31. Proximal suture line constructed with three continuous sutures. Note the "shallower" aortotomy stopping above the sinus ridge.

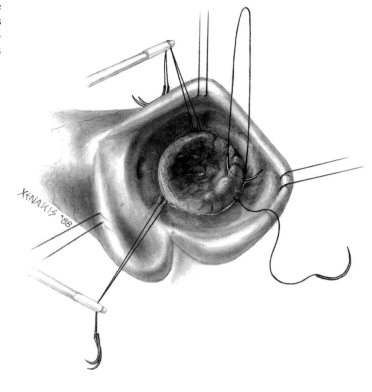

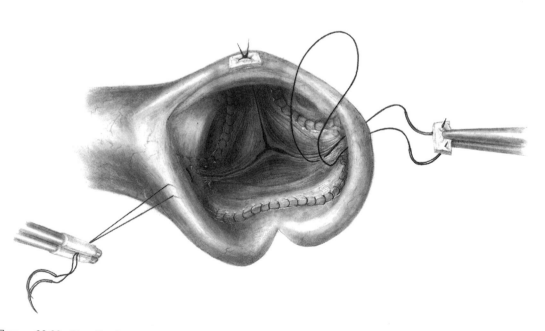

FIGURE 32.32. The distal suture line of the non-coronary sinus runs just below the aortotomy. The pillars are fixed to pledgets outside the native aorta. Additional suture to obliterate space behind allograft scallop can be placed through flange and non-coronary sinus (not shown).

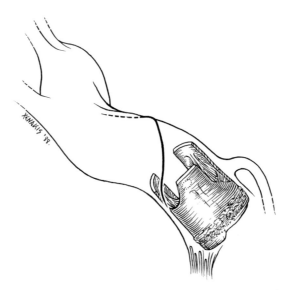

FIGURE 32.33. Position of the allograft within the aortic root, demonstrating retention of the pillar architecture.

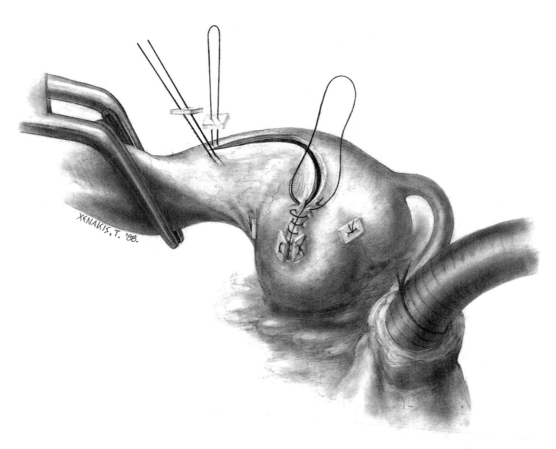

FIGURE 32.34. Aortotomy closure independent of the distal allograft suture line.

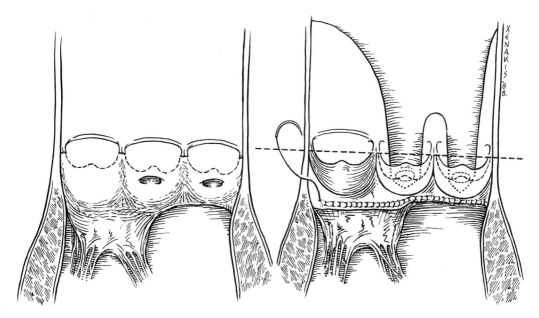

FIGURE 32.35. The dotted line is at the sinus ridge. Allograft pillars are "hitched" higher than the native pillars.

applications such as an extended aortic root replacement with Konno, as described by Clarke and associates,[9,10] rotation is mandatory. Barratt-Boyes recommended complete scalloping of all three sinuses and 120° rotation of the allograft (i.e., classic technique).[5] Minor degrees of rotation to account for cusp asymmetry and coronary ostia asymmetry are an essential part of the technique (*vida infra*).

Barratt-Boyes' aortotomy appears similar to ours with perhaps a slightly less exaggerated transverse component. He also emphasized the subannular suturing of the proximal suture line. Like Ross and Yacoub, we have found this step not to be essential except when the native coronary ostia are very close to the fibrous attachment of the semilunar cusps.[11] In these cases subannular placement of the proximal suture line is critical (*vida infra*). Also, Barratt-Boyes has emphasized *not* utilizing monofilament suture material as he believes it tends to slice through homograft tissue (personal communication). Others have used an interrupted proximal suture line technique for both aortic root replacements and freehand aortic valve replacements.[12] We recommend the continuous suture technique with the freehand aortic valve replacement for aortic insufficiency (where

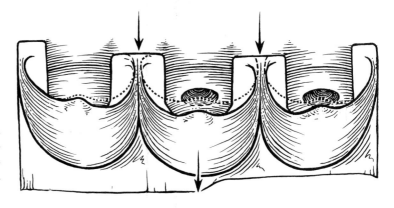

FIGURE 32.36. Sagging of the commissures when the pillar suspension is not maintained. The dotted lines indicate the optimal leaflet edge positions.

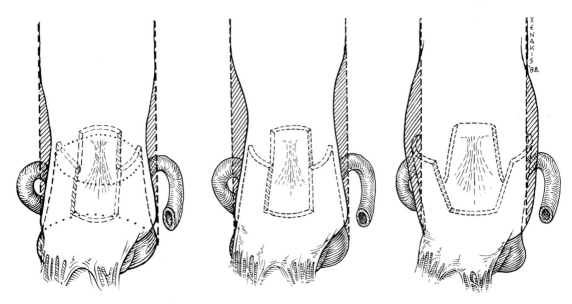

FIGURE 32.37. The sinus ridge is reconstructed at a diameter up to 20% less than the base but should never exceed the diameter of the cylinder base at the proximal suture line. If the pillars converge, or splay, the distortion can alter semilunar function, resulting in insufficiency.

aorta and annulus were dilated) because of the speed and hemostasis, but we use the interrupted technique for aortic root replacement, and for small aortic roots.

Barratt-Boyes has emphasized reduction aortic root tailoring involving excision of a wedge of aortic root to avoid splaying of the commissural post, which leads to central incompetence when transplanting allografts into dilated aortic roots.[13] Avoidance of splaying or sagging is critically important, being one of the keys to the success of the procedure (Figure 32.37).[14] Bailey has recommended a technique to avoid splaying of the sinus ridge region of the allograft by leaving this portion of the graft intact until final sutures are placed.[15] We have not used this technique as it appears cumbersome; our delaying the excision of the allograft sinuses until completion of the proximal suture line (similar to Ross) accomplishes the same important geometric goal.

References

1. Barratt-Boyes BG, Roche AH. A review of aortic valve homografts over a six and one-half year period. Ann Surg 1969;170:483–492.

2. Kunzelman KS, Grande KJ, David TE, Cochran RP, Verrier ED. Aortic root and valve relationships. Impact on surgical repair. J Thorac Cardiovasc Surg 1994;107:162–170.

3. Barratt-Boyes BG. Homograft aortic valve replacement in aortic incompetence and stenosis. Thorax 1964;19:131–150.

4. Karp RB. The use of free-hand unstented aortic valve allografts for replacement of the aortic valve. J Card Surg 1986;1:23–32.

5. Barratt-Boyes BG. A method for preparing and inserting a homograft aortic valve. Br J Surg 1965; 52:847–856.

6. Ross DN. Application of homografts in clinical surgery. J Card Surg 1987;2:175–183.

7. Doty DB. Replacement of the aortic valve with cryopreserved aortic valve allograft: considerations and techniques in children. J Card Surg 1987;2:129–136.

8. Doty DB. Aortic homograft technique. In Cardiac Surgery. Chicago: Yearbook 1986:12–15.

9. Clarke DR. Extended aortic root replacement for treatment of left ventricular outflow tract obstruction. J Card Surg 1987;2:121–128.

10. McKowen RL, Campbell DN, Woelfel GF, Wiggins JW, Clarke DR. Extended aortic root replacement with aortic allografts. J Thorac Cardiovasc Surg 1987;93:366–374.

11. Ross D, Yacoub MH. Homograft replacement of the aortic valve. A critical review. Prog Cardiovasc Dis 1969;11:275–293.

12. Moreno-Cabral CE, Miller DC, Shumway NE. A simple technique for aortic valve replacement using freehand allografts. J Card Surg 1988;3:69–76.

13. Barratt-Boyes BG, Roche AH, Subramanyan R, Pemberton JR, Whitlock RM. Long-term follow-up of patients with the antibiotic-sterilized aortic homograft valve inserted freehand in the aortic position. Circulation 1987;75:768–777.

14. Frater RW. Aortic valve insufficiency due to aortic dilatation: correction by sinus rim adjustment. Circulation 1986;74:I136–I142.

15. Bailey WW. A modified free-hand technique for homograft aortic valve replacement. J Card Surg 1987;2:193–197.

33
The Small Aortic Root: Surgical Techniques for Annulus Enlargement

Richard A. Hopkins

Indications

Usually placement of a mechanical prosthetic valve smaller than 21–23 mm is not recommended because of the risk of inducing prosthetic aortic stenosis.[1,2] Allograft aortic valves have superior hydraulic performance. Hemodynamically, a 17 mm allograft functions better than a 21 mm prosthesis. In the presence of a small aortic annulus, enlargement can be accomplished with techniques similar to that used for prosthetic valves, but the use of allograft tissue simplifies the technique. Aortic annulus enlargement can be used for absolute size increases as well as for altering the rotational geometry of the aortic root (*vida infra*). This technique can also be used for aortic valve replacement in children so that an adult-sized aortic valve can be positioned into which the child may "grow." The Appendix, which gives aortic valve diameters, is a good guide to the need for aortic annulus enlargements. If a patient of body surface area (BSA) 1.6 m² (or one who is expected to grow to that size) has a native annulus of 19 mm or less, he or she should not be left with an allograft smaller than 17 mm or risk the creation of aortic stenosis hemodynamics. As a practical matter, a BSA 2.0 m² individual, as a large adult, has a 20 to 24 mm diameter aortic valve. Thus we rarely leave a patient with a valve smaller than 19–20 mm. Conversely, except in small children, it is usually possible to place a 17 mm or larger aortic valve allograft with the techniques described below.

"Manouguian" Technique

The method described by Manouguian and Seybold-Epting for prosthetic valve placement and enlargement utilizing a pericardial patch sutured into the anterior leaflet of the native mitral valve can be adapted to a technique applicable to freehand allograft insertion.[3] The aortotomy is extended somewhat more posteriorly than usual through the region of the native commissure above the midpoint of the anterior leaflet of the mitral valve (Figure 33.1). The depth of the incision into the left atrium and mitral valve is determined by the amount of enlargement necessary but can extend for a distance of 4–8 mm. The incision into the roof of the left atrium is closed with pledgetted sutures.

The defect in the anterior leaflet of the mitral valve is filled with a shallow piece of residual anterior mitral valve leaflet left on the allograft (Figure 33.2). When a relatively deep V is created in the anterior leaflet of the mitral valve, these sutures are placed as horizontal interrupted 4-0 monofilaments until the level of the true annulus is reached (Figure 33.3). At this point, an additional suture is placed on either side, tied, and used as a running suture. A third suture is placed underneath the right coronary ostia of both the allograft and the native valves. The valve is inverted into the ventricular cavity and the proximal suture line constructed by running each suture toward the middle (Figure 33.4). Unless there is a very bulbous root, the flange technique is usually used for the distal aortic closure (Figure 33.5).

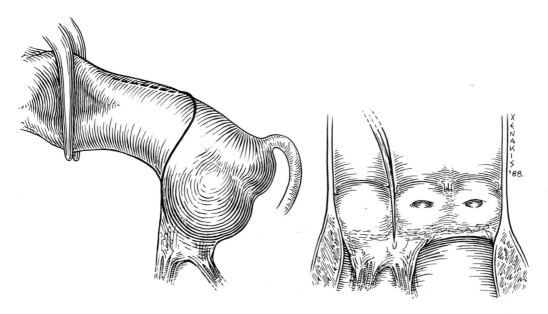

FIGURE 33.1. Aortotomy for enlargement of the annulus when using the Manouguian approach.

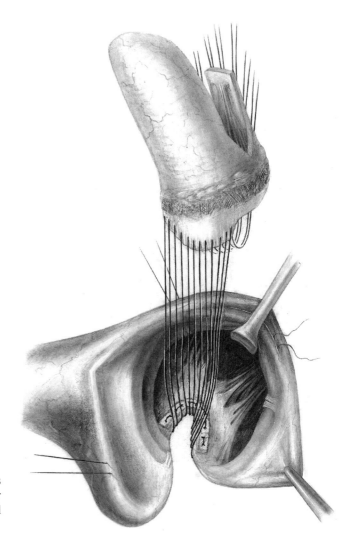

FIGURE 33.2. Enlargement of the annulus by filling the incision into the anterior leaflet of the mitral valve with mitral valve tissue of the allograft.

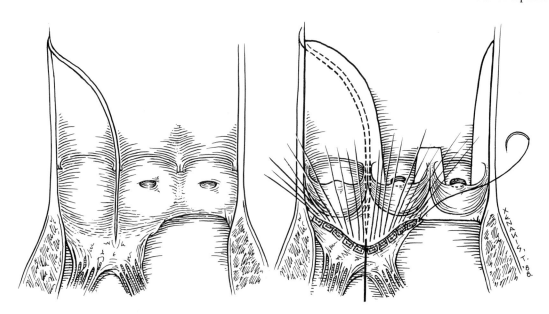

FIGURE 33.3. Pledgetted technique used for mitral to mitral valve tissue closure. Running sutures are used for the remainder of the proximal suture line.

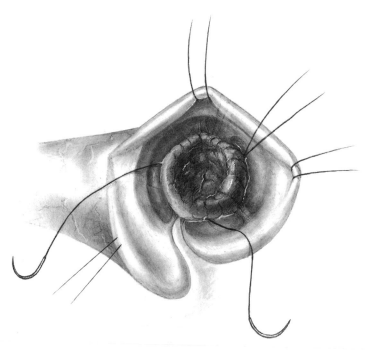

FIGURE 33.4. Proximal suture line with three running sutures. The third suture is begun at a point equidistant from the two begun near the fibrous trigones, where the mitral pledgetted sutures stop.

FIGURE 33.5. Closure after annulus enlargement usually requires augmentation aortoplasty.

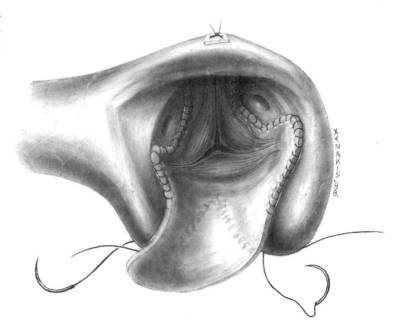

"Nicks" Technique

The method of Nicks and coworkers can be adapted for use with allografts.[4] It is an incision similar to that originally described by Barratt-Boyes.[5] The incision across the annulus is made to the right of the commissure between the left and noncoronary sinuses of the native aortic root and extended into the anterior leaflet of the mitral valve (Figure 33.6). It is posterior to the bundle of His. If only a small amount of

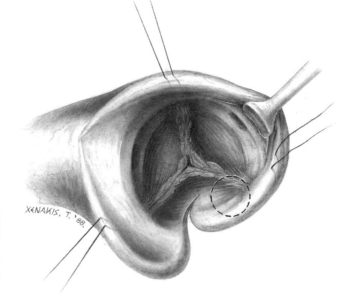

FIGURE 33.6. Enlargement of the annulus by extension of the aortotomy across the annulus anterior to the native commissure and posterior to the membranous septum. Dotted circle indicates the region of the AV node.

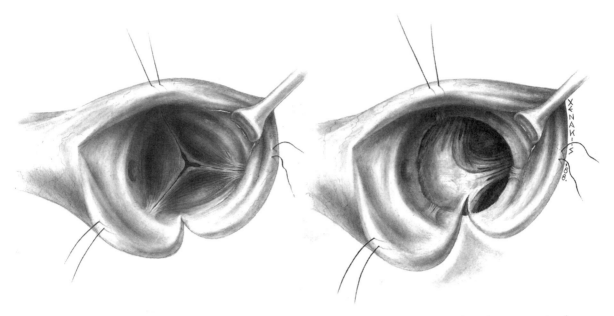

FIGURE 33.7. Incision into the annulus without entering the left atrium (on the left) and a more extensive annulus enlargement into the mitral valve behind the right fibrous trigone.

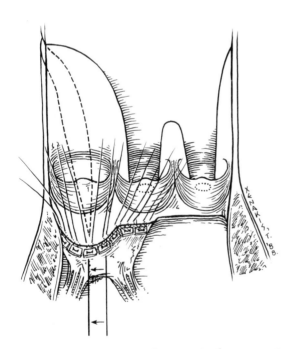

FIGURE 33.8. Annulus enlargement when a more anterior extension of the incision into the mitral valve is chosen. Care is taken to remain posterior to the AV node.

enlargement is necessary, the annulus is simply "nicked," which allows an enlargement of 1–2 mm without actually entering the left atrium (called by us as a "nicked Nicks"). If additional enlargement is necessary, the incision is continued into the anterior leaflet of the mitral valve and reconstruction is accomplished in a manner similar to the Manouguian technique, utilizing the anterior leaflet of the allograft mitral valve (Figure 33.7). In this case, interrupted sutures are place; the remnant of mitral valve tissue is somewhat asymmetric and not in the middle of the leaflet but rather slightly displaced toward the non-coronary sinus (Figure 33.8). It is usually simplest to use the flange technique for the distal suture line, but the classic method can also be used. Whichever method is chosen, care must be taken to symmetrically reestablish the non-coronary sinus.

References

1. Teoh KH, Fulop JC, Weisel RD, et al. Aortic valve replacement with a small prosthesis. Circulation 1987;76:II123–II131.

2. Kirklin JW, Barratt-Boyes BG. Cardiac Surgery, Second Edition: Volume 1. New York: Churchill Livingstone, Inc. 1993.

3. Manouguian S, Seybold-Epting W. Patch enlargement of the aortic valve ring by extending the aortic incision into the anterior mitral leaflet. J Thorac Cardiovasc Surg 1979;78:402–412.

4. Nicks R, Cartmill T, Bernstein L. Hypoplasia of the aortic root. The problem of aortic valve replacement. Thorax 1970;25:339–346.

5. Barratt-Boyes BG. A method for preparing and inserting a homograft aortic valve. Br J Surg 1965; 52:847–856.

34
Aortoplastic Techniques for Problematic Aortic Root Geometry

Richard A. Hopkins

Indications and Contraindications

One of the major reasons for failure of free-hand aortic valve implants is lack of attention to aortic root geometry and its effect on the functional anatomy of the allograft. Barratt-Boyes and associates clearly demonstrated the problem of native aortic root dilatation causing failure.[1] Aortoplastic techniques can be applied to both dilated and constricted aortic roots, and they are also applicable to the "normal" aortic root for which closure of the aortotomy would result in narrowing at the sinus ridge level. Contraindications to aortic root tailoring include connective tissue disease and grossly distorted roots with asymmetric sinuses; the latter is best treated with root replacement.

Functional Aortic Valve Anatomy

As has been reviewed by many authors, the aortic valve function depends on semilunar valvular anatomy. This design function depends on leaflet suspension to maintain apposition to the other two leaflets.[2] In an allograft, it depends on adequate suspension of the pillars to maintain the semilunar mechanism and avoidance of splaying, which causes central incompetence or convergence of the pillars, which in turn can result in sagging of the cusps (Figures 32.35, 32.36, 34.1 and 34.2). As has

been pointed out by Frater,[3] the intercommissural distance at the sinus rim level must be maintained and seen to approximate the cylindrical diameter of the fibrous skeleton of the heart forming the base of the aortic root (Figure 34.3). Tyrone David and colleagues have pointed out that the parallel anatomy of the pillars must be maintained but that the optimal sinus ridge diameter is up to 20% narrower than the aortic root diameter as originally suggested by Leonardo DaVinci as critical for creating eddy currents for accelerating closure of the coronary valve leaflets.[4] If these geometric principles are recreated with the freehand technique, the semilunar aortic valve mechanisms is preserved and valve competence is maintained. If the suspension of the semilunar valve is lost owing to incorrect placement of the pillars, sagging, or distortion, incompetence results from prolapse of a valve leaflet. Some technical adjustment to aortic root anatomy has been required in 30% of our cases.

Reduction Aortoplasty

Barratt-Boyes[5] and Ross and associates[6] have emphasized the role of aortic root reduction, or "tailoring," to reduce the size of the aortic root. One of the major reasons cited for failure in Barratt-Boyes' 1987 review was dilated aortic root. His group advised against placement of an allograft in a root larger than 30 mm in diameter, although they did recommend placement if the aortic root could be tailored to a diameter

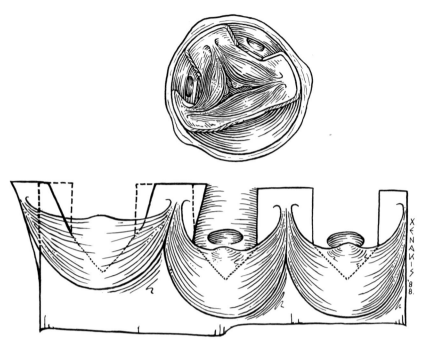

FIGURE 34.1. Effect of splaying and convergence of pillars on semilunar valve function. One of the major technical errors leading to early insufficiency is deviation of the allograft pillars off the long axis of the aortic outflow.

of 30 mm or less. We basically use his technique, as published in 1965, for reduction aortoplasty.[5]

The aortotomy is extended just into the mitral leaflet posterior to the right fibrous trigone, which is similar to the incision location of Nicks and associates.[7] Native aorta is excised, and the aortotomy is closed to "reef" the excess aortic root tissue, thereby reducing the diameter of the aortic cylinder between the aortic base and the top of the new sinus ridge (Figure 34.4).

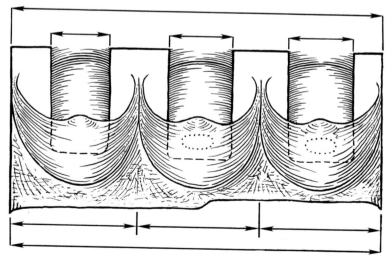

FIGURE 34.2. Relation of aortic base to sinus ridge.

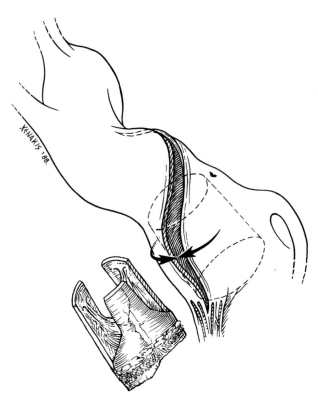

FIGURE 34.3. Closure of the aortic root following freehand aortic valve insertion must maintain the cylindrical relation of the sinus ridge, pillars and fibrous base of the aortic valve with a slight waist being created at the level of the sinus ridge.

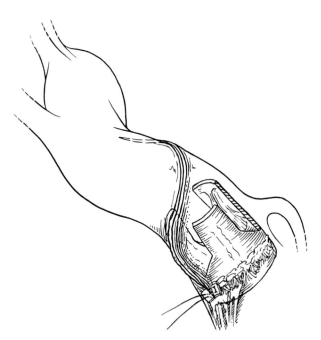

FIGURE 34.4. Reduction aortoplasty required for excess aortic tissue due to postvalvular dilatation. Extra aorta can be excised during closure.

FIGURE 34.5. Sutures are placed at the base of the aortotomy and are tied when beginning the final aortotomy closure.

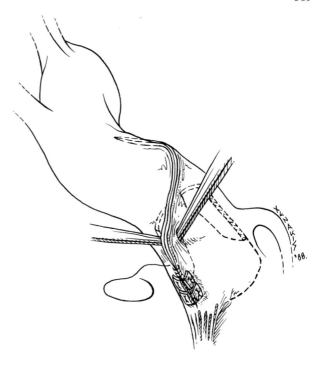

Interrupted sutures are placed at the base of this incision prior to beginning the allograft implant. This measure allows later tying of these sutures after placement of the allograft (Figure 34.5). Two to three such sutures may be required. It is important when reducing the size of the aortic root in the region of the non-coronary sinus, that compensation for pillar positioning is performed so as to avoid splaying the allograft pillars toward the reduction aortoplasty. The base of the pillars is relatively orthotopic, but the line of pillar suturing must be deviated away from the reduction aortoplasty rather than being parallel to the native commissural line. If desired, the stay sutures at the top of the pillars can be passed through the native aorta at selected points to test the orientation prior to freehand suturing of the distal suture line.

Augmentation Aortoplasty

When the postvalvular aortic root is small, the aorta can be enlarged to maintain the diameter of the proximal root and new sinus ridge after allograft implantation. With a small or deformed aortic root, it is obvious that this step must be done and can be accomplished either with Dacron of PTFE material, a separate piece of allograft, or using an aortoplastic technique that utilizes a flange of allograft left attached (preferred technique). Augmentation is always necessary in the "normal" aortic root when allografts are used for aortic valve replacement, as the aortotomy cannot be closed without displacing orthotopically positioned pillars on either side of the non-coronary sinus, as would occur, for example, during aortic valve replacement for acute bacterial endocarditis in a young patient.

The allograft is sewn with a standard proximal suture line, and the right and left coronary ostia are aligned as usual. The pillars are placed on either side of the non-coronary sinus but deviated toward the aortotomy and not parallel to native commissures. The non-coronary sinus is closed with an oval patch of Dacron or free patch of allograft aortic wall (Figure 34.6).

A perhaps easier and more aesthetically pleasing method is the flange technique, which leaves the non-coronary portion of the allograft aorta intact and uses it to enlarge the aorto-

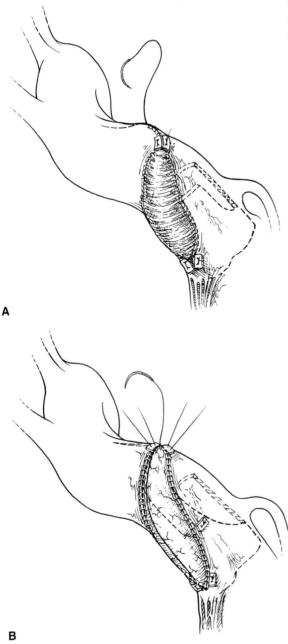

A

B

FIGURE 34.6. Aortic root geometry and the size of the non-coronary sinus are maintained using the classic technique plus augmentation for a small aortic root. Direct closure of the non-coronary sinus would have deformed and converged the pillars toward the aortotomy suture line. Use of a Dacron patch (A) and the flange aortoplasty technique (B).

tomy to the point of the transverse component (*vida supra*). When it is obvious at the time of analysis that this enlargement, or augmentation, of the non-coronary sinus is required, this portion of the allograft is not trimmed. The right and left coronary sinuses are constructed in the usual way, but the top of the pillars on either side of the non-coronary sinus are completed by suturing the running suture from the bottom of the coronary sinus to the stay sutures, which have been brought through the aortic wall and tied over by a pledget. The aortotomy is then closed by starting a pledgetted suture at the base of the aortotomy to the outside of the allograft aortic annulus. This suture is tied and each limb run superiorly along the inside of the aortotomy to the allograft flange. The suturing is completed to the point where the transverse aortotomy turns superiorly; the flange fills the proximal aortotomy (Figure 34.6). It augments the aortic root and, in addition, maintains the geometry of the allograft aortic root. It should now be clear why the original aortotomy is so important. The lower portion of the incision should cross the sinus ridge and go to the annulus parallel to the long axis, thereby providing the correct orientation for any necessary augmentation.

Augmentation Aortoplasty with Concomitant Annulus Enlargement

Aortic root augmentation aortoplasty can be combined with an annuloplasty to place a larger aortic allograft inside a small aortic root while maintaining accurate aortic root geometry. When annulus enlargement is required, an augmentation aortoplasty is usually necessary to maintain aortic root geometry. The original aortotomy is extended across the annulus toward the mitral valve.[8] It can then be extended into the mitral leaflet, as originally suggested by Nicks and Barratt-Boyes, using the more posterior incision of Manouguian. If only another 2mm of circumference is required, this incision does not need to enter the left atrium. The left atrial tissue is reflected

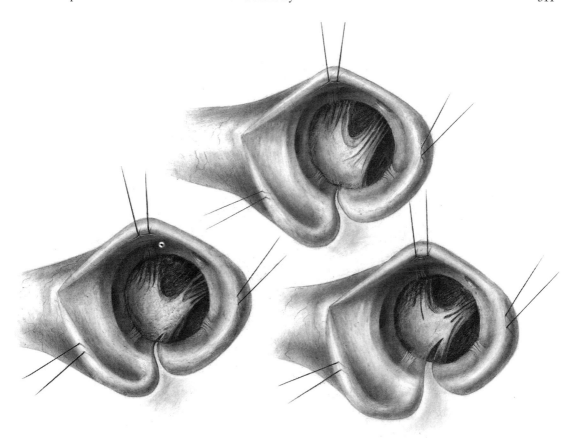

FIGURE 34.7. Extent of the incision across the annulus depends on the amount of annuloplasty required. Demonstrated are incisions into the annulus (top) and through the annulus (bottom left). The bottom right drawing represents a formal extension well into the mitral leaflet.

off the aortic-mitral region into the anterior leaflet of the mitral valve, as described above for the annuloplasty technique (Figure 34.7). The defect in the mitral valve leaflet is then filled by leaving a portion of the allograft anterior leaflet attached (Figure 34.8). The enlargement of the non-coronary sinus is continued by utilizing the flange technique of aortic root augmentation (Figure 34.9). When using this technique, the alteration in the pillar positions on either side of the right and left coronary sinuses needs to be carefully analyzed when the first three proximal sutures are placed because although the enlargement is obtained within the non-coronary sinus it is partly transferred to the coronary sinuses by parallel shifting of the pillars toward the surgeon.

Management of Complicating Coronary Anatomy

In the idealized aortic valve, the sinuses are of equal size, and the right and left coronary ostia are at 120° angles.[9] Techniques have been described as though one perfectly symmetric valve is always inserted into another symmetric annulus. However, just as the ancient concept of the idealized human fitting into a perfect circle was wrong, rarely is the human aortic valve so symmetric. The pathology of aortic insufficiency and stenosis further alters the native symmetry. These alterations in coronary ostia and sinus relations must be accounted for in the freehand aortic valve insertion surgical technique.

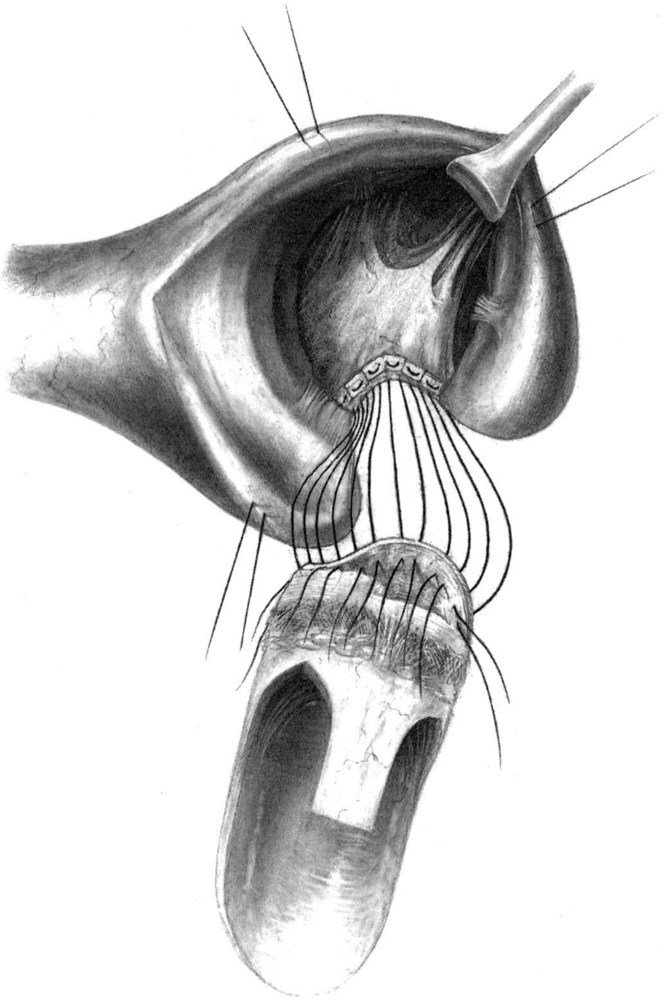

FIGURE 34.8. Annulus enlargement with an allograft mitral leaflet.

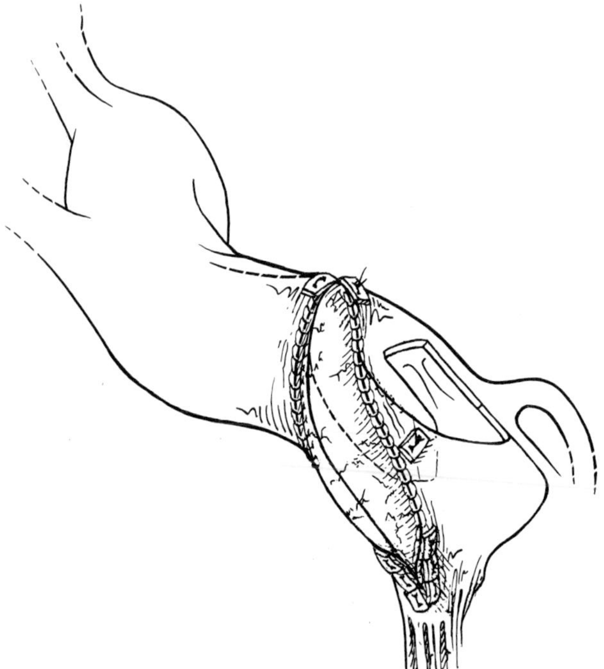

FIGURE 34.9. Enlargement of the root using the flange technique.

As was pointed out by McAlpine, the sinuses are variable in size; in general the disparity in annular circumference encompassing the various sinuses can be as great as 20–25% in "normal" valves.[8] The order of size, from large to small, is right, left, and non-coronary. In addition, asymmetric placement of the coronary ostia within the coronary sinuses increases the problem for the surgeon performing the freehand suturing. A methodical approach to placing the first three sutures allows management of these geometric problems in virtually all cases.

Asymmetric Placement of Coronary Ostia Within Native Sinuses: Mini-Rotation

A common geometry involves rotational displacement of the right coronary orifice to the right within its sinus such that the right and left coronary ostia begin to approach 180° (Figure 34.10). Occasionally, asymmetry of the allograft sinuses allows management by rotating sinuses (e.g. allograft left to recipient right). Usually placement of an allograft inside this geometry requires a slight rotation, placing the left coronary ostia closer to the pillar between the left and non-coronary sinuses such that the pillar

between the right and non-coronary sinuses is shifted away from the native coronary ostia and the extremely close native commissure. Placing the allograft in the orthotopic position and utilizing the placement of the first three sutures as the architectural guide assists in this "minirotation." The first suture is placed through the native aortic annulus at a point immediately underneath the left coronary ostia. The suture is then passed as a simple suture through the annulus of the allograft at a point counterclockwise from the bottom of the sinus, which then "sets up" the minirotation. The second suture is then placed below the native right coronary ostia and passed as a simple suture through the annulus of the allograft at a point in the right coronary sinus that allows suturing around the native coronary ostia and effects a similar minirotation of the anterior pillar to the right. The third suture for the proximal suture line is placed at a point equidistant between the first two sutures on both the allograft and the native annulus. The allograft is inverted into the ventricle and the suture lines completed in the usual manner, avoiding tilting of the allograft pillars. A somewhat similar asymmetry can occur when the right coronary sinus of the native aorta is small even without rightward displacement of the right coronary ostia but with leftward displacement of the pillar. The allograft pillar is sutured to the surgeon's side of the native pillar (Figure 34.11). The principle

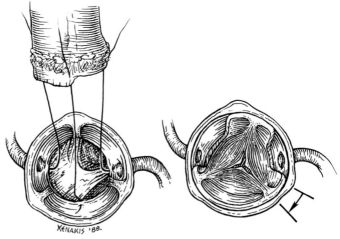

FIGURE 34.10. Placement of sutures to manage coronary ostia approaching 180° orientation. Arrow indicates the "minirotation" of the allograft within the root.

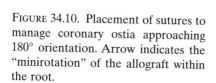

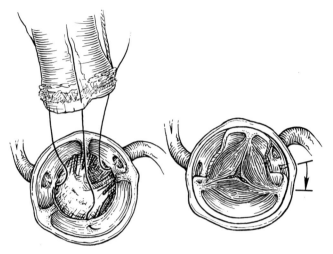

FIGURE 34.11. A small right recipient sinus requires suturing an allograft pilar to the surgeon's side of the native commissural post. The "rotation" to move the pillar is at the level of the annulus.

of aligning the new pillar parallel to the recipient commissural post is followed.

Both Coronaries Arising from a Single Sinus

A variation on the asymmetry problem occurs when both right and left coronary ostia arise from the left coronary sinus of the recipient aortic root. The native left coronary sinus is usually larger, and the problem is to place a smaller allograft valve inside the native annulus without splaying the pillars on either side of the dual coronary ostia. This problem can be solved by combining the techniques of rotation with augmentation aortoplasty. It is done by enlarging the non-coronary sinus with an augmentation aortoplasty (*vida supra*), which enlarges the total aortic root and allows a larger allograft to be inserted (Figure 34.12).

The largest sinus (or the left sinus when they are relatively equal) of the allograft valve is then selected to match the native left coronary sinus and the three guide sutures are placed. The first suture is placed at the bottom of the native left coronary sinus to the bottom of the allograft sinus. The other two sutures are then placed at 120° angles from the first and the pillars allowed to rotate to their imperative positions. The augmentation aortoplasty can be done either with prosthetic material or an allograft (flange technique).

Bicuspid Aortic Valve with 180° Coronary Ostia

In a situation where the coronary ostia are at 180° angles from each other in the native aortic root, simple orthotopic placement of a trileaflet valve would be defeated. Once again, if the allograft aortic valve is clearly the optimal choice for the patient, it can be managed with enlargement of the non-coronary sinus region of the native aortic root with or without an annuloplasty. Most often, an annuloplasty is also required that rotates the native coronary

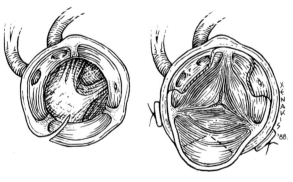

FIGURE 34.12. Large native left coronary sinus with origins of both coronary ostia. Note the small coronary artery arising from the right sinus. A large allograft is placed to accommodate the large left sinus using the combined technique of annulus enlargement plus augmentation aortoplasty.

FIGURE 34.13. Management of a bicuspid aortic valve with 180° coronary ostia by combining the techniques of annulus enlargement with aortoplasty to rotate the right coronary ostium to the left while maintaining aortic root geometry.

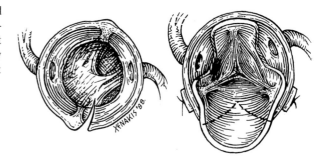

ostia toward each other (Figure 34.13). When the aortic root is significantly dilated, this technique can be combined with an incision between the right and left coronary ostia on the left side of the aorta, which is then sutured with a pledgetted technique (Figure 34.14). This measure further rotates the coronary ostia toward each other and, with the enlargement of the aortic root on the non-coronary side, allows displacement of the 180° coronary ostia into the right and left coronary sinuses of the allograft. The pillar borders hug the non-coronary side of each ostia. An alternate solution is aortic root replacement with suturing of the coronary buttons to the right and left coronary sinuses.

Coronary Ostia Arising Low in the Sinuses

When the native coronary ostia are low in their sinuses and are close to the leaflet attachment, placement of the proximal suture line must be more in the subleaflet position, as originally described by Barratt-Boyes.[5,10] If the proximal

suture line is displaced 2–3mm below the leaflet attachment, there is ample room for the proximal suture line to "roll" the allograft aortic wall below the coronary ostia of the recipient aorta (Figures 34.14 and 34.15).

Coronary Ostia Arising High in the Sinuses

In the case of the coronary ostia arising high in the sinuses, the problem for the surgeons is simplified. Resection of the allograft coronary sinus can be minimized, and the proximal suture line placed conveniently at the bottom of the sinus at the level of the native leaflet attachment (Figure 34.16). The distal suture line is comfortably created around the coronary orifice. Note that the proximal suture line does not follow the semilunar cusp attachment superiorly but, rather, crosses the base of the pyramid of the commissural pillars. The "annulus" of the aortic valve is not a true circular fibrous ring like an atrioventricular (AV) valve annulus.

FIGURE 34.14. Counterincision in the aortic root, posterior to the commissural region between the right and left coronaries. This incision does *not* extend to the annulus but takes advantage of post-stenotic dilatation of the aortic root to "pull" the coronary ostia toward each other.

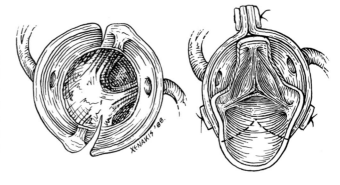

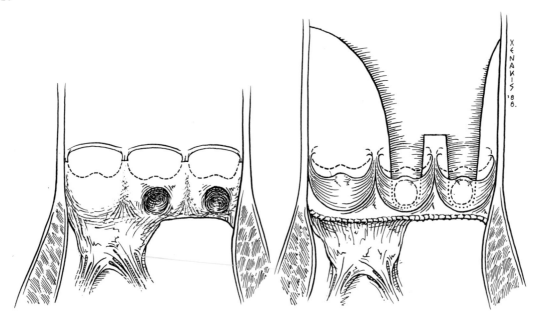

FIGURE 34.15. The proximal suture line is place underneath the origin of the native leaflets in a "subannular" position to maintain a subcoronary distal suture line.

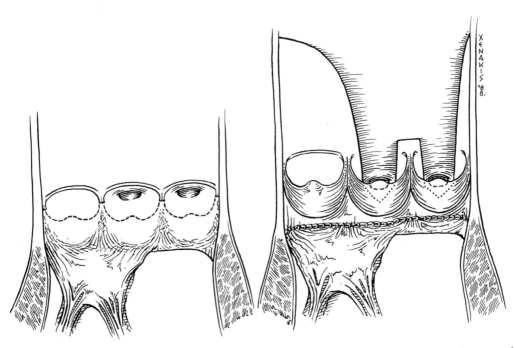

FIGURE 34.16. The proximal suture line is at the level of the base of the native leaflet attachments when coronary ostia are relatively high in their sinuses.

References

1. Barratt-Boyes BG, Roche AH, Subramanyan R, Pemberton JR, Whitlock RM. Long-term follow-up of patients with the antibiotic-sterilized aortic homograft valve inserted freehand in the aortic position. Circulation 1987;75:768–777.

2. McAlpine WA. Heart and Coronary Arteries. New York: Springer-Verlag 1975.

3. Frater RW. Aortic valve insufficiency due to aortic dilatation: correction by sinus rim adjustment. Circulation 1986;74:I136–I142.

4. David TE, Feindel CM, Bos J, Sun Z, Scully HE, Rakowski H. Aortic valve replacement with a stentless porcine aortic valve. A six year experience. J Thorac Cardiovasc Surg 1994;108:1030–1036.

5. Barratt-Boyes BG. A method for preparing and inserting a homograft aortic valve. Br J Surg 1965;52:847–856.

6. Virdi IS, Monroe JL, Ross JK. Eleven-year experience of aortic valve replacement with antibiotic sterilized aortic homograft valves in Southampton. J Thorac Cardiovasc Surg 1986;34:277–282.

7. Nicks R, Cartmill T, Bernstein L. Hypoplasia of the aortic root. The problem of aortic valve replacement. Thorax 1970;25:339–346.

8. McAlpine WA. Heart and Coronary Arteries. New York: Springer-Verlag 1975.

9. Doty DB. Aortic homograft technique. In Cardiac Surgery. Chicago: Yearbook 1986:12–15.

10. Barratt-Boyes BG. Homograft aortic valve replacement in aortic incompetence and stenosis. Thorax 1964;19:131–150.

35
Aortic Root Replacement with Aortic Allograft Conduit

Richard A. Hopkins

In certain left ventricular outflow tract reconstructions, one encounters abnormalities extending beyond that of the native valvular leaflets or severe distortion of the aortic root, which are best treated with total aortic root replacement. The solution for this spectrum of difficulties was introduced by Ross, Yacoub, and colleagues.[1–3] Aortic root replacement is indicated for reconstruction of the left ventricular outflow tract in which diffuse hypoplasia coexists with the valvular abnormality or in children, where it is desirable to place an adult-sized aortic outflow tract into which the child may grow. Aortic root replacements involve moving the coronary ostia on buttons. Complex coronary anatomy can also be managed by aortic root replacement.

In many ways, an aortic root replacement with reimplantation of the coronary ostia is a simpler technique than the freehand aortic valve replacement. Nevertheless, we do not recommend it as the routine allograft replacement technique. There are some concerns about later re-replacement in such a setting, although such operations have been reported without difficulty by groups in New Zealand, London, and other centers.[4] Aortic root replacement is indicated for bacterial endocarditis in which loss of aortic continuity with the heart offers a technical challenge. The aortic allograft is a superb prosthetic choice in this setting. Aortic root replacement is also useful in patients with greatly deformed aortic roots in which severe aortic stenosis coexists with asymmetric bulbar dilatations of the aortic sinuses, causing horrendous difficulties in the freehand technique.

In the latter anatomic situation, a mechanical prosthesis or xenograft should be placed or an aortic root replacement utilized. We have found that when an aortic root replacement is used for hypoplastic aortic stenosis complex, a myomectomy is almost always required.

Indications

Aortic root replacement may be indicated for: (1) complex multilevel aortic stenosis (valvular, subvalvular, supravalvular) in which the subvalvular component is moderate or can be relieved with an accompanying myomectomy—there is always a relatively hypoplastic annulus; (2) aortic valvular stenosis with hypoplastic annulus; (3) aortic valve stenosis—the "solution" for severely distorted valvular anatomy for which freehand allograft valve replacement cannot be done but in a patient in whom it is preferred that an allograft be positioned;[5] (4) aortic root replacement in children, allowing an adult-sized valve to be placed into which the child can grow (e.g. tunnel aortic stenosis, subacute bacterial endocarditis); (5) a possible solution for aortic insufficiency with proximal aortic root dilatation in which distortion makes simple reduction aortoplasty accompanying a freehand aortic valve replacement difficult (in the absence of Marfan's syndrome or other connective tissue disorders); (6) possible solution for complex coronary anatomy such as 180° coronary ostia in bicuspid aortic stenosis; and (7) bacterial endocarditis with destruction of aortic-ventricular continuity.

Although connective tissue disorders such as Marfan's syndrome have been listed as contraindications for the use of allografts for free-hand aortic valve replacement, allografts have been used for aortic root replacement with suture-line reinforcement using Teflon felt or Dacron graft material to prevent later distortion.[6] It remains to be seen whether splinting an allograft in such disorders prevents the later development of aortic insufficiency, as was seen in the early experience of Barratt-Boyes and associates.[5,7]

Sizing

Aortic root replacement solves some of the problems inherent in a hypoplastic left ventricular outflow tract. Excision of the aortic root down to the fibrous skeleton and onto the septum allows "expansion" of the ventricular outflow orifice. A myomectomy, as in the Morrow operation for idiopathic hypertrophic subaortic stenosis (IHSS), can be added to further enlarge the left ventricular outflow in the presence of a markedly hypertrophied septum.[8] Once excision of the native aorta has been accomplished, the outflow tract can be sized with Hegar dilators and the same-sized internal diameter allograft chosen. It can be "upsized" for children in whom it is desirable to place an adult-sized allograft. For example, if the outflow tract measures 20 mm, a 20 mm (ID) allograft is selected. In children over 15 kg it is usually possible to place an 18 mm or larger allograft. If further enlargement is necessary, a Manouguian-type maneuver can be performed onto the anterior leaflet of the patient's mitral valve, which allows further enlargement of 2–4 mm. If additional enlargement of the subvalvular outflow trach is necessary, an aortoventriculoplasty must be performed (see next section).

Preparation and Choice of Allograft

We perform aortic root replacement with an aortic allograft, although a pulmonary allograft would not offer technical problems. The valve is thawed in the usual way, and the aortic conduit is left long, to the point of the allograft innominate artery takeoff, where it is transected. The muscle is trimmed and the anterior leaflet of the mitral valve excised 3 mm below the annulus, unless a portion of it is necessary for a Manouguian maneuver.

Surgical Technique for Standard Aortic Root Replacement

As Ross originally devised, we use an interrupted proximal suture line technique.[4,5] The aortic root is excised and the native coronary ostia left on large buttons of aortic tissue (Figures 35.1, 35.2, and 35.3). An additional septal myomectomy is performed if necessary (Figure 35.4). The allograft is then oriented in the orthotopic position, with the left coronary ostia comfortably positioned toward the button of the native left coronary ostia. The proximal suture line is constructed of a series of interrupted 4-0 Tycron sutures on a half-circle taper-point needle, placed 1.0–1.5 mm apart as simple sutures (Figure 35.5). The allograft is sutured to the fibrous skeleton of the heart at the hinge point of the anterior leaflet of the native mitral valve, and the suture line is brought medially over the top of the membranous septum. A remnant of recipient aortic root is usually left counterclockwise from this region so as to avoid any encroachment in the region of the AV node, but then the dissection is brought down to the septum. The simple sutures are continued throughout the circumflex and placed in individual rubber-shod clamps. A narrow strip of Teflon felt is then inserted through the middle of the simple sutures so that as they are tied down the Teflon felt is positioned as a caulking gusset outside the allograft cardiac anastomosis (Figure 35.6). The sutures are sequentially tied. Fibrin glue can be used for additional hemostasis.

Now it is easy to see where the coronary buttons need to positioned on the allograft. The are brought to the region of the allograft coronary ostia, which are excised (Figure 35.7). These excision buttonholes should be enlarged

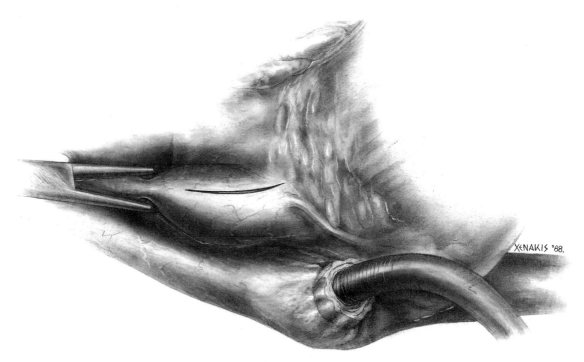

FIGURE 35.1 The initial incision of aortic root replacement is vertical and deviated to the left of the right coronary ostia.

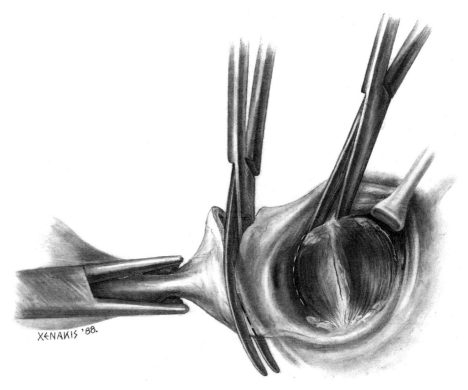

FIGURE 35.2 The aorta is divided, avoiding leaving too long an aortic remnant, to allow some "suspension" of the aortic root transplant.

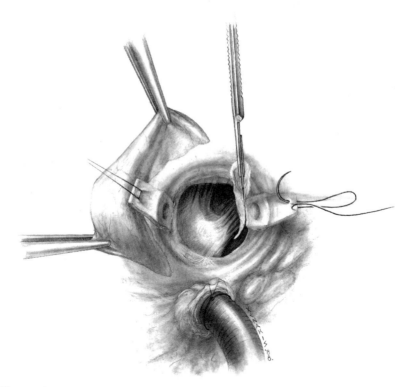

FIGURE 35.3 The aortic root is excised, leaving elliptical large coronary buttons. The fibrous skeleton is excised over the septum up to, but not into, the left fibrous trigone. The area of the conduction system is not violated. Once the fibrous base is partially excised, the left ventricular outflow orifice expands.

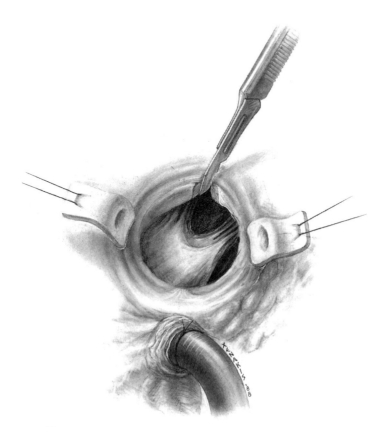

FIGURE 35.4 A hypertrophied septum can be incised or a myotomy performed to further enlarge the outflow tract. The rest of the septum is not incised.

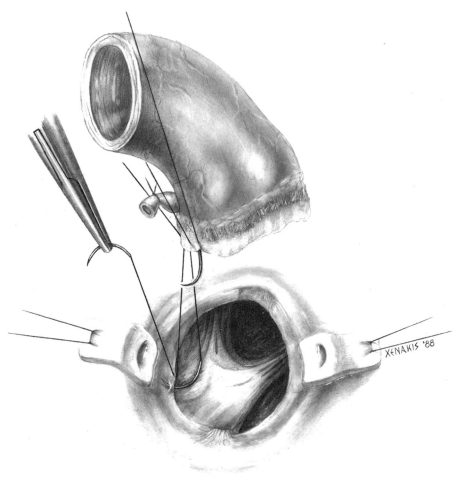

FIGURE 35.5 Proximal suture line constructed of many simple interrupted braided sutures. Each is placed as in individual rubber-shod clamp.

superiorly so that the tendency is to slightly "stretch" the native coronary ostia up to the orifices to avoid kinking. The patient's buttons are made large to protect the ostia. The stretching to a higher position within the sinus is particularly important when shifting the position of the native coronary ostia in a rotational direction (i.e., moving a bicuspid 180° right coronary ostia slightly to the left into the allograft right coronary sinus). This trick was learned during arterial switch operations for transposition and is also applicable in this setting to avoid coronary kinking. The coronary buttons are sewn to their respective orifices in the allograft utilizing the running 5-0 polypropylene suture technique.

The distal aortic suture line is constructed after checking the length of the allograft. It should usually be cut longer than first appears with a slight anterior posterior bevel (Figure 35.8). The suture line is accomplished with a running 4-0 polypropylene suture technique utilizing a Teflon felt strip buttress. De-airing maneuvers are performed, and the aortic cross-clamp is removed.

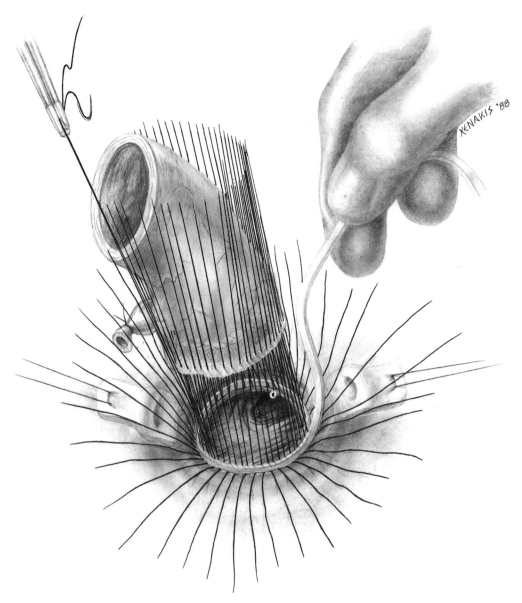

FIGURE 35.6 Usually around 40 interrupted sutures are placed and then tied over a strip of Teflon felt, which is placed within the circle of sutures *after* seating the allograft, so that it lies external to the tissue closure.

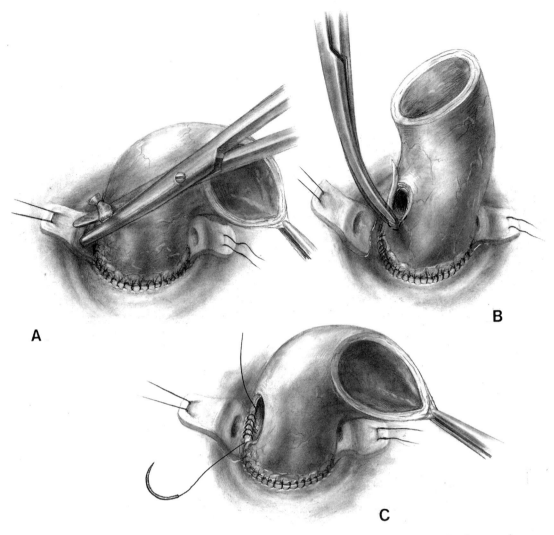

FIGURE 35.7 Preparation and suturing of the coronary buttons. Stay sutures on the buttons improve exposure for the preceding steps as well as the manipulations at this stage.

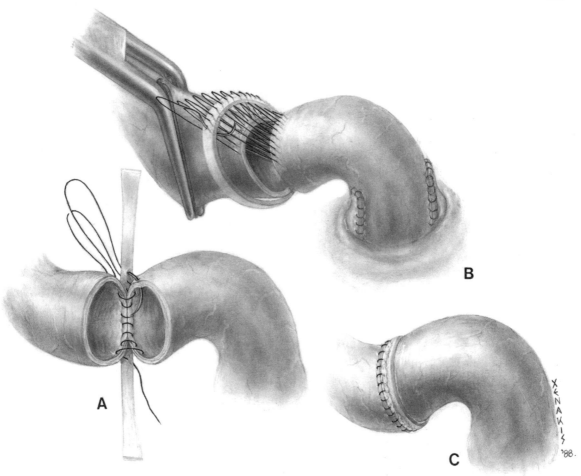

FIGURE 35.8 Distal suture line of an allograft aortic root replacement. Note the Teflon felt strip positioned on the allograft side.

Hints

Helpful hints include very high cannulation of the aorta or the use of femoral artery cannulation in adults. In addition, the native aorta should be fully mobilized. Left ventricular venting is always used.

Continuous suture lines have been advocated by some, but we find that the interrupted technique provides better visibility and allows placement of a larger aortic root on top of a smaller heart by spreading the dissimilarity over the entire circumference of the root. Similar reasoning has been advocated by Ross.

We recommend a soft-braided suture rather than monofilament for the interrupted proximal suture line to reduce the risk of cutting through the allograft tissues. Horizontal pledgetted mattress sutures utilized for standard prosthetic valve replacements are discouraged in this setting because the tendency is to narrow the circumference of the native left ventricular outflow orifice. Such narrowing is not a problem in the presence of aortic insufficiency in a large outflow tract for which aortic root replacement has been chosen; but in the usual situation, in which the surgery is done because of a hypoplastic left ventricular outflow tract, this technique is less desirable.

If a pledgetted horizontal mattress suture technique is utilized, pledgets should be placed on both sides of the suture line to prevent narrowing when tying each knot. A variation of this technique has been recommended by the

Polish group utilizing Teflon felt strips to stabilize the aortic root in patients with Marfan's syndrome in order to avoid later dilatation of the base of the aorta.[6]

References

1. Somerville J, Ross D. Homograft replacement of aortic root with reimplantation of coronary arteries. Results after one to five years. British Heart Journal 1982;47:473–482.

2. Gula G, Ahmed M, Thompson R, et al. Combined homograft replacement of the aortic valve and aortic root with reimplantation of the coronary arteries. Circulation 1976;53/54(suppl):II150.

3. Thompson R, Knight E, Ahmed M, Somerville W, Towers M, Yacoub M. The use of "fresh: unstented homograft valves for replacement of the aortic valve: analysis of 6½ years experience. Circulation 1977;56:837–841.

4. Ross DN. Application of homografts in clinical surgery. J Card Surg 1987;2:175–183.

5. Okita Y, Franciosi G, Matsuki O, Robles A, Ross DN. Early and late results of aortic root replacement with antibiotic-sterilized aortic homograft. J Thorac Cardiovasc Surg 1988;95:696–704.

6. Dziakowiak A, Pfitzner R, Andres J, et al. Modified techniques for subcoronary insertion of allografts. In Yankah AC, Hertzer R, Miller DC, et al. (eds). Cardiac Valve Allografts 1962–1987. New York: Springer-Verlag 1988:141–147.

7. Barratt-Boyes BG, Roche AH, Subramanyan R, Pemberton JR, Whitlock RM. Long-term follow-up of patients with the antibiotic-sterilized aortic homograft valve inserted freehand in the aortic position. Circulation 1987;75:768–777.

8. Tamura K, Jones M, Yamada I, Ferrans VJ. A comparison of failure modes of glutaraldehyde-treated versus antibiotic-preserved mitral valve allografts implantedin sheep. J Thorac Cardiovasc Surg 1995;110:224–238.

36
Aortoventriculoplasty with Aortic Allograft

Richard A. Hopkins

Indications

In some hearts the entire left ventricular outflow tract is hypoplastic, involving subvalvular, valvular, and even supravalvular stenosis. These patients have various degrees of tunnel aortic stenosis and are typically managed with multiple operations. The final operation usually involves a Konno-type annulus enlargement. Clarke and colleagues have described the extended aortic root replacement for such situations, and we have found it most satisfactory. It combines the concept of the aortoventriculoplasty as described by Konno, Rastan, and their associates with the aortic root replacement of Ross.[1-6] This procedure is indicated for tunnel aortic stenosis where the annulus is hypoplastic and extensive fibromuscular obstruction involves the subvalvular region. Coexisting supravalvular stenosis may also be excised and replaced with allograft aorta using this technique. Isolated subvalvular aortic stenosis is managed by traditional resection. If complex and extensive subvalvular stenosis is present yet the aortic annulus and valve leaflets are normal, the modified subvalvular operation, as described by Kirklin and Barratt-Boyes, is applicable.[7] If the obstruction involves only a hypoplastic annulus with or without sinus/leaflet abnormalities, treatment is with either simple aortic root replacement or aortic valve replacement, with annulus enlargement and augmentation aortoplasty as necessary (*vida supra*).

Indications for surgical correction of multi-level aortic stenosis are traditional and are performed for onset of symptoms or for gradients exceeding 50–75 torr. Small children may undergo temporizing procedures with subvalvular resections, valvuloplasty, and so on to reduce gradients until body size has increased such that an adult-sized outflow tract can be constructed (15–20 kg or more).

Surgical Techniques

The heart is cannulated for cardiopulmonary bypass utilizing ascending aortic cannulation relatively high near the innominate artery and dual vena caval cannulas. Prior to aortic cross-clamping, the aorta and pulmonary artery are fully mobilized. There are usually adhesions from previous operations. After induction of cardioplegic arrest, a vertical aortotomy is performed, begun anteriorly and directed slightly to the left of the right coronary ostia (Figure 36.1).

The aortotomy is retracted with two stay sutures, and the valve and subvalvular region are examined. If the valve annulus is more than two standard deviations smaller than is normal for that age, it is necessary to enlarge it to an adult size. If the subvalvular obstruction cannot be reasonably handled with a conservative resection, extended aortic root replacement (aortic root–Konno procedure) is performed. The incision in the aorta is extended into the annulus at the point between the left and right

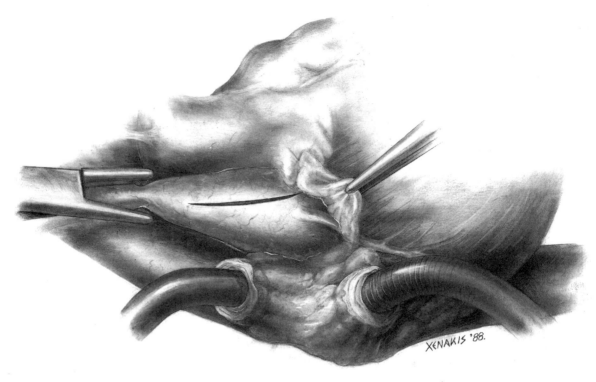

FIGURE 36.1. Aortotomy for aortic root–Konno reconstruction.

coronary ostia, where the commissure is or normally would be. An oblique incision is then made in the right ventricular outflow tract meeting the aortotomy. It is angled toward the apex to avoid the base of the pulmonary valve. These incisions combine to open the top of the septum to view. The septum, which by definition is thick, is incised vertically toward the apex, and the incision is extended until the left ventricular outflow tract is widely open (Figure 36.2).

The coronary ostia are excised on large buttons and the aorta transected at or above (if narrowed) the level of the sinus ridge. The remainder of the proximal aortic root is excised, however, leaving the fibrous aortic tissue intact just above the membranous septum and not violating the aortic mitral continuity (Figure 36.3). The incision into the septum allows enlargement to the desired size, which is accomplished with Hegar dilators. The goal is to place, at the minimum, a 19mm human aortic allograft, which means that a size 21 Hegar should fit generously into the opened left ventricular outflow tract.

The prepared allograft has been trimmed at its base, but coronary windows are not excised at this point. Pledgetted 4-0 monofilament sutures are placed with the pledgets on the ventricular side of the septal incision and passed as horizontal mattress sutures through the anterior leaflet of the mitral valve, the entirety of which is used to fill the septal defect. These sutures are sequentially placed until the level of the "true" annulus is reached (Figure 36.4).

At this point the suture technique is changed to 3-0 braided interrupted sutures in the manner of the aortic root replacement, as described by Ross. They are placed 1–2mm apart, circumferentially through the annulus of the allograft and recipient. They are not placed as horizontal mattress sutures but, rather, as simple sutures (Figure 36.5). Particular care is taken at the transition from the septal horizontal mattress sutures to the interrupted simple sutures at the left side of the septal incision so as to ensure excellent hemostasis (Figure 36.6). Two additional horizontal mattress sutures are placed with the pledget on the right side of the ventricular septotomy and then through the

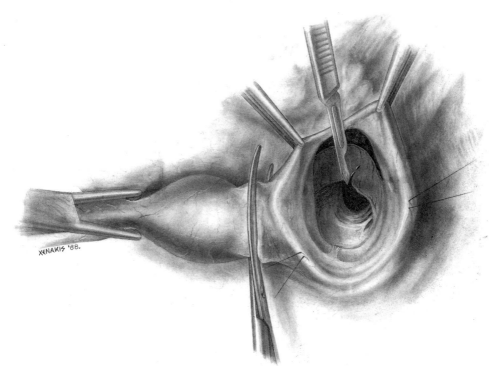

FIGURE 36.2. The incision in the aorta is extended across the annulus to the left of the right coronary ostia and then aimed apically down the free right ventricular wall away from the pulmonary valve. The septum is then incised and excised to open the left ventricular outflow tract.

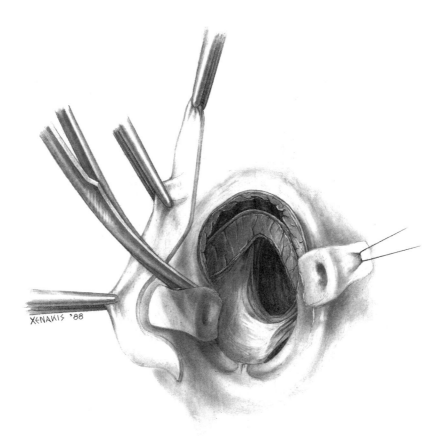

FIGURE 36.3. The aortic root is excised, leaving coronary buttons.

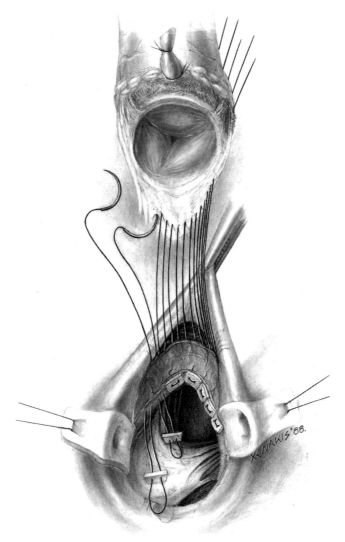

FIGURE 36.4. The septal defect is filled with the entire anterior leaflet of the mitral valve, fixed with pledgetted horizontal mattress sutures of 4-0 polypropylene monofilament.

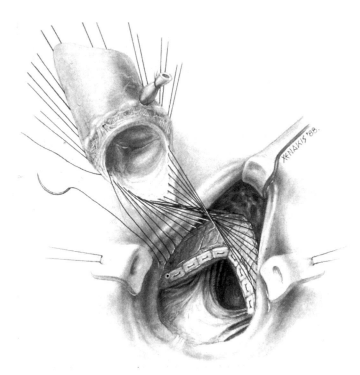

FIGURE 36.5. Once the "annulus" is reached with the monofilament mattress sutures, the interrupted braided sutures are used as for simple root replacement.

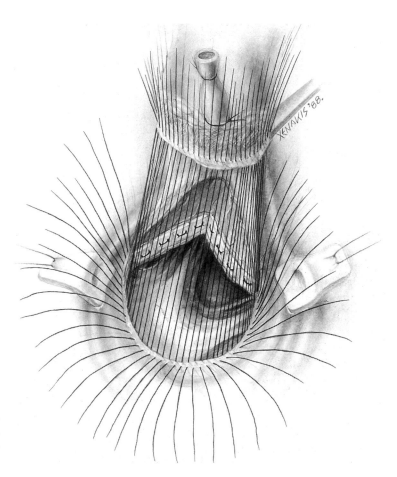

FIGURE 36.6. Usually about 30–40 interrupted braided sutures are required for the proximal suture line.

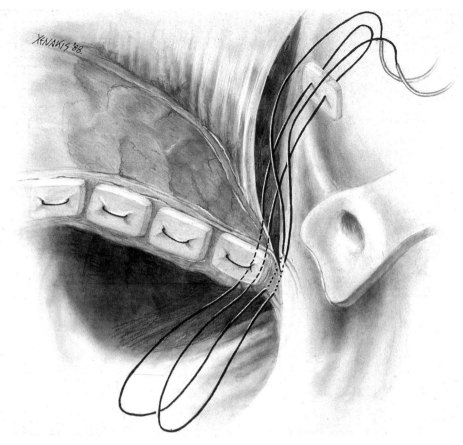

FIGURE 36.7. Additional sutures placed at both triangulation points are tied and then later used for the right ventriculotomy pericardial patch.

allograft; they are later passed through the pericardial patch closure of the right ventriculotomy and tied, which secures the triangulation points of the closure (Figure 36.7). All sutures are then sequentially tied, thereby positioning the allograft over the left ventricular outflow. The septal sutures are tied first (Figure 36.8).

Clarke recommended a running polypropylene suture technique and a double suture technique on the septal portion of the repair.[1] We have not found that necessary and prefer the interrupted technique with multiple pledgetted sutures on the ventricular septum. The allograft mitral leaflet is sutured to the right side of the septum so that the "depth" of the septum contributes to enlargement of the left ventricular outflow tract.

The coronary sinuses are then excised from the allograft to accept the large buttons of the native coronary ostia. The allograft right coronary stump is suture-ligated, as it has been rotated 120° into the non-coronary sinus region. The coronary buttons are made large and usually slightly higher than would be anatomic in order to maintain length and stretch to avoid kinking. The buttons are sutured to the oval defects with running 5-0 monofilament sutures (Figures 36.9 and 36.10).

The left ventricular vent is shut off and the left ventricle gradually allowed to fill while the distal aortic suture line is constructed with running 4-0 monofilament suture. This suture line is buttressed with a strip of felt (Figure 36.11). Because the native curve of the allograft

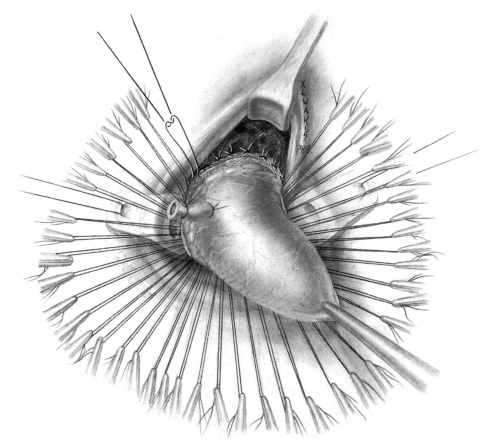

FIGURE 36.8. After seating the allograft, the sutures are sequentially tied, beginning with the mattressed septal sutures. The simple interrupted sutures are buttressed with a strip of Teflon felt.

is in a direction reversed from normal, the distal allograft aorta is usually beveled posteriorly. It is also helpful to keep the allograft ascending aortic root relatively short, but of course the incision needs to be above the sinus ridge (Figure 36.12). Native supravalvular ascending aortic pathology must be excised.

The reconstruction is completed after de-airing the aortic root and removing the aortic cross-clamp. As in the Konno operation, the right ventricular free wall defect is repaired with a patch (Figure 36.13). Clarke recommended a piece of homograft. We have tended to use pericardium for this patch, suturing it to the defect with a running 4-0 or 5-0 polypropylene suture. The suturing along the annulus of the allograft is, of course, nontrans-

mural, and these sutures need to be carefully placed.

Postoperative Management

Postoperative care is similar to that for any aortic valve replacement. Anticoagulation, if not necessary for other reasons, is limited to daily aspirin (81 mg). The patient is followed, especially looking for murmurs indicating insufficiency. Echocardiography with Doppler is performed prior to discharge for a baseline reading; it is repeated every 6 months for 1 year and then done yearly. Routine prophylaxis for subacute bacterial endocarditis is recommended for all indications, as noted in the

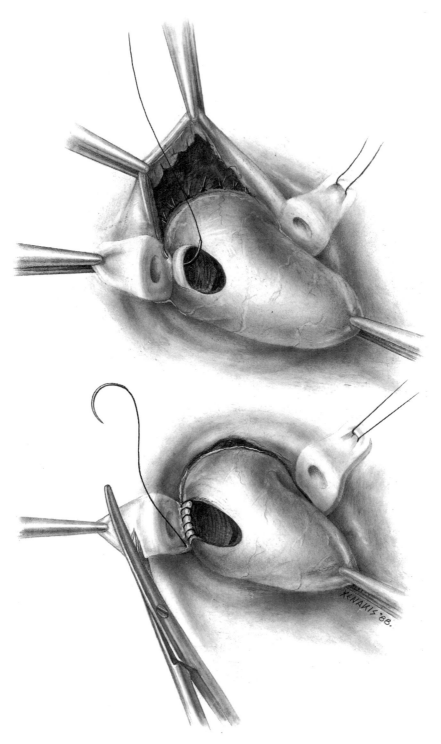

FIGURE 36.9. Coronary "buttons" sutured with 5-0 polypropylene.

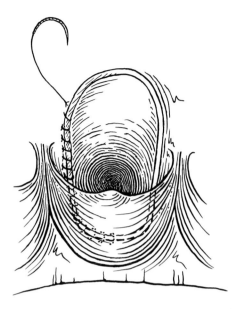

FIGURE 36.10. Large coronary buttons sutured within their new sinuses.

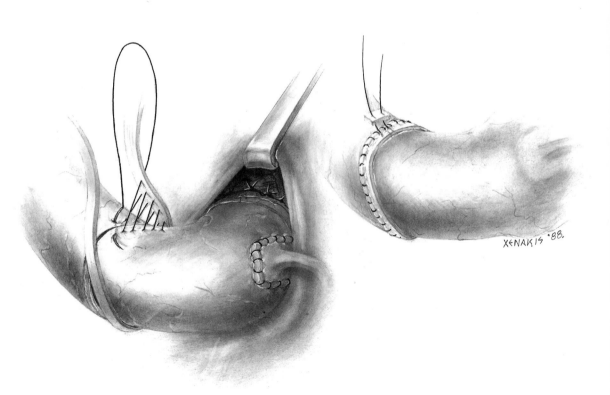

FIGURE 36.11. Distal suture line buttressed with a Teflon felt strip.

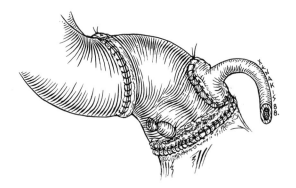

FIGURE 36.12. A beveled distal suture line is used to increase the anastomosis size and smooth the curvature of the new aortic root.

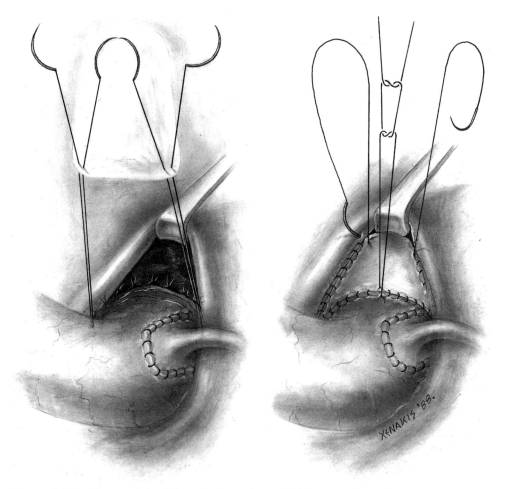

FIGURE 36.13. Closure of the right ventricular free wall defect completes the reconstruction.

prosthetic heart valve guidelines of the American Heart Association.

References

1. Clarke DR. Extended aortic root replacement for treatment of left ventricular outflow tract obstruction. J Card Surg 1987;2:121–128.
2. McKowen RL, Campbell DN, Woelfel GF, Wiggins JW, Clarke DR. Extended aortic root replacement with aortic allografts. J Thorac Cardiovasc Surg 1987;93:366–374.
3. Konno S, Iai I, Iida Yea. A new method for prosthetic valve replacement in congenital aortic stenosis associated with hypoplasia of the aortic valve ring. J Thorac Cardiovasc Surg 1976;70:909–917.
4. Rastan H, Koncz J. Aortoventriculoplasty: a new technique for the treatment of left ventricular outflow tract obstruction. J Thorac Cardiovasc Surg 1976;71:920–927.
5. Rastan H, Abu Aishah N, Rastan D, et al. Results of aortoventriculoplasty in twenty-one consecutive patients with left ventricular outflow tract obstruction. J Thorac Cardiovasc Surg 1978; 75:659–669.
6. Somerville J, Ross D. Homograft replacement of aortic root with reimplantation of coronary arteries. Results after one to five years. British Heart Journal 1982;47:473–482.
7. Kirklin JW, Barratt-Boyes BG. Modified Konno operation. In Kirklin JW, Barratt-Boyes BG (eds). Cardiac Surgery. New York: Wiley 1986: 996–998.

37
"Miniroot" Replacement Techniques

Neal D. Kon and A. Robert Cordell

Aortic insufficiency and aortic stenosis are mechanical problems of the heart that result in left ventricular dysfunction. Among patients with severe cases treated medically only, 80% are no longer alive after eight years.[1-3]

Survival is considerably improved with surgical treatment. Expected survival at eight years with either a mechanical heart valve or a stented porcine bioprosthetic heart valve is 80%.[4,5] However, these survival curves do not approach normal life expectancy. The reduced life expectancy is multifactorial, but probably involves factors that relate to the presence of a prosthetic heart valve.

Prosthetic heart valves may have significant associated problems. The first among these is hydraulic dysfunction. Placing a prosthetic heart valve with a sewing ring inside the left ventricular outflow tract is obstructive.[6] The result may be not only a measurable gradient across the prosthetic valve but also a change in flow pattern across the valve from laminar to turbulent. Return to normal left ventricular dimensions is thereby inhibited. Turbulent flow also causes microabrasions and deposition of platelets, which may result in a prosthetic valve more prone to thromboembolic complications and endocarditis. The need for anticoagulants with a mechanical heart valve and the tendency for calcific degeneration of a stented xenograft valve are clear disadvantages and additional explanations of why life expectancy is still diminished even after successful replacement of a diseased aortic valve with a mechanical or stented bioprosthetic valve.

Many of the problems addressed above can be averted with the use of an aortic allograft heart valve to replace the diseased aortic valve. The hemodynamic performance of a properly placed allograft is clearly superior to that of a stented xenograft or a mechanical valve.[6] Not only are discernable gradients absent, but flow patterns are laminar. Echocardiographic results are indistinguishable from those in patients with normal heart valves. Avoidance of anticoagulation not only has benefits related to longevity but also results in a significantly improved lifestyle. Resistance to infection in the early postoperative phase (1 to 12 months) also makes the use of aortic allograft heart valves more attractive.[7]

Even though the first clinical allograft valve replacements were performed in 1962,[8,9] only a few centers acquired significant experience with them. The simplicity of inserting either a mechanical heart valve or a stented xenograft based on a single ring, and the wide availability of the xenografts made those the choice operations of most surgeons around the world. Not until O'Brien reported 10-year follow-up data with no structural deterioration when cryopreserved aortic allografts were used did enthusiasm develop in many other centers for inserting allograft heart valves.[10] In addition to their superior durability, other advantages of cryopreserved valves included indefinite storage time and ready availability.

As enthusiasm increased for the use of cryopreserved allograft heart valves once the Brisbane experience became known, the biggest drawbacks to the use of allografts became their limited availability and technical demands of implantation. Regional tissue banks specializing in cryopreservation helped alleviate some of the demands for human heart valves. However, the technical demands of implantation as manifested by difficult learning curves remained a most important hurdle.[11]

Surgeons at centers where allografts had been implanted since the early 1960s were very experienced with the freehand subcoronary technique of insertion and therefore had little trouble placing a competent aortic valve. This was not true for inexperienced allograft surgeons, and at many centers, after a rather short, unhappy experience, allografts were no longer used.

The primary reason for the lack of success with the subcoronary freehand technique is that when the sinuses of Valsalva are scalloped to accommodate a distal suture line beneath the coronary arteries, the valve mechanism is violated and the valve is no longer competent. For the valve to become competent again, the commissures must be suspended appropriately in a foreign (host) aortic root. If the host aortic root is symmetrical and the host sinus rim is within 2 mm of the diameter of the host aortic annulus, it is not difficult to make an appropriate size allograft competent within its new aortic root. Unfortunately, appropriately sized allograft is not always available, and distortion of part or all of the root is generally present in patients with aortic valvular heart disease. Therefore, techniques that rely less on altering the host's root geometry and more on utilizing the allograft's root geometry evolved.

The term "miniroot" will not be further used since it has been used to describe different techniques in the allograft literature: O'Brien and colleagues used "miniroot" to describe an inclusion root replacement technique that allowed them to place an allograft in a host annulus that was greater than 30 mm;[12] others have used the term to describe a short total-root replacement, which includes replacement the sinuses of Valsalva and the sino-tubular ridge and reimplanting the coronary arteries.[13] Our "miniroot" is best described as an intra-aortic cylinder technique. We will use the terms

"intra-aortic cylinder" to describe in inclusion type root techniques and "total root replacement" to describe a free standing root replacement (short or otherwise).

As stated previously, the freehand subcoronary technique of aortic allograft implantation has some associated drawbacks. Many inexperienced allograft surgeons lack the confidence in their ability to implant a competent valve, and it has been difficult for some relatively experienced allograft-implanting surgeons to use this technique for all types of aortic root pathology. To help apply the use of aortic allografts for aortic valve replacement to all types of root pathology, O'Brien and colleagues described three separate techniques of allograft implantation.[12] 1) The subcoronary technique, with inversion of the valve during implantation, was applicable to cases in which the annulus was 21 to 29 mm and the overall root geometry was asymmetrical. 2) For the small aortic root, interrupted sutures were used and the valve was not inverted. 3) For the large aortic annulus and the aneurysm aortic root, root-replacement techniques in which the entire allograft valve mechanism was kept intact were used.

Techniques

The inclusion-root technique, or intra-aortic cylinder technique, is used primarily in the patient whose annulus is 30 mm or larger. By using the allograft valve with its intact aortic sinuses as a small cylindrical tube, competence is assured. For this technique, the selected allograft should have an internal diameter 1–2 mm less than that of the host aortic annulus. The allograft aorta is transected 2 to 4 mm above the sino-tubular ridge; the allograft is trimmed, leaving a 2- to 3-mm cuff below the leaflets; the muscle bar is thinned as much as possible to limit obstruction of flow and to facilitate placement of the suture (Figure 37.1). Superiorly, the aortic wall of the allograft is transected approximately 5 mm above the top of the commissures, which leaves room for it to be cut again to appropriate length when the distal suture line is established. After the cardiopulmonary bypass and cardioplegic arrest of the heart are

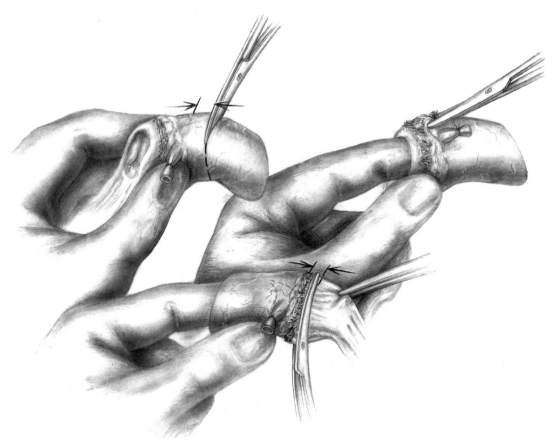

FIGURE 37.1. Trimming of the aortic allograft.

established, exposure is gained through an oblique, or transverse, aortotomy incision, the choice depending on the surgeon's preference. We prefer a transverse aortotomy that encircles three fourths of the aorta 4mm above the sinus rim (Figure 37.2A, B). The proximal suture line can be established with either a continuous or interrupted suture technique. We prefer an interrupted technique with no inversion of the valve (Figure 37.3A). Sutures are placed in a single plane beneath the aortic valve (Figure 37.3B). The sinus walls around the left and right coronary ostia of the allograft are excised to create appropriate holes for the left and right coronary arteries. Coronary anastomoses are performed with continuous 5-0 Prolene sutures (Figures 37.4 and 37.5). At this stage, the allograft may appear distorted because it is tethered to the host wall in two places. For the distal suture line, three simple 4-0 Prolene sutures are used to approximate the top of the allograft commissures against the host aorta at the sino-tubular ridge. Excess allograft aorta distal to the commissures is excised, and the sutures are then tied, making allowance for the aortotomy. If the aortotomy is extended into the non-coronary sinus, it can be closed up to the sino-tubular ridge at this point. Each suture at the top of the commissure is then run inside the aorta at the level of the sino-tubular ridge to the adjacent commissure to complete the inclusion root replacement (Figure 37.6). Before the aortotomy is completely closed, one or two mattress sutures may be applied to the non-coronary sinus to minimize or obliterate dead space between the layers. The rest of the aortotomy is then closed with a continuous 4-0 Prolene suture.

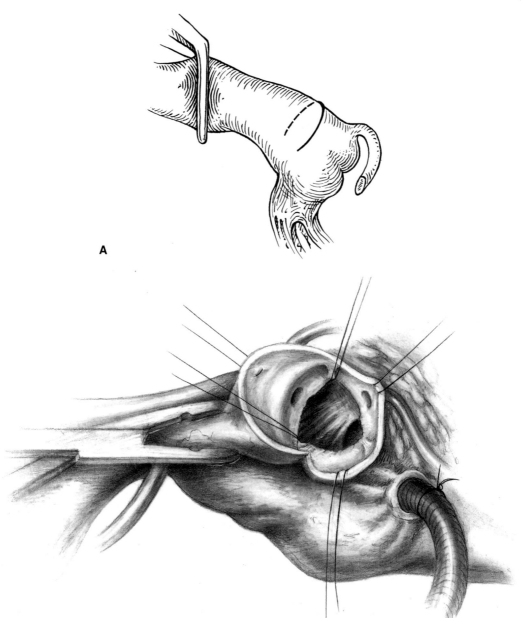

FIGURE 37.2. (A) Transverse aortotomy encircles three-quarters of the aorta above the sinus rim. (B) Strategic stay sutures are applied to display the aortic valve and right coronary ostium.

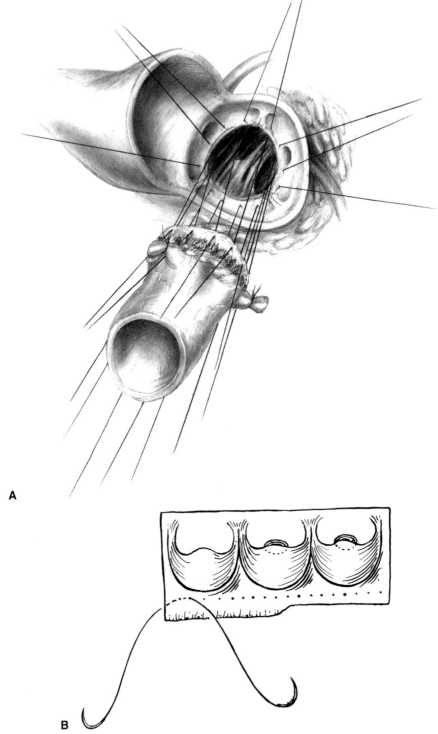

FIGURE 37.3. (A) Interrupted suture technique is used to establish the proximal connection of the allograft to the left ventricular outflow tract. (B) Sutures are place in a single plane beneath the aortic valve.

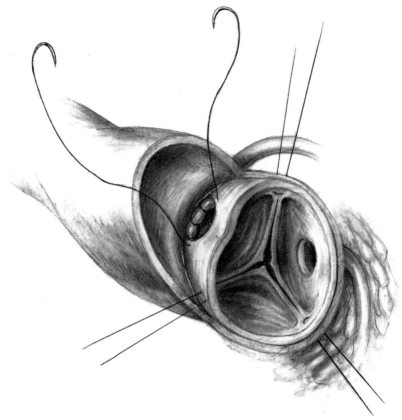

FIGURE 37.4. The left coronary anastomosis is accomplished with a continuous 5-0 polypropylene suture.

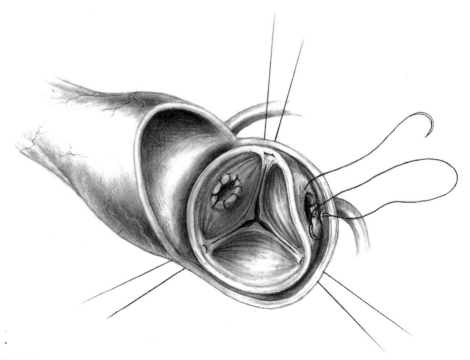

FIGURE 37.5. The right coronary anastomosis is accomplished with a continuous 5-0 polyproplylene suture.

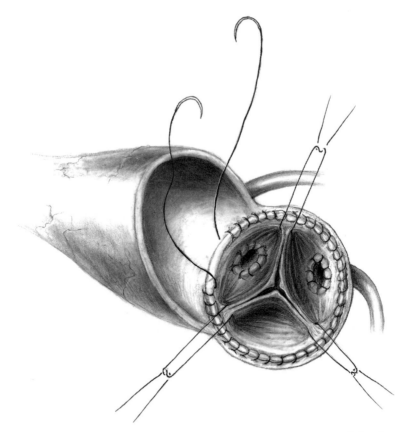

FIGURE 37.6. Inclusion distal suture line is accomplished with a semi-continuous 5-0 polypropylene suture.

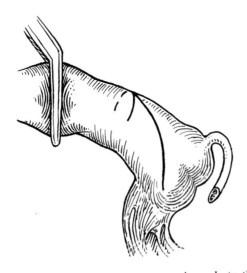

FIGURE 37.7. A T-shaped aortotomy is made to the base of the non-coronary sinus to expose the aortic root.

In another approach to the problem of the early onset aortic insufficiency seen with the scalloped, subcoronary allograft valve replacement technique, Angell and associates described a partial-inclusion, aortic root replacement technique.[14] A T-shaped longitudinal aortotomy is made to the base of the non-coronary sinus to expose the aortic root (Figure 37.7). A proximal interrupted suture line orients the allograft root anatomically to the host root and fixes the annulus of the allograft to the host annulus. To facilitate exposure and placement of the proximal sutures, the allograft is split posteriorly into the left sinus of Valsalva and the left coronary ostium (Figure 37.8A, B). Simple running-suture lines are carried around both coronary ostia, and the posterior split in the graft is re-approximated. The posterior portion of the graft is then secured from just above the left coronary ostium medially and laterally to the superior ends of the superior portion of the T-shaped aortotomy (Figure 37.9). The anterior graft length is trimmed appropriately as the distal suture line is completed to re-establish vascular continuity (Figures 37.9 and 37.10). The cross clamp can be removed at this point, which allows the surgeon to observe the allograft in the distended configuration and to check for bleeding points before closing the allograft completely

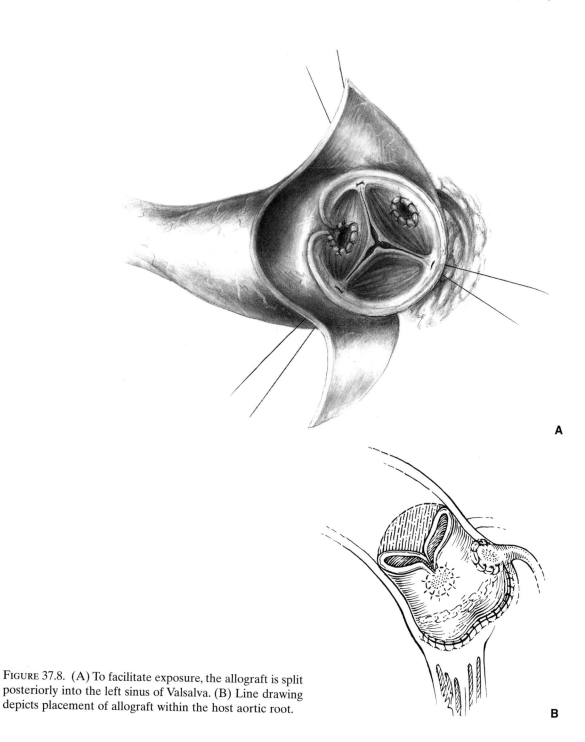

A

B

FIGURE 37.8. (A) To facilitate exposure, the allograft is split posteriorly into the left sinus of Valsalva. (B) Line drawing depicts placement of allograft within the host aortic root.

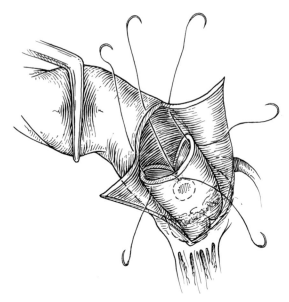

FIGURE 37.9. The posterior portion of the allograft is secured to host aortic wall. Anterior sutures are placed to establish vascular continuity prior to completion of the host aortotomy closure.

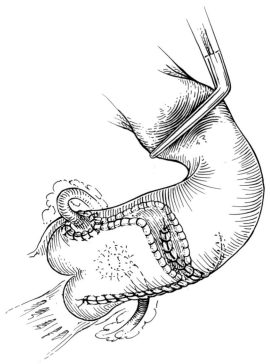

FIGURE 37.10. Line drawing depicting the completion inclusion root replacement.

within the host aorta. It also allows the surgeon to close the aorta in a fashion that does not compromise the allograft in any way. The surgeon could also choose not to close the aorta completely around the allograft. Thus, with this technique, unlike the intra-aortic cylinder approach, the valve assumes the shape of the donor rather than being placed in the host root prior to distention with blood and pressure. There is also no need to secure the commissures to the host aorta. As a result, all of the elements that determine final configuration of the allograft are those of the donor unrestricted by the host root.

Inclusion techniques have several advantages. The entire allograft valve mechanism is left intact, thereby assuring aortic valve competence. The host sinuses are also left intact, and thus, if early or late valve failure should occur, the entire allograft valve could be removed and a mechanical or bioprosthetic valve put in its place.

Inclusion techniques also have disadvantages. They are probably the most cumbersome techniques to perform. Each of the coronary suture lines is established with more limited exposure.

When the coronary arteries lie at 180° it is difficult to implant them into the corresponding sinus of Valsalva. The intra-aortic cylinder technique also suffers from problems similar to those of the Bentall mechanical valve conduit inclusion-root replacement. It is difficult to tell exactly how the allograft will distend within the aortic root and thus any malalignment will put added stress on the coronary suture line. Two of our patients have experienced such problems, and, in one, part of the distal suture line pulled loose. In this patient, we had placed an allograft with three sinuses of Valsalva into a truly bicuspid root with only two sinuses of Valsalva and one coronary ostium. Although this allograft valve has not been insufficient and shows only a mild degree of stenosis, the turbulent flow across the aortic root is much greater than that we have seen with most of our inclusion intra-aortic cylinder allograft valve replacement. The other patient developed a fistulous tract between the left coronary anastomosis and the layers between the allograft root and the host root.

Finally, with the inclusion techniques, if there is bleeding from the coronary artery suture lines but the source cannot be seen, the bleeding has to be controlled by wrapping the aorta. Theoretically, hematomas between the layers can alter valve function and produce obstruction.

Perhaps the most significant disadvantage of using an intra-aortic cylinder technique is that these replacements are innately more obstructive than free-standing root replacements in which the entire host root is excised except for the coronary ostia. With the inclusion technique, the surgeon must, in some fashion, "stuff" one entire aortic root inside another.

We, and some others,[13,15] now prefer the free-standing total aortic root replacement with a cryopreserved aortic allograft for all patients requiring aortic valve replacement, regardless of aortic root pathology.

Total-root replacement is accomplished in uncomplicated aortic valve disease by establishing cardioplegic arrest and then transecting the aorta just above the sinotubular ridge (Figure 37.11). The thawed allograft is prepared by removing the anterior leaflet of the mitral valve and redundant outflow tract muscle beneath the valve, leaving a 2- to 3-cm remnant beneath the lowers point of each sinus of Valsalva. This remnant will be used for placement of the proximal suture line. The allograft aorta is initially transected 5 to 6 cm above the sinus rim, leaving adequate room to cut it again when connecting the allograft to the distal aorta. Adequate amounts of the left and right sinuses of Valsalva are excised to accommodate the left and right coronary arteries.

Attention is then turned back to the host aortic root. Both host coronary arteries are mobilized from the aortic root on generous buttons of aortic wall, and the remaining tissue of each of the right and left sinuses of Valsalva, as well as the non-coronary sinus of Valsalva, is excised (Figure 37.12). The aortic valve is removed and all calcium in the annulus and outflow tract is debrided. The proximal or inflow anastomosis is accomplished using a 28 to 35 simple interrupted sutures of 3-0 braided Dacron tied around a 1-mm strip of Teflon felt (Figure 37.13). We use this trip of Teflon felt not

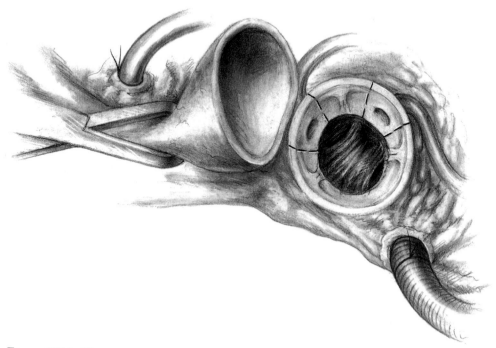

FIGURE 37.11. The aortic root is exposed by transecting the aorta 2–5 mm above the sinus rim.

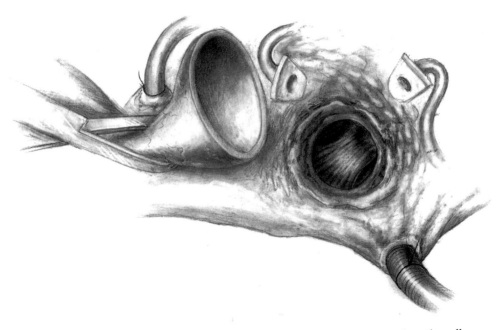

FIGURE 37.12. The coronary ostia are mobilized on generous buttons of aortic wall.

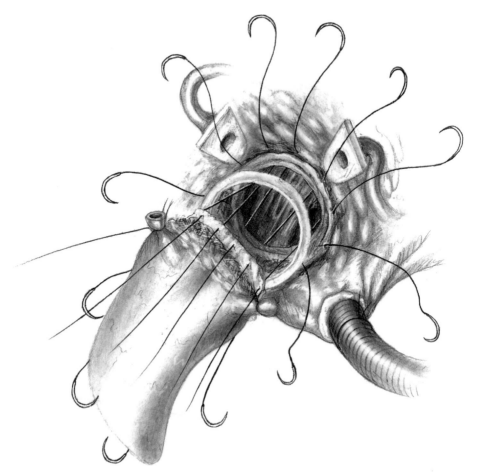

FIGURE 37.13. The proximal anastomosis is accomplished using 28 to 35 simple interrupted sutures of 3-0 braided Dacron tied around a 1 mm strip of Teflon felt.

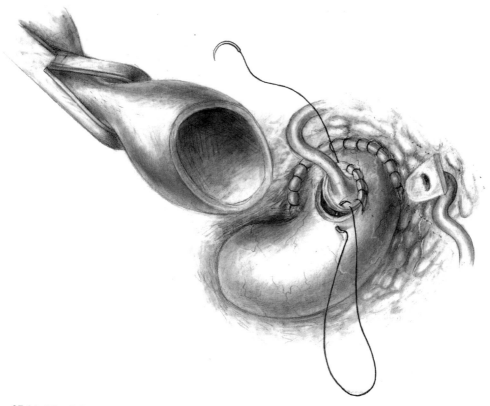

Figure 37.14. The left coronary artery on a generous button of aortic wall is sewn end-to side to the left sinus of the allograft with a continuous 5-0 polypropylene suture.

only to aid in hemostasis, but also to prevent sutures from tearing through the allograft muscle bar when the knots are tied. The coronary arteries on their buttons of aortic wall are sewn end-to-side to the corresponding sinus of Valsalva of the allograft with a continuous 5-0 polypropylene suture (Figures 37.14 and 37.15). The distal end of the allograft, which is usually cut just above the sinus rim, is then sewn to the host aorta end-to-end with a continuous 5-0 polypropylene suture to complete the root replacement (Figures 37.15 and 37.16).

If the host aorta is considerably larger than the allograft aorta, an appropriately sized "V" can be cut out of the distal aorta and the edges re-approximated with running 5-0 Prolene suture prior to establishing the end-to-end anastomosis.

When the host annulus is dilated greater than 28 mm, we use the largest allograft we can find (23 mm or greater) and fix the size of the host annulus with a 1 mm thick Dacron ring 4 mm greater in diameter than the size of the allograft. When the host annulus is nearly normal in size, we try to use an allograft with an internal diameter as close to that of the aortic annulus as possible.

Several recently published studies have also favored using a free-standing total-root graft for all aortic-root replacements with a stentless valve, whether it be a xenograft, an allograft, or an autograft.[13,15–17] The major theoretical disadvantage of the free-standing root replacement technique is the perceived radical nature of the procedure, even though several series have demonstrated a similar operative risk for both techniques under elective circumstances.[18–20] Reimplantation of coronary arteries theoretically risks the development of coronary ostial complications, but we and others have not seen such complications, either early or late.[13,15–18,20,21] The best way to prevent late problems with calcification in the region of the coronary ostia is to use generous buttons of native aortic wall

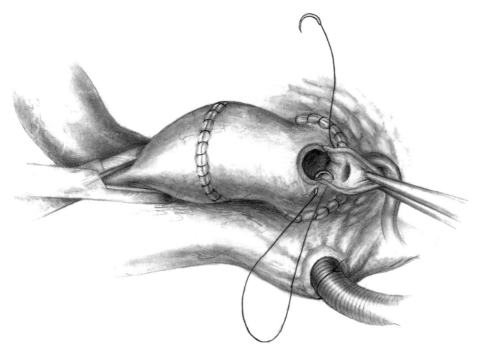

FIGURE 37.15. The site on the allograft for the right coronary anastomosis is selected after the distal aorta-to-allograft suture line is completed and the aortic root is distended. This maneuver limits the possibility of torquing the reimplanted right coronary.

around the coronary ostia at the initial operation.[21] Excessive bleeding at the proximal suture line has not occurred with the technique described.

A risk of constant concern is the potential problem of reoperation after a free-standing root replacement. We and others have not found this to be a serious problem, albeit numbers are still small.[13,15–18,20,21] Simple mechanical valves placed within allograft roots at the time of reoperation, repeat allograft root replacements, or mechanical valve root replacements have been accomplished without unexpected mortality.

Our experience at North Carolina Baptist Hospital/Bowman Gray School of Medicine over the past six years also supports the use of a short total aortic root replacement for aortic valve replacement in all cases. The first 12 left ventricular outflow tract reconstructions we performed were of the freehand subcoronary type (Table 37.1). By 18 months, three have been removed for severe aortic insufficiency

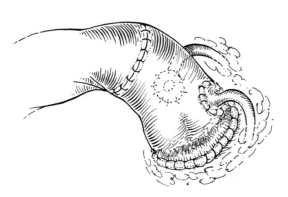

FIGURE 37.16. Line drawing depicts the completed free-standing total aortic root replacement.

TABLE 37.1. Results of 12 Freehand Reconstructions.

Incidence of Postoperative AI		
0–1+	2+	3–4+
1	8	3

Mean peak gradient—22.05 ± 11.75 mmHg.
Three valves were removed before 1.5 years for severe.
AI without leaflet abnormalities.
AI = aortic insufficiency.

TABLE 37.2. Twenty-three Intra-Aortic Cylinders.

Incidence of Postoperative AI		
0–1+	2+	3–4+
21	1	1

Mean peak gradient—17.19 ± 6.38 mmHg.
One valve was removed before 3.5 years for severe.
AI from endocarditis with leaflet destruction.
AI = aortic insufficiency.

and eight of the remaining nine had 2+ aortic insufficiency on the latest echocardiogram; the ninth had 1+ aortic insufficiency. The mean peak systolic echo gradient in this group was 22.05 ± 11.75 mmHg. On the basis of these results, we turned to the intra-aortic cylinder technique and closely followed 23 of those patients with echocardiography (Table 37.2). We believed that using a technique that maintains all of the donor valve mechanism would ensure valvular competence, and the lower incidence of postoperative aortic regurgitation in this group has proved that point. One patient developed 2+ to 3+ aortic insufficiency, but it turned out to be secondary to a paravalvular leak; one patient developed severe aortic insufficiency secondary to endocarditis with destruction of the leaflets; 21 patients have only had a stable course with 2+ aortic insufficiency. The mean peak systolic gradient in this group is 17.19 ± 6.38 mmHg.

During the time we were performing the intra-aortic cylinder technique, we performed a significant number of total root replacements. Initially, these were in patients with endocarditis and root abscess, ascending aortic aneurysms, or small aortic roots. The total root replacement was simpler to perform, took less time than placement of the intra-aortic cylinder, and was applicable to every type of aortic root disease. Total root replacement also maintained the entire valve mechanism of the allograft, and thus became our choice for replacement.

We have followed echocardiographically 87 patients total root replacements (Table 37.3). One patient has had severe aortic insufficiency, but that was the result of recurrent endocarditis. There was no evidence of active infection at the time of reoperation, so we placed a St. Jude valve inside his allograft root after excising the destroyed, insufficient valve leaflets. He continues to do well with no signs of recurrent infection. Two patients have had 2+ aortic insufficiency, and the remaining 84 patients have 1+ aortic insufficiency or less. Also, as would be expected, the mean peak systolic echocardiographic gradient in this group is the lowest of the three (10.47 ± 6.40).

Total root replacement is also our technique of choice for endocarditis with annular abscess, whether from a host aortic valve or a prosthetic aortic valve.[22,23] This technique allows all abscess material to be debrided extensively and drained into the pericardium outside the circulation. After the left ventricular outflow tract has been debrided thoroughly, excess tissue on the allograft provides ideal material for repair. Much of the anterior leaflet of the mitral valve can be left on the allograft to fill in defects along the aorto-mitral membrane. The proximal suture line on the allograft may also be placed deep to draining abscess material in the left ventricular outflow tract. If one or both of the coronary ostia are involved in abscess material, it (they) can be ligated. The coronary blood supply is then re-established with appropriate saphenous vein bypass grafts (Figure 37.17).

In conclusion, we believe that a total root replacement technique is the technique of choice for all patients undergoing aortic valve replacement with a cryopreserved aortic allograft. The technique is easily reproducible by cardiac surgeons and a competent valve is assured at the time of surgery. The allograft sinuses of Valsalva are unrestricted and free to distend at the completion of the procedure, thereby avoiding obstruction and turbulent flow. The potential hazards of increased

TABLE 37.3. Eighty-seven Total (Freestanding) Root Replacements.

Incidence of Postoperative AI		
0–1+	2+	3–4+
84	2	1

Mean peak gradient—10.97 ± 6.40 mmHg.
One valve was removed at 7 months for severe AI from recurrent endocarditis with leaflet destruction.
AI = aortic insufficiency.

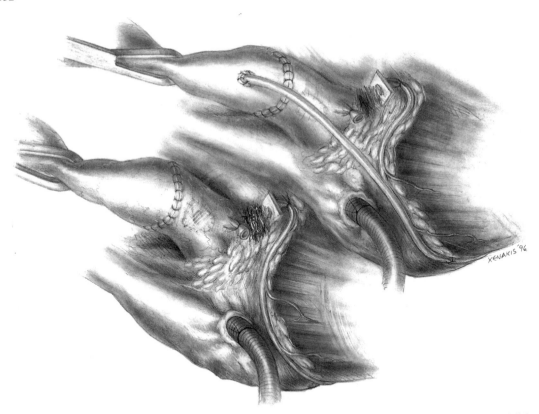

FIGURE 37.17. When endocarditis and root abscess involve the coronary ostia, the root replacement can be accomplished by ligating one or both coronary ostia. Coronary blood supply is then re-established with appropriate saphenous vein bypass grafts.

bleeding at the initial operation have not been realized, and options at reoperation are not restricted to only redoing the root replacement. The technique is also easily applied to cases of complicated root anatomy; i.e. 180 degree coronary arteries, a large aortic annulus, and major discrepancies in size between the aortic annulus and the sinus rim. The best early valve results appear to be obtained with this approach. Thus, by inference, enhanced long term durability of aortic allografts performed as root replacements, compared to already very good results with freehand subcoronary implantation,[24] may be attainable.

References

1. Wood P. Aortic stenosis. Am J Cardiol 1958;1: 553–571.
2. Frank S, Ross JJ, Jr. The natural history of severe, acquired valvular aortic stenosis. Am J Cardiol 1967;19:128–129.
3. Grant RT. After histories for ten years of a thousand men suffering from heart disease: A study in prognosis. Heart 1933;16:275.
4. Arom KV, Demetre MN, Kersten TE, et al. Ten year's experience with the St. Jude Medical Valve prosthesis. Ann Thorac Surg 1989;47:831–837.
5. Jamieson WRE, Munro AI, Miyagishima RT, et al. Carpentier-Edwards standard porcine bioprosthesis: Clinical performance to seventeen years. Ann Thorac Surg 1995;60:999–1007.
6. Jaffe WM, Coverdale HA, Roche AH, Whitlock RM, Neutze JM, Barratt-Boyes BG. Rest and exercise hemodynamics of 20 to 23 mm allograft, Medtronic Intact (porcine), and St. Jude Medical valves in the aortic position. J Thorac Cardiovasc Surg 1990;100:167–174.
7. Ivert T, Dismukes W, Cobbs C, Blackstone E, Kirklin J, Bergdahl L. Prosthetic valve endocarditis. Circulation 1984;69:223–232.

8. Ross DN. Homograft replacement of the aortic valve. Lancet 1962;2:487.

9. Barratt-Boyes BG. Homograft aortic valve replacement in aortic incompetence and stenosis. Thorax 1964;19:131–150.

10. O'Brien MF, Stafford EG, Gardner MA, Pohlner PG, McGiffin DC. A comparison of aortic valve replacement with viable cryopreserved and fresh allograft valves, with a note on chromosomal studies. J Thorac Cardiovasc Surg 1987;94:812–823.

11. Jones EL. Freehand homograft aortic valve replacement—the learning curve: a technical analysis of the first 31 patients. Ann Thorac Surg 1989;48:26–32.

12. O'Brien MF, McGiffin DC, Stafford EG. Allograft aortic valve implantation: techniques for all types of aortic valve and root pathology. Ann Thorac Surg 1989;48:600–609.

13. Daicoff G, Botero L, Quintessenza J. Allograft replacement of the aortic valve versus the miniroot and valve. Ann Thorac Surg 1993;55:855–859.

14. Angell WM, Pupello DF, Bessone LN, et al. Implantation of the unstented bioprosthetic aortic root: An improved method. J Card Surg 1993;8:466–471.

15. O'Brien MF, Finney RS, Stafford EG, et al. Root replacement for all allograft aortic valves: Preferred technique or too radical? Ann Thorac Surg 1995;60:S87–S91.

16. Elkins RC, Santangelo K, Stelzer P, et al. Pulmonary autograft replacement of the aortic valve: An evolution of technique. J Cardiac Surg 1992;7:108.

17. Kouchoukos NT, Davila-Roman VG, Spray TL, Murphy SF, Perrillo JB. Replacement of the aortic root with a pulmonary autograft in children and young adults with aortic-valve disease. New Eng Journ Med 1994;330:1–6.

18. Kon ND, Westaby S, Pillae R, Amaresena N, Cordell R. Comparison of implant techniques using freestyle stentless porcine aortic valve. Ann Thorac Surg 1995;59:857–862.

19. Blundell PE, MacFarlane JK, Sutherland NG, Scott HJ. Heterotransplantation of the aortic valve in calves. J Thorac Cardiovasc Surg 1967;54:616–21 passim.

20. Yacoub M, Rasmi NRH, Sundt TM, Lund Oea. Fourteen-year experience with homovital homografts for aortic valve replacement. J Thorac Cardiovasc Surg 1995;110:186–194.

21. Sundt TM, III, Rasmi N, Wong K, et al. Reoperative aortic valve operation after homograft root replacement: Surgical options and results. Ann Thorac Surg 1995;60:S95–S100.

22. Glazier JJ, Verwilghen J, Donaldson RM, Ross DN. Treatment of complicated prosthetic aortic valve endocarditis with annular abscess formation by homograft aortic root replacement. J Am Coll Cardiol 1991;17:1177–1182.

23. Kirklin JK, Kirklin JW, Pacifico AD. Aortic valve endocarditis with aortic root abscess cavity:surgical treatment with aortic valve homograft. Ann Thorac Surg 1988;45:647–657.

24. O'Brien MF, Stafford EG, Gardner MA, et al. Allograft aortic valve replacement: Long term follow-up. Ann Thorac Surg 1995;60:S65–S70.

38
Stentless Xenograft Valves

Richard A. Hopkins

Stentless porcine heterografts for aortic valve replacement are now commercially available. Three such valves have now been approved by the FDA for use in humans. One is a scalloped valve designed for a standard subcoronary insertion ("Toronto SPV Valve", St. Jude Medical, St. Paul, MN) and two others (Medtronic "Freestyle" and Edwards "Prima Plus") are prepared as a root and can be trimmed for insertion as either a miniroot, root or subcoronary scalloped technique. All three valves are glutaraldehyde fixed. The current version of the Medtronic valve is also treated with an anticalcification method (alpha amino oleic acid).[1] The Edwards valve is also prepared with an anti-calcification treatment and utilizes low-pressure fixation. All porcine valves share the need for a Dacron support as a consequence of the muscle bar below the right coronary cusp which exists in pigs but is not present in humans. All three appear to share the hydraulic engineering advantage of stentless valves with reduced energy dissipation across the valve, lower effective gradients, less inertial effects, ability to flex during cardiac motion and apparently result in improved hemodynamics both short term and medium term.[2-4] There appear to be advantages similar to homograft and autograft insertions in terms of regression of left ventricular hypertrophy, reduction in valve gradients over time and improved diastolic properties of the left ventricle.[2,5] Stentless valves may be especially appropriate for patients over age 60, with significant LVH and small aortic annuli.[6,7]

Insertion methods for the stentless xenografts are natural derivatives of the lessons learned from homograft valve replacement surgery. Many of the same concerns are present including careful sizing, a range of techniques for assuring architectural symmetry and the need for assessing and reconstructing as necessary the left ventricular outflow at all three levels of subvalvular, annular and supra-annular (sinus ridge). Care in reconstructing the entire outflow tract to optimize the performance of the stentless valves is as critical as in homograft insertions. However, there are a number of differences. The glutaraldehyde treatment results in a valve complex which is more rigid and in some ways easier to insert as the architecture is better maintained by the prosthesis during insertion. The Dacron support at the base in association with rigidity makes continuous proximal suturing techniques more appealing than with fresh or cryopreserved homografts and autografts. On the other hand, this rigidity prevents inversion of the stentless porcine heterografts into the left ventricle and reduces the plasticity for the reconstructions.

A significant range of implantation techniques are available for this category of valve.[8] These include the scalloped subcoronary inclusion method, cylinder inclusion or miniroot techniques and a complete aortic root replacement (Figure 38.1). As discussed elsewhere in this chapter, aortoplastic techniques are occasionally necessary for tailoring of aortic root geometry and the presence of subvalvular

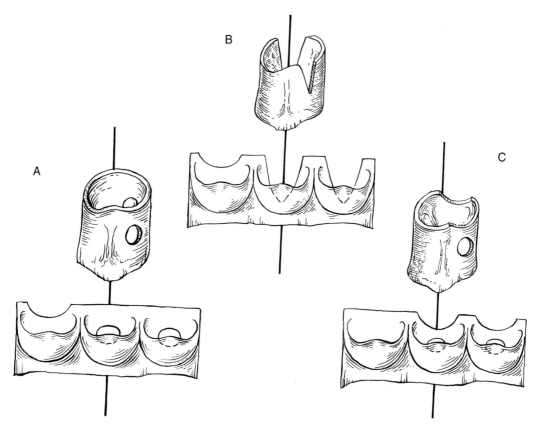

FIGURE 38.1. This demonstrates three alternative methods for insertion of stentless porcine valves. The middle figure demonstrates the scalloped sub-coronary inclusion method which is useful for the pre-cut Toronto valve or the surgeon-contoured intact root valves. Cylinder inclusion can be performed as on the right and the total root replacement on the left.

stenosis may require attention to that portion of the outflow tract as well.

Sizing

Sizing is performed differently for the currently available valves. The Toronto SPV Valve is sized based upon the sino-tubular junction of the recipient (if normal or as altered by aortoplasty if abnormal). For the Medtronic and Baxter versions, the sizing is performed at the annulus level, using the manufacturers' sizers which reflect the "outside" diameter of the prosthesis (not internal diameter as in homografts). Especially for valves inserted as "roots," a bias towards upsizing is encouraged as opposed to the downsizing bias when using fresh or cryopreserved homografts.

Surgical Technique for Scalloped Subcoronary Insertion

The scalloping of the valve is either accomplished by the manufacturer or can be performed by the surgeon prior to or after the proximal suture line has been accomplished.

Aortotomy is performed in one of two ways depending upon whether the ascending aorta at the level of the sinus ridge is of the diameter desired at the conclusion of the repair or is enlarged. A transverse aortotomy is performed above the level of the sinus ridge if the sinus ridge anatomy appears appropriate where as a "Lazy S" incision is performed which crosses the sinus ridge anatomy into the non-coronary cusp of the recipient if tailoring of the aortic root is required (Figure 38.2).

The native valve is excised with decalcification of the annulus as necessary (Figure 38.3). The stentless porcine heterograft has already been prepared on the back table with rinsing and is presented onto the operating field. The proximal suture line is accomplished with interrupted 2-0 or 3-0 braided sutures. These sutures can be placed further apart than used for fresh or cryopreserved homografts as a consequence of the rigidity of the glutaraldehyde Dacron reinforced base. These are placed as simple sutures through the subcoronary annulus or subannular base of the aortic root, thence through the base of the heterograft (Figure 38.4). Each suture is clipped with a small hemostat which is placed on an Allis clamp for safekeeping in order. Between 14 and 26 sutures are

required. The heterograft is then seated and the sutures sequentially tied. Alternatively, a continuous suture of 2-0 polypropylene on a semi-circular tapered needle is utilized and, depending upon surgeon preference, this can be accomplished with a single running suture or with three sutures placed at equidistant points and each then tied to each other (Figure 38.5). The running technique is currently preferred when feasible.

Upon completion of the proximal suture line, the right and left coronary sinuses may be excised depending upon the insertion technique. They may simply be scalloped if not already performed by the manufacturer. If an oblique vertical aortotomy has been performed into the non-coronary sinus, then scalloping of the non-coronary sinus sometimes allows better realignment of the aortic root via a reduction aortoplasty. The sinus ridge diameter should be no larger than the base annulus, and preferably 10–20% smaller to encourage "eddy currents" in the sinuses. If this portion of the aortic root

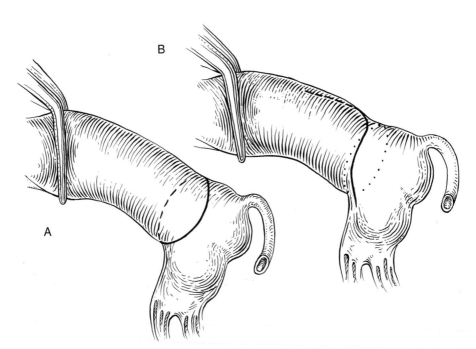

FIGURE 38.2. Aortotomies can be performed in a multitude of ways. The easiest access is with a transverse aortotomy (A). The remaining ascending aorta should be kept relatively short to provide suspension to the stentless valve root. If the subcoronary method is used, then native aorta is reattached to native aorta.

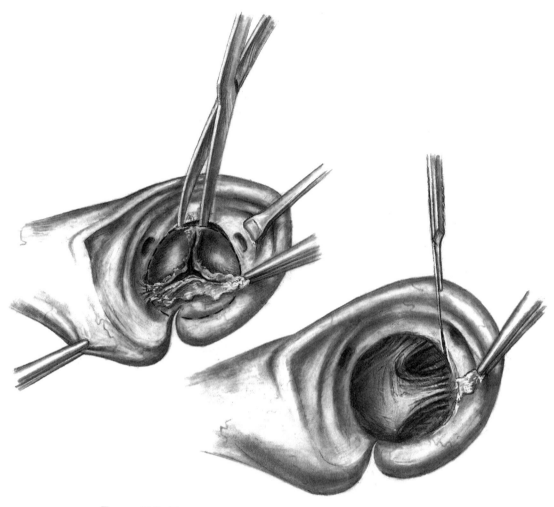

FIGURE 38.3. The native valve is excised and the annulus decalcified.

does not require alteration, then leaving the non-coronary sinus intact is very appropriate. If the scallop technique is utilized, suturing is begun below the left coronary ostia with a running 5-0 polypropylene suture and brought to the top of each pillar on either side. Exiting the aorta at this point, tension is maintained while a similar suture is placed beginning at the base of the sinus below the right coronary ostia up to the top of the pillars on either side (Figure 38.6). These sutures are tied outside of the aorta over a pledget of either Teflon felt or autologous pericardium. If a transverse aortotomy has been performed, a tacking suture or two are placed to the non-coronary cusp, once again with sutures being tied outside to obliterate any

potential "dead space" (Figure 38.7). For a transverse aortotomy, the distal suture line is now accomplished either at the level of the top of the pillars or above the level of the pillar placements with a running 3-0 or 4-0 polypropylene continuous suture technique. Care is taken throughout to assure suspension of the pillars, usually a little higher than the native pillars were suspended. In addition, the sinus ridge is maintained at a diameter 10 to 20% smaller than the aortic annulus base diameter (Figure 38.8). If a ostial cut-out technique is performed, then the distal suture line throughout its circumference includes the top of the heterograft, the proximal native aorta and the distal aorta (Figure 38.9). If the scallop

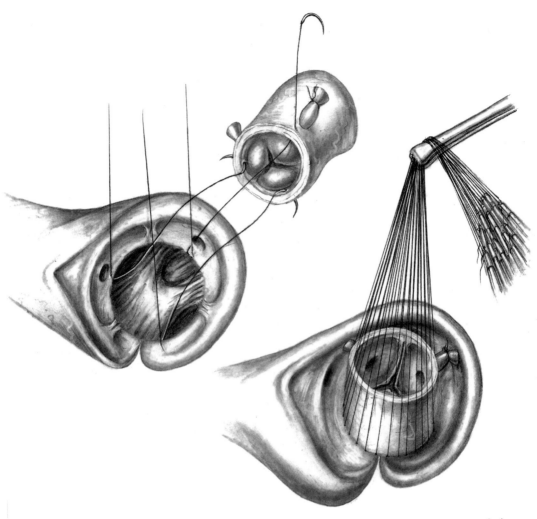

FIGURE 38.4. Proximal suture line is created with either interrupted or continuous suture techniques.

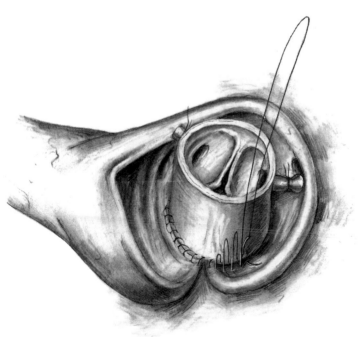

FIGURE 38.5. Demonstrates a continuous suture technique with a cylinder inclusion method.

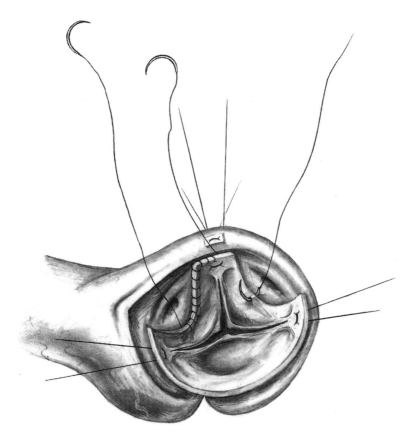

FIGURE 38.6. Demonstrates subcoronary suturing technique very similar to inserting a homograft.

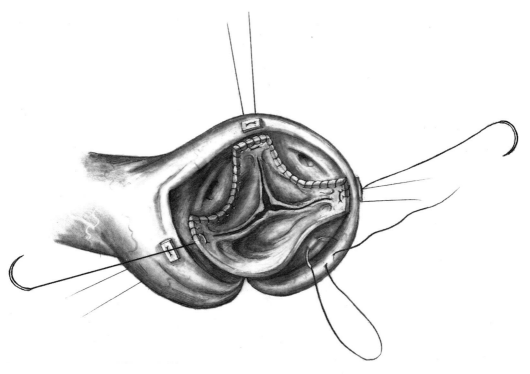

FIGURE 38.7. Sutures are placed to obliterate any potential dead space between retained sinus wall of the xenograft.

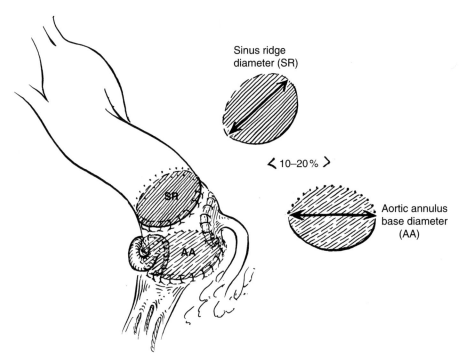

FIGURE 38.8. The sinus ridge should be reconstructed to be narrower than the aortic annulus by approximately 15%.

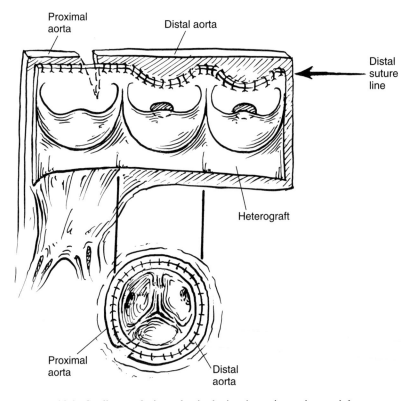

FIGURE 38.9. Scallop technique for inclusion insertion using ostial cut-out.

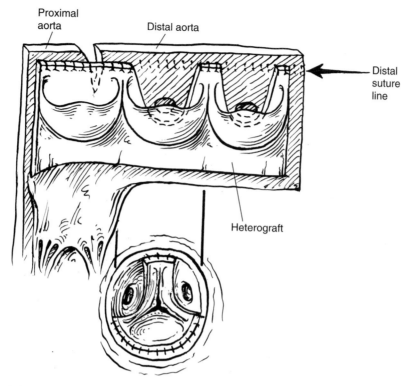

FIGURE 38.10. Subcoronary insertion method where the distal suture line incorporates the top of the pillars.

techniques have been performed, then the distal suture line only includes the top of the pillars and the top of the heterograft if the non-coronary cusp is left intact (Figure 38.10). If the sinus ridge intact with cut-out technique is utilized, then the suture line again incorporates the top of the aortic wall of all three sinuses (Figure 38.11).

Aortic Root Replacement with Stentless Porcine Heterografts

For complex aortic root anatomy or for infected aortic roots, it is sometimes preferable to completely replace the entire aortic root rather than using a miniroot or subcoronary scallop technique. In this case, the operation is very similar to that described for the aortic root replacement with a homograft.

Sizing is accomplished utilizing either Hegar dilators or sizers provided by the companies. Only the intact aortic root heterograft prosthe-ses are suitable for this technique. The size of the aortic root base after excision of the native valve can be matched to the internal diameter of the heterograft equivalently. There is usually enough tolerance that upsizing by 2mm is also feasible. Downsizing by 2mm can also be accomplished but is not recommended.

All tissue is excised leaving the coronaries on buttons (Figure 38.12). Any subvalvular septal incisions can be made at this time (Figure 38.13). The proximal suture line can be accomplished with either interrupted simple techniques of 2-0 or 3-0 braided sutures (Figure 38.14) but does not need reinforcement with Teflon felt as with homografts, or can be accomplished with a running suture technique utilizing 3-0 polypropylene suture (Figure 38.15). The left coronary button is sutured first to the aortic root complex after completion of the proximal suture line. This can be accomplished in one of two ways. Either a circular button is excised or preferably a large "U" shaped wedge is excised from the left coronary sinus of the

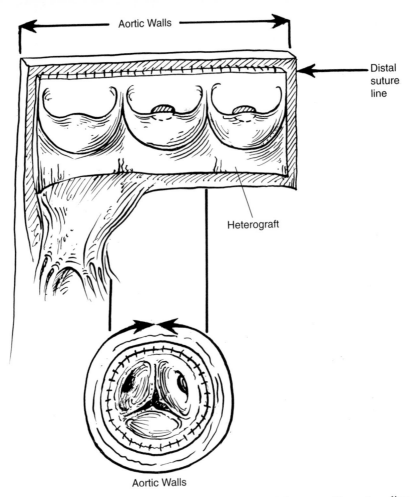

FIGURE 38.11. Sinus ridge of xenograft left intact with coronary ostial cut-out. Top suture line may incorporate native aortic wall into the stentless distal aortic anastomosis, across all three sinuses.

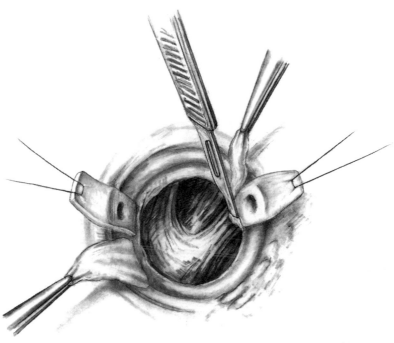

FIGURE 38.12. Aortic root method requires removal of all the native aortic root tissue except the coronary buttons.

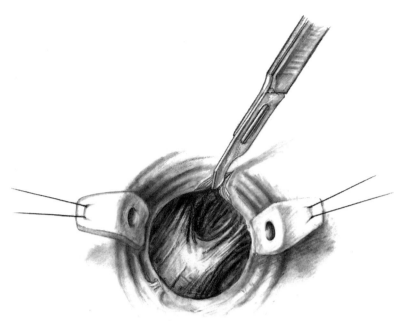

FIGURE 38.13. Subvalvular muscular stenosis can be relieved with a myotomy in the usual location, such as is used for IHSS. The aortic root proximal suture line can be accomplished either with interrupted or continuous suture methods. Proximal suture line accomplished with a continuous polypropylene suturing technique. This is safer with the manufactured stentless valves than with homografts as the tissue is stiffer and will not be damaged by tugging and pulling to seat the valve.

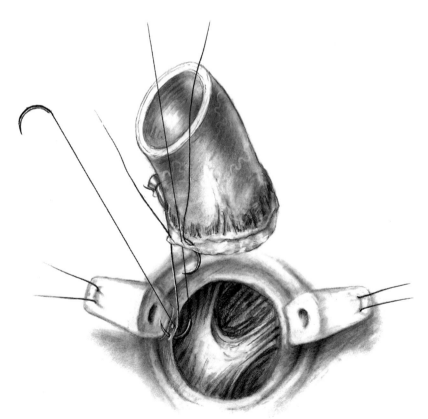

FIGURE 38.14. The proximal suture line can be accomplished with an interrupted simple technique, preferably utilizing braided sutures, in a manner analogous to aortic root replacement with homo- grafts. The thicker tissue and stronger material properties of the xenograft mitigates the need for a Teflon felt strip as is used with homografts.

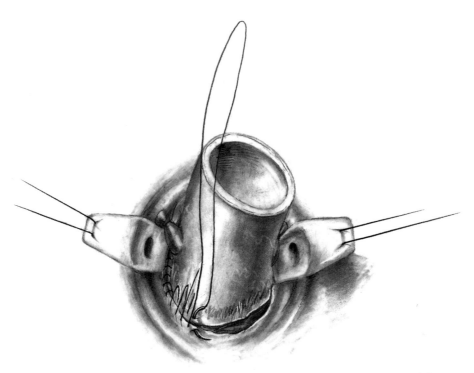

FIGURE 38.15. A running suture technique with either 2-0 or 3-0 polypropylene suture is often a faster and easier way of constructing the proximal suture line with the manufactured xenograft stentless valves. The more robust material properties of the treated valves allows for more tugging and pulling to seat the xenograft utilizing the running suture method. This is particularly appropriate for aortic insufficiency.

heterograft and the large coronary ostial "U" shaped "button" inserted with a running 5-0 polypropylene suture technique in either case (Figure 38.16). It is usually better to place the left coronary button higher than it had been positioned in the native aortic root to avoid kinking. Often, this is facilitated by the "U" shaped replacement technique as opposed to the circular button technique. The distal suture line is then accomplished with a running 3-0 or 4-0 polypropylene technique. This allows more accurate placement of the right coronary ostia which is usually placed somewhat above the coronary stump of the heterograft as the coronary positions in the pig are somewhat different than in the human (Figure 38.17). This can often be placed as a circular button. If it appears that the placement should be performed higher so that the top of the coronary button will be involved in the distal suture line, then it is easier to perform this portion prior to beginning the distal suture line (Figure 38.18).

De-airing maneuvers are performed and the aortic cross-clamp removed. We like to leave an aortic root vent above the level of the distal aortic anastomosis throughout rewarming of the patient for continuous suction and evacuation of any air that may become apparent (Figure 38.19). Intraoperative TEE facilitates evaluation of residual intracavity air. CO_2 flooding of the field is helpful as well. Additional cardiopulmonary bypass techniques include both retrograde and antegrade blood cardioplegia and the use of a left ventricular vent.

Aortoplasty technique can be combined with insertion of a stentless valve including annulus enlargement with a patch of bovine pericardium or woven collagen impregnated Dacron. Either a Manouguian type enlargement can be accomplished with a patch extending from the mitral valve leaflet of the recipient and coming above for tailored enlargement of the aortic root (Figure 38.20). If this technique is utilized then it is best to secure the sutures of the patch enlargement at the level just below the sinus ridge for later completion after insertion of the heterograft. Reduction aortoplasties are more often required in the patients receiving stentless heterografts and this can be accomplished by either resection of a piece of aortic root (Figure 38.21) or by simply closing the vertical portion of the aortotomy with significant overlay (Figure 38.22). If a transverse aortotomy has been performed and enlargement or reduction of the non-coronary cusp region of the aortic root outflow is required, then a "T" incision can be performed

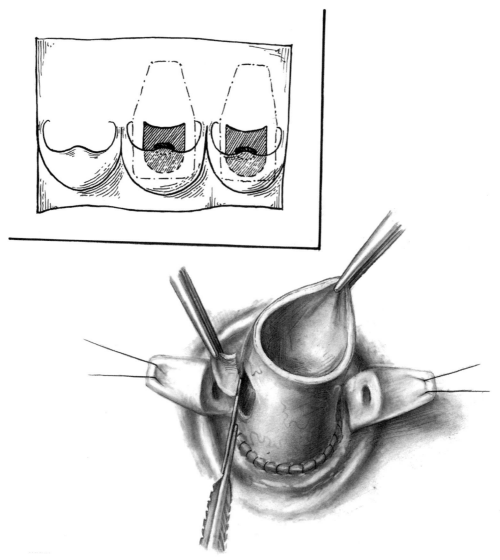

FIGURE 38.16. Aortic root replacement with stentless porcine heterograft. Coronary buttons are sutured to the respective sinuses. Mobilization of the right coronary button allows it to often be placed in the region of the new right sinus by removing the xenograft right coronary ostia. These buttons are made large and occasionally can extend up to the top of the suture line.

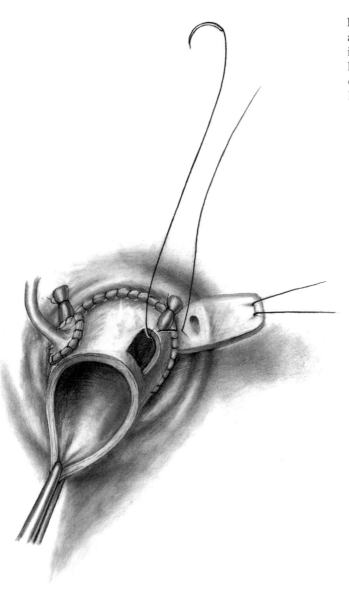

FIGURE 38.17. The coronary ostia are in slightly different locations in the pig aortic root than in the human, which occasionally mandates placing the coronary ostia higher than the native pig origins.

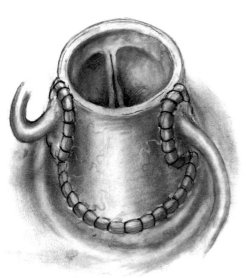

FIGURE 38.18. It is often useful to place the coronary buttons somewhat high in the xenograft root.

FIGURE 38.19. De-airing is performed. In this case it is shown with a "hockey stick" type aortotomy in which the distal suture line is placed inside the reconstructed ascending aorta as an inclusion technique. Aortic cross-clamp not shown.

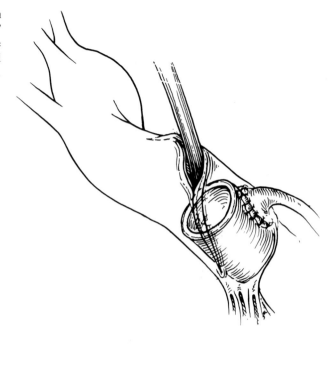

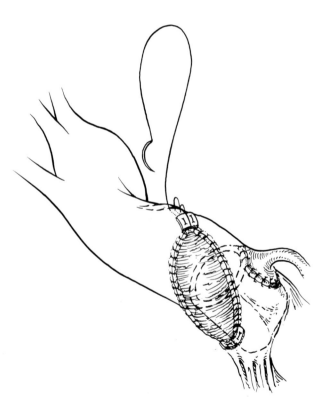

FIGURE 38.20. If the ascending aorta is too small or requires a larger stentless valve then an oval patch can be positioned to enlarge the aortotomy.

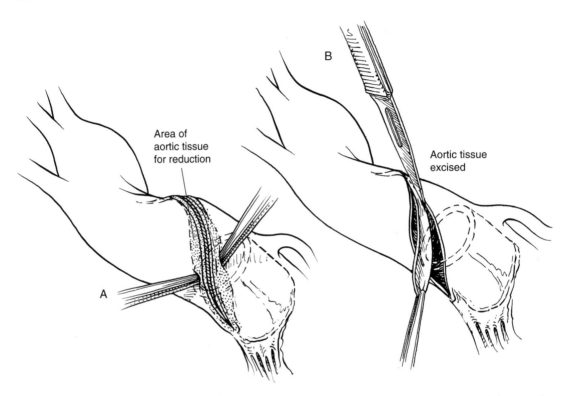

FIGURE 38.21. In older patients the ascending aorta is often moderately aneurysmal and should be reduced to reestablish a normal ascending aortic diameter. (A) Assessing excess tissue. (B) Resection of excess tissue.

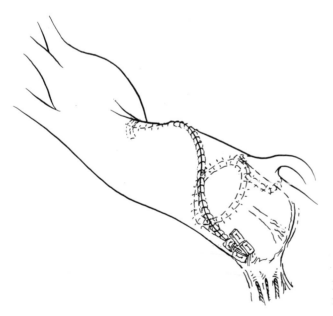

FIGURE 38.22. Closure of the aortotomy following stentless aortic root inclusion.

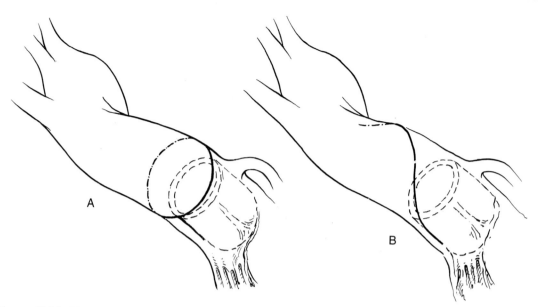

FIGURE 38.23. If transverse aortotomy has been performed and aortic root tailoring is required, then a "T" incision can be performed as demonstrated in **A**. If this is perceived by the surgeon prior to performing the aortotomy, then the "Lazy S" aortotomy is often easier to use when tailoring (**B**).

(Figure 38.23A). But usually this is apparent prior to performing the aortotomy and the "Lazy S" aortotomy can be chosen in these cases (Figure 38.23B).

References

1. Gott JP, Chih P, Dorsey L, Jay J, Jett GK, Schoen FJ et al. Calcification of Porcine Valves: A Successful New Method of Antimineralization. Ann Thorac Surg 1992;53:207–216.
2. Kunzelman KS, Grande KJ, David TE, Cochran RP, Verrier ED. Aortic root and valve relationships. Impact on surgical repair. J Thorac Cardiovasc Surg 1994;107:162–170.
3. Vesely I, Krucinski S, Campbell G. Micromechanics and mathematical modeling: an inside look at bioprosthetic valve function. J Card Surg 1992; 7:85–95.
4. Walther T, Falk V, Autschbach R, Scheidt A, Baryalei M, Schindewolf K et al. Hemodynamic assessment of the stentless Toroto SPV bioprosthesis by echocardiography. J Heart Valve Dis 1994; 3:657–665.
5. Jin XY, Zhang Z, Gibson DG, Yacoub MH, Pepper JR. Effects of valve substitute on changes in left ventricular function and hypertrophy after aortic valve replacement. Ann Thorac Surg 1996; 62:683–690.
6. Sintek CF, Fletcher AD, Khonsari S. Stentless Porcine Aortic Root: Valve of Choice for the Elderly Patient with Small Aortic Root? J Thorac Cardiovasc Surg 1995;109:871–876.
7. Jones EL, Shah VB, Shanewise JS, Martin TD, Martin RP, et al. Should the Freehand Allograft be Abandoned as a Reliable Alternative for Aortic Valve Replacement? Ann Thorac Surg 1995;59:1397–1404.
8. Kon ND, Westaby S, Pillae R, Amaresena N, Cordell R. Comparison of implant techniques using freestyle stentless porcine aortic valve. Ann Thorac Surg 1995;59:857–862.

Section X
Surgical Techniques:
Ross Operation and Variants

39
Indications: Ross Operation

Richard A. Hopkins

Since the first report of the pulmonary autograft procedure by Donald Ross in the *Lancet*, 1967, there has been a slow but steady increase in its acceptance as a procedure of choice for specific patient subsets.[1–8] As the advantages have been gradually delineated, the procedure has been expanded to include not only children, but neonates, and in patients with significant distortion of the left ventricular outflow tract.[9–12] The durability of the pulmonary valve appears to be excellent once initial technical difficulties have been overcome. The advantages are that the valve is a living and potentially growing valve, and as a consequence, it has the ability to respond to stresses and repair itself.[11] There are no immunological issues. In most patients, the geometric match is appropriate with the pulmonary valve being slightly larger than the native aortic annulus. Studies suggest that the long-term durability is extraordinary with the potential that the most patients might never need another aortic outflow tract procedure.[5] In addition, the patients do not require anticoagulation and the hemodynamics are superior to any others that have been measured.

Currently this is the aortic valve replacement of choice in my practice for patients under the age of 55 years who have relatively well maintained ventricular function, have a potential life expectancy greater than 20 years and particularly for those with some additional contraindication to anticoagulation such as being a young female entering the pregnancy years, a competitive athlete, or a child trying to live a normal life. We have combined it with other procedures such as coronary bypass grafting, complex congenital reconstructions (*vida infra*) and AV valve reconstructions.

As delineated in the following sections, the Ross procedure requires attention to detail and the ability to visualize the outflow tract as a total reconstruction. As such, the lessons learned from homograft valve reconstructions of the left ventricular outflow tract are to a great extent translatable to the Ross operation. The Ross operation has replaced the homograft as our replacement valve of choice for appropriate younger patients with most indications except for complex combined multilevel outflow tract disease, coexisting pulmonary valve pathology, connective tissue disease, severe destructive endocarditis, or when other indications for anticoagulation coexist. We never utilize the procedure in patients older than 60.

There are many important technical details that need to be learned that lead to consistently successful use of the pulmonary valve autotransplant. Yet, the operation and its principles solve many difficult issues even in complex neonatal reconstructions. Thus, a significant amount of space in this book has been allocated to a refined and complete presentation of the many applications of the "Ross procedure."

References

1. Ross DN. Replacement of the aortic and mitral valve with a pulmonary valve autograft. Lancet 1967;2:956–958.

2. Somerville J, Saravalli O, Ross D, Stone S. Long term results of pulmonary autograft for aortic valve replacement. British Heart Journal 1979; 42:533–540.

3. Matsuki O, Okita Y, Almeida RS, McGoldrich JP, Hooper TL, Robles A, Ross DN. Two decades experience with aortic valve replacement with pulmonary autograft. J Thorac Cardiovasc Surg 1988;95:705–711.

4. Joyce F, Tingleff J, Pettersson G. Expanding indications for the Ross Operation. J Heart Valve Dis 1995;4:352–363.

5. Ross D, Jackson M, Davies J. Pulmonary Autograft Aortic Valve Replacement: Long-Term Results. J Card Surg 1991;6:529–533.

6. Gerosa G, McKay R, Ross DN. Replacement of the aortic valve or root with a pulmonary autograft in children. Ann Thorac Surg 1991;51: 424–429.

7. Ross D, Jackson M, Davies J. The pulmonary autograft–a permanent aortic valve. EJCTS 1992; 6:113–6; discuss.

8. Gerosa G, McKay R, Davies J, Ross DN. Comparison of the aortic homograft and the pulmonary autograft for aortic valve or root replacement in children. J Thorac Cardiovasc Surg 1991;102:51–60; discus.

9. Elkins RC, Knott-Craig CJ, Ward KE, Lane MM. The Ross Operation in Children: 10 year experience. Ann Thorac Surg 1998;65:496–502.

10. Sievers HH, Leyh R, Loose R, Guha M, Petry A, Bernhard A. Time course of dimension and function of the autologous pulmonary root in the aortic position. J Thorac Cardiovasc Surg 1993; 105:775–780.

11. Elkins RC, Knott-Craig CJ, Ward KE, McCue C, Lane MM. Pulmonary autograft in children: realized growth potential. Ann Thorac Surg 1994;57:1387–1394.

12. David TE, Omran A, Webb G, et al. Geometric Mismatch of the aortic and pulmonary root causes aortic insufficiency after the Ross procedure. J Thorac Cardiovasc Surg 1996;112:1231–1239.

40
Surgical Anatomy: Ross Operation

Patricia A. Penkoske and Robert H. Anderson

The early morbidity and mortality of the Ross Procedure was attributed mainly to hemorrhage and to problems in harvesting the pulmonary autograft or implanting the pulmonary homograft. Arrhythmias were attributed to injury to the first septal perforator. Since the very early experience of Dr. Ross[1] there have been remarkably few reports of similar problems with this area. We will concentrate of four areas: the anatomy of the right ventricular outflow tract, aortic/pulmonary valve relationships, coronary artery anatomy in normal hearts, and coronary artery anatomy in hearts with aortic stenosis.

To this end, 45 autopsy specimens were examined at the Children's Hospital of Pittsburgh: 20 normal hearts being compared with 25 from patients with valvar aortic stenosis with or without insufficiency.

Anatomy of the Right Ventricular Outflow Tract

Before describing variations in coronary arterial anatomy, it is imperative to have a clear understanding of the anatomy of the pulmonary valve, specifically of the components of the pulmonary infundibulum (Figure 40.1). Excellent work in this area was published many years ago,[2,3] and will be amplified here.

The pulmonary valve is, in most cases, a trileaflet valve supported by a muscular infundibulum. The infundibulum has two components, a free-standing component existing in a plane superior to the muscle of the right ventricular (RV) wall and an "internal" component below the surface of the RV wall. The pulmonary valve therefore, sits higher than the RV mass, since it is supported by this free-standing infundibulum. When excising the autograft, the dissection is carried down from superiorly and stops when the RV mass is encountered. The height of this free-standing infundibulum is remarkably consistent, both in normal hearts and those with aortic pathology, ranging from 5 to 10 mm in length (5 mm—20%, 6 mm—30%, 7 mm—30%, 8–10 mm—20%). There were no differences in this anatomy between the two groups.

The pulmonary valve has not received as much interest as the aortic valve, but it's interrelationships and anatomy are crucial to both the Ross procedure and also the arterial switch operation. As already discussed, the pulmonary valve is, in most cases, a trileaflet valve. Its suitability as a systemic valve should always have been assessed preoperatively using an echocardiograph.

The three leaflets are right and left facing relative to the right and left coronary leaflets of the aortic valve, and the non-facing or lateral leaflet (Figure 40.2). In both the normal and abnormal hearts examined, these leaflets were equal in their circumferential extent. As with the aortic valve,[4] there is no true basal collagenous annulus supporting the valvar subcomponents. Instead the overall structure is similar to the aortic valve, with sinuses, leaflets and a

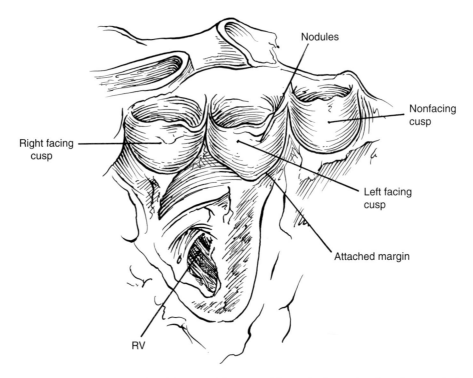

FIGURE 40.1. The infundibulum of the right ventricle opened from the front showing the morphology of the pulmonary valve.

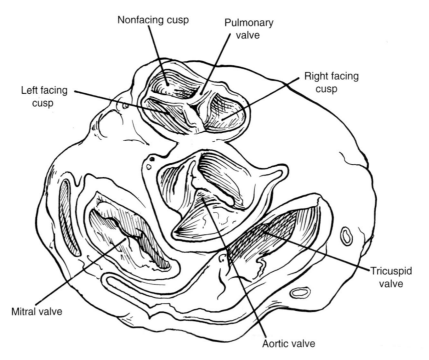

FIGURE 40.2. The atrioventricular junction viewed from its atrial aspect after removal of the atrial chambers and great arteries. It shows the relationship of the leaflets of the pulmonary valve and aortic valve. Two leaflets of these valves always face each other, permitting the normination of right-facing and left-facing leaflets of the pulmonary valves.

supporting infundibulum with three fibrous interleaflet triangles. The free surface of the leaflets is thickened at the point of coaptation to form a lunula. This is not as discrete a structure as in the aortic valve, nor is there such a well-developed sino-tubular ridge. A possible explanation for this is the lower pressures to which the right ventricular outflow tract is exposed, or the more proximal bifurcation of the pulmonary tract.

Aortic/Pulmonary Valvar Relationship

In performing the Ross procedure, plane must be developed first between the aortic and pulmonary valves, and then posterior to the pulmonary infundibulum. This extends 4 to 5 mm below the edge of the left facing and lateral pulmonary valvar leaflets during the harvesting of the autograft. The first area contains dense connective tissue, which must be sharply divided, but then one encounters a well developed plane of cleavage in the region of the free-standing pulmonary root. This plane is particularly well developed in neonates and young children.

Coronary Arterial Anatomy in Normal Hearts

Critical for safe excision of the autograft is a knowledge of the anatomy of the left coronary artery. The main stem of the left coronary has been reported to vary in length from 2–20 mm.[5] In the hearts examined, its length was from 1 to 8 mm. The first branch of the left anterior descending may be a infundibular branch, completing the "ring of Vieussens," but the descending artery gives off from 3 to 6 perforating arteries.[6] There is some discussion over whether all are similar in size, or whether the first is the largest. In our hearts, the latter was the case. This first perforator courses at right angles to the descending artery (Figure 40.3) and enters the septum 1 to 6 mm beneath the endocardium. It supplies the proximal part of the septomarginal trabecula (septal band) and a portion of the right and left bundle branches. Injuring the proximal descending artery would undoubtedly be a fatal event, with the resulting arrhythmias and cardiac dysfunction almost certainly occurring secondary to injury to the first septal perforator.

An understanding of the relationship of this perforator to the pulmonary valvar leaflets is helpful during harvesting of its autograft. A

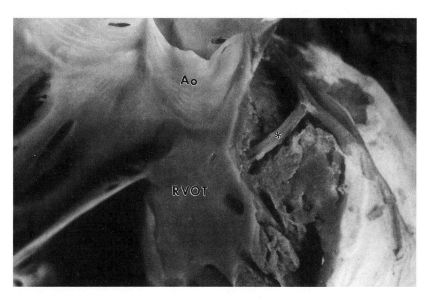

FIGURE 40.3. Demonstration LAD/septal perforator normal heart. Asterisk (*) marks the large first septal perforator coursing behind the right ventricular outflow tract in a normal heart (Ao = aorta; RVOT = right ventricular outflow tract).

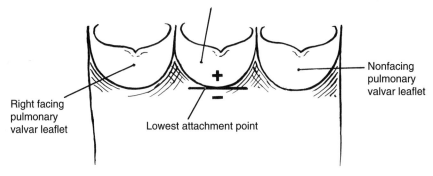

FIGURE 40.4. Line drawing of measurements made in right ventricular outflow tract. A+ indicates the level of the septal perforator was above the level of the left pulmonary cusp attachment and a negative number below.

wide variation has been described in normal hearts, with 30% showing a proximal origin above the pulmonary root, 25% at the level of the root and 45% below the pulmonary root. For our analysis, as a reference point we took the zone of apposition (in old terms the commissure) between the left facing and lateral pulmonary valvar leaflets. We have measured the level of the perforator by comparing it to the lowest portion of attachment of the left pulmonary valvar leaflet (Figure 40.4). A positive number means the perforator was above the lowest point of attachment of the valvar leaflets and a negative number, below. In normal hearts, 75% of cases showed the first septal perforator arising 1 to 2 mm before this junction, in other words directly posterior to the left leaflet of the pulmonary valve. In 15% of cases, the first septal perforator originated at the commissure and, in the remaining 10%, 0 to 3 mm, lateral to the commissure or in the region of the lateral pulmonary valvar leaflets. In the superior/inferior axis, 35% of the first perforating arteries originated superior to the lowest point of the attachment of the pulmonary valvar leaflet and 65% at or lower than that attachment.

Coronary Arterial Anatomy in Hearts with Aortic Stenosis/Insufficiency

In the hearts examined with aortic valvar pathology, the main stem of the left coronary artery was much shorter, being 1 to 2 mm in all cases. In the hearts with aortic stenosis, therefore, the artery that begins to course towards the posterior surface of the pulmonary artery is actually the anterior descending that lies 2 to 3 mm behind the pulmonary artery in the region of the free-standing pulmonary root. It is surrounded by fatty tissue in this area.[7] Concerning its relationships, in 60% of cases the first septal perforator originated 1 to 3 mm medial to the "commissure" between the left facing and non-facing sinus, and in 40% of cases it was either found at the "commissure" or lateral to it, findings similar to those seen in normal hearts (Figure 40.5).

The superior/inferior relationships to the inferior attachment of the left pulmonary artery leaflet were also comparable to normals, with the perforator being inferior to the leaflet attachment in 60% and superior in 40%.

In excising the autograft, therefore, the danger point can be localized to an area 3 mm on either side of the commissure between the left and lateral pulmonary valvar leaflets and, in the superior/inferior axis from 2 to 3 mm above and below the inferior attachment of the left pulmonary valvar leaflet. This is also the area that is at risk when suturing on the new homograft.

The most remarkable finding in examining all the hearts with aortic stenosis was the paucity and hypoplasia of the septal perforating arteries (Figures 40.6 and 40.7). It has been mentioned,[8] although not documented, that with the hypertrophy of the septum present in aortic stenosis, one would expect very large septal

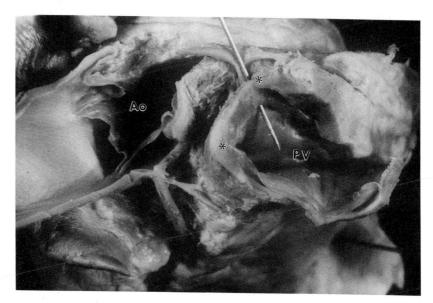

FIGURE 40.5. Origin of the first septal perforator in a normal heart demonstrating relationship to pulmonary valve (Ao = aorta; PV = pulmonary valve, * = commissure).

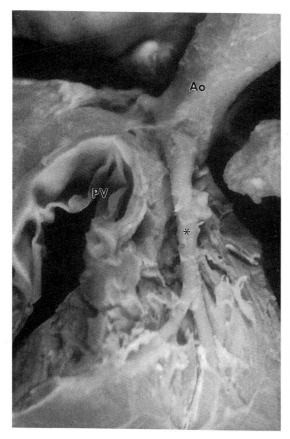

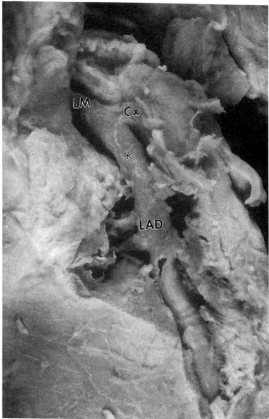

FIGURE 40.6. Relationship of left main coronary artery to pulmonary root in a heart with aortic stenosis. The asterisk (*) shows the region where the septal perforators originated in normal hearts. There are a paucity of these vessels (Ao = aorta; PV pulmonary valve).

FIGURE 40.7. Detailed coronary anatomy in a heart with aortic stenosis—there are virtually no septal perforators in the area posterior to the right ventricular outflow tract (LM = left main coronary artery; Cx = circumflex coronary artery; LAD = left anterior descending coronary artery; * = area behind right ventricular outflow tract.

perforators. We were surprised to find these consistently tiny vessels, but this may explain the paucity of recently reported problems with harvesting of autografts. Care should still be taken since the anterior descending artery itself is also at risk. Bleeding would be problematic in this area, and assessment should be made by instilling cardioplegia prior to reconstructing the RV outflow tract with the homograft.

A recent study in patients with idiopathic hypertrophic subaortic stenosis has suggested that purposeful ablation of the first septal perforator by alcohol injection in the catheterization laboratory not only was not harmful, but lead to a reduction in septal mass and a decrease in gradients. This finding suggests the first septal perforator may not be as vital a structure as previously thought and may explain the paucity of recently reported cases of fatalities with the Ross procedure.

References

1. Kouchoukos NT, David TE, Elkins RC, Ergin A, Luciani GB. Discussion: Session I—Ascending Aorta. Ann Thorac Surg 1999;67:1853–1856.

2. Geens M, Gonzales-Lavin L, Dawbarn C, Ross DN. The surgical anatomy of the pulmonary artery root in relation to the pulmonary valve autograft and surgery of the right ventricular outflow tract. Thoracic and Cardiovascular Surgeon 1972;62:262–267.

3. Gonzales-Lavin L, Geens, Ross DN. Aortic valve replacement with a pulmonary valve autograft: Indications and surgical techniques. Surgery 1970; 68:450–455.

4. Sutton JP, Ho SY, Anderson RH. The forgotten interleaflet triangles: a review of the surgical anatomy of the aortic valve. Annals of the Thoracic Surgery 1995;59:419–427.

5. McAlpine WA. Heart and Coronary Arteries. New York: Springer-Verlag 1975.

6. Stelzer P, Elkins RC. Pulmonary autograft: An American experience. J Carciac Surg 1987;2: 429–433.

7. Grondin C. Surgical Anatomy of the coronary arteries. In Baue A, Geha AS, Lako H, Hammond GL, Naunheim KS (eds). Glenn's Thoracic and Cardiovascular Surgery. New York, NY: Appleton and Lang 1996:2057–2066.

8. Sigwart U. Non-surgical myocardial reduction for hypertropic obstructive cardiomyopathy. Lancet 1995;346:221–214.

41
Surgical Technique: Ross Operation

Richard A. Hopkins

The median sternotomy is performed in the usual way. Cannulation is accomplished as high on the ascending aorta as possible or as femoral artery cannulation. We use a single atrial return cannula but bicaval cannulation is preferred by some authorities or by us when other reconstructive procedures are needed in the patient.[1-3] Left ventricular venting is accomplished via the right superior pulmonary vein. Mild total body hypothermia is used with cardioplegic arrest supplemented by topic slush cooling. Multiple doses of cold blood cardioplegia are delivered antegrade at 20 minute intervals via direct coronary cannulas and retrograde as well. We use a high-dose aprotinin protocol and heparin bonded cardiopulmonary circuits (Carmeda) for Ross operations.

After cannulation and cooling has begun, the outside of the heart is examined. Measurements are made at the base of the pulmonary artery trunk and the base of the aorta to give a rough estimate of external size to compare to the measurements being made with the transesophageal echocardiography probe. Examination of the aorta and pulmonary artery externally gives some idea as to whether there might be distortions that would prevent Ross type reconstructions. Once the heart is empty and cooling has progressed, the pulmonary artery dissection is begun. The pulmonary artery is separated from the aorta with blunt and sharp dissection, preferably performed as much as possible with the electrocautery (Figure 41.1). This dissection is relatively extensive and extends down to the base of each great

vessel. Care is taken to identify the origin of the right coronary artery and to get a feel for the external position of the left main coronary artery, although not necessarily completely exposing it at this stage. The pulmonary artery is transected just below the bifurcation and the pulmonary valve inspected (Figure 41.2). At this stage, the operation can be abandoned if there are congenital or acquired abnormalities of the pulmonary valve that would preclude its use for a Ross operation. We do this prior to cross-clamping the aorta so that cross-clamp time has been saved if alternative prostheses are needed (eg. homograft, stentless valve, etc.). The aorta is now cross-clamped and the heart is stilled with an infusion of cold blood cardioplegia (if there is severe aortic insufficiency, the heart is stopped with retrograde cold cardioplegia first and then the aorta opened. Antegrade cardioplegia is now delivered if necessary via direct soft cardioplegia cannula. The aortotomy is selected based on the intended backup plan (if the Ross procedure is not utilized). Thus, a transverse aortotomy is performed if a stentless porcine valve insertion is envisioned. If a root replacement with a porcine root is envisioned, then any type of aortotomy can be performed. We tend to use a modified "hockey stick" incision if a backup plan for a traditional manufactured prosthesis is contemplated (Figure 41.3). The aortic valve is now examined and excised. The annulus of the pulmonary artery is measured with Hegar dilators internally, carefully placed inside the valve leaflets and then matched to the aortic size. Alterna-

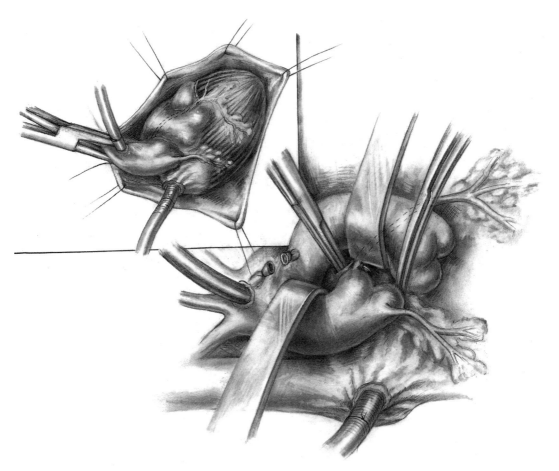

FIGURE 41.1. Dissecting the pulmonary artery from the aorta. Inset emphasizes LAD coronary.

tively manufacturers' valve sizers can be used with the intent of assessing whether the pulmonary artery is the same or larger than the aorta. The best repairs appear to be with the pulmonary valve internal annulus size being at least two millimeters larger than the aortic internal diameter. If the aortic annulus is more than 6mm larger than the pulmonary artery diameter, then we do not use aortic annulus reduction techniques but instead abandon the Ross operation. Although David, Elkins and others have reported annulus adjustment techniques, we have avoided their use except in the most compelling of circumstances and as such have yet to have late aortic insufficiency develop in a Ross procedure due to acute or gradual annular dilatation.[4-6] If there is significant calcification of the aortic annulus, then

geometric mismatch is even less tolerable as the ability to reduce the aortic annulus is less. Enlargement of the aortic annulus is easily accomplished with Manouguian or Nicks type of techniques but reduction in size can be fraught with late failure.[7]

If the geometric match appears appropriate then attention is turned to excising the pulmonary valve. An incision is made in the right ventricular outflow tract, well below the level of the valve. There is usually a muscular clear space where no fat is present which is marker for the infundibulum well beneath base of the pulmonary valve. Our incision begins at that point and is angled up towards the annulus on either side (Figure 41.4). The incision is brought around the right side of the pulmonary trunk to the back of the annulus at which time the left

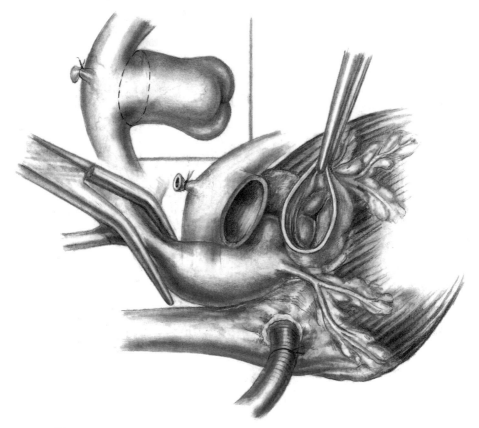

FIGURE 41.2. Pulmonary artery transected. Pulmonary valve inspected.

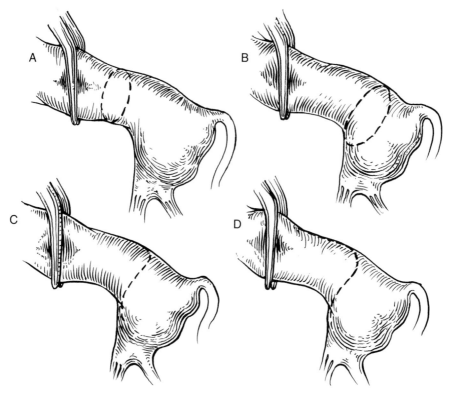

FIGURE 41.3. Aortic incision is determined by the backup operations. Ross procedure is best with high transverse.

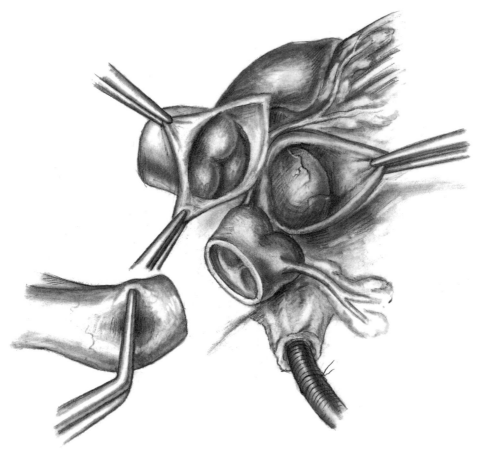

FIGURE 41.4. Incision in the right ventricular outflow tract to excise pulmonary valve.

coronary artery is visualized in the bed of fat behind the pulmonary artery and bluntly dissected away from the pulmonary trunk (Figure 41.5). The dissection of the left side of the pulmonary artery resection is now performed extremely carefully, keeping the scissors in a cephalocaudad orientation and parallel to the floor. This helps the operator stay away from the first septal perforator artery (Figure 41.6). If the septal artery can be visualized, then it can easily be avoided. Often it cannot be visualized and by staying very close to the pulmonary annulus, damage is avoided. As the final separation is accomplished, the pulmonary valve complex is retracted towards the patient's left knee and the incision is brought across the posterior fibrous connection, keeping the left coro-

nary artery cephalad and posterior to the incision (Figure 41.7).

Cardioplegia is usually repeated at this point and the coronary buttons excised. These buttons are excised as large sinus buttons. They can always be trimmed smaller later on as necessary (Figure 41.8). Minimal dissection is performed at the base of the right and left coronary artery to increase their mobility. Stay sutures are applied to the top of each and retracted away from the aortic root as the aortic root is being excised (Figure 41.9). Debridement of the annulus is performed. Care is taken to avoid any damage to the mitral valve. Incision down to the level of the muscle for at least a part of the aortic root excision at the left anterior septal portion of the dissection ensures the

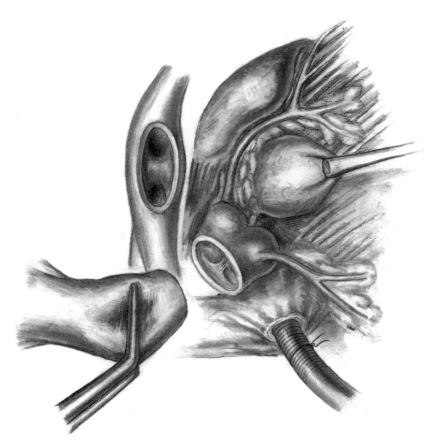

FIGURE 41.5. Dissection behind pulmonary root, in the fat plane.

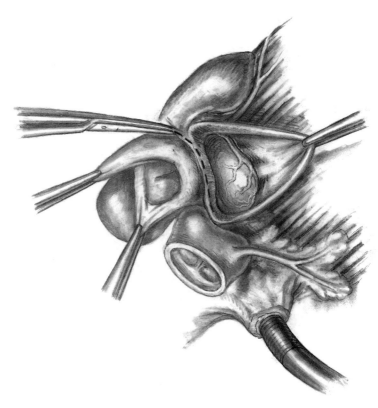

FIGURE 41.6. Pulmonary valve retracted superiorly gives access to posterior base in muscle.

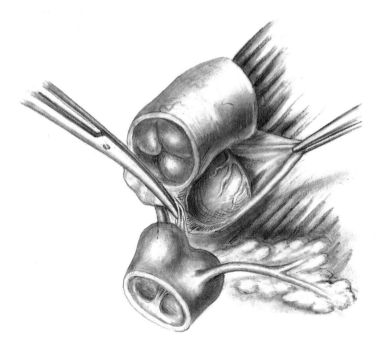

FIGURE 41.7. Final separation of pulmonary valve complex.

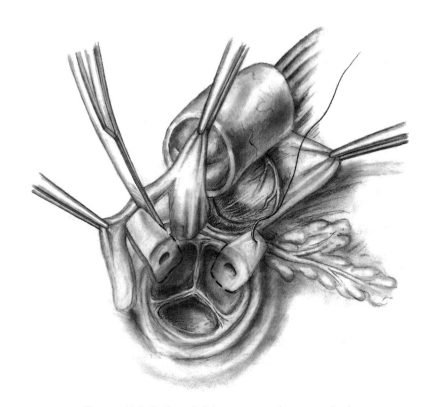

FIGURE 41.8. Left and right coronary sinuses excised.

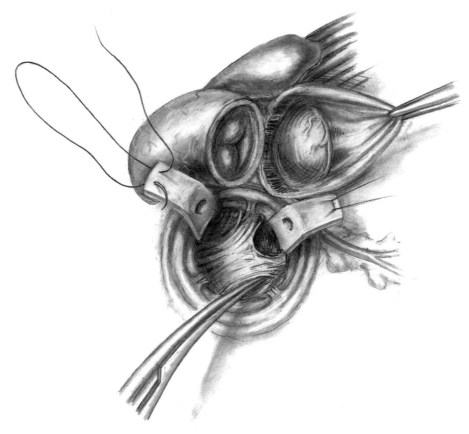

FIGURE 41.9. Aortic root "removed."

aortic root expands slightly. Alternatively, if the annulus size is "perfect" then some fibrous tissue on the aortic root base cylinder can be left circumferentially to aid in suture placement.[8–11]

Sutures are placed as simple sutures through the aortic annulus base and then through the base of the pulmonary valve. We tend to work from the left side along the posterior row first, working towards the surgeon on the right side of the table (Figure 41.10). Once the posterior 180° has been accomplished, the final clamp is clipped inside the jaws of the Allis clamp and can be laid down on the drapes superiorly, thus keeping the posterior row of sutures in order.

The orientation of the pulmonary valve complex is made by definition with the placement of this posterior suture row by committing the middle portion of the larger sinus of the pulmonary valve to the left coronary sinus region with an eye to simplifying placement of the left coronary button. It is preferable to plan to place the left coronary button slightly higher than it originally was on the aorta, but with minimal distortion in any other direction (Figure 41.11). Given good placement, stretching the left main coronary artery more than 1 mm cephalad is not necessary. The anterior row of simple sutures is placed, once again working from the patient's left side to the right side and thus working toward the surgeon (Figure 41.12). Once all sutures have been placed, a strip of Teflon felt, 2 mm in width, is slipped through the sutures as the autograft is parachuted down into the base of the aortic outflow. The Teflon is dampened with saline containing

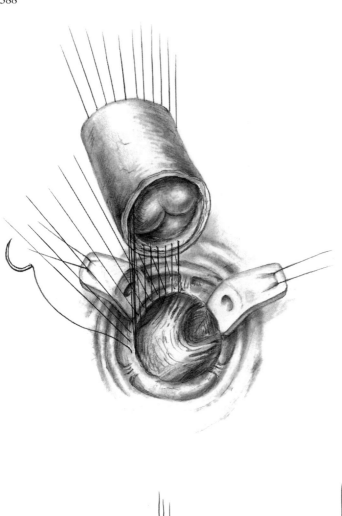

FIGURE 41.10. Figure of posterior row simple sutures. Each suture is placed in its own clamp and slipped over an Allis clamp to maintain orientation.

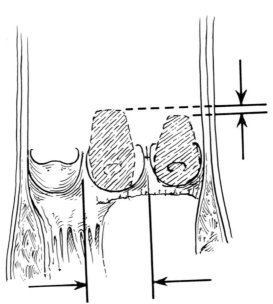

FIGURE 41.11. Alignment of left coronary button to its new sinus of the autograft.

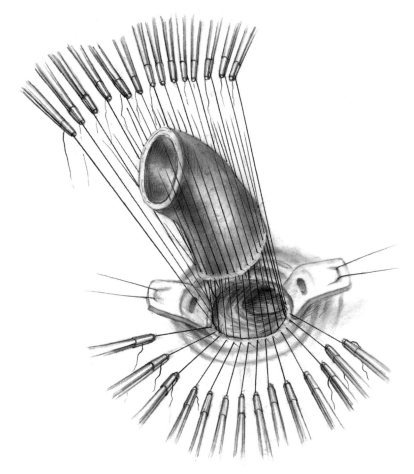

FIGURE 41.12. Proximal suture line.

antibiotics to help in its caulking function (Figure 41.13).

The sutures are sequentially tied, working sequentially from the surgeon's side and tying each suture sequentially moving from right to left. We prefer to tie the posterior row so that the inside "seating" can be checked. The anterior row is completed and the sutures tied. Our preference for suture material is 3-0 (in adults) or 4-0 (in children and neonates), coated braided suture (Tycron©: on the Tycron brand suture material we prefer the T16 needle). The left coronary button is sutured to its position on the posterior sinus. A small button of autograft tissue is excised. A somewhat larger button of aortic wall tissue is left around the coronary ostia and sutured to the orifice with a running

5-0 polypropylene suture technique, either working from posteriorly or occasionally working from inside the autograft, whichever is simpler (Figure 41.14). Usually at this point, we similarly place the right coronary button in its respective sinus. There is usually a bit more "play" with the right button. We take care to more it superiorly and then either to the right or the left as is necessary to avoid tension. If it is difficult to arrange the button, then the distal suture line can be accomplished first and then the button sutured. The advantage of suturing the right coronary button prior to the distal anastomosis is that damage to the pulmonary valve leaflet can be avoided and that suturing can be accomplished from both inside and outside as necessary. For smaller children or

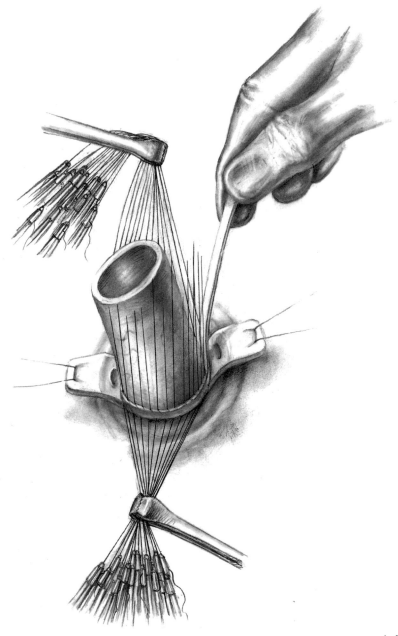

FIGURE 41.13. Seating of autograft. Felt inside suture loops, outside neo-aortic base.

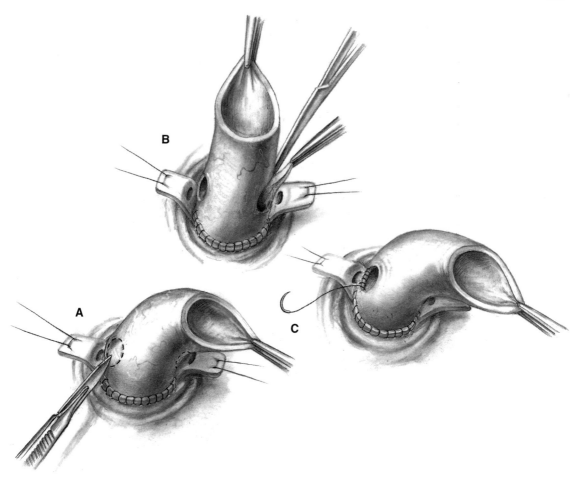

FIGURE 41.14. Coronary buttons being sutured.

neonates, we use 6-0 or 7-0 polypropylene for the buttons (Figure 41.14). The distal suture line is accomplished with a running polypropylene suture reinforced with a strip of Teflon felt. The suture is usually 4-0 polypropylene for adults and 5-0 for children. The reinforcement Teflon felt is helpful as the distal pulmonary artery autograft tissue is often quite thin. The elasticity of the pulmonary artery leads to great flexibility in this distal anastomosis, but as necessary, incisions in the aorta or plication to tailor its size is sometimes necessary (Figure 41.15).

Restoration of the right ventricular outflow tract is accomplished. A homograft has been thawed of appropriate size. We prefer a pul-monary valve but do not hesitate to use an aortic valve homograft if necessary. The valve graft is sized to be the size of the patient's own valve or larger. There is significant expansion of the right ventricular outflow orifice as a consequence of the "V" infundibular incision and thus it is often easier to select a homograft larger than the native; we routinely "upsize" the RVOT valve in pediatric Ross operations.[12,13]

The distal anastomosis of the homograft to the pulmonary artery just below the bifurcation is accomplished with a running 5-0 (adult) or 6-0 (pediatric) polypropylene suture (Figure 41.16). No Teflon felt is used in this anastomosis. It is our preference to accomplish this anas-

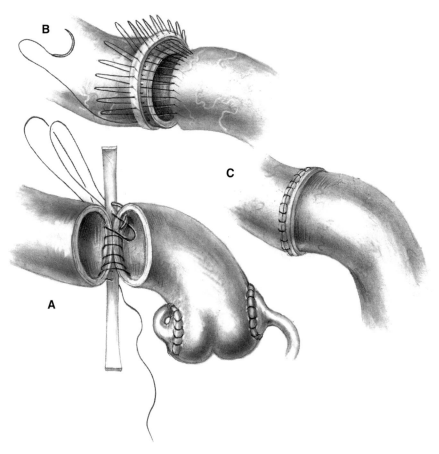

Figure 41.15. Technique for distal anastomosis. Continuous suture with felt strip.

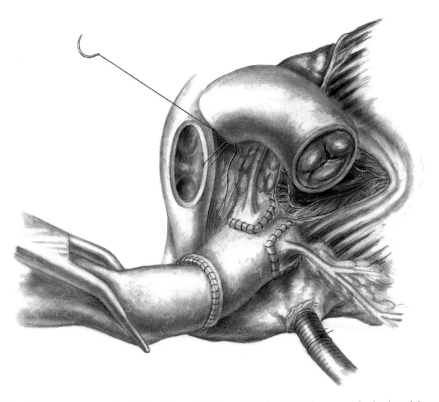

Figure 41.16. PA anastomoses distal first. Length (for clarity) of PA homograft depicted longer than is typical. Should keep segment short to "suspend" semilunar pulmonary valve complex.

FIGURE 41.17. Beginning the posterior RVOT suture line.

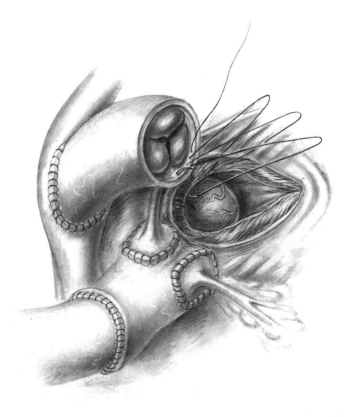

tomosis prior to removing the cross clamp. Cardioplegia can be delivered via the aortic root needle which is in the aortic root above the level of the distal anastomosis at this stage which allows for checking of the integrity of all of the aortic suture lines. We initiate this with cold cardioplegia which continues the myocardial protection while additional sutures are placed in the aorta or distal pulmonary artery anastomosis. This step also allows visualization of any coronary arterial leaks in the muscle of the right ventricular outflow tract which can be easily electrocauterized for hemostasis. Once hemostasis is felt to be adequate, then cardioplegia is changed to warm (hot shot) cardioplegia for five minutes as the suturing of the proximal pulmonary artery homograft is accomplished. This suturing is begun left and posteriorly in the region of the first septal perforator which allows the most accurately placed sutures (Figure 41.17). A strip of Teflon felt is placed at the posterior base of the right ventricular orifice and the sutures are place either through or around this as the base of the homo-

graft is sutured to the right ventriculotomy. These sutures are the secured at either end of the posterior suture line with additional sutures. Suture material is polypropylene of a 3-0 size for adults and, 4-0 size for children and 5-0 in neonates and infants. Once the posterior suture line of the right ventricular outflow tract has been secured, the aortic cross-clamp is removed. De-airing maneuvers are performed. Throughout the rewarming phase of the patient, continuous suction is applied to an aortic root vent. The anterior reconstruction of the pulmonary outflow tract is completed. There is often enough ventricular myocardium that the suture line can be continued anteriorly with muscle to the annulus of the homograft (Figure 41.18A). Augmentation of the right ventricular outflow tract connection to the anterior base of the homograft results in a smoother reconstruction and aids in upsizing the homograft. A piece of PTFE fashioned from a tube graft slightly larger than the homograft (Figure 41.18B), is used for this "gusset" or "hood."

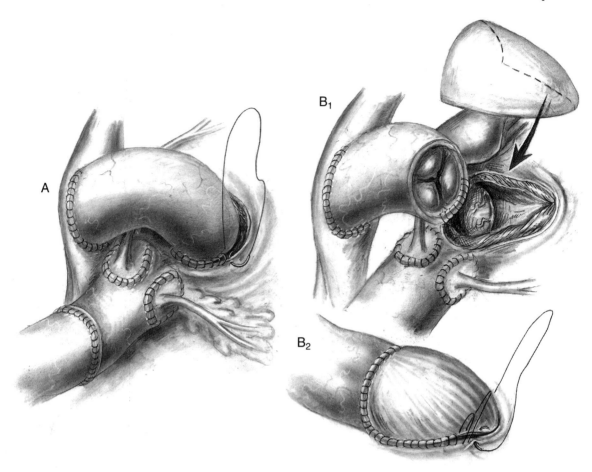

FIGURE 41.18. Completion. (A) Direct suturing of the muscle to the base of the homograft in the right ventricular outflow tract. Panel (B) PTFE "hood" added to ventricular outflow.

The patient is weaned from cardiopulmonary bypass after full rewarming. The decannulation is performed in the usual fashion. The pericardium is not closed in these patients. Hemostasis has been excellent especially after initiating the aprotinin protocol (*vida infra*).

Prior to separation from cardiopulmonary bypass, transesophageal echocardiography is performed to look for any gross malfunction of either the pulmonary or aortic valves (*vida infra*). The patient is weaned from cardiopulmonary bypass and transesophageal echocardiography repeated. Direct palpation of both the base of the aortic and pulmonary arterial reconstructions is performed and the absence of bruits correlates with absence of insuffi-

ciency. Blood pressures are maintained at around 100 Torr. In many cases, blood transfusions are not necessary. If there is oozing, then fibrin glue, either home made or manufactured, can be utilized to reinforce the hemostasis of the suture lines.

Postsurgical Management

Vigorous exercise, especially associated with the Valsalva maneuver, is avoided for the first six to eight weeks.[3] Patients are anticoagulated with aspirin only. Echocardiography follow up every six months for the first two years is required and then yearly thereafter.

References

1. Joyce F, Tingleff J, Pettersson G. Expanding indications for the Ross Operation. J Heart Valve Dis 1995;4:352–363.
2. Matsuki O, Okita Y, Almeida RS, McGoldrich JP, Hooper TL, Robles A, Ross DN. Two decades experience with aortic valve replacement with pulmonary autograft. J Thorac Cardiovasc Surg 1988;95:705–711.
3. Oury JH, Maxwell M. An appraisal of the Ross Procedure: Goals and Technical Guidelines. OTCTS 1997;2:289–301.
4. David TE, Omran A, Webb G, et al. Geometric Mismatch of the aortic and pulmonary root causes aortic insufficiency after the Ross procedure. J Thorac Cardiovasc Surg 1996;112:1231–1239.
5. Elkins RC, Knott-Craig CJ, Howell CE. Pulmonary autografts in patients with aortic annulus dilatation. Ann Thorac Surg 1996;61:1141.
6. Elkins RC. The Ross operation in patients with dilatation of the aortic annulus and of the ascending aorta. OTCTS 1997;2:331–341.
7. Daenen W, Conte S, Eyskens B, Gewillig M. Ross Procedure with Enlargement Annuloplasty. OTCTS 1997;2:318–330.
8. Ross DN. Replacement of the aortic and mitral valve with a pulmonary valve autograft. Lancet 1967;2:956–958.
9. Sievers HH, Leyh R, Loose R, Guha M, Petry A, Bernhard A. Time course of dimension and function of the autologous pulmonary root in the aortic position. J Thorac Cardiovasc Surg 1993;105:775–780.
10. Pettersson G, Joyce F, Tingleff J. The Pulmonary autograft (Ross Operation) for Aortic Valve Endocarditis. OTCTS 1997;2:302–317.
11. Gerosa G, McKay R, Ross DN. Replacement of the aortic valve or root with a pulmonary autograft in children. Ann Thorac Surg 1991;51:424–429.
12. Elkins RC, Knott-Craig CJ, Ward KE, McCue C, Lane MM. Pulmonary autograft in children: realized growth potential. Ann Thorac Surg 1994;57:1387–1394.
13. Ross D, Jackson M, Davies J. The pulmonary autograft—a permanent aortic valve. EJCTS 1992;6:113–116; discuss.

42
The Role of Transesophageal Echocardiography During the Ross Procedure

Arthur A. Bert and Scott F. MacKinnon

Introduction

Pulmonary autograft replacement of the aortic valve, the "Ross procedure," involves transplantation of the native pulmonary valve into the aortic position and reconstruction of the right ventricular outflow tract with a cryopreserved pulmonary or aortic homograft. In any surgeon's hands this operation is technically challenging and successful performance of the Ross procedure requires strategies to avoid coronary artery and myocardial injury and optimize post-transplantation pulmonary autograft architecture. Transesophageal echocardiography (TEE) can be instrumental in guiding surgical management of these patients.

Assessment of Pulmonary and Aortic Annuli Geometric Mismatch

It is now well delineated that geometric mismatch between the diseased aortic valve and the normal pulmonary valve is a common cause of significant aortic insufficiency and ultimately surgical failure after the Ross procedure. TEE is an excellent tool to assess both the aortic and pulmonary valve diameters and determine surgical feasibility of the Ross procedure prior to dissection and harvesting of the pulmonary autograft. The aortic valve can be visualized in a variety of TEE imaging planes. For measurement of the aortic valve annulus diameter and the aortic root we prefer the longitudinal plane (90°), basal short-axis view (transducer tip

25–30 cm from the incisors). With an omniplane transducer the preferred imaging plane is between 110°–130° (Figure 42.1). Longitudinal imaging at this level visualizes both the aortic valve annulus and 5–10 cm of the ascending aorta in the near field. Brief 2D imaging will recognize annuloaortic ectasia of Marfan's syndrome or an aortic root aneurysm. Most surgeons will not perform the Ross procedure if the aortic root diameter measures greater than 45–50 mm, whatever its etiology. In the absence of such pathology the aortic annulus diameter is measured from the "hinge" points where the posterior (non-coronary cusp) and anterior (right coronary cusp) leaflets attach to the walls of the left ventricular outflow tract (LVOT). The annulus is measured during diastole with the optimal plane for measurement being that which demonstrates the widest leaflet separation in systole. In heavily calcified valves the insertion sites of the leaflets may be difficult to image and the annulus is measured at the end of the LVOT.

TEE imaging and measurement of the pulmonary valve diameter is less reliable for a number of reasons. While the pulmonary valve can be visualized in a variety of scanning planes, it is most reliably imaged using the longitudinal plane, right ventricular outflow tract view which is obtained slightly above and with counterclockwise rotation from the aortic valve view in this plane. With an omniplane transducer the optimal plane is usually between 70°–80° (Figure 42.2). In this plane (and others) the pulmonary valve is imaged in the far field

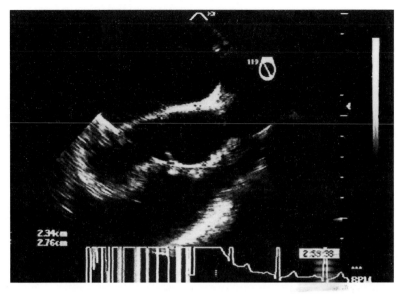

FIGURE 42.1. Left ventricular outflow tract (LVOT). Depicted here, markers are at annulus and sino-tubular junction.

where detail is often lost. Nevertheless the valve diameter is measured with 2-D echocardiography in this view, while color flow Doppler imaging is used to screen for any incompetence in the native valve. We will not harvest a native pulmonary valve that demonstrates even mild pulmonary regurgitation. The pulmonary valve diameter is again measured during diastole where the leaflets insert to the RVOT walls. This measurement often varies a few millimeters from the surgeon's sizer-derived diameter. The explanation for this observation may be related to the pulmonary valve's lack of a discrete annulus. The leaflets are partly attached to

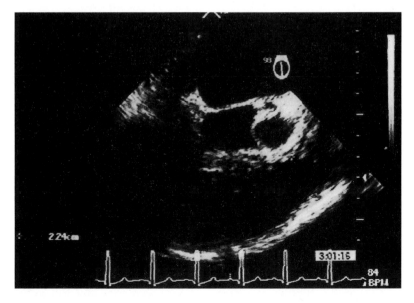

FIGURE 42.2. RVOT. Markers are placed at origin of pulmonic valve leaflets.

the relatively thin muscle of the infundibulum and partly to the pulmonary arterial wall. In vivo the pulmonary "annulus" is distensible and its diameter varies depending on the right ventricular stroke volume. When sized directly by standard cylindrical dilators one can easily stretch the pulmonary valve over a "larger" sizer. Nevertheless with close attention to these nuances, the TEE derived pulmonary valve diameter rarely varies from the "sized" diameter by more than 3 mm.

Geometric mismatch of the aortic and pulmonary annuli is the most common source of aortic insufficiency after the Ross procedure and at the extreme remains a contraindication to the procedure. Similar to the experience of Stelzer et al.,[1] we consider an aortic to pulmonary annulus discrepancy of 10 mm or more a contraindication to the Ross procedure. This magnitude of discrepancy is reliably determined by TEE and obviates dissection of the pulmonary artery trunk. Lesser degrees of valve size mismatch are reported to the surgeon and often helps direct the surgical plan. Our operative experience in a patient population of teenagers and young adults (age range 13 to 50 years) is not dissimilar from that of David and colleagues[2] in that the mean aortic annulus is 3 mm larger than the mean pulmonary anulus. We have not yet found a patient whose pulmonary valve diameter was larger than the aortic annulus. Use of an undersized pulmonary autograft in a dilated aortic annulus invites aortic insufficiency and compromises long-term outcome. Many surgeons[2,3] will perform some technique of aortic root tailoring when the aortic annulus diameter is 2–3 mm larger than the pulmonary anulus. TEE will usually alert the surgeon that the surgical plan is likely to require such a technique prior to initiation of cardiopulmonary bypass.

Evaluation of Ventricular Function

On-line assessment of ventricular function can be particularly useful during the Ross procedure since this surgery carries potential for injury to coronary arteries and the myocardium. Harvesting of the pulmonary autograft requires meticulous surgical dissection to avoid injuring the first septal perforator branch of the left anterior descending artery, whose origin lies precariously close to the base of the pulmonary valve. The preferred method of transplantation of the pulmonary autograft is the root inclusion technique because of its superiority in maintaining valve architecture. This technique requires reimplantation of the native coronary arteries into the autograft and both inadvertent coronary artery ligation or post-implant "kinking" have been reported as complications. Finally the complexity and extensive nature of the Ross procedure results in prolonged periods of iatrogenic cardiac arrest demanding optimal myocardial preservation to avoid myocardial injury. Despite improved operative techniques, myocardial failure remains the primary etiology of surgical mortality in the modern era.

The relationship between regional wall-motion abnormalities (RWMA) and myocardial ischemia is well described. In animal models of coronary artery occlusion the myocardium first contracts weakly (hypokinesis), then contracts not at all (akinesis) and finally bulges outward during systole (dyskinesis) following ligation of its supplying coronary artery. Based on acute changes in regional wall motion, cardiologists and anesthesiologists have used TEE to detect ischemic and infarcted myocardium reliably. During intraoperative TEE, the transgastric mid-papillary transverse-plane cross section of the left ventricle is a useful plane for regional wall motion assessment since this view visualizes myocardium perfused by all three coronary arteries and the majority of left ventricular contraction (80%) occurs along this short axis. This imaging plane is also a reliable monitor of left ventricular preload, in fact more reliable than pulmonary artery catheter pressures. Injury to the left main coronary artery or a large septal perforator branch would be readily identified by new RWMA following the Ross procedure. Inadequate myocardial preservation will also be readily identified and will present most often as a global diminution in endocardial excursion and wall thickening in comparison to pre-arrest myocardial wall motion.

TEE imaging at the basal short axis, transverse plane slightly above the aortic valve will reliably visualize the left main coronary ostia and initial few centimeters of the coronary artery. Using color flow Doppler, the anastomosis of the left coronary button can be assessed following transplantation of the pulmonary autograft. The color flow should demonstrate blood flow into the left coronary ostia and proximal artery. In the presence of anterior wall and interventricular septal hypokinesis or akinesis the absence of blood flow identifies this anastomosis as the culprit. The right coronary button is not as reliably imaged and obstruction of blood flow at this ostia is inferred by new wall motion abnormalities inferiorly and posteriorly.

Evaluation of Pulmonary Autograft Function

Following transplantation of the pulmonary autograft, TEE evaluation of the autograft function is critical to assess immediate surgical adequacy and predict the long-term results. In their retrospective series of 145 Ross operations Stelzer et al.[1] noted the consistent absence of any significant pressure gradient across the autograft on early and late follow-up echocardiographic examination. In this series and others, a tiny central jet of aortic regurgitation (AR) is commonly seen. Mild autograft regurgitation intraoperatively or in the early postsurgical period does not correlate with progression to more than mild regurgitation or the need for reoperation at follow-up. More than mild aortic regurgitation of the pulmonary autograft is problematic. While their reoperation rate for progressive autograft regurgitation was low (3.8%), Stelzer noted that all five patients were among the nine patients with more than mild aortic regurgitation on the initial echo evaluation. Most surgeons performing the Ross procedure today believe that more than mild regurgitation of the transplanted pulmonary autograft will likely be progressive over time and will jeopardize the long-term success of the surgery.

The detection of aortic regurgitation and quantification of its severity is reliably accomplished with TEE. Because the severity of valvular regurgitation cannot be assessed reliably with 2D echocardiography alone, we screen for pulmonary autograft regurgitation in the transverse five-chamber view with color flow Doppler (CFD). The presence of a mosaic-colored jet on the left ventricular outflow side of the aortic valve in diastole confirms the presence of regurgitation (Figure 42.3; see color insert). A quick and validated semiquantitative method of assessing aortic regurgitation is based on the measurement of the regurgitant jet width relative to the width of the LVOT. The AR jet width is measured nearest its origin as possible, usually about 5mm from the valve leaflets in this plane. Both measurements are based on those images with the maximal demonstrable AR jet and LVOT diameter and multiple planes of the five-chamber view must be imaged to avoid underestimates. Using this method, aortic regurgitation is quantified as follows: proximal jet width/ LVOT width <30% is mild AR, 30–65% is moderate AR and >65% is severe AR. This method has been demonstrated to be a good predictor of the angiographic AR severity. One disadvantage of this imaging plane is that highly eccentric regurgitant jets are often inaccurately assessed.

The decay of the AR jet velocity is a quantitative method that can used to confirm the transverse five-chamber view or assess the severity of an eccentric jet. With this technique a transgastric, long axis image (transverse plane) must be obtained (Figure 42.4; see color insert). Continuous wave Doppler (CWD) is used to obtain a maximum velocity waveform of the regurgitant jet across the aortic valve. As the size of the regurgitant orifice increases, the interval of time required for aortic pressure to equilibrate with ventricular pressure will decrease. Therefore the rate at which the AR jet velocity approaches zero can be used to evaluate the severity of regurgitation. This rate of decay of the AR jet velocity can be measured by either the slope or pressure half-time (the time interval for the peak velocity to decline to

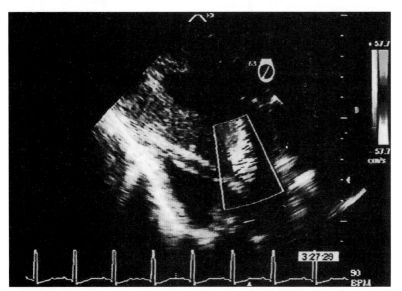

FIGURE 42.3. Deep, transgastric five chamber view permits accurate assessment of competency of newly placed autograft. In this picture, minimal insufficiency is noted.

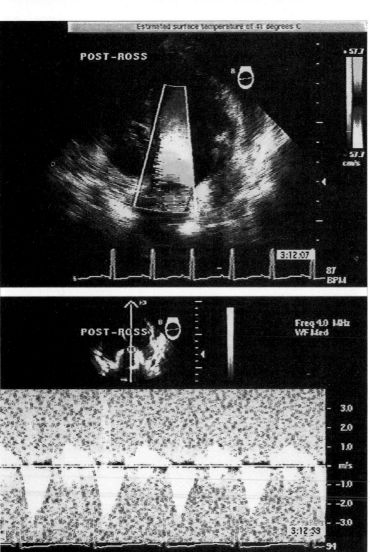

FIGURE 42.4. Deep, transgastric five chamber view of LVOT. Again, this orientation will permit adequate assessment of residual regurgitation. Using continuous wave Doppler, one can also assess a potential gradient.

the peak velocity divided by the square root of 2). Mild AR jets have a pressure half-time of greater than 400 msec, while severe AR jets are characterized by pressure half-times of less than 250 msec. The disadvantage of this technique is that image and maximum velocity waveform can be difficult to acquire, and its poorer correlation with angiographic AR severity. Nevertheless we use both techniques to assess post-transplant autograft function. Regurgitation greater than mild severity is considered an unacceptable surgical result.

References

1. Stelzer P, Weinrauch S, Tranbaugh RF. Ten years experience with the modified Ross procedure. J Thorac Cardiovasc Surg 1998;115:1091–1100.
2. David TE, Omran A, Webb G, et al. Geometric Mismatch of the aortic and pulmonary root causes aortic insufficiency after the Ross procedure. J Thorac Cardiovasc Surg 1996;112:1231–1239.
3. Durham LA, desJardins SE, Mosca RS, Bove EL. Ross procedure with aortic root tailoring for aortic valve replacement in the pediatric population. Ann Thorac Surg 1997;64:482–486.

43
Guidelines for Use of Aprotinin with the Ross Procedure

Arthur A. Bert

While the clinical indications and surgical techniques of the Ross procedure continue to evolve, present-day success is focused on three areas: architecture of the pulmonary autograft, optimal myocardial protection and meticulous hemostasis. Aprotinin is a pharmacologic agent that has proven highly effective in reducing blood loss and the need for homologous blood product transfusions after cardiac surgical procedures requiring cardiopulmonary bypass. However, aprotinin safety in certain types of cardiac surgery is still being defined and its expense is substantial. In addition, alternative pharmacologic agents (aminocaproic acid; Amicar and tranexamic acid; Cyklokapron) have been demonstrated to be effective in reducing blood loss under similar circumstances. The decision of when to utilize aprotinin requires active participation of the entire cardiac surgical care team.

We have made the use of aprotinin an integral part of our surgical strategy to obtain optimum hemostasis during the Ross procedure. This monograph is intended to provide clinical guidelines based on recent data on efficacy and dosing after the decision to use aprotinin has been made by the responsible physicians and to serve as a resource when considering its use in any cardiac surgical patient.

Pharmacology

Aprotinin (Trasylol; Bayer AG) is a serine proteinase inhibitor isolated from bovine lung. Its potential to inhibit protease enzymes with serine residues as their active site varies with dosing. For example, a plasma concentration of 50 KIU/ml (Kallikrein inactivator units) is required to inhibit plasmin and 200 KIU/ml to inhibit plasma kallikrein. The activator of plasminogen derived from endothelium (i.e. tissue-type plasminogen activator or t-PA) is a serine protease, as is urokinase, but both are not inhibited by aprotinin at extremely high concentrations (^{3} 25,000 KIU/ml) not likely to be found clinically. Because the plasma half-life of aprotinin is short (about 1 hour), a continuous infusion is required to maintain inhibitor activity.

Aprotinin is renally metabolized and excreted. Functional changes in renal perfusion, glomerular filtration rate, diuresis and electrolyte excretion all occur after aprotinin use. Aprotinin is a comparatively weak immunogen yet aprotinin-specific antibodies can be found in human sera during and after treatment. Additionally an IgE mediated anaphylactic reaction has been confirmed. Rapid intravenous injection should be avoided as well since the high basicity of the molecule may activate the complement system and precipitate an anaphylactoid reaction. Anaphylactic and anaphylactoid reactions, life-threatening in this population, have been reported to occur rarely (0.5–0.7%) with first-time exposure but much more frequently (6–10%) with subsequent exposure. A test dose (1 ml = 10,000 KIU) is always given prior to the start of aprotinin dosing.

Dosage

Aprotinin dosing and timing are critical to achieve its beneficial effects. Notwithstanding a recent multicenter, double-blind, placebo-controlled study of three different dosing regimens in patients undergoing first-time CABG surgery, lower aprotinin dosing regimens have not consistently reduced post-bypass blood loss over non-medicated controls. Studies indicate that platelet adhesive capacity is specifically damaged by the first pass of blood through the extracorporeal circuit and therapeutic plasma levels of aprotinin need to be achieved by this time.

The most consistently used blood-sparing dose of aprotinin, now commonly referred in the literature as "high-dose" or the "Hammersmith" regimen, was originally formulated to achieve a plasma concentration of 200 KIU/ml or a level theoretically derived to inhibit plasma kallikrein, and has been proven efficacious by numerous studies. It is delivered as a loading dose of 2 million KIU, started after surgical incision and infused over a twenty minute period, followed by a 500,000 KIU/hr continuous infusion. The extracorporeal circuit is primed with an additional 2 million KIU to overcome the dilutional effects of 2 liters of crystalloid prime, and the maintenance dose infusion is continued during the CPB period and stopped when the patient is transferred to the ICU. Most studies report an average adult total dose in the range of 6 million KIU. Presently the Rhode Island Hospital pharmacy purchases Trasylol as 200 ml glass bottles with a aprotinin concentration of 10,000 KIU/ml. The cost of one bottle is $310. Thus a 6 million KIU dose per patient (3 bottles) will cost a hospital approximately $930.

A number of studies have investigated the efficacy of lower aprotinin dosing regimens in various cardiac surgical populations. Some studies have not demonstrated significant blood transfusion sparing with the lower doses. The most significant exceptions are the recently reported[1] multicenter study of standard "high-dose", "low(half)-dose" and "pump prime only" regimens versus non-medicated controls in a surgical population (primary CABG) at low risk for bleeding. This study reported significant efficacy of all aprotinin dosing regimens versus placebo. However the mean red blood cell transfusion "saving" was only 1 unit in all the aprotinin groups over the controls in this low-risk population. Levy and associates[2] tested the high, low, and pump-prime only dosing regimens versus placebo in nearly 300 redo-CABG patients. In that study both the high- and low-dose aprotinin groups had significantly less bleeding and transfusion requirements compared to controls, but the low-dose aprotinin was less blood-sparing. "Pump prime only" and "Ultra-low dose" regimens have not proven efficacious in reducing transfusion requirements in cardiac surgical patients.

Efficacy

Numerous studies have conclusively demonstrated less blood loss in aprotinin treated cardiac surgical patients in the post-bypass period when compared to non-medicated controls. The mean difference in blood loss between aprotinin treated and control patients undergoing a primary elective CABG procedure is in the region of 200–400 ml. At those institutions utilizing conservative transfusion "triggers" (i.e. Hgb ≤ 9.0 g/dl) use of homologous blood products usually is not significantly different between treated and control patients in the primary elective CABG population. In those studies where aprotinin has significantly reduced red blood cell transfusion requirements in this population the mean "blood-sparing" effect has been one unit of packed red blood cells. In studies comparing high-dose aprotinin with aminocaproic acid (Amicar) or tranexamic acid (Cyklokapron) in patients undergoing isolated, first-time CABG surgery, neither postoperative blood losses nor transfusion requirements differed significantly between the groups. Given the prohibitive cost of aprotinin and the availability of alternate, lower-cost, effective blood-sparing pharmacologic agents as well as effective blood conservation techniques (i.e. good surgical hemostasis, normovolemic hemodilution, use of Heamonetic Cell-Saver or hemoconcentration), the use of aprotinin is not recommended in primary CABG or single valve replacement procedures unless the patient's clinical circumstances places them at high-risk for bleeding due to platelet dysfunction or unable to accept blood product transfusions (i.e. Jehovah's Witness).

Historically, patients undergoing repeat cardiac surgery through a prior median sternotomy were the first group of patients who received the described "high-dose" regimen.[3] The original study reported a mean blood loss of 1509 ml in the non-treated control population, all of whom (11 patients) required blood transfusions (total 41 units PRBC). Only 4 of 11 aprotinin treated patients received blood transfusions (total 5u PRBC) and had a mean blood loss of 286 ml. In subsequent studies aprotinin has proven highly efficacious in reducing patient exposure to transfused homologous blood products and in reducing postop bleeding in this group of patients. The Cleveland Clinic experience[4] in redo CABG patients reported a mean blood loss of 1121 ml and blood transfusion of 4 units of red cells in the placebo group compared with a 720 ml blood loss and 2 unit red cell transfusion in a "high-dose" aprotinin group. Other studies of "high-dose" aprotinin therapy in this cardiac surgery population consistently report a mean red cell transfusion requirement of 2–3 units less in treated patients. A recent multicenter, prospective and randomized study of aprotinin in patients undergoing repeat CABG surgery[2] found both "high-dose" and "low-dose" (one-half of Hammersmith regimen) to be equally blood-sparing versus a control group and a pump-prime (2 million KIU) group. Incidences of perioperative MI and renal dysfunction were similar among all groups. Patients undergoing repeat cardiac surgeries are at higher risk for bleeding, and aprotinin therapy routinely saves at least 2 units of transfused red cells during redo procedures, so that these patients are appropriate candidates for aprotinin therapy.

Patients undergoing surgical procedures utilizing deep hypothermic circulatory arrest (DHCA) historically suffer significant bleeding and therefore are a population which might benefit from the use of aprotinin. At this time there is no prospective, randomized trial of aprotinin versus placebo in this population and not likely to be one until a thoracic aorta surgery center engages in such a project which will require a few years. What exists in the literature is a disturbing number of case reports and retrospective series of adverse and often fatal thrombotic events in DHCA patients treated with aprotinin. Kouchoukos and colleagues[5] compared 20 patients enrolled in an ongoing study of aprotinin in complex surgery who underwent DHCA for surgery of the thoracic aorta with 20 age-matched controls undergoing similar procedures during DHCA without aprotinin. The aprotinin group did not have less bleeding or blood transfusion requirements, but did have a dramatically greater incidence of postop renal dysfunction (65% vs. 5%) and renal failure requiring hemodialysis (25% vs. none) than the matched controls. There was also a trend of greater thrombotic complications (MI, stroke) in the aprotinin-treated patients and a significantly greater mortality rate. Autopsies of patients who died revealed diffuse intravascular platelet-fibrin thrombi in the microvasculature of multiple organs in the aprotinin group not seen in the deceased non-treated group. Westaby et al.[6] reported on 80 consecutive patients operated on for acute Type A aortic dissections over a six year period utilizing DHCA with and without aprotinin (per physician preference). Aprotinin-treated patients did not benefit from any reduction in bleeding or blood product transfusions in this population, and sustained more fatal thrombotic events.

The Columbia Presbyterian Medical Center experience[7] in patients undergoing complex aortic procedures utilizing DHCA with aprotinin has been more favorable. In a retrospective comparison with a historical control group they found no difference in thrombotic complications and a lower overall mortality rate in the aprotinin group (34 patients). They found small reductions in postop blood product transfusion needs in the aprotinin group but they did report an increased incidence of postop renal dysfunction in the aprotinin-treated patients. Regragui et al.[8] reported 95% survival without major neurologic or cardiac adverse events in a small group of patients undergoing aortic surgery under DHCA with aprotinin therapy. As noted all of these reports are retrospective and suffer from serious design flaws. The efficacy and safety of aprotinin therapy during DHCA is unlikely to be answered outside of a prospectively randomized trial. Until further data is forthcoming, there is little evidence that aprotinin is efficacious in patients undergoing surgical procedures requiring DHCA and controversy over its safety exists in this setting. It is not possible to make firm conclusions based on the limited and conflicting clinical experiences about the efficacy and safety of aprotinin with DHCA. For the Ross procedure DHCA is not utilized and one is not faced with this dilemma. At the present time, our cardiac surgical team is not employing aprotinin routinely in DHCA cases.

Safety and Toxicity

One of the principal safety concerns associated with the use of aprotinin is the potential for thrombotic complications including early saphenous vein closure and perioperative MI and stroke. Cosgrove et al.[4] reported a trend toward an increased incidence of MI in aprotinin treated redo-CABG patients. Although not statistically significant, the incidence of Q-wave infarction was 17.5% in a "high-dose" aprotinin group versus 8.9% in a control group. In addition, autopsies of seven patients who died in the early postop period revealed thrombi in 6 of 12 vein grafts of aprotinin-treated patients compared with none of 5 grafts in control patients. This led to a caution that aprotinin may be capable of inducing a hyper-coagulable state and thrombotic complications. The extensive European experience (over 10,000 treated patients by 1991) has not reported increased mortality, stroke, MI or graft occlusion with the use of high-dose aprotinin. Bidstrup et al.[9] using MRI to assess early saphenous vein graft patency, found no differences in incidence of graft occlusion between 90 patients randomized to aprotinin or placebo and evaluated within 10 days of surgery. Other prospective, randomized and placebo-controlled studies[2,10–12] designed to evaluate the safety of "high-dose" aprotinin did not find an increased incidence of perioperative MI or stroke in the aprotinin-treated patients (strokes appear to be consistently less in the aprotinin groups[13]) but suffered in study design from relatively few patients. Using either repeat coronary angiography or ultrafast computed tomography to evaluate graft patency in the early postop period, these studies confirm similar graft patency between controls and aprotinin-treated patients. Most recently, a much larger multi-centered prospective study randomized over 800 primary CABG patients and studied mammary arterial and saphenous vein graft patency using early postoperative coronary angiography.[14] The overall results of this graft patency study found an increased incidence of saphenous vein occlusion, but not internal mammary artery occlusion, in aprotinin-treated patients when analyzed on both per-patient and per-graft basis. Secondary analyses revealed that female patients, patients with distal vessels less than 1.5 mm in diameter and those with poor quality distal vessels were predisposed to graft occlusion when aprotinin was administered. In surgical patients with coronary arteries with these "high-risk" characteristics, the blood sparing benefits of aprotinin must be weighed against the greater incidence of early vein graft occlusion. For the Ross procedure, severe coronary artery disease is a relative contraindication and its presence should determine a more straightforward valve implantation procedure be used. If a saphenous vein graft is to be part of the planned Ross procedure, one needs to weigh the total benefits and risks of aprotinin use. At our institution we favor the use of aprotinin in this situation.

Allergic reactions have been anticipated because aprotinin is an animal-derived peptide. IgE-mediated anaphylaxis to aprotinin has been documented. Aprotinin-specific IgG antibodies have also been found in patients suffering severe or fatal anaphylaxis on re-exposure. Large clinical experiences or trials have consistently reported allergic reactions of 0.5% on first exposure to aprotinin. The majority of serious allergic reactions have been reported during the second exposure to the drug. The frequency of hypersensitivity reactions after repeated aprotinin administration has been reported as high as 10% in Germany where the drug has been available and used for a variety of indications for 40 years. Because of the severity of these reactions some centers recommend initiation of aprotinin infusion only after sternotomy when the institution of CPB may be accomplished to assist with resuscitation.

As aprotinin is selectively taken up by renal tissues, specifically the proximal convoluted tubule, there is concern that the current "high-dose" regimen may result in nephrotoxicity. Evaluating clinically significant renal dysfunction by either changes in serum creatinine levels or the need for hemodialysis large clinical trials of aprotinin in non-DHCA procedures have not found significant differences in postop renal function between treated and non-treated patients. Postoperative serum creatinine level increases of more than 0.5 mg/dl over preoperative levels occur in 8–10% of patients undergoing primary cardiac procedures and receiving either high-dose or low-dose aprotinin, an incidence not significantly different from those not treated with aprotinin.

Monitoring of Anticoagulation

When celite is used as the contact-activating agent (Hemochron, International Technodyne Co.), there will be a prolongation of the ACT that is independent of heparin concentration. At concentrations of aprotinin achieved clinically with the "high-dose" regimen, activated factors in the intrinsic coagulation cascade (XIIa, XIa, XIa, VIIIa) are partially inhibited. Dietrich et al.[15] demonstrated that aprotinin acts as an anticoagulant by inhibiting prothrombin activation during CPB. Some of the confusion in the assessment of the role of ACT in monitoring anticoagulation in the presence of aprotinin is caused by interchanging the terms "anticoagulation" and "heparinization." When aprotinin is present, the celite-activated ACT reflects not only the AT-III dependent heparin anticoagulation, but the anticoagulation induced by aprotinin.

Heparin administration based on celite ACT values and dosed to maintain standard ACT times of ≥400 seconds, may result in inadequate anticoagulation. Alternate monitoring strategies include direct measurement of heparin levels by titration with protamine (Hepcon, Medtronic Hemotec) keeping the heparin concentration near 3 IU/ml, or use of kaolin-activated ACT monitoring and maintenance of standard ACT values. If kaolin is used as the activator, the ACT is not prolonged by aprotinin. At Rhode Island Hospital we utilize kaolin-activated ACT monitoring with prolongation to 480 seconds the "safe" level of anticoagulation. Of note is that the "Hammersmith" aprotinin dosing regimen has been shown to result in a prolonged activated partial thromboplastin time (aPTT) to about twice control values in the early postop period (6–12 hours) rendering this test useless for monitoring residual heparin after surgery.

Clinical Use Summary

Test dose 1 cc given prior to surgery

Loading dose 2 million KIU (200 cc) over 20 minutes prior to cardiopulmonary bypass

Maintenance infusion of 500,000 KIU (50 cc) per hour through bypass until end of surgery

Priming dose 2 million KIU (200 cc) placed in extracorporeal circuit prime.

References

1. Lemmer JH, Jr., Dilling EW, Morton JR, Rich JB, Robicsek F, Bricker DL, Hantler CB, et al. Aprotonin for primary coronary artery bypass grafting: a multicenter trial of three dose regimens. Ann Thorac Surg 1996;62:1575–1577.
2. Levy JF, Pifarre R, Schaff HV, Harrow JC, Albus R, Spiess B, et al. A multicenter, double blind, placebo controlled trial of aprotinin for reducing blood loss and the requirement for donor blood transfusion in patients undergoing repeat coronary artery bypass grafting. Circulation 1995;92: 2236–2244.
3. Royston D, Bidstrup BP, Taylor KM, Sapsford RN. Effect of aprotonin on need for blood transfusion after repeat open heart surgery. Lancet 1987;2:1289–1291.

4. Cosgrove DM, Heric L, Lytle BW, Taylor PC, Novoa R, Golding LA, Stewart RW, et al. Aprotonin therapy for reoperative myocardial revascularization: a placebo controlled study. Ann Thorac Surg 1992;54:1031–1038.

5. Sundt TM, Kouchoukos NT, Saffitz JE, Murphy SF, Wareing TH, Stahl DJ. Renal dysfunction and intravascular coagulation with aprotinin and hypothermic circulatory arrest. Ann Thorac Surg 1993;55:1418–1424.

6. Westaby S, Forni A, Dunning J, Diannopoulos N, O'Regan D, Drossos G, Pillai R. Aprotinin and bleeding in profoundly hypothermic perfusion. EJCTS 1994;8:82–86.

7. Goldstein DJ, DeRosa CM, Mongero LB, Michler RE, Rose EA, Oz NC, Smith CR. Safety and efficacy of aprotinin under conditions of deep hypothermia and circulatory arrest. J Thorac Cardiovasc Surg 1995;110:1615–1622.

8. Regragui IA, Bryan AJ, Izzat MB, Wisheart JD, Hutter JA, Angelini G. Aprotinin use with hypothermic circulatory arrest for aortic valve and thoracic aortic surgery: renal function and early survival. J Heart Valve Dis 1995;4:669–673.

9. Bidstrup BP, Underwood SR, Sapsford RN. Effect of aprotinin (Trasylol) on aorta-coronary bypass graft patency. J Thorac Cardiovasc Surg 1993;105:147–153.

10. Kalangos A, Tayyareci G, Pretre R, DiDio P, Sezerman O. Influence of aprotinin on early graft thrombosis in patients undergoing myocardial revascularization. EJCTS 1994;8:651–656.

11. Havel M, Grabenwoger F, Schneider J, Laufer G, Wolenek G, Owen A, Simon P, et al. Aprotinin does not decrease early graft patency after coronary artery bypass grafting despite reducing post operative bleeding and use of donated blood. J Thorac Cardiovasc Surg 1994;107:807–810.

12. Lemmer JH, Stanford W, Bonney SL, Breen JF, Chomka EV, Eldredge WJ, Holt WW, et al. Aprotinin for coronary bypass operations: efficacy, safety, and influence on early saphenous vein graft patency. J Thorac Cardiovasc Surg 1994;107:543–553.

13. Murkin JM, Lux J, Shannon NA, Guiraudon GM, Menkis AH, McKenzie FN, Novick RJ. Aprotinin significantly decreases bleeding and transfusion requirements in patients receiving aspirin and undergoing cardiac operations. J Thorac Cardiovasc Surg 1994;107:554–561.

14. Alderman EL, Levy JH, Rich JB, Nili M, Vidne B, Schaff H, Utretzky G, et al. Analysis of coronary graft patency after aprotinin use: results from the international multicenter aprotinin graft patency experience (image) trial. J Thorac Cardiovasc Surg 1998;116:716–730.

15. Dietrich W, Dilthey G, Spannagl M, Jochum M, Braun SL, Richter JA. Influence of high-dose aprotinin on anticoagulation, heparin requirement, and celite- and kaolin-activated clotting time in heparin-pretreated patients undergoing open heart surgery: a double blind, placebo controlled study. Anesthesiology 1995;83:679–689.

44
Ross-Konno Procedure

V. Mohan Reddy, Doff B. McElhinney, and Frank L. Hanley

Pulmonary autograft aortic valve replacement (the Ross procedure) is increasingly being considered for application in pediatric patients with a wide spectrum of congenital abnormalities of the left ventricular outflow tract.[1–6] However, the establishment of this procedure increases our therapeutic choices for many pediatric patients with *complex left ventricular outflow tract obstruction*, thereby forcing us to re-evaluate more traditional treatment protocols for a number of patient subsets.[6–9] Such patients fall into the following diagnostic groups.

1. The physiologically compensated older pediatric patient (beyond infancy) with aortic stenosis, a hypoplastic annulus and/or long segment subaortic stenosis with our without insufficiency who may have previously undergone one or more surgical or balloon procedures on the aortic valve.

2. The neonate or infant with critical aortic stenosis who has an unacceptable result following surgical valvotomy or balloon valvuloplasty. These patients often have a relatively small aortic root and may also have long segment subaortic stenosis.

3. The neonate with borderline hypoplastic left heart syndrome who is being considered for a two-ventricle repair rather than the Norwood procedure.

Patients in the first two groups have typically been managed conservatively through infancy and childhood by repeated valvotomy or balloon dilatation, often with the acceptance of significant residual obstruction and/or insufficiency. These residual lesions have been considered acceptable because no reasonable alternative options existed until recently. Prosthetic aortic valve replacement with a mechanical or allograft valve, along with concomitant enlargement of the subaortic left ventricular outflow tract and the aortic annulus is eventually required. However, this procedure is commonly delayed until the patient either reaches full somatic growth or shows signs of severe decompensation. In the past, this approach made sense because the problems of prosthetic aortic valve replacement in children are numerous.

Patient Selection

In neonates and infants with critical aortic stenosis the initial intervention is usually balloon or surgical valvotomy.[10] If valvotomy achieves an acceptable result (≤ mild aortic stenosis and/or regurgitation), the patient is followed closely to detect any early progression of stenosis or regurgitation. If progression of residual lesions is documented, these patients undergo a Ross or Ross-Konno operation. If the patient has ≥ moderate aortic stenosis or insufficiency following valvotomy, a Ross or Ross-Konno operation is performed immediately.

A similar approach is taken in older infants and children with greater than moderate isolated aortic stenosis or regurgitation, or mixed disease of a moderate degree. In addition, in selected patients with borderline hypoplastic left heart syndrome, the Ross-Konno procedure along with extensive resection of endocardial fibroelastosis and arch reconstruction is offered as a two-ventricle alternative to the Norwood procedure. In this subset of patients, those with adequate mitral valve size and function are most likely to benefit.

Surgical Technique

Standard techniques of neonatal and pediatric cardiopulmonary bypass are used, including bicaval cannulation, moderate hypothermia, and cardioplegia. After initiation of cardiopulmonary bypass, the pulmonary autograft is harvested along with an extension of attached infundibular free wall muscle (Figure 44.1). Special care should be taken not to injure the first septal perforator branch. In neonates and infants the dissection is carried in the plane

anterior to the left anterior descending coronary artery. The autograft infundibular muscle can generally be peeled off the muscular septum in this group of patients if the correct plane is identified.

The ascending aorta is then cross-clamped and cardioplegia is administered into the aortic root (except in cases with severe insufficiency, in which case the aorta is opened and cardioplegia is administered directly into the coronary ostia). In patients with mild to moderate aortic regurgitation, the initial dose of cardioplegia is administered into the root after placement of a left ventricular vent to prevent left ventricular distention. The aorta is then transected at the level of the sino-tubular junction. The coronary arteries are explanted with large coronary buttons comprising almost the entire wall of the sinus of Valsalva. The remaining aortic root tissue is then excised along with the aortic valve leaflets. In older patients, the non-coronary sinus wall is preserved (Figure 44.2) The interventricular septum is incised in a

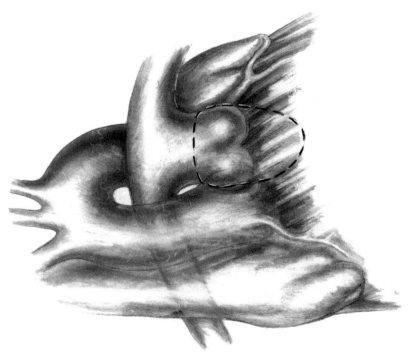

FIGURE 44.1. Technique of Ross-Konno. The dashed lines indicate the lines of incision along which the autograft pulmonary valve is harvested, transected, and coronary buttons are developed.

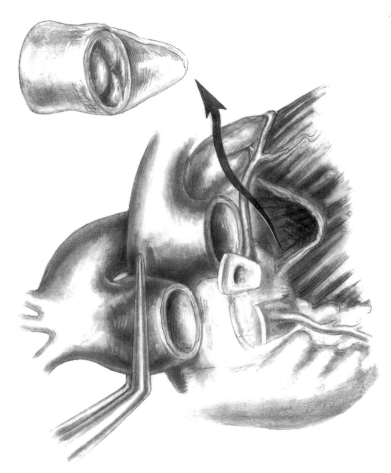

FIGURE 44.2. The pulmonary autograft is harvested. Large coronary buttons are developed and diseased aortic valve is excised up to the annulus. Septal incision is made to enlarge the aortic annulus and if necessary the subaortic region.

fashion similar to that used in a Konno aortoventriculoplasty procedure (Figure 44.3).[11] Additional ventricular myectomy is performed if it is deemed necessary. The pulmonary autograft is seated with the infundibular muscle extension fitting into the Konno incision in the interventricular septum. The autograft is then sutured to the native aortic annulus with continuous monofilament absorbable suture beginning at the posterior midpoint (Figure 44.3). This is then continued onto the infundibular muscle extension which is sutured to the septal incision and reinforced with non-absorbable interrupted pledgetted mattress sutures. The coronary buttons are then anastomosed to the appropriate sinuses of the autograft using running 7-0 absorbable monofilament suture (Figure 44.4). The right ventricular outflow tract is reconstructed with an allograft valved conduit (Figure 44.5). The allograft can be sutured directly to the right ventricular infundibular muscle with or without the use of any additional patching material. We prefer a pulmonary allograft that is substantially oversized relative to the patient's size. The patient is separated from bypass in the usual manner and transesophageal echocardiography is performed.

UCSF Experience

Between June 1992 and June 1997, we have performed the Ross-Konno procedure in 14 patients ranging in age from 7 days to 17 years (median 1.7 years). All patients have valvar aortic stenosis and subvalvar obstruction was present in 11 patients. In 9 patients there was associated mild to moderate aortic insufficiency. There were no early or late deaths in this

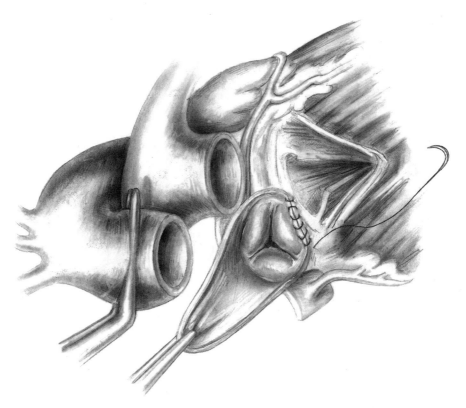

FIGURE 44.3. Pulmonary autograft is seated with the suture line starting posteriorly continuing along the annulus and onto the interventricular septum.

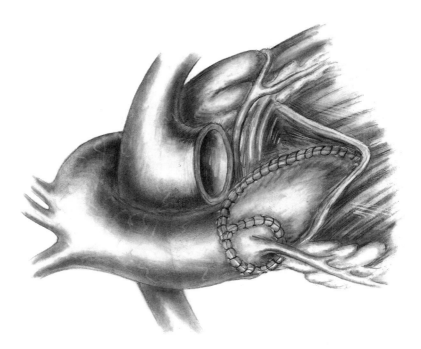

FIGURE 44.4. The pulmonary autograft in place with reimplantation of the coronary artery buttons.

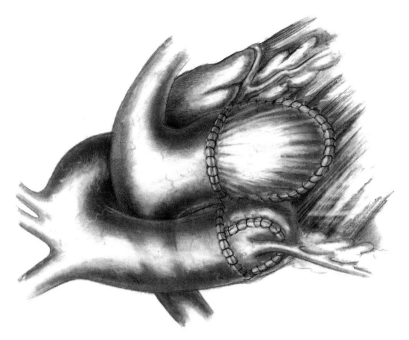

FIGURE 44.5. The allograft conduit is sutured directly to the right ventricle without the use of additional patch material.

group of patients and no patients have required reintervention at follow-up ranging from 1 to 55 months.

In four additional patients with borderline hypoplastic left heart syndrome, a Ross-Konno procedure was performed as part of a more extensive operation that also included resection of endocardial fibroelastosis. Three of these patients died due to inadequate mitral valve function (inflow obstruction and/or regurgitation) despite a normal left ventricular outflow tract and good ventricular function. The surviving patient has good autograft and ventricular function 28 months postoperatively.

Advantages of the Ross-Konno Procedure

The pulmonary autograft seems to be the ideal valve for aortic valve replacement in the pediatric population. Several reports have documented autograft growth in older children, with excellent mid-term results. Adaptation of the pulmonary autograft for aortoventriculoplasty incorporates the principles of both aortic root replacement and aortoventriculoplasty, and is similar to extended aortic root replacement with allografts. Among our patients in whom the contiguous infundibular free wall flap was used for the septal patch, there have been no cases in which right ventricular function was compromised.

The encouraging short- and mid-term results achieved in our experience suggest that approaches to managing small patients (especially neonates and infants) with critical aortic stenosis should be re-assessed. Balloon or surgical valvotomy should probably remain the procedures of choice. However, in a substantial subset of patients, these approaches result in significant residual stenosis and progressive left ventricular hypertrophy or dilation. Without valve replacement, some of these patients do not survive long term, while others do survive but at the cost of compromised left ventricular function. Timely use of the Ross or Ross-Konno procedure will maximally preserve left ventricular function in this population. Similarly, the practice of conservatively managing patients with aortic stenosis into the teen years because they are clinically "compensate" in spite of significant residual lesions should be reassessed if left ventricular function is to be maximally preserved. In this group as well, earlier use of the Ross or Ross-Konno procedure is likely to allow for maximal preservation of the left ventricle. Finally, the Ross-Konno procedure offers a two-ventricle alternative to the Norwood procedure for certain selected patients with borderline hypoplastic left heart syndrome. The criteria for performing the Ross-Konno in the population are still evolving.

One drawback of the Ross-Konno procedure in neonates and young infants is that reoperations will inevitably be necessary to replace the small allograft conduits that are used for reconstruction of the right ventricular outflow tract. We believe, however, that this disadvantage is outweighed by the early normalization of left ventricular dynamics.

In summary, the pulmonary autograft can be modified for use in the aortoventriculoplasty procedures for the management of complex left ventricular outflow tract obstruction, even in neonates and infants, with excellent short- and mid-term results. However, long-term follow up will be necessary to completely define the timing and indications of this procedure.

Alternate Approaches

Left ventricular outflow tract obstruction with a hypoplastic aortic annulus and/or diffuse subaortic stenosis has been a challenging lesion to manage in neonates and small infants. Standard approaches such as balloon or surgical valvotomy are only palliative and often leave the patient with substantial residual stenosis and/or insufficiency.[10] Many of these patients will eventually require an annular enlargement procedure or aortoventriculoplasty. The tendency to postpone these procedures until the patient is much older with the hope of placing an adult size prosthesis is a common practice. However, substantial left ventricular dysfunction due to the long standing aortic stenosis or

insufficiency is an important concern when this approach is taken.[12] In addition, there are other drawbacks to aortoventriculoplasty using a prosthetic valve. Mechanical valves generally warrant chronic anticoagulation and the attendant complications.[13] Bioprosthetic valves have a high rate of degeneration and calcification requiring replacement.[14] Both mechanical and bioprosthetic valves may also result in thromboembolism and hemolysis. In young children, any sort of non-autologous prosthetic valve will inevitably require replacement as the patient outgrows the fixed-diameter valve. Efforts to insert larger prosthesis in younger children may result in compression of the right coronary artery with fatal consequences.

Early extended aortic root replacement using allograft valved conduits avoids the complications of anticoagulation, thromboembolism and hemolysis. However, rapid degeneration of allografts is a serious drawback, especially in infants and younger children.[15] In selected patients, another potential option is a "valve sparing" Konno procedure, in which the native aortic valve is repaired and the outflow tract is enlarged by performing a septal ventriculoplasty.[16] However, this option is limited to the small group of patients with significant obstruction at the subvalvular level but not at the valve.

References

1. Elkins RC, Santangelo D, Randolph JD, Knott-Craig CJ, Stelzer P, Thompson WM, Razook JD, Ward KE, Overholt ED. Pulmonary Autograft Replacement in Children: the ideal solution? Ann Surg 1992;216:363–371.
2. Kouchoukos NT, Davila-Roman VG, Spray TL, Murphy SF, Perrillo JB. Replacement of the aortic root with a pulmonary autograft in children and young adults with aortic-valve disease. New Eng Journ Med 1994;330:1–6.
3. Schoof PH, Cromme-Dijkhuis AH, Bogers AJJC, Thijssen HJM, Witsenburg M, Hess J, Bos E. Aortic root replacement with pulmonary autograft in children. J Thorac Cardiovasc Surg 1994;107:367–373.
4. Gerosa G, McKay R, Davies J, Ross DN. Comparison of the aortic homograft and the pulmonary autograft for aortic valve or root

replacement in children. J Thorac Cardiovasc Surg 1991;102:51–60; discus.

5. Elkins RC, Knott-Craig CJ, Ward KE, McCue C, Lane MM. Pulmonary autograft in children: realized growth potential. Ann Thorac Surg 1994;57:1387–1394.

6. Cartier PC, Metras J, Cloutier A, Dumesnil JG, Raymond G, Doyle D, Desaulniers D, Lemieux MD, Lentini S. Aortic valve replacement with pulmonary autograft in children and adults. Ann Thorac Surg 1995;60:S177–S179.

7. Daenen W. Repair of complex left ventricular outflow tract obstruction with a pulmonary autograft. J Heart Valve Dis 1995;4:364–367.

8. Reddy VM, Rajasinghe HA, Teitel DF, Haas GS, Hanley FL. Aortoventriculoplasty with the pulmonary autograft: the "Ross-Konno" procedure. J Thorac and Cardiovasc Surg 1996;111:158–167.

9. Starnes VA, Luciani GB, Wells WJ, Allen RB, Lewis AB. Aortic root replacement with the pulmonary autograft in children with complex left heart obstruction. Ann Thorac Surg 1996;62:442–449.

10. Kirklin JW, Barratt-Boyes BG. Congenital aortic stenosis. In Kirklin JW, Barratt-Boyes BG (eds).

Cardiac Surgery. New York: Church Livingstone 1993:1195–1237.

11. Konno S, Iai I, Iida Y et al. A new method for prosthetic valve replacement in congenital aortic stenosis associated with hypoplasia of the aortic valve ring. J Thorac Cardiovasc Surg 1976;70: 909–917.

12. Hoffman JIE. Effects of outflow tract obstruction on total and regional coronary blood flow, and tis influence on ventricular function. Adv Cardiol 1976;17:13–19.

13. Bradley SM, Sade RM, Crawford FA, Stroud MR. Anticoagulation in children with mechanical valve prostheses. Ann Thorac Surg 1997;64: 30–36.

14. Geha AS, Laks H, Stensel HC et al. Late failure of porcine valve heterografts in children. J Thorac Cardiovasc Surg 1979;78:351–364.

15. McKowen RL, Campbell DN, Woelfel GF, Wiggins JW, Clarke DR. Extended aortic root replacement with aortic allografts. J Thorac Cardiovasc Surg 1987;93:366–374.

16. Cooley DA, Garrett JR. Septoplasty for left ventricular outflow obstruction without aortic vavle replacement: a new technique. Ann Thor Sur 1986; 42:445–448.

45

Methods for Avoiding Technical Errors in Performing the Autograft Pulmonary Valve Transplant

Erle H. Austin, III

The primary concern of surgeons and cardiologists with the outcome of the Ross procedure is the development of insufficiency of the pulmonary autograft (neo-aortic valve). Although mild insufficiency is commonly noted following pulmonary autograft technique, the potential for development of severe or progressive neo-aortic insufficiency requiring reoperation has dissuaded many surgeons from including this operation in their surgical repertoire. Present evaluation of reported results of the Ross procedure indicate that the development of aortic insufficiency can be separated into at least two time-defined categories. Early insufficiency is discovered less than six months after the operation, while late insufficiency develops after this period of time. Although early insufficiency is most likely secondary to a technical imperfection at the time of surgery, late insufficiency may simply be related to the insertion of a low-pressure valve in a high-pressure position. The technical details of pulmonary autograft insertion, however, may have as important an effect on the development of late valve insufficiency as on the occurrence of early insufficiency.

Incidence of Aortic Insufficiency After the Ross Procedure

The incidence of aortic insufficiency after the Ross procedure is not well known, primarily due to the limited amount of published experience in this regard. Of course, the initial experience with this technique was that of Mr. Ross himself. Long-term follow-up of Ross' experience was reported in 1991 and included 339 patients beginning with his first patient in 1967.[1] The mean follow-up was 11.8 years and maximum follow up was 24 years. In that entire group of patients, the number of patients requiring reoperation for pulmonary autograft insufficiency was 33 patients. Of those 33 patients, it was felt that the neo-aortic insufficiency resulted from technical failure in 19 cases, from endocarditis in 9 cases, and from "degeneration" in 5 cases. The linearized incidence of autograft insufficiency in Ross' report was 0.8% per patient-year. It is noteworthy that in the vast majority of Ross' patients the subcoronary implantation technique was utilized. An actuarial analysis of a subset of Ross' experience (National Heart Hospital, London) is depicted in Figure 45.1, showing a 25 year freedom from autograft replacement of 69%. These remarkable long-term results attest to the potential for excellent durability of the pulmonary autograft. It is unfortunate that none of Ross' contemporaries embraced his operation and provided a comparative series with similar long-term follow-up.

To collect more results, the Ross Procedure International Registry was developed as a clearinghouse for surgeons around the world performing this operation. In 1996, the Ross Registry reported a total of 1,976 operations performed by 126 surgeons from 1987 through 1995.[2] In this analysis, mean follow-up was 2 years with a maximum follow-up of 8 years.

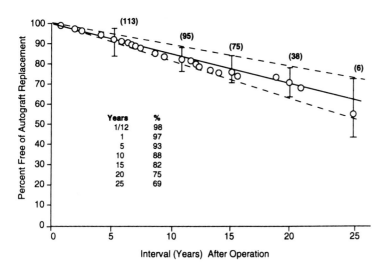

FIGURE 45.1. Actuarial freedom from autograft removal in 131 consecutive patients at the National Heart Hospital, 1967 to 1984. Follow-up was 95% complete. Reprinted from *Annals of Thoracic Surgery*, Vol 62, Elkins et al, "Pulmonary autograft reoperation: incidence and management," 450. © 1996, with permission from Elsevier.

Out of this number of operations, 56 patients required reoperation for autograft insufficiency, a linearized incidence of 1.5% per patient-year. Among patients for whom the information was available, the percentage of patients undergoing root replacement as the implantation technique was 66%, whereas 23% underwent subcoronary implantation and 11% underwent the inclusion technique. The exact reasons for reoperation were not detailed, but of the 56 patients the reason for reoperation was categorized as mechanical for 27, endocarditis for 15, technical for 8 and other pathology for 6. Out of a group of 49 autograft failures, it was remarkable that 36 were sub-

coronary implantations. Only 5 of the autograft failures were inclusion roots and only 8 were root replacements. Although registry information of this type is helpful because of the larger numbers generated, follow-up is likely to be inconsistent, incomplete and potentially inaccurate, and thus must be interpreted with caution.

Probably the most closely studied group of patients undergoing the Ross procedure in the present era has been that of Elkins and associates. In 1996, Elkins reported his experience with 196 consecutive patients operated on between 1986 and 1995.[3] The mean follow-up was 2.4 years and maximum follow up was 9.3

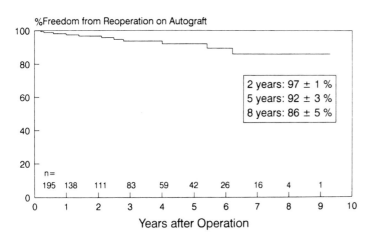

FIGURE 45.2. Actuarial freedom from reoperation on pulmonary autograft valve in Elkins series, 1986–1995. Follow-up was 100%. Reprinted from *Seminars in Thoracic and Cardiovascular Surgery*, Vol 8, Ross D, "The pulmonary autograft: history and basic techniques," 354. © 1996, with permission from Elsevier.

years. Eleven patients underwent reoperation for autograft insufficiency for a linearized incidence of 2.4% per patient-year. The life-table analysis is depicted in Figure 45.2 showing an 8 year freedom from reoperation of 86%. One hundred and sixteen of the 196 procedures were done using the root replacement technique and out of that group, only four re-operations occurred. Of the 25 patients who underwent the subcoronary implantation technique, 3 reoperations were required, and of the 55 who underwent the inclusion technique, four required reoperation. Of the three patients who developed early failure, one was secondary to persistent endocarditis, and two patients developed aortic insufficiency from technical errors. In one case, there was poor subcoronary alignment with a subcoronary implantation, and the other was a significant mismatch between the pulmonary and aortic roots. Of the eight patients requiring reoperation after one year, one patient developed endocarditis, one patient had systemic lupus erythematosus, and one patient developed prolapse of a valve leaflet with adherence to a ventricular septal defect patch. The other five patients experienced progressive dilatation of the pulmonary autograft. In 3 of these 5 patients, there was a mismatch between the size of the pulmonary root and the left ventricular outflow tract. In two of the patients, however, the pulmonary autograft appeared to correctly match the size of the aortic root. Using univariate and multiple logistic regression analysis, Elkins identified several factors associated with freedom from autograft insufficiency. These included the presence of aortic stenosis preoperatively ($p = 0.01$) and implantation technique, with root replacement better than the inclusion technique and the inclusion technique better than subcoronary implantation ($p = 0.01$). The history of a previous median sternotomy also appeared to decrease the incidence of neo-aortic insufficiency ($p = 0.05$).

In addition to the findings cited by Ross, Elkins and other surgeons, other causes for aortic insufficiency after the Ross procedure have been identified and included recurrent rheumatic fever[4] and juvenile rheumatoid arthritis[5]. Most of these reports, however, are anecdotal. The incidence of autograft failure in patients with a history of rheumatic heart disease is not known but may be significantly higher than in other patients.

Currently, the development of aortic insufficiency after the Ross procedure appears to have several potential causes. The subcoronary implantation technique appears to increase the risk of insufficiency (except in Ross' experience). This is most likely related to imperfect positioning of the pulmonary valve in the aortic root. A second major cause of aortic insufficiency is a mismatch between the pulmonary valve and the aortic valve. A third factor appears to be the development of dilatation of the pulmonary autograft. This often occurs at the annular level but may also occur at the sinotubular level. Endocarditis continues to pose a risk to the pulmonary autograft, as to other inflammatory processes, such a systemic lupus erythematosus, rheumatic fever and juvenile rheumatic arthritis.

Techniques to Minimize Aortic Insufficiency

Taking these findings into account, several technical aspects may be important in minimizing the development of aortic insufficiency after the Ross procedure. The experience of Ross would suggest that implanting the pulmonary valve inside the aortic root might have significant merit. Certainly, the potential for dilatation of the aortic root would be minimized if the pulmonary valve is sewn freehand in a subcoronary position or placed inside the aortic root as a cylinder (inclusion technique). The subcoronary implantation technique, however, introduces the potential for misalignment of the commissures, a problem that surgeons other than Ross have experienced. The inclusion cylinder technique may minimize commissural misalignment but discrepancies between the pulmonary and aortic roots often make it difficult to insert one within the other.

Presently most surgeons prefer to transfer the pulmonary valve as a complete root replacement. With this approach, natural align-

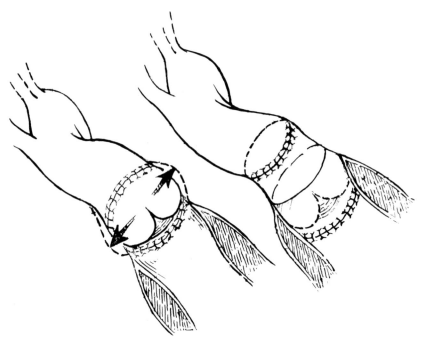

FIGURE 45.3. Attaching the pulmonary autograft root above the annulus of the original aortic valve bed may result in dilatation and neo-aortic insufficiency. Reprinted from Ross DN: Aortic Root Replacement with a Pulmonary Autograft—Current Trends. *The Journal of Heart Valve Disease* 3:360, 1994, with permission.

ment of the commissures is assured, resulting in a low incidence of early insufficiency. The thin wall of the pulmonary root, however, is susceptible to dilatation and subsequent aortic insufficiency. The technical details of root implantation, therefore, must take into account this potential.

Mr. Ross has stressed the importance of implanting the annulus of the pulmonary root within the annulus of the aortic valve (Figure 45.3). At this level, the fibrous skeleton of the heart and the muscular portion of the left ventricular outflow tract provide external support at the ventriculoaortic junction. Other surgeons have suggested providing a more complete external support by wrapping the pulmonary root in pericardium[6] or mesh (Figure 45.4).

A technical aspect of the procedure used by some surgeons and demonstrated in this text is the preservation of the entire aortic sinus surrounding each coronary ostium to replace the corresponding sinus of the pulmonary root (large buttons). The non-coronary aortic sinus is left *in situ* to externally buttress the resultant non-coronary sinus of the autograft (Figures 45.5, 45.6, and 45.7). With this technique, most of the patient's own aortic wall makes up the circumference of the neo-aortic root. As such, the amount of thin pulmonary root exposed to high intra-aortic pressure is minimized.

Accurate matching of the pulmonary autograft to the left ventricle outflow tract appears to importantly affect early and late results. Drs. David and Elkins have independently recognized the importance of this size match and have devised techniques to adjust the left ventricular outflow tract to match the size of the pulmonary autograft.[7,8] First, it is important to assess the size of the pulmonary autograft and compare it to that of the left ventricular outflow tract. Preoperative echocardiography can often prepare the surgeon for any major size discrepancy. Hegar dilators or standard valve

FIGURE 45.4. Technique described by Pacifico and colleagues involves placing pulmonary autograft root on a Hegar dilator and wrapping the root with a cylinder of bovine pericardium. From Pacifico AD, Kirklin JK, McGiffin DC, et al: The Ross Operation—Early Echocardiographic Comparison of Different Operative Techniques. *The Journal of Heart Valve Disease* 3:336, 1994.

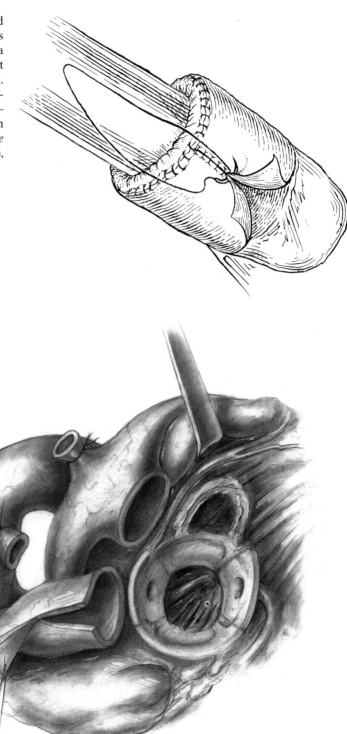

FIGURE 45.5. Technique of Hanley and colleagues preserves most of the aortic sinus around each coronary ostia and leaves the non-coronary aortic sinus *in situ*. Reprinted from *Annals of Thoracic Surgery*, Vol 60(5), Black et al, "Modified pulmonary autograft aortic root replacement: The sinus obliteration," 1434. © 1995, with permission from Elsevier.

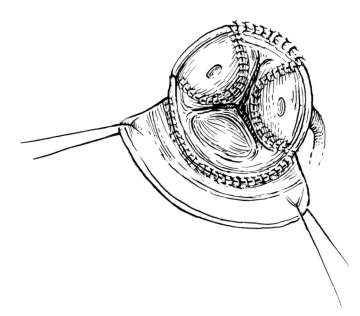

FIGURE 45.6. After the pulmonary autograft is sutured in place the corresponding sinus are replaced with the aortic coronary sinuses and the non-coronary sinus of the autograft is externally buttressed with the preserved non-coronary sinus. (A) As a result, most of the circumference of the neo-aortic root at the sinotubular junction is made up of or is reinforced by native aortic tissue (B) Reprinted from *Annals of Thoracic Surgery*, Vol 60(5), Black et al, "Modified pulmonary autograft aortic root replacement: The sinus obliteration," 1434. © 1995, with permission from Elsevier.

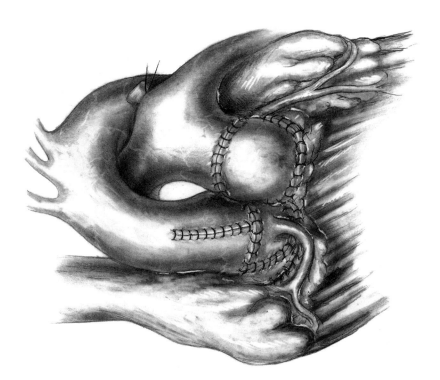

FIGURE 45.7. The completed pulmonary autograft root replacement using Hanley's sinus obliteration technique. Reprinted from *Annals of Thoracic Surgery*, Vol 60(5), Black et al, "Modified pulmonary autograft aortic root replacement: The sinus obliteration," 1434. © 1995, with permission from Elsevier.

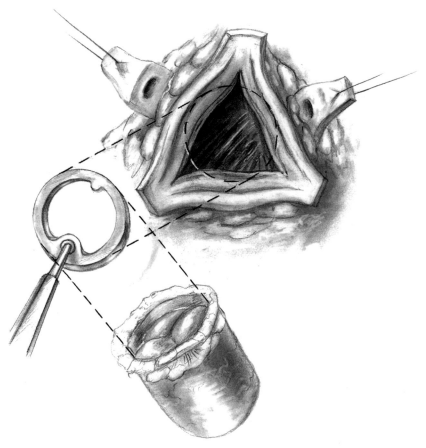

FIGURE 45.8. Determining the relative sizes of the left ventricular outflow tract and pulmonary autograft is important to avoid significant mismatch. Standard prosthetic valve sizers can be used.

Reprinted from *ACC Current Journal Review*, Vol 5, Doty DB, "Aortic valve replacement with the pulmonary autograft: The Ross procedure," 49. © 1996, with permission from Elsevier.

sizers are used to make the intra-operative comparison (Figure 45.8). The surgeon should recognize that the sizers and dilators have a tendency to stretch the tissues, particularly the pulmonary autograft. This can be done by closing the commissures between the left and non-coronary cusps and between the non-coronary and right coronary cusps (Figure 45.9).[7] When a large discrepancy exists, the technique described by Elkins may be preferable. Two parallel 3-0 polypropylene purse string sutures are placed around the full cir-

cumference of the left ventricular outflow tract and tightened to achieve a size that matches the autograft (Figure 45.10).[8] The autograft is then sewn into place.

Once proper size matching has been achieved, the potential for late dilatation should be addressed. Although a complete wrap of the pulmonary autograft may prevent dilatation, most surgeons prefer to buttress the proximal suture line with a strip of Dacron, pericardium, or Teflon felt to fix the diameter of the ventriculoaortic junction (Figure 45.11).

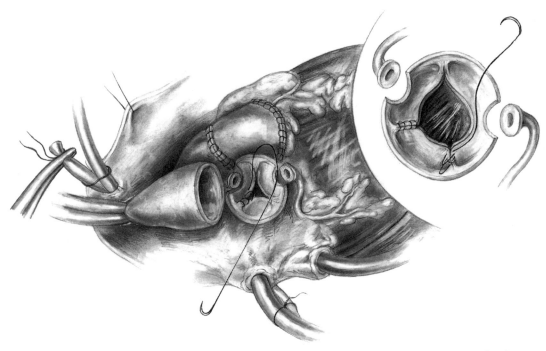

FIGURE 45.9. An oversized aortic annulus can be reduced by placating the fibrous tissue beneath the commissures. Reprinted from *Journal of Thoracic and Cardiovascular Surgery*, Vol 112(5), David et al, "Geometric mismatch of the aortic and pulmonary roots causes aortic insufficiency after the Ross procedure," 1233. © 1996, with permission from Elsevier.

Patients with aortic valve disease requiring valve replacement often have a dilated ascending aorta. Therefore, a size mismatch often exists between the ascending aorta and the pulmonary autograft root. In this circumstance the dilated ascending aorta must be corrected down to a size that matches that of the pulmonary autograft. This is done by removing a wedge of the ascending aorta to reduce its circumference to match that of the pulmonary autograft (Figure 45.12A, B). A cuff of Teflon felt or Dacron may also be used to reinforce the anastomosis at this level.

Summary

Aortic insufficiency after the Ross procedure is an uncommon but serious complication. Current data suggests that aortic insufficiency occurs at a rate of 1 to 3% per patient-year. The development of aortic insufficiency can be minimized by careful patient selection, appropriate attention to the size match of the aortic and pulmonary roots and reinforcement of suture lines to prevent dilatation. As more experience is obtained with this operation the long-term results should continue to improve.

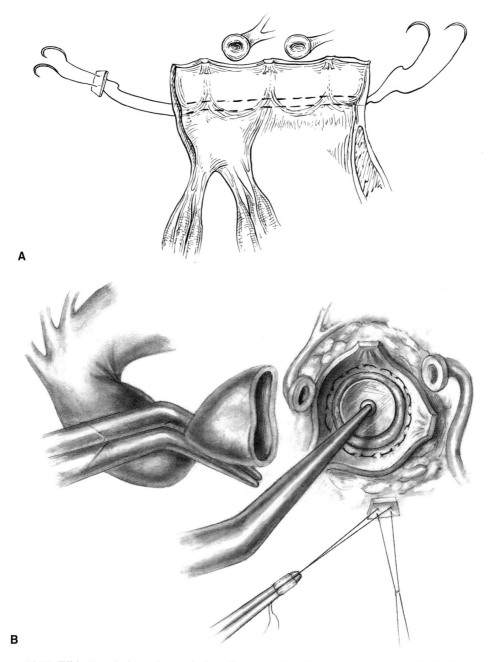

A

B

FIGURE 45.10. Elkins' technique for reducing the size of the left ventricular outflow tract. Two parallel polypropylene sutures are placed around the aortic annulus and passed through a felt pledget placed outside of the non-coronary sinus. (A) The sutures are then tied over a predetermined valve sizer (B). Reprinted from *Annals of Thoracic Surgery*, Vol 61, Elkins, et al, "Pulmonary autografts in patients with aortic annulus dysplasia," 1143. © 1996, with permission from Elsevier.

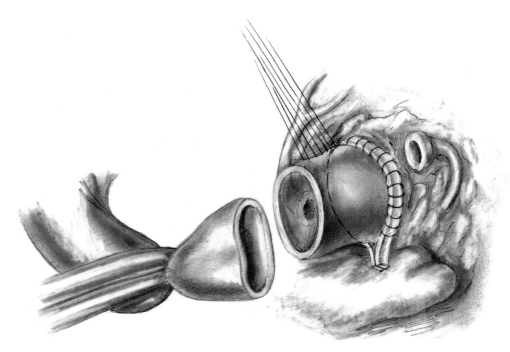

FIGURE 45.11. Reinforcement of proximal suture line with 3 to 4mm strip of Dacron to fix the diameter of the pulmonary autograft at the ventriculo-aortic level. Reprinted from *Annals of Thoracic* *Surgery*, Vol 61, Elkins, et al, "Pulmonary autografts in patients with aortic annulus dysplasia," 1143. © 1996, with permission from Elsevier.

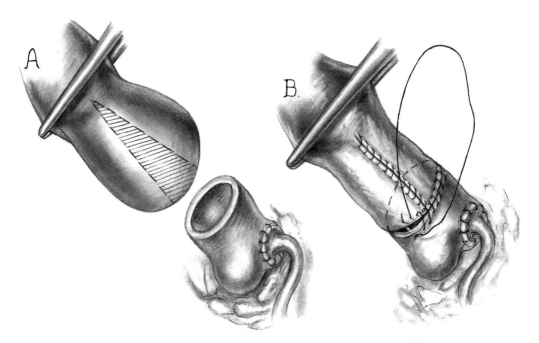

FIGURE 45.12. When significant size discrepancy exists between the ascending aorta and the pulmonary autograft, a reduction aortoplasty is performed by excising a wedge of the anterior wall of the aorta. Reprinted from *Cardiac Surgery: Operative Technique*, Doty D, 249. © 1997, with permission from Elsevier.

References

1. Ross D, Jackson M, Davies J. Pulmonary Auto-graft Aortic Valve Replacement: Long-Term Results. J Card Surg 1991;6:529–533.
2. Ross Procedure International Registry. Summary: The Ross Procedure International Registry at St. Patrick Hospital. Ross Procedurel International Registry. [April 1993 to April 1996]. 1009. Missoula, Montana.
3. Elkins RC, Lane MM, McCue C. Pulmonary Autograft Reoperation: Incidence and Management. Ann Thorac Surg 1996;62:450.
4. Al-Halees Z, Zumar N, Gallo R, Gometza B, Duran CMG. Pulmonary autograft for aortic valve replacement in rheumatic disease: a caveat. Ann Thorac Surg 1995;60:172.
5. Van Suylen RI, Schoof PH, Bos E, Frohn-Mulder OME, den Hollander JC, Herzbergerten CR, Thijssen HJM. Pulmonary autograft failure after aortic root replacement in a patient with juvenile rheumatoid arthritis. Eur J Cardiothorac Surg 1992;6:571.
6. Schoen FJ, Levy RJ. Pathology of substitute heart valves: new concepts and developments. J Card Surg 1994;9 (Suppl):222–227.
7. David TE, Omran A, Webb G, et al. Geometric Mismatch of the aortic and pulmonary root causes aortic insufficiency after the Ross procedure. J Thorac Cardiovasc Surg 1996;112:1231–1239.
8. Elkins RC, Knott-Craig CJ, Howell CE. Pulmonary autografts in patients with aortic annulus dilatation. Ann Thorac Surg 1996;61:1141.

Section XI
Surgical Techniques:
Complex Reconstructions

46

Management of Transposition with Complex Systemic Ventricular Outflow Tract Reconstruction: Rastelli's Operation and Aortic Root Translocation

Pedro J. del Nido

Rastelli's Operation: Applications and Techniques

The surgical management of complex forms of transposition of the great arteries with ventricular septal defect continues to present a challenge to the cardiac surgeon due to the wide variability in anatomy and the disappointing late results with current approaches. For this reason, several techniques have been proposed. However, Rastelli's operation remains the most widely applied procedure for surgical repair of transposition of the great arteries, ventricular septal defect and left ventricular outflow tract obstruction. The goal of the procedure is to divert left ventricular blood flow through the ventricular septal defect to the anteriorly positioned aorta. Right ventricle to pulmonary artery continuity is then achieved by insertion of a conduit. Although several modifications have been described, the procedure itself has remained relatively unchanged since it was first described in 1969.

Anatomy

The essential defect in transposition is discordant connection between the ventricles and the great vessels. In the subgroup that includes left ventricular outflow tract obstruction (LVOTO),

usually there is an associated ventricular septal defect, which can vary in size but is most frequently adjacent to the pulmonary valve. With an outlet type ventricular septal defect, the nature of the LVOTO is usually due to posterior deviation of the outlet septal defect, the mature of the LVOTO is usually due to posterior deviation of the outlet septum causing a muscular and occasionally tunnel-like obstruction in the subpulmonary region. Frequently, the pulmonary valve annulus is hypoplastic and the pulmonary valve itself can be dysplastic. In older children, commonly there is a fibrous ridge present on the outlet septum leading to progressive and more fixed obstruction. Conduction tissue, in the presence of a cono-ventricular VSD that reaches the tricuspid valve, resides in the posterior and inferior margin of the VSD. Therefore, muscular resection can be done safely if confined to the outlet septum or the antero-superior border of the VSD.

An important feature of all forms of transposition is the presence of an infundibulum supporting the anterior positioned aorta. This infundibulum is analogous to that in normally related great vessels supporting the pulmonary valve. This feature is important when considering translocation of the aortic root into the left ventricular outflow tract in that the entire aortic root can be excised similarly to a pulmonary autograft in a heart with normally related great vessels.

Indications for Rastelli Operation

Left ventricular outflow tract obstruction can be dynamic or fixed and this must be determined preoperatively in order to decide whether an arterial switch procedure with VSD closure is sufficient to correct the anatomic defect or whether alternative procedures are required. If the pulmonary valve annulus is of adequate size, then serious consideration should be given to the arterial switch approach since the outlet septum will shift towards the right ventricle once the left ventricle is connected to the systemic circulation and the right ventricular pressures fall. Partial resection of the outlet septum can be accomplished through the neo-aortic root in cases where there is concern that the LVOTO is fixed.

When there is both annular hypoplasia of the pulmonary valve with subpulmonary obstruction and there is a VSD present, then a Rastelli type of procedure can be performed. The VSD may be restrictive and this should be reviewed at the time of surgery since enlargement of the VSD is often required. In cases where there is no VSD, the defect is small, or the defect remote from the cono-ventricular septum, then other alternatives to the Rastelli operation should be considered. These include aortic root translocation and enlargement of the LV outflow tract by septal myotomy (Konno procedure).

Surgical Technique

Moderate to deep hypothermia is used in all cases with cannulation for bypass being achieved with an arterial cannula placed distally at the level of the innominate artery or beyond to permit wide mobilization of the ascending aorta. A single venous cannula in the atrial appendage is usually adequate. In most cases the procedure can be performed without a period of circulatory arrest other than for closure of the interatrial communication. Once on bypass, access to the left ventricular outflow tract is accomplished through a right ventriculotomy that is slightly oblique in orientation just below the aortic root aimed towards the left of the right ventricular outflow (Figure 46.1). Care must be taken to start the ventriculotomy well below the aortic root since the base of the sinus of Valsalva can extend below the visible edge of ventricular muscle. The distal end of the ventriculotomy should end no more than 4–5 mm away from the left main coronary

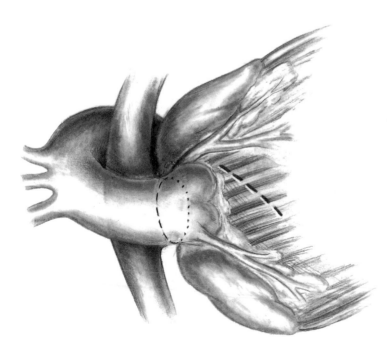

FIGURE 46.1. Depicts the relationship of the great vessels in transposition with the aorta arising from the infundibulum of the right ventricle. The infundibular incision is denoted by the dashed line. Transection of the main pulmonary trunk posterior to the aorta is also shown (dashed circle). Note the position and course of the left main coronary artery and left anterior descending coronary with respect to the right ventricular infundibulum and ventriculotomy.

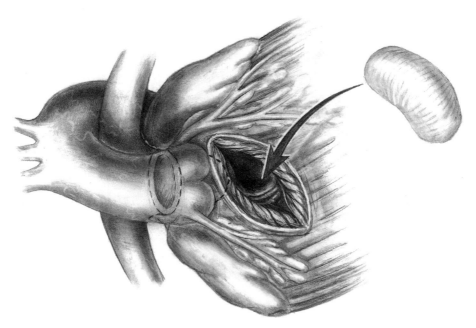

FIGURE 46.2. Once the infundibular incision is made, the ventricular septal defect can be seen in the outflow segment of the left ventricle. Through the ventriculotomy, the outlet septum can be inspected and septal resection with enlargement of the ventricular septal defect can be performed.

to permit insertion of the conduit and suturing without compromising the coronary. This approach gives direct access to the ventricular septal defect, outlet septum and anterior portion of the septum (Figure 46.2). The size of the VSD must be compared to the size of the aortic root and if necessary, enlargement of the VSD should be carried out to prevent left ventricular outflow tract obstruction. VSD enlargement can be done by partial resection of the outlet septum between the aortic and pulmonary valves and by excising the anterior superior edge of the VSD extending to the anterior free wall ventricle. Once the VSD is of adequate size, the main pulmonary trunk can be transected and the proximal end is oversewn to include the dysplastic pulmonary leaflets. The branch pulmonary arteries are dissected with mobilization extended to include upper lobe branches on both sides. This permits mobilization of the transected pulmonary trunk towards the left, facilitating connection to a conduit (Figure 46.3).

Diversion of left ventricular blood flow to the aorta requires creation of a roof to tunnel the LV flow from the VSD up to the anterior edge of the aortic valve annulus or superior edge of the ventriculotomy. The dimensions of the patch and contour should be such that a uniform diameter tunnel is created from the edges of the VSD up to the aorta (Figure 46.3). This is most easily accomplished by using part of the tube graft, which is tailored to reach around the lateral edges of the outlet septum and aortic annulus. Care, however, must be taken not to create too large a baffle for the LV outflow since this will restrict right ventricular outflow through the ventriculotomy. The VSD patch should be attached to the ventricle wall close to the aortic annulus since trabeculations are frequently present in the infundibulum. Care must be taken to exclude these trabeculations from the intraventricular tunnel since they can lead to residual ventricular septal defects if not closed (Figure 46.3).

Right ventricle to pulmonary artery continuity is then established by conduit insertion (Figure 46.4). We prefer to use a homograft, either aortic or pulmonary. The posterior portion of the annulus of the homograft is sewn

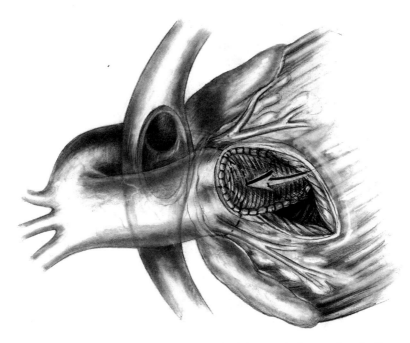

FIGURE 46.3. Diversion of the left ventricular outflow through the VSD using a tunnel shaped synthetic patch that accommodates to the contour of the outflow tract. Note that the patch extends from the edge of the VSD up to the aortic valve annulus. Once the left ventricular outflow is diverted to the aorta through the VSD, the pulmonary arteries are mobilized so that the transected main pulmonary trunk is to the left of the aorta.

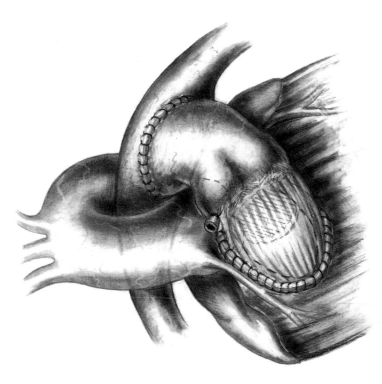

FIGURE 46.4. Continuity between the right ventricle and pulmonary trunk is achieved by use of a homograft interposition conduit. The posterior edge of the homograft is sewn directly to the distal portion of the ventriculotomy. The anterior roof of the connection is created with the attached mitral valve leaflet or preferably with the use of glutaraldehyde treated autologous pericardium or prosthetic material.

to the distal one-third of the ventriculotomy. The proximal connection is covered by either a portion of the anterior leaflet of the mitral valve of an aortic homograft, with a patch of autologous glutaraldehyde treated pericardium or a portion of the homograft wall, if available. The distal end of the homograft is then connected to the main pulmonary trunk by direct anastomosis, preferably to the left of the aorta. Since the homograft conduit arises from the anterior-most portion of the ventricle, this places it directly underneath the sternum so that diverting the conduit towards the right would lead to further compression. In our experience, placing the conduit to the right of the aorta is an independent risk factor for mortality and morbidity in the Rastelli operation. In cases where the pulmonary artery arises rightward of the aorta, extensive mobilization of the branch PAs permits shifting of the main pulmonary trunk towards the left. Extending the pulmonary arteriotomy into the left pulmonary artery branch may also facilitate this anastomosis (Figure 46.4). Extensive mobilization of the pericardium including an incision of the diaphragmatic reflection anteriorly, towards the apex of the heart permits shifting of the conduit towards the left minimizing compression with sternal closure.

Early Complications

The potential sources of early morbidity from a Rastelli operation are most frequently related to anatomic features which restrict the intraventricular baffle, conduit obstruction, and injury to conduction tissue. In a recent review of out experience[1] with 101 patients having the Rastelli procedure from 1973 to 1998, risk factors for hospital mortality were the presence of prior surgery (systemic to pulmonary artery shunt), use of circulatory arrest for the repair, longer cardiopulmonary bypass times, the presence of complete AV block postoperatively, and placement of the right ventricle to pulmonary artery conduit to the right of the aorta. The incidence of complete AV block was 6% and the most frequently observed arrhythmia was junctional ectopic tachycardia, which occurred in 11% of the patients. Delayed sternal closure

due to mediastinal edema or compression of the conduit was required in 5% of the patients.

In-hospital mortality decreased over the 25 year period of the study from 10% in the period prior to 1989 to 0% during the most recent seven year period. Risk factors for early mortality included complete AV block requiring pacemaker insertion, longer cardiopulmonary bypass and cross-clamp times. Anatomic risk factors included the presence of straddling tricuspid valve. Significantly, weight and age at the time of surgery were not risk factors for early mortality.

Late Results

Actuarial survival was 93% at one year, 81% at five years, 79% at ten years, and 52% at 20 years. The incidence of late reoperations increased significantly over time with the most frequent indication being right ventricular outflow tract obstruction from conduit or pulmonary artery stenosis. Left ventricular outflow tract obstruction was the second most common indication for reoperation. Freedom from reoperation was 71% at five years and 47% at ten years.

Aortic Root Translocation and Arterial Switch for Transposition and Left Ventricular Outflow Obstruction

Several alternative techniques to the Rastelli operation have been described with varying results. Atrial level repair (Mustard or Senning Operation) with closure of ventricular septal defect and resection of LV outflow with or without a conduit is associated with a very high late mortality and is currently rarely done. Aortic root translocation posteriorly with resection of outlet septum was originally proposed by Nikaidoh. He described direct mobilization of the aortic root and attached coronaries. The main limitation of this procedure was the potential for coronary artery obstruction particularly if applied to younger children.

An alternative procedure we have utilized applies the concept of a pulmonary autograft to this anatomic defect. The advantages of this approach are that it can be used in infants as well as older children and since it does not require the presence of a VSD, it can be applied to anatomic variants with absent, severely restrictive VSD, or in cases where the VSD it remote from the ventriculo-arterial connection.

Surgical Technique

For this procedure, cardiopulmonary bypass is utilized in the same way as for the Rastelli operation. Obtaining a significant length of the ascending aorta by more distal insertion of the arterial cannula facilitates resection of the aortic root. Once the ascending aorta is cross-clamped and the heart arrested with cardioplegia, the ascending aorta is transected above the level of the commissures. Similarly, a transverse ventriculotomy is then done as performed in the Rastelli procedure except that the aim is to resect the aortic root including infundibular muscle similar to that done for a pulmonary

autograft in normally related great vessels (Figure 46.5).

The coronary arteries are then excised as circular buttons and an effort is made to maintain the ring of ascending aorta above the sinuses of Valsalva intact to prevent the distortion of the aortic root. Once the coronaries are mobilized, similar to an arterial switch procedure, the aortic root is then excised by completing the circumferential incision in the right ventricular infundibulum (Figure 46.6). The main pulmonary artery is then transected above the level of the pulmonary valve and an incision is then made across the anterior portion of the pulmonary annulus extending towards the ventricular septal defect, if present, or towards the anterior septum similar to a Konno procedure. This permits enlargement of the left ventricular outflow tract by insertion of a triangular shaped VSD patch to accommodate the larger aortic root. The aortic root autograft is then rotated 180° so that the defects from the coronary buttons are anterior. The subvalvar portion of the autograft is then sewn to the left ventricular outflow by attaching it directly to the pul-

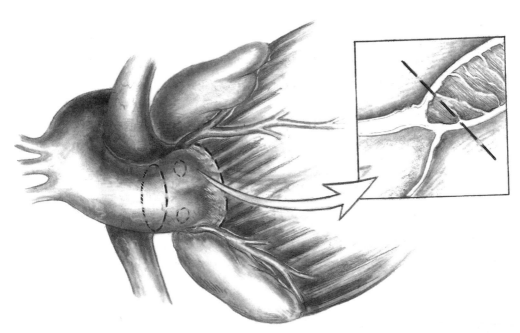

FIGURE 46.5. The ventricular and aortic incisions required for aortic autograft excision are depicted. Note that the infundibular incision is circumferential just below the aortic valve annulus. The coronary ostia are excised as circular buttons from the respective sinuses of Valsalva.

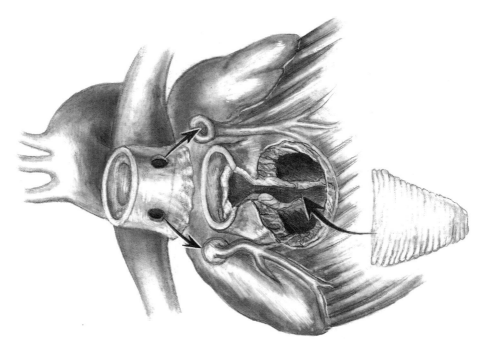

FIGURE 46.6. Once the aortic autograft is excised and the coronaries mobilized, the main pulmonary trunk is transected and an incision is extended across the pulmonary valve annulus and outlet septum con-necting to the ventricular septal defect, if present. Enlargement of the left ventricular outflow tract is then accomplished by insertion of a triangular shaped VSD patch.

monary valve annulus posteriorly and to the distal edge of the VSD patch anteriorly. The junction between the VSD patch, ventricular edge of LV outflow and the aortic autograft must be reinforced since this is a frequent site of bleeding. The distal orifice of the aortic auto-graft is then sewn to the ascending aorta after the branch pulmonary arteries are mobilized anterior to the aorta (Lecompte maneuver) similar to an arterial switch procedure (Figure 46.7). Re-implantation of the coronaries is done into the neo-aortic root at the side of the defects from the excision of the coronary buttons or more distally in the aorta if the aortic root is too low into the base of the left ventricle. Right ventricle to pulmonary artery continuity is then established by inserting an interposition homograft sewn directly to the right ventricular infundibulum (Figure 46.8). Posteriorly, the homograft must be attached to the distal edge of the VSD patch since this is now the posterior wall of the right ventricular outflow tract. Further reinforcement of the

junction between the VSD patch, right ventric-ular infundibulum and homograft must be done with additional sutures to prevent bleeding from the site.

In cases where the pulmonary artery and aorta are in a side-by-side arrangement, then anterior mobilization of the pulmonary branches is not necessary and the right ventri-cle to pulmonary artery homograft conduit can be positioned either to the right or to the left of the aorta. Since part of this procedure involves shifting the ascending aorta posteri-orly, this provides substantial room for the conduit, minimizing the risk of conduit com-pression from sternal closure.

Early and Late Results

Experience with this procedure is much more limited when compared to the Rastelli opera-tion. However, sources of morbidity and mor-tality may be similar to those of the Rastelli operation. Preliminary results indicate

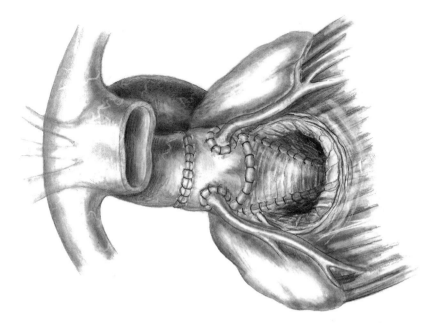

FIGURE 46.7. The aortic autograft is re-inserted into the LV outflow. The coronaries are then re-implanted anteriorly. Prior to re-establishing ascending aortic continuity, the branch pulmonary arteries are mobilized and brought anterior to the aorta (Lecompte Maneuver) in preparation for RV outflow reconstruction.

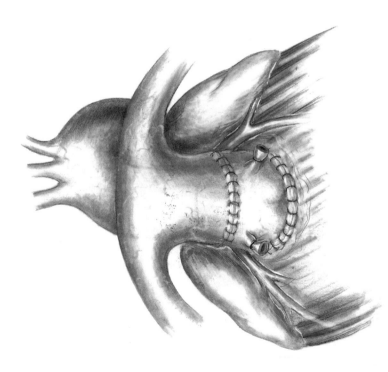

FIGURE 46.8. Right ventricle to pulmonary artery continuity is achieved by insertion of an interposition homograft connecting the RV infundibulum to the pulmonary trunk.

however, that there is a tendency towards less left and right ventricular outflow tract obstruction with this procedure compared to the Rastelli operation due to the more favorable position of the left ventricular outflow reconstruction as well as the right ventricle to pulmonary artery conduit.

Reference

1. Kreutzer C, Gauvreu K, de Vivie J, Oppido G, Kreutzer J, Freed M, Mayer JE, Jonas RA, del Nido P. Twenty-five year experience with Rastelli repair for transposition of the great arteries. J Thorac Cardiovasc Surg 1999; IN PRESS.

47
Homograft Variant of the Nikaidoh Procedure

Richard A. Hopkins

In 1984, Hisashi Nikaidoh reported a novel procedure for management of transposition of the great arteries associated with ventricular septal defect and pulmonary stenosis.[1] Subsequent experience with the Ross, the switch and homograft operations have made this an even more attractive operation for management of transposition with a large aortic outflow and a hypoplastic left ventricular outflow. We have performed the operation with restitution of right ventricular continuity of the pulmonary circulation with a separate homograft which differs from Nikaidoh's original operation where the PA was attached to the aorta directly.

The operation is performed with single atrial cannula, distal aortic arch cannulation, hypothermia with periods of low flow.

As described by Nikaidoh, the aortic root is mobilized with minimal mobilization of the coronary arteries (Figure 47.1).

The aortic root is separated from the ventricle and the pulmonary artery transected (Figure 47.2).

A portion of the outflow septum is resected which fully opens the left ventricular outflow tract (Figure 47.3). The VSD is closed with a patch of double velour Dacron sutured up to the edge of the anterior border of the resected base of the aorta. This gives a very large outflow tract which is then sutured to the base of the aorta with a continuous running 4-0 polypropylene suture that incorporates the patch anteriorly (Figure 47.4).

The right ventricular outflow tract continuity with the pulmonary artery is now re-established with an aortic or pulmonary homograft. This can be accomplished with an aortic homograft in which the right ventriculotomy is performed lower down on the anterior right ventricle and the outflow curvature augmented with a hood of thin wall PTFE (Figure 47.5).

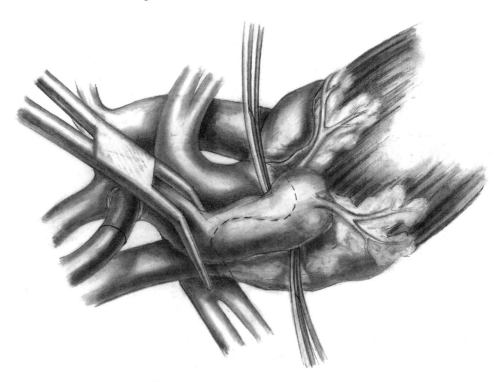

FIGURE 47.1. Aortic root is mobilized.

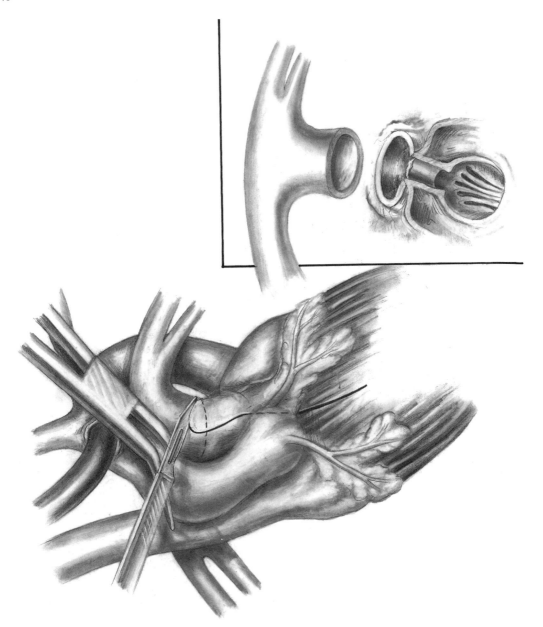

FIGURE 47.2. The main pulmonary artery is transected posteriorly and an incision prepared from the pulmonary artery across the fibrous ring and into the outflow septum.

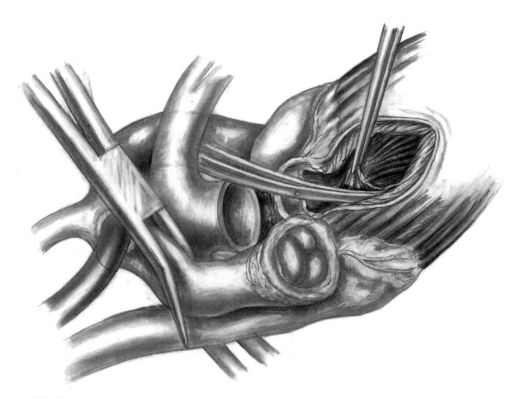

FIGURE 47.3. The incision across the pulmonary annulus is extended to the level of the VSD. Muscle tissue is carefully excised from the infundibular septum to enlarge the left ventricular outflow. In our one case, heart block did not develop.

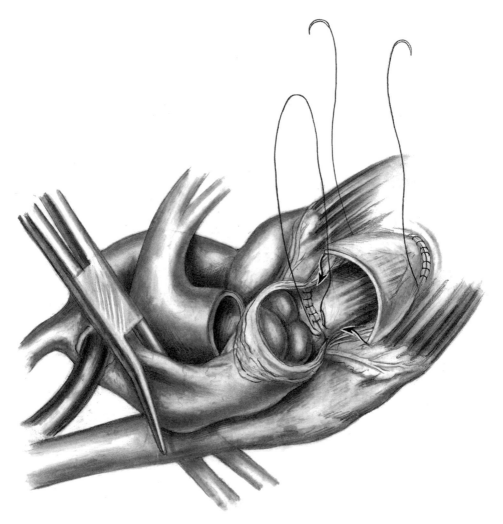

FIGURE 47.4. The difference in our technique and the Nikaidoh technique is that the VSD patch is actually brought to the edge of the ventricular muscle, which opens up the whole outflow tract beautifully. It is sutured, not with interrupted sutures, but with a continuous running suture for both the VSD patch as well as the aorta on top of the outflow portion.

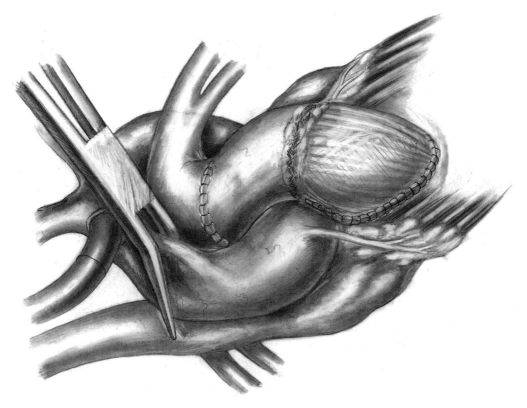

FIGURE 47.5. This figure shows completion with the homograft.

Reference

1. Nikaidoh H. Aortic translocation and biventricular outflow tract reconstruction: a new surgical repair for transposition of the great arteries associated with ventricular septal defect and pulmonary stenosis. J Thorac Cardiovasc Surg 1984; 88:365–372.

48
Application of the Principle of Creation of Double Outlet Systemic Ventricle for Hypoplastic Aortic Outflow

Richard A. Hopkins and Gary K. Lofland

Homograft tissue can be used in creative ways to reconstruct systemic outflow by dedicating the pulmonary valve to the systemic ventricle, using nonvalved homograft tissue to augment the neo-LVOT outflow, and re-establishing with a second homograft, pulmonary ventricle to pulmonary continuity, or in the case of single ventricle, performing a variation on the Norwood operation.

Double Outlet Right Ventricle with Transposition of the Great Arteries and Hypoplastic Aorta with Either Interrupted Aortic Arch or Severe Coarctation

Figure 48.1 demonstrates the anatomy. The distal arch may involve a severe coarctation (Figure 48.1). The operation is performed under deep hypothermia and total circulatory arrest and incisions are made as demonstrated in Figure 48.2 after closing the ventricular septal defect via right ventriculotomy. Closure of the VSD in this fashion diverts the left ventricular outflow to both the hypoplastic aortic valve and the large pulmonary valve. An aortic homograft of appropriate size (usually an 8 or 10mm) is then tailored as demonstrated in Figure 48.3. The repair is completed by suturing the proximal nonvalved homograft to the proximal native pulmonary artery above the sino-tubular ridge of the pulmonary valve. The distal anastomosis is accomplished to a long Norwood-like incision in the transverse and distal aortic arch. The homograft anastomosis is continued well down to the descending aorta to avoid any late re-coarctation (Figure 48.4). Double outflow from left ventricle is accomplished and a standard RVOT to pulmonary artery homograft reconstruction completes the repair.

Transposition of the Great Arteries, Ventricular Septal Defect, Interrupted Aortic Arch and Subaortic Stenosis

This operation is performed similarly to the double outlet variety. The patch for closure of the ventricular septal defect is constructed so as to deviate all the left ventricular outflow into both the hypoplastic aorta and pulmonary artery. The subaortic stenosis is ignored (Figure 48.5). The interrupted aortic arch is managed with an end-to-end anastomosis to the homograft conduit and then a slit (Figure 48.6) made along the top to suture the head vessels as an on-lay patch to the top of the homograft. The proximal anastomosis to the pulmonary artery above the native pulmonary valve completes the left ventricular double outflow.

The operation can be performed also in the presence of a coarctation by not utilizing two separate anastomoses to the aortic components (Figure 48.7). The operation is then completed with a pulmonary or aortic homograft reconstruction of the right ventricular outflow tract.

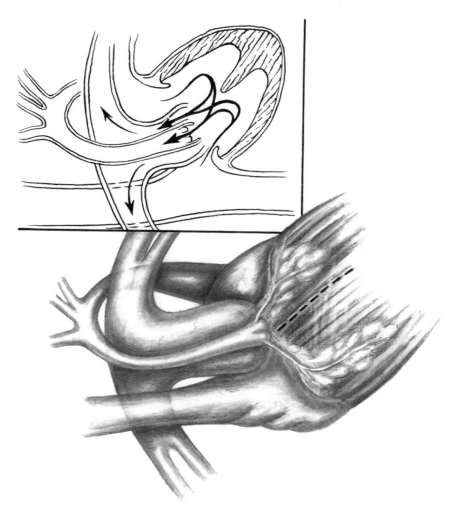

FIGURE 48.1. This demonstrates the anatomy of double outlet right ventricle with transposition of the great arteries and severe coarctation with hypoplas-tic ascending aorta. Repair is only mildly different if an interrupted aortic arch is present. Dotted line marks incision site.

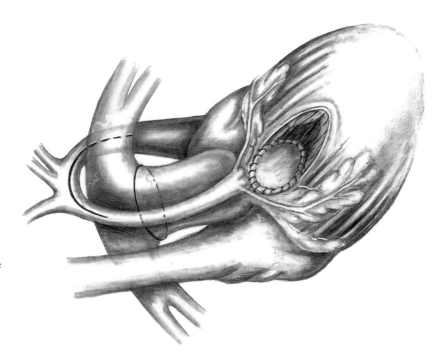

FIGURE 48.2. Incisions for correction of double outlet right ventricle with transposition of the great arteries with hypoplastic aortic outflow by creating double outlet left ventricle.

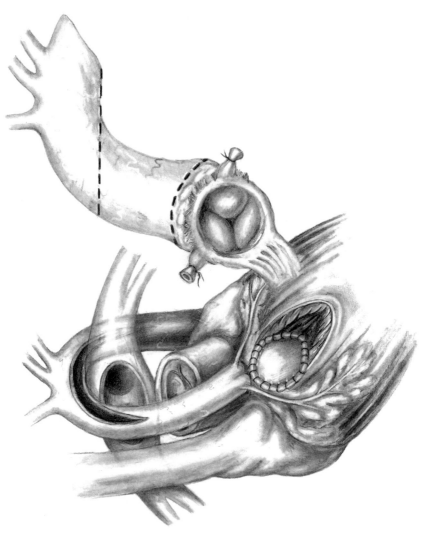

FIGURE 48.3. The homograft aortic valve is excised and a severely oblique distal end of the homograft is created for the repair.

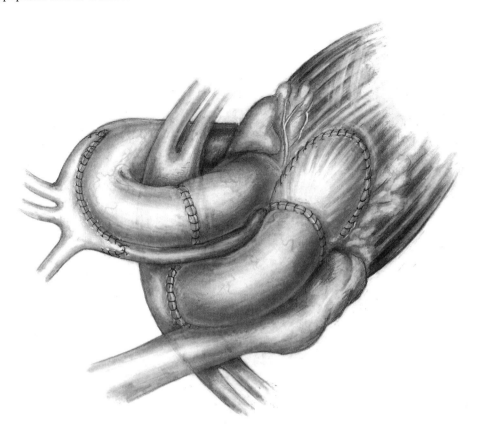

FIGURE 48.4. Completion of repair for double outlet right ventricle with transposition of the great arteries and hypoplastic ascending aorta utilizing the principle of the creation of double outlet left ventricle. The valved conduit for the right ventricular homograft reconstruction is up-sized as much as possible and is brought to the right side of the systemic outflow reconstruction in most cases.

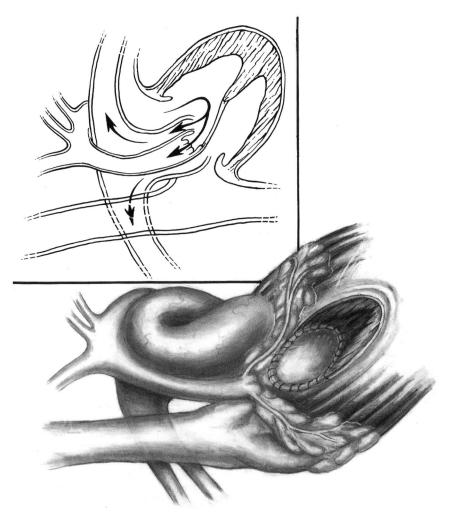

FIGURE 48.5. Transposition great arteries, VSD, interrupted aortic arch and subaortic stenosis.

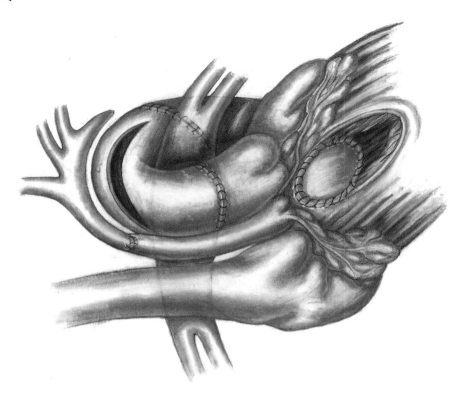

FIGURE 48.6. The head vessels are sutured as a "patch" to the top of the homograft.

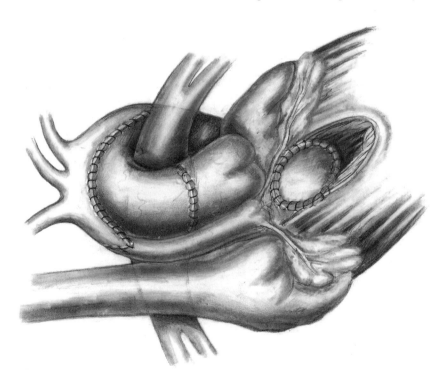

FIGURE 48.7. Creation of double outlet left ventricle for transposition of the great arteries, ventricular septal defect, subaortic stenosis with severe coarcta- tion (not interruption) with ascending aortic hypoplasia by not utilizing two separate "distal" aortic anastomoses.

Single Ventricle, Transposition of the Great Arteries, Hypoplastic Aorta (Interrupted Aortic Arch or Coarctation)

Application of the approach described for the two ventricle repairs can also be used in the single ventricle (Figure 48.8) in a fashion similar to a classic Norwood (Figure 48.9). In this case, where there is hypoplasia of the aorta, there is some opportunity for growth of the native ascending aorta, but the anastomoses are made in a similar fashion (Figure 48.10).

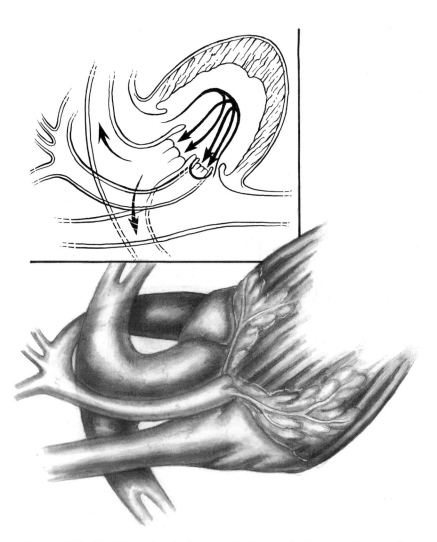

FIGURE 48.8. Double outlet single ventricle for repair (Norwood concept).

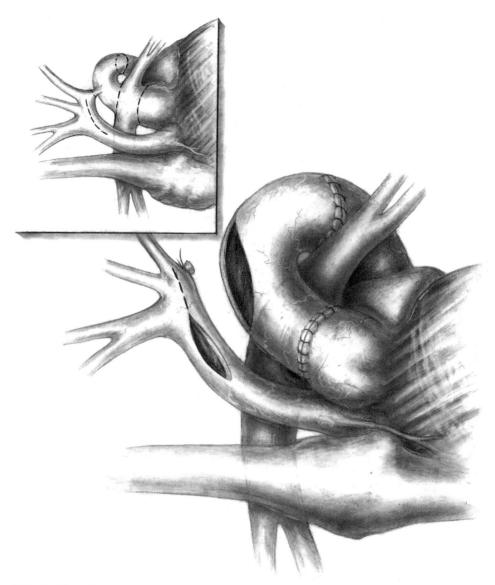

FIGURE 48.9. Incisions for reconstruction for single ventricle, transposition great arteries, hypoplastic aortic valve and ascending aorta. All ductal tissue is discarded.

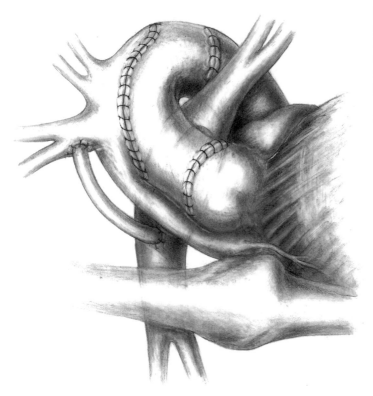

FIGURE 48.10. Application of arch reconstruction with homograft utilizing the Norwood principle. Two separate "distal" anastomoses are fashioned. This figure demonstrates patching of the main pulmonary artery where it has been divided from the heart. A systemic to pulmonary artery shunt completes the repair.

Section XII
Surgical Techniques: Right Ventricular Outflow Tract Reconstructions

49
Indications: Right Ventricular Outflow Reconstructions

Richard A. Hopkins

The development of the extracardiac conduit for reconstruction of "blue" ventricle to pulmonary artery continuity has revolutionized the surgery of many complex congenital defects.[1-5] In infants with anomalies such as tetralogy of Fallot, non-valved reconstruction of the right ventricular outflow has been well tolerated with a low early reoperation rate (e.g., 100% reoperation-free at 4 years in the Boston Children's Hospital series).[6] However, patients developing progressive right ventricular dilatation have required later replacement with a valved prosthesis. Other anatomic situations, particularly that of pulmonary atresia or pulmonary atresia accompanying other defects (e.g., corrected transposition) that have usually been repaired during childhood rather than infancy, have done best with right ventricular outflow tract reconstructions utilizing valved conduits (Rastelli concept). There are neonatal and infant reconstructions that are optimally accomplished with valved conduits (e.g., truncus arteriosus, absent pulmonary valve syndrome). The allograft has become the conduit of choice for all right ventricular outflow tract reconstructions.[7]

Symptoms of progressive right ventricular failure due to pulmonary insufficiency include fluid retention, fatigue, and exercise intolerance. Once right ventricular dilatation progresses to the point that tricuspid regurgitation occurs, symptomatology advances rapidly. Right ventricular function has been demonstrated to improve following placement of a pulmonary valve.[8] Tricuspid insufficiency is important as a marker for deteriorating right ventricular function and as a potent hemodynamic burden in the presence of outflow tract abnormalities. As the San Francisco experience has demonstrated, once tricuspid incompetence develops rapid and persistent right ventricular failure follows that is difficult to mitigate medically.[9] There is marked improvement with restoration of pulmonary sufficiency even if a murmur or mild tricuspid regurgitation persists.[10] If pulmonary valve replacement is postponed and tricuspid regurgitation progresses, the reconstructive surgery must include restoration of tricuspid competence.

Performance of most models of mechanical valves in the right side of the heart has been relatively poor, and in general either bioprostheses or allografts have been recommended. In the series from Chicago, more than one-third of the patients developed prosthetic pulmonary valvular dysfunction less than 1 year following insertion of a mechanical prosthesis.[11] Thus despite the issue of accelerated failure, if an allograft is not available a porcine prosthesis is probably the optimal choice for the right ventricular outflow tract position.

Ideally, anticoagulation in children is avoided. Unfortunately, porcine prostheses have not fared well in the right-sided circulation, although they have done somewhat better in older children and young adults.[12] Mechanical prostheses are associated with a significant rate of dysfunction in the right-sided position.[13] Synthetic right heart *conduits* have been noted to require replacement 100% of the time by 10 years following insertion, although initial early results are good.[6]

Fontan and colleagues have reported on more that 100 allograft aortic valve conduits with only one replacement for allograft valve dysfunction and no thromboembolism or hemolysis; in the same series, a pressure gradient (13–85 mmHg, mean 39 mmHg) was present in only 14 ventricle-dependent conduits.[14] In this series from France, gradients across the allograft conduits occurred at three sites in the pre-valvular region, five sites in the valvular or undetermined region, and five sites in the postvalvular (presumably distal anastomosis) region.[15] In the United States Kirklin and associates have demonstrated a 94% actuarial freedom from reoperation for obstruction in cryopreserved allograft conduits at 3.5 years.[15]

A functioning right ventricular outflow valve is recommended for either primary or secondary reconstructions where there is (1) symptomatic right ventricular dysfunction, (2) fixed pulmonary hypertension, (3) hypoplastic pulmonary arteries, (4) pulmonary insufficiency with right ventricular dilatation, (5) tricuspid regurgitation, (6) echocardiographic evidence of small right ventricular volume or poor performance, (7) absent pulmonary valve syndrome, (8) peripheral pulmonary stenoses, (9) highly reactive pulmonary circulation (e.g., neonatal truncus).[16]

If there were a perfect valve substitute that could grow or be of adult size when placed in the pulmonary position, it could be argued that a valved reconstruction of the right ventricular outflow tract could be applicable in all cases to (1) protect against the long-term effects of pulmonary insufficiency including right ventricular dysfunction and dilatation, (2) accomplish right ventricular outflow tract reconstruction without relative obstruction, and (3) prevent or mitigate tricuspid dysfunction. At present, we do *not* recommend universal application, e.g., for routine primary tetralogy of Fallot repairs.[17] However, a proportion of patients with non-valved conduits or transannular patches return with progressive right ventricular dysfunction, especially when additional preload or afterload lesions are present, and require reconstruction with an allograft.[18]

References

1. Rastelli GC, Ongley PA, Davis GD, Kirklin JW. Surgical repair for pulmonary valve atresia with coronary-pulmonary artery fistula: Report of a case. Mayo Clin Proc 1965;40:521–727.
2. Ciaravella JM, Jr., McGoon DC, Danielson GK, Wallace RB, Mair DD, Ilstrup DM. Experience with the extracardiac conduit. J Thorac Cardiovasc Surg 1979;78:920–930.
3. McGoon DC, Danielson GK, Puga FJ, et al. Late results after extracardiac conduit repair for congenital cardiac defects. Am J Cardiol 1982;49:1741–1749.
4. Moore CH, Martelli V, Ross DN. Reconstruction of right ventricular outflow tracts with a valve conduit in seventy-five cases of congenital heart disease. J Thorac Cardiovasc Surg 1976;71:11–19.
5. Weldon CS, Rowe RD, Gott VL. Clinical experience with the use of aortic valve homografts for reconstruction of the pulmonary artery, pulmonary valve, and outflow portion of the right ventricle. Circulation 1968;37:II51–II61.
6. Jonas RA, Freed MD, Mayor JE, Castaneda AR. Long term follow-up of patients with synthetic right heart conduits. Circulation 1985;72 (Suppll. 2):II77–II83.
7. Kay PH, Ross DN. Fifteen years' experience with the aortic homograft: the conduit of choice for right ventricular outflow tract reconstruction. Ann Thorac Surg 1985;40:360–364.
8. Bove EL, Kavey REW, Byrum CJ, et al. Improved right ventricular function following late pulmonary valve replacement for residual pulmonary insufficiency or stenosis. J Thorac Cardiovasc Surg 1985;90:50–55.
9. Ebert PA. Second operations for pulmonary stenosis or insufficiency after repair of tetralogy of Fallot. In Engle MA, Perloff JK (eds). Congenital heart disease after surgery: Benefits, residua, sequela. New York: Yorke 1983:202–209.
10. Ebert PA. Second operations for pulmonary stenosis or insufficiency after repair of tetralogy of Fallot. Am J Cardiol 1982;50:637–640.
11. Ilbawi MN, Idriss FS, DeLeon SY, et al. Factors that exaggerate the deleterious effects of pulmonary insufficiency of the right ventricular after tetralogy repair. J Thorac Cardiovasc Surg 1987;93:36–44.

12. Ilbawi MN, Idriss FS, DeLoin SY, et al. Long-term results of porcine valve insertion for pulmonary regurgitation following repair of tetralogy of Fallot. Ann Thorac Surg 1986;41: 478–482.

13. Ilbawi MN, Idriss FS, DeLeon SY, et al. Valve replacement in children: guidelines for selection of prosthesis and timing of surgical intervention. Ann Thorac Surg 1987;44:398–403.

14. Fontan F, Choussat A, DeVille C, et al. Aortic valve homografts in the surgical treatment of complex cardiac malformations. J Thorac Cardiovasc Surg 1984;87:649–657.

15. Kirklin JW, Blackstone EH, Maehara T, Pacifico AD, Kirklin JK, Pollock S, Stewart RW. Inter-mediate-term fate of cryopreserved allograft and xenograft valved conduits. Ann Thorac Surg 1987;44:598–606.

16. Ebert PA. The role of valves in pulmonary conduits. In Dunn JM (ed). Cardiac Valve Disease in Children. New York: Elsevier 1988:147–152.

17. Hopkins RA. Right ventricular outflow tract reconstructions: the role of valves in the viable allograft era. Ann Thorac Surg 1988;45:593–594.

18. Finck SJ, Puga FJ, Danielson GK. Pulmonary valve insertion during reoperation for tetralogy of Fallot. Ann Thorac Surg 1988;45:610–613.

50
Right Ventricle to Pulmonary Artery Aortic Allograft Conduits in Children and Infants

Richard A. Hopkins

Sizing

Usually an adult-sized right ventricular conduit (19 to 26 mm aortic allograft) is placed, except in small infants (see Appendix: Valve Diameters). It is generally possible in the patient weighing 3.5–5.0 kg to place a 12-mm conduit whereas in those weighing less than 3 kg an 8- to 10-mm conduit may be required (See appendix). A 14 to 16 mm conduit is used in patients who weigh 5–10 kg. These weight guidelines are similar to those used by Kirklin and colleagues; they reported the use of 9 to 12 mm allografts for infants with body surface area (BSA) of 0.2–0.3 m², 12 to 14 mm allografts for infants with BSA 0.3–0.4 m², and 15 to 17 mm allografts for children with BSA 0.4–0.5 m². Once a child weighs 15–20 kg it is almost always possible to place a 20 mm or larger conduit in the right ventricular outflow tract position. The distal anastomosis can be enlarged by sewing obliquely (beveled); the size in the neonates is restricted primarily by the maximum ventriculotomy that can be achieved and secondarily by thoracic volume. Conduit compression by the anterior chest is usually easily avoided.

Interestingly, Mercer presented data suggesting that a 12 mm (inside diameter; ID) pulmonary annulus (not conduit) results in only a 50% reduction in cross-sectioned area and might result in acceptably low gradients even as the child approaches 10 years of age.[1] The 12-mm synthetic conduit has been shown to give superb early results in infants but always results

in gradients requiring later replacement; it is also a more difficult material with which to avoid kinking, compression, and so on.[2] An 18-mm or larger allograft is usually free of significant obstruction and is a perfectly adequate size into which a child can grow. This implant is achievable in most children exceeding 15 kg in weight. This discussion presupposes a ventricular-supported pulmonary circulation; atrial-dependent pulmonary circulations require pulmonary inflow geometry to approximate normal tricuspid valve areas in order to avoid obstructive hemodynamics.

Principles

A number of principles are emphasized to optimize the result of allograft insertions for right ventricular outflow tract reconstructions:[3] (1) avoidance of the use of synthetic tubular grafts on either end of the conduit; (2) placement that avoids compression by the sternum; (3) use of nonrestrictive ventriculotomy; (4) use of a PTFE hood extension to the anterior leaflet of the mitral valve to complete the exit from the ventriculotomy into the conduit; (5) oblique suturing of the distal suture line with polypropylene monofilament surgical technique; (6) slight "stretching" of the conduit to enhance semilunar suspension (i.e. keep conduit short as possible); and (7) avoiding an excessively long ventriculotomy, which tends to flatten the anterior mitral leaflet closure and distort the new outflow valve.

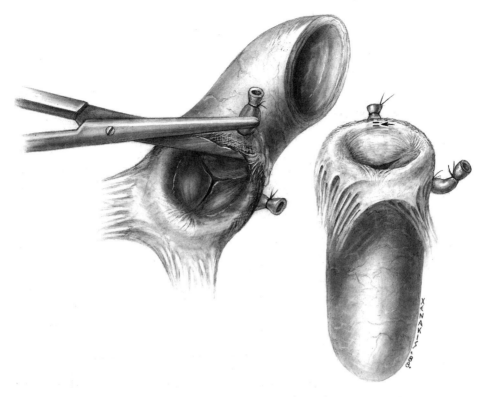

FIGURE 50.1. Trimming the allograft. Note the 2-mm remnant (arrow) underneath the right coronary cusp. Care must be taken when debulking the muscle in this region.

If extensions of the conduit are necessary, they should usually be constructed at the proximal end with pericardium. (We rarely have to use this procedure.) If an allograft pulmonary valve is used rather than an aortic valve, it should be recognized that the postvalvular segment of the allograft is shorter.[4] When so used, the pulmonary allograft requires a patch of pericardium to close the ventriculotomy in order to avoid distortion of the valve (analogous to use of the aortic allograft anterior mitral leaflet).

Technique

Patients are placed on cardiopulmonary bypass utilizing dual caval cannulation. Hypothermia and cardioplegic cardiac arrest allow optimal visualization of the pulmonary arteries for reconstruction during the distal anastomosis. The proximal anastomosis is usually accom-

plished during rewarming. The conduit is selected and thawed. It is trimmed, debulking the muscle and leaving the anterior leaflet of the mitral valve attached. Care is taken underneath the right coronary ostia where the right leaflet base is usually close to the muscle being trimmed (Figure 50.1).

A ventriculotomy is performed high in the infundibulum, placed so as to avoid the coronary arteries and to minimize right ventricular dysfunction. It is extended out the main pulmonary artery when the artery is in continuity with the base of the heart. When there is no main pulmonary artery continuity with the base of the heart, the confluence or whatever element of the main pulmonary artery is present is opened longitudinally and the incision extended toward the confluence or into either, or both, right and left pulmonary arteries if necessary to relieve a stenosis. The length of the conduit is adjusted so that the annulus of the allograft valve seats at the upper edge of

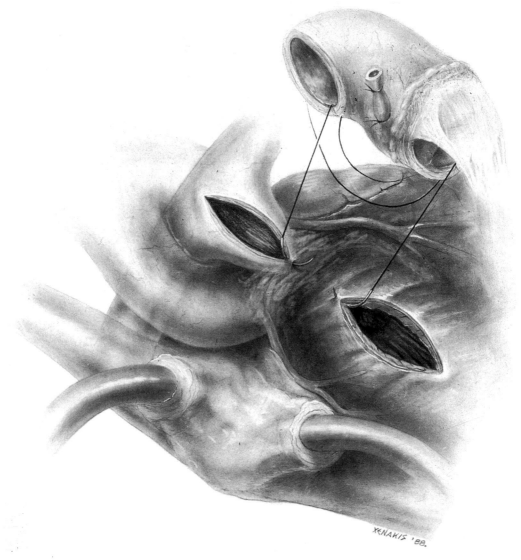

FIGURE 50.2. Distal anastomosis of aortic allograft (conduit) is performed in an oblique fashion to the pulmonary artery for pulmonary atresia when the main pulmonary artery is reasonably well developed.

the right ventriculotomy. The distal anastomosis is accomplished with a running 5-0 or 6-0 polypropylene suture or with an oblique or beveled fashion (Figure 50.2). An end-to-end distal technique can be used when the main pulmonary artery is of adequate caliber and there is pulmonary valve atresia or side-to-side technique when bypassing a hypoplastic but competent pulmonary valve that exits the pulmonary ventricle (i.e., some continuity exists) (Figures 50.3 and 50.4). If the native pulmonary valve exits the systemic ventricle, complete division is performed and the stump oversewn.

The proximal anastomosis is accomplished with either a running 4-0 or 5-0 polypropylene suture technique. The allograft should be trimmed of excessive muscle to the point that the fibrous skeleton can be seen. The attached portion of the anterior leaflet of the donor mitral valve is partially preserved, but chordal insertions and tags are all excised. This anterior leaflet mitral valve provides a filling point for the PTFE hood which is used to enlarge and smooth the outflow. The membranous septum is usually retained on the allograft. The suture line is begun posteriorly and run to the corner of the anterior leaflet of the mitral valve at either side of the annulus and secured. The hood of PTFE is then obtained from an appro-priate sized tube graft (usually the size of the annulus or 2–6 mm larger). The PTFE gusset is fashioned and sutured at the far corner away from the surgeon at the point that the annulus and ventriculotomy and anterior leaflet of the mitral valve meet. This is secured with a running polypropylene suture which is then run across the top of the anterior leaflet of the mitral valve securing the PTFE gusset (Figure 50.4). As the other fibrous trigone is reached at

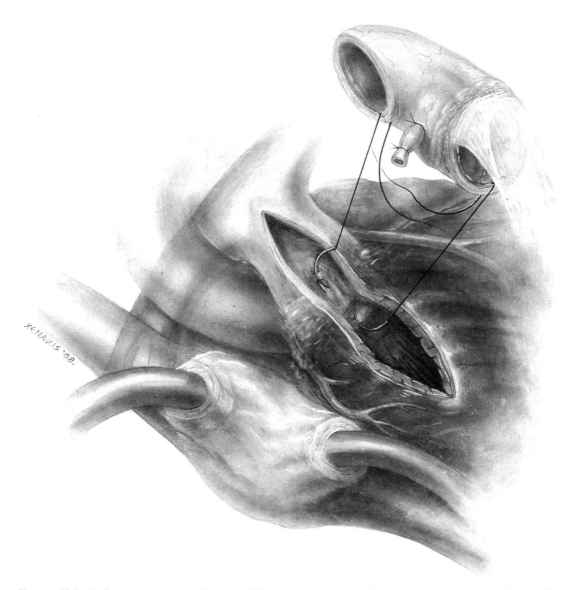

FIGURE 50.3. End-to-end anastomosis in an oblique manner when pulmonary ventricular-arterial continuity is present (e.g., valvular atresia).

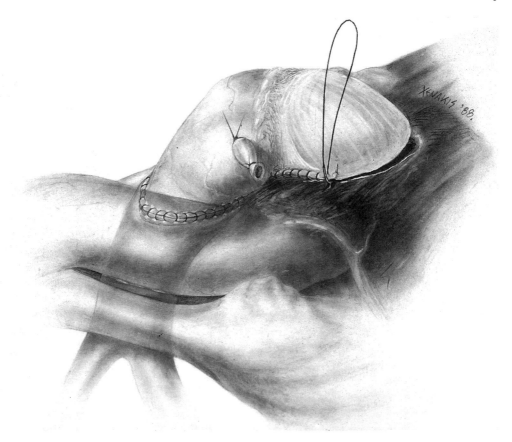

FIGURE 50.4. Proximal anastomosis completed with a single running polypropylene suture. Note the tie on the coronary stump.

the ventriculotomy point meeting the allograft annulus, the continuous suturing is briefly interrupted while any trimming and tailoring of the PTFE hood is required. The suture line is then completed to the edge of the ventriculotomy where it is secured with an additional polypropylene suture which then leaves a limb of that suture to be continued as continuous suture along the PTFE hood and ventriculotomy edge meeting the other suture coming around from the far side.

When there is a native pulmonary annulus, even hypoplastic (e.g., normally related great arteries), the posterior allograft annulus is inset and sewn at the level of the recipient "annulus" (Figure 50.5). Otherwise, the ventriculotomy is made high on the infundibulum, and the proximal anastomosis is accomplished between ventricular muscle and allograft (Figure 50.6). The ventriculotomy is not made so long that there is flattening of the entrance into the allograft. It is kept generous so that the outflow area is slightly larger than the annulus of the transplanted allograft valve. This is achieved by augmenting the anterior leaflet of the mitral valve with a patch of PTFE gusset obtained from an appropriate sized tubular graft. This technique allows the allograft aortic valve to "sit up" leaving a wide open outflow from the ventricle (Figure 50.7). Retention of the allograft membranous septum enhances this orientation (Figure 50.8). If there is marked hypertrophy of the ventricular muscle, undercutting can enlarge the orifice without lengthening the ventriculotomy (Figure 50.9).

When operating on such lesions as truncus arteriosus, a pledget is often placed in the suture line beginning at the middle posteriorly, as there is often a relative deficiency of myocardial tissue and sutures have been place nearby for ventricular septal defect closure (Figure 50.10).

As with the use of Dacron conduits, positioning is arranged to minimize sternal compression. When necessary, the left pericardium can be incised to allow rotation of the heart to the left. In any case, some sternal compression is much better tolerated by the allograft tissue than rigid Dacron conduits, and it rarely seems to present postoperatively as the heart size decreases.

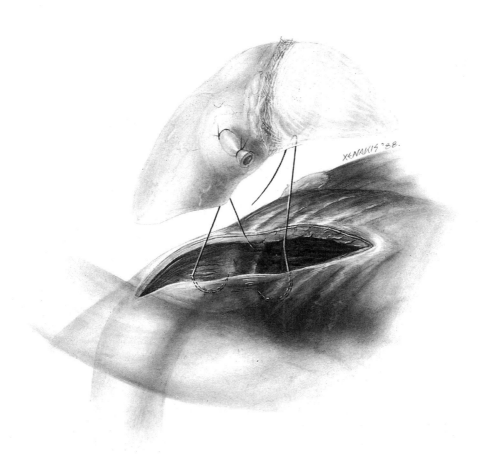

FIGURE 50.5. Positioning the allograft at the outlet from the ventricle when an annular remnant is present. The posterior location of the sutures beginning both proximal and distal anastomoses are shown.

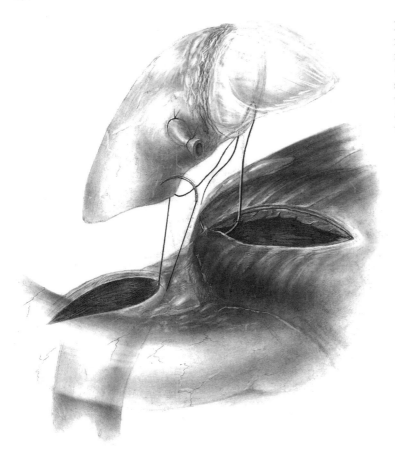

FIGURE 50.6. Proximal anastomosis to ventriculotomy when no pulmonary annulus is present (conduit). The distal anastomosis is shown here as an end-to-end one. The pulmonary arteriotomy is deviated down the left pulmonary artery.

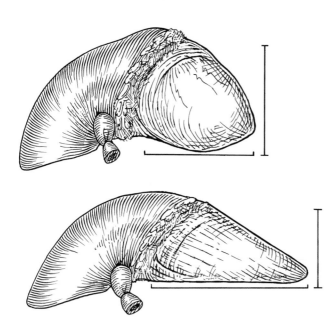

FIGURE 50.7. This drawing demonstrates the narrowing and flattening of the ventricular outflow orifice that occurs when the ventriculotomy is made too long. The horizontal lines represent the dimensions of the ventriculotomy and the ventricle lines the height in the anteroposterior diameter of the allograft valve. PTFE is helpful to construct a hood to lengthen and enlarge the circular outflow to prevent compression of the annulus and narrowing of the ventricular outflow into the allograft.

FIGURE 50.8. Blow-up view demonstrating the membranous septal
remnant, which can be used to enlarge
the proximal anastomosis.

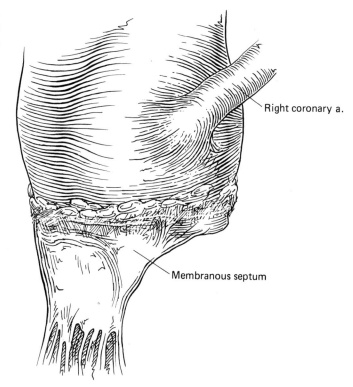

Right coronary a.

Membranous septum

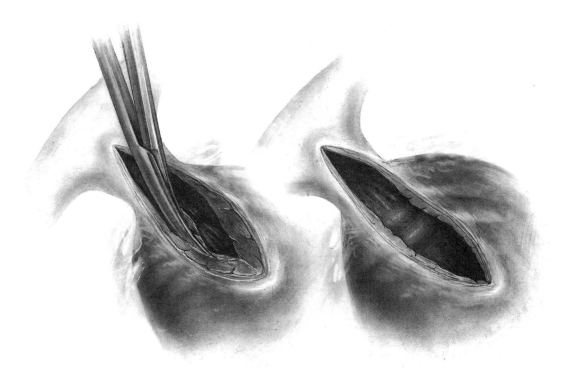

FIGURE 50.9. Enlargement of the ventricular outflow by resecting hypertrophied anterior ventricular myocardium.

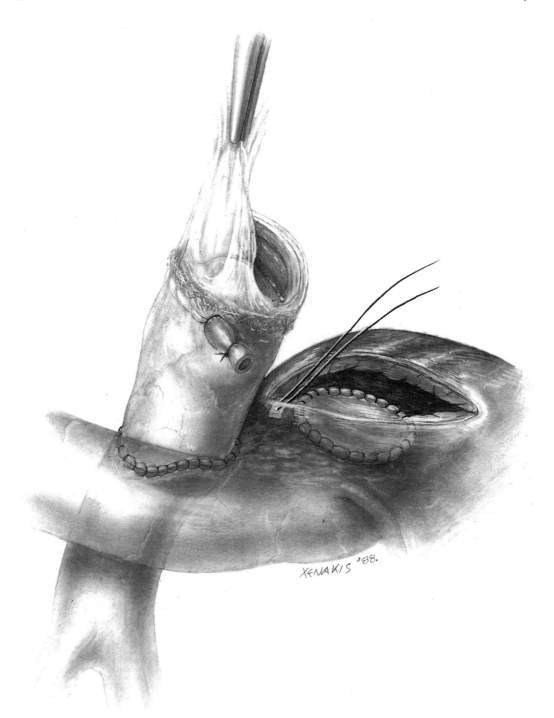

FIGURE 50.10. Use of a pledget at the start of the ventricular anastomosis when there is minimal muscular tissue remaining. Alternatively, the allo- graft can be sutured directly to the VSD patch at the midpoint of the proximal anastomosis.

References

1. Mercer JL. Acceptable size of the pulmonary valve ring in congenital cardiac defects. Ann Thorac Surg 1975;20:567–570.
2. Boyce SW, Turley K, Yee ES, et al. The fate of the 12mm porcine valved conduit from the right ventricle to the pulmonary artery: a ten year experience. J Thorac Cardiovasc Surg 1988;95: 201–207.
3. Bull C, Macartney FJ, Horvath P, et al. Evaluation of long-term results of homograft and heterograft valves and extracardiac conduits. J Thorac Cardiovasc Surg 1987;94:12–19.
4. Bailey WW. Cryopreserved pulmonary homograft valved external conduits: early results. J Card Surg 1987;2:I199–I204.

51
Pulmonary Valve Replacement in Adults

Richard A. Hopkins

Indications

Pulmonary valve replacement is usually contemplated in adults in the setting of previous right ventricular outflow tract surgery for pulmonary hypoplasia or atresia. In most cases valve insertion is for symptomatic pulmonary insufficiency that has resulted in right ventricular dysfunction with incipient or manifest tricuspid insufficiency (e.g., tetralogy of Fallot).[1-6]

Sizing

Sizing is easy in adult pulmonary valve replacements. There is a broad tolerance in the size of aortic allografts that can be placed. An allograft of 22–26 mm is usually selected (see Appendix: Valve Diameters). In general, the tendency is to upsize. The conduit is chosen to allow a large oblique distal anastomosis, and the ventriculotomy is made to accommodate the chosen allograft. If there are any pulmonary arterial stenoses, they are managed at the time of the same operation.

Technique with Aortic Allograft

The patient is placed on cardiopulmonary bypass usually with dual caval cannulas, but a single right atrial cannula can also be used if the only operation to be performed is pulmonary valve replacement. In the absence of septal defects, cardioplegia is contemplated on the branch pulmonary arteries. The right ventricular outflow tract is approached initially with an incision in the proximal pulmonary artery, which is extended across the region of the annulus. The incision is extended into the right ventricular muscle for a short distance (approximately 3–4 cm). Any residual valve leaflet tissue is excised. The incision is then extended for a distance of approximately 5 cm distally on the pulmonary artery (Figure 51.1).

The prepared aortic allograft is positioned. The distal anastomosis is accomplished in an oblique end-to-end fashion with a running 5-0 or 4-0 polypropylene suture technique (Figure 51.2). The allograft is positioned so that the allograft annulus is at the level of the native pulmonary annulus. When the recipient annular region is dilated, the positioning is similar to the "inlay" technique of Meisner, Hagl, and Sebening.[7]

The proximal anastomosis is then accomplished with a single running suture begun posteriorly. Each suture is run along the annulus to the surface of the right ventriculotomy, which usually approximates the fibrous trigone on each side of the allograft (Figure 51.3). If the allograft sits higher than this point, the anterior leaflet of the mitral valve can be deviated so as to cover a portion of this region, requiring then an additional piece of pericardium or PTFE to enlarge the outflow and avoid flattening.

The suture line is continued to the right and left fibrous trigones of the allograft where they are each secured to a horizontal mattress of the

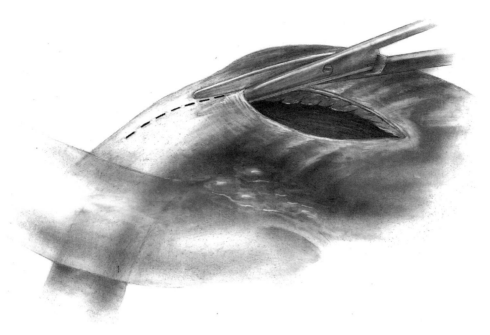

FIGURE 51.1. Incision extending from the ventriculotomy out the pulmonary artery for pulmonary valve replacement.

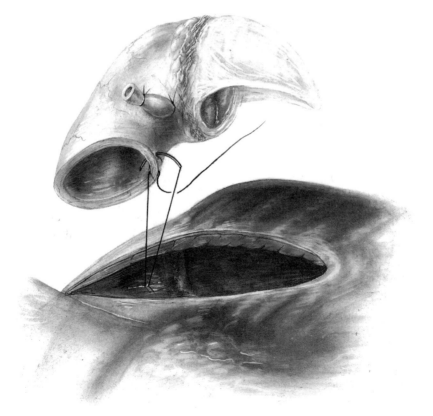

FIGURE 51.2. Distal anastomosis for pulmonary valve replacement with an aortic allograft.

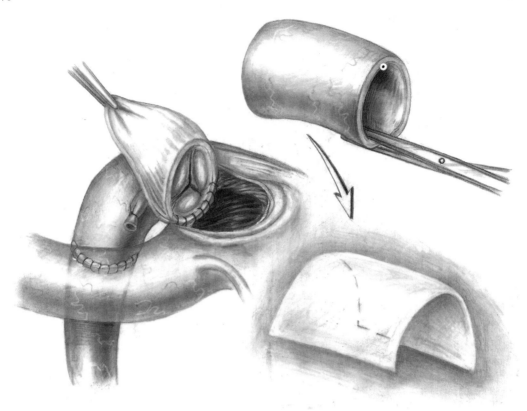

FIGURE 51.3. Proximal anastomosis is begun at mid-point posteriorly or annulus to annulus "away" from surgeon and suture line run posteriorly toward surgeon. Hood of proximal "outflow" is constructed from PTFE and mitral leaflet remnant and shaped as a chevron or shield configuration.

same size polypropylene sutures. This maintains tension on the suture line while the architecture of the outflow gussett is created by the surgeon. A PTFE tube graft of the same size or 2–4 mm larger than the annulus of the allograft is selected and a gusset obtained. The anterior leaflet of the mitral valve is allowed to bow slightly anteriorly to fully open the pathway to the neo-pulmonary valve and it is divided at that point as a suture line to be constructed with the gusset near the annulus of the allograft. The PTFE hood gusset is then sutured to the far corner with the polypropylene horizontal mattress suture which is tied. The arms of the sutures are then used as continuous suturing limbs, one taking the PTFE gusset to the far edge of the ventriculotomy and the other coming across the anterior leaflet of the mitral valve edge to PTFE and completing the suture line at the level of the other fibrous trigone of

the allograft (Figure 51.4). When the allograft is replacing a previously positioned Dacron conduit, the latter is always completely removed when feasible. Occasionally adherence to the region of the left anterior descending coronary artery prevents full removal and residual Dacron can be left undisturbed and the suture line brought underneath to the myocardium directly.

Technique with Pulmonary Allograft

Pulmonary allografts can be used as conduits or orthotopic valve replacements.[8] The technique is similar to aortic allograft in the pulmonary position except that the role of the anterior leaflet of the mitral valve is replaced with a trapezoidal patch of pericardium. This patch is kept generous so as to not deform the annulus of the pulmonary valve with tightening during ventricular contractions (Figure 51.5). The distal anastomosis is usually not as oblique as with an aortic allograft, as the amount of conduit available distal to the sinus ridge (tops of commissures) of the pulmonary valve is not as great and the elasticity and diameter of the pulmonary allograft is usually greater. Thus the arteriotomy in the main pulmonary artery is kept shorter and closer to the heart than when an aortic allograft is utilized.

The pulmonary valve allograft appears to function well in the right ventricular outflow position.[9] Autotransplants to the aortic position have been reported by Ross and others to function well and with excellent durability. Thus portending even better durability in the low pressure position.[10,11] Both Ross and McGrath have noted that implantation of the allograft pulmonary valve into both the pulmonary and the aortic positions is, if anything, technically easier than with an aortic allograft: There is less bulk at the proximal suture line, and the wall is thinner. An extensive series has yet to be reported that supports the use of the allograft pulmonary valve in the aortic position. In fact, some authorities believe that the use of a cryopreserved allograft pulmonary valve in the aortic position is contraindicated. Pieces of cryoreserved allograft pulmonary artery tissue

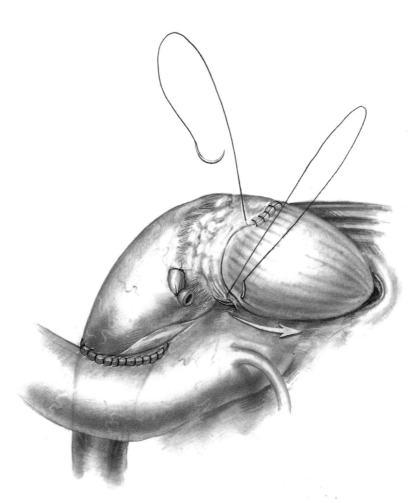

Figure 51.4. Proximal completed. PTFE to leaflet can be at homograft annulus or anywhere in the "hood" that is convenient.

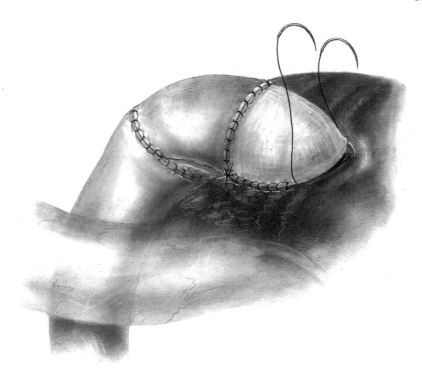

FIGURE 51.5. Pulmonary allograft in an orthotopic position. Ventriculotomy is completed with a pericardial patch. End-to-end distal anastomosis for pulmonary artery in continuity with ventricle.

have been used to augment recipient pulmonary arteries during reconstructions of the pulmonary artery bifurcation and, as reported by Ziemer and colleagues, can be combined with an allograft pulmonary valve to accomplish total right ventricular outflow tract reconstructions with allograft pulmonary tissue. The most common use of pulmonary allografts is now for replacement of the pulmonary valve when the native pulmonary valve has been used for autograft procedures (See Section X for discussion of the Ross operation and its variants).

References

1. Bove EL, Kavey REW, Byrum CJ, et al. Improved right ventricular function following late pulmonary valve replacement for residual pulmonary insufficiency or stenosis. J Thorac Cardiovasc Surg 1985;90:50–55.
2. Ebert PA. Second operations for pulmonary stenosis or insufficiency after repair of tetralogy of Fallot. Am J Cardiol 1982;50:637–640.
3. Ilbawi MN, Idriss FS, DeLeon SY, et al. Factors that exaggerate the deleterious effects of pulmonary insufficiency of the right ventricular after tetralogy repair. J Thorac Cardiovasc Surg 1987;93:36–44.
4. Misbach GA, Turley K, Ebert PA. Pulmonary valve replacement for regurgitation after repair of tetralogy of Fallot. Ann Thorac Surg 1983; 36:684–691.
5. Bove EL, Byrum CJ, Thomas FD, et al. The influence of pulmonary insufficiency on ventricular function following repair of tetralogy of Fallot. J Thorac Cardiovasc Surg 1983;85:691–696.
6. Ilbawi MN, Lockhart G, Idriss FS, et al. Experience with St. Jude medical valve prosthesis in children: A word of caution regarding right-sided placement. J Thorac Cardiovasc Surg 1987;93: 73–79.
7. Meisner H, Hagl S, Sebening F. Technique of inlay allografts into the RVOT to prevent pulmonary insufficiency. In Yankah AC, Hetzer R, Miller DC (eds). Cardiac Valve Allografts. New York: Springer-Verlag 1987:205–213.
8. Bailey WW. Cryopreserved pulmonary homograft valved external conduits: early results. J Card Surg 1987;2:I199–I204.

9. McGrath LB, Gonzalez-Lavin L, Graf D. Pulmonary homograft implantation for ventricular outflow tract reconstruction: early phase results. Ann Thorac Surg 1988;45:273–277.

10. Wain WH, Greco R, Ignegeri A, Bodnar E, Ross DN. 15 years experience with 615 homograft and autograft aortic valve replacements. Int J Artif Organs 1980;3:169–172.

11. Gonzales-Lavin L, Robles A, Graf D. The Ross operation: the autologous pulmonary valve in the aortic position. J Card Surg 1988;3:29–43.

52
Corrected Transposition

Richard A. Hopkins

The relief of associated pulmonary stenosis or atresia in the anomaly of corrected transposition (atrioventricular discordance and ventriculoarterial discordance) requires attention to special anatomic features. The correction is usually but not always associated with closure of a ventricular septal defect.[1] The position of the conduction system mandates a different technique for closure of a ventricular septal defect, as well as care when performing the ventriculotomy for relief of the pulmonary outflow obstruction from the morphologic left ventricle.[2] In general, we close the ventricular septal defect through the defect with sutures placed on the morphologic right side.[2] It is usually accomplished through the ventriculotomy. The emphasis of this section is on the correct performance of the ventriculotomy and construction of the allograft pathway to the pulmonary arteries.

The conduction bundle courses anterior to the pulmonary artery just below the annulus. Thus a ventriculotomy placed high on the morphologic left ventricle (pulmonary ventricle) places the conduction bundle at risk. In addition, retraction of the superior border of the ventriculotomy can induce conduction blocks. There are usually large coronary arteries from the circumflex coronary artery coursing across the upper portion of this anterior (but morphologically left) ventricle that must be avoided (Figure 52.1).

Technique

The patient is placed on cardiopulmonary bypass with bicaval cannulation. Hypothermic cardioplegic arrest is induced. The best way to create the ventriculotomy is to place a finger through the mitral valve so as to palpate the location of the papillary muscles (Figure 52.2) and perform the ventriculotomy relatively low on the ventricle, cutting to the surgeon's finger (Figure 52.3). The anterior papillary muscle is usually located just to the right of this ventriculotomy.[3] This technique is designed to protect the mitral valve support, the conduction system, and to allow adequate egress from the pulmonary ventricle. An allograft aortic valve conduit must be selected that is of adult size and that has a long conduit (6cm or more), at least to the level of the innominate artery (Figure 52.4). An allograft this large can usually be placed without the addition of prosthetic material. The direct suturing of the aortic allograft to the ventriculotomy is thus placed in a relatively low position, where the heart is curving away from the sternum, and there is rarely difficulty with compression of the prosthesis. The ventriculotomy is positioned adjacent and fairly far apically. Ventriculotomy is begun and then, under direct vision, enlarged to the point that, for a typical-sized patient, a 22 to 24mm allograft valve can be sewn to the

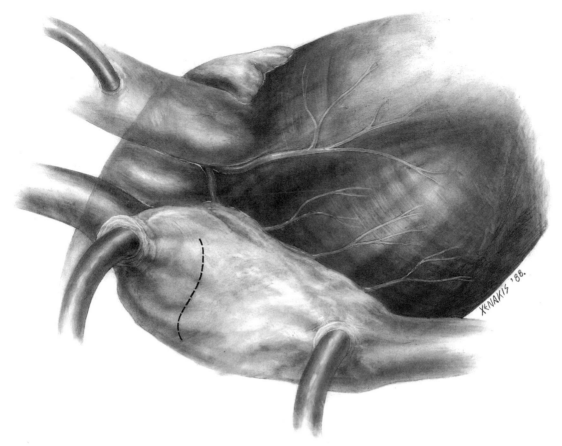

FIGURE 52.1. Cannulation and atriotomy for corrected transposition. Note the location of the coronary arteries.

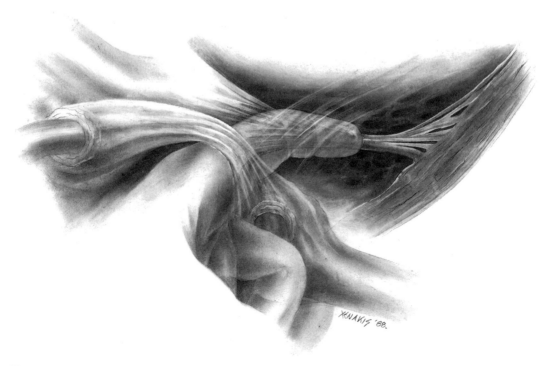

FIGURE 52.2. Mitral papillary muscle is located by a finger placed through the atrium into the ventricle.

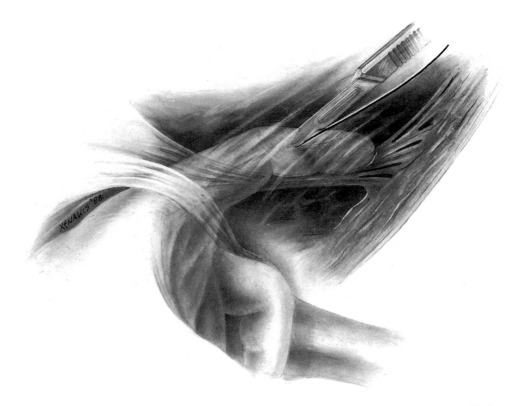

FIGURE 52.3. Ventriculotomy is made toward the apex, cutting to the surgeon's finger to avoid the atrioventricular subvalvular apparatus.

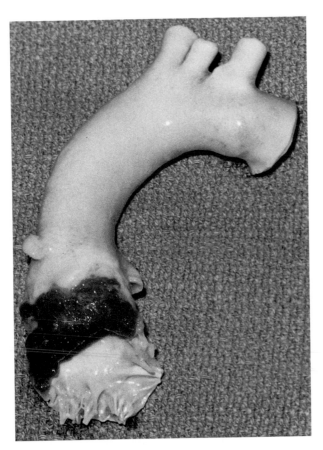

FIGURE 52.4. Aortic allograft conduit is chosen with a long segment to avoid use of prosthetic extensions. Courtesy of LifeNet Tissue Services.

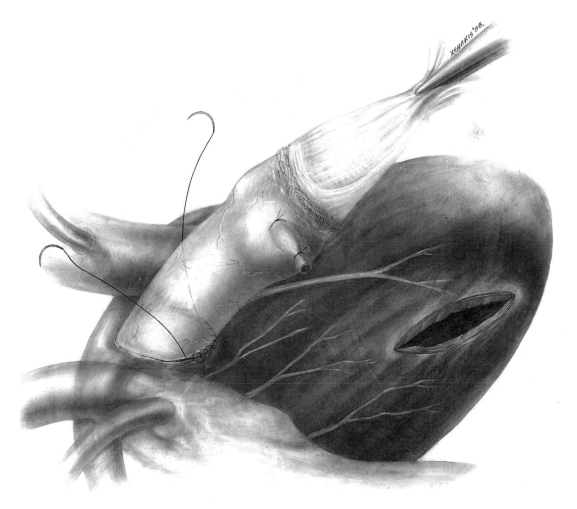

FIGURE 52.5. Distal native pulmonary artery to allograft anastomosis is performed first.

ventriculotomy. The ventricular septal defect is then closed as described by de Leval and associates.[2]

The allograft is prepared, leaving the anterior leaflet of the mitral valve attached but with all chordae and thin valve excised. Trimming of the muscular base of the allograft valve is relatively vigorous, but tissue underneath the fibrous skeleton of the valve is usually left to a distance of 2mm. The membranous septum is left attached to the allograft. This additional material, with the remnant of anterior leaflet of the mitral valve in association with an additional piece of PTFE allows suturing of the allograft complex to the ventriculotomy in such a way that it "sits up" on the ventriculotomy, thereby avoiding flattening of the annulus

and enlarging the ventricular outflow proximal to the valve.

The length of the allograft required between the ventriculotomy and the pulmonary arteriotomy is assessed. If there is continuity between the pulmonary artery and the pulmonary ventricle, an end-to-side anastomosis is utilized to the main pulmonary artery in an oblique fashion. If there is complete pulmonary valvular atresia, an end-to-end oblique anastomosis is accomplished.

The distal anastomosis is accomplished first with a running 5-0 polypropylene suture line (Figure 52.5). The conduit is cut at the appropriate length to allow an easy reach to the ventriculotomy. It has not been necessary, in our experience, to extend it into the midarch of the

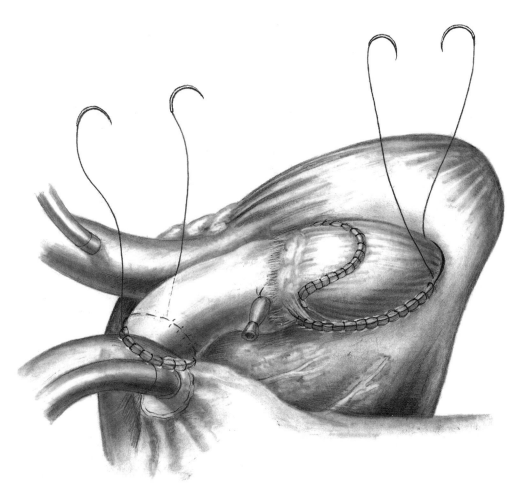

FIGURE 52.6. Proximal anastomosis in corrected transposition. This depiction illustrates retention of some allograft mitral tissue.

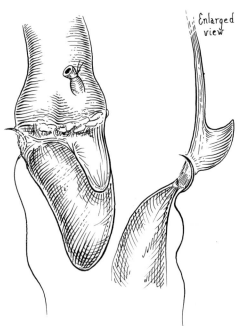

FIGURE 52.7. Angle of entry for the needle to take advantage of both the inner fibrous base underneath the valve cusps and the fibrous rim externally on the aortic root, which is higher than the base of the leaflet insertions.

allograft. Such extension is certainly possible, when necessary, to avoid synthetic material extensions. We have never needed to extend conduits proximally or distally, purely for length reasons as our procurement team usually obtains the allograft aortic valve with aorta complete to the distal arch.

After the distal suture line is completed, we normally remove the aortic cross-clamp, perform de-airing maneuvers, and begin rewarming. The proximal anastomosis is accomplished with a running 5-0 polypropylene suture technique utilizing the anterior leaflet of the mitral valve augmented with a semicircular tubular gussett of PTFE (Figure 52.6). Some subvalvular muscle tissue may be left on the allograft to provide bulk to the suturing. However, care is taken with all suture bites to enter fibrous material (Figure 52.7).

References

1. Danielson GK, McGoon DC, Wallace KB, et al. Surgery of corrected transposition. In Anderson RH, Shinebourne EA (eds). Pediatric Cardiology 1977. Edingurgh: Churchill Livingstone 1978:224–230.
2. De Leval MR, Bastos P, Stark J, et al. Surgical technique to reduce the risks of heart block following closure of ventricular septal defect in atrioventricular discordance. J Thorac Cardiovasc Surg 1979;78:515–526.
3. Danielson GK. Atrioventricular discordance. In Stark J, deLeval M (eds). Surgery for congenital heart defects. London: Grunen Stratton 1983: 387–395.

53
Reconstruction of Right Ventricular Outflow with Abnormal Pulmonary Arteries

Richard A. Hopkins

Stenoses in Confluent Pulmonary Arteries

Proximal Stenosis

If a short stenosis is present near or at the midpoint of the pulmonary artery bifurcation, reconstruction of the confluence can be accomplished with primary anastomosis of the distal allograft to the pulmonary artery. The pulmonary artery is split through the level of the stenosis (Figures 53.1 and 53.2). The distal end of the allograft is slightly rounded (Figure 53.3). The allograft is sutured to the native pulmonary arterial tissue, with the mid-point of the allograft being shifted to the point of greatest stenosis. This anastomosis is accomplished with running 5-0 monofilament suture technique (Figure 53.4). Alternatively, the distal anastomosis can be enlarged by cutting the distal allograft somewhat obliquely in the transverse plane to provide a "tongue" of tissue to extend the distal anastomosis laterally. During this procedure care must be taken to align the allograft so the mitral leaflet is positioned anteriorly (Figure 53.5).

The "height" of the reconstructed pulmonary artery bifurcation is also accomplished by utilizing an allograft that is large (in diameter) for the patient (e.g., 23 mm allograft for a 1.5-m^2 BSA individual) and by making the conduit slightly long. This reconstruction of the bifurcation with the distal conduit avoids any interposition of foreign material. A conduit length distal to the aortic valve of around 6 cm is usually required for this kind of reconstruction, and even longer conduit lengths are needed for large individuals. By selecting longer conduits, a proximal anastomosis can be accomplished *without* the need for augmentation with prosthetic material.

Distal Stenoses

When stenoses occur beyond 1–2 cm from the mid-point of the pulmonary artery confluence, deviation of the distal anastomosis to cover the stenoses becomes difficult. After splitting through the length of the stenosis (Figure 53.6), the pulmonary artery is enlarged with a patch of pericardium constructed so as to develop both height and width to the stenosed pulmonary artery (Figure 53.7).

Pericardium is usually sutured with 5-0 or 6-0 monofilament suture to the pulmonary artery. The sutures are tied at the points at which the "hood" leaves the native pulmonary artery (Figure 53.8).

The distal aortic allograft is fashioned so as to adapt to this augmentation patch, but the allograft cutback is not exaggerated; rather, that edge is slightly rounded (Figure 53.9), which contributes to the height of the reconstruction as well as bringing the allograft conduit back to the midline. The distal anastomosis is accomplished with a two-suture running technique.

The initial suturing is begun by placing a horizontal mattress suture at the junction of the

FIGURE 53.1. Stenosis extending to the origin of the right pulmonary artery involving the confluence. The incision completely opens the stenotic area.

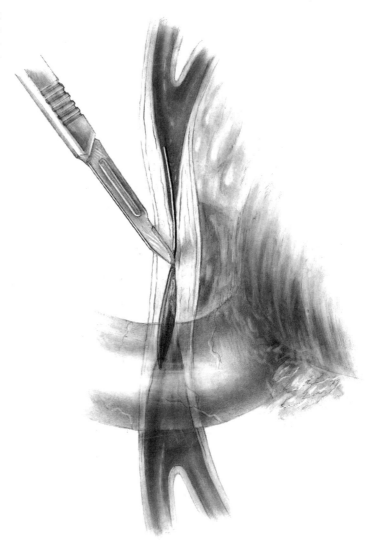

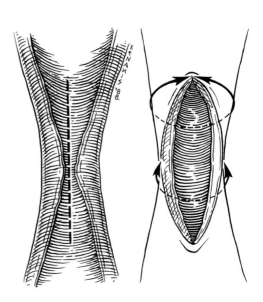

FIGURE 53.2. The incision opens the stenosis. Note that there is less native tissue circumferentially at the stenotic region (arrows).

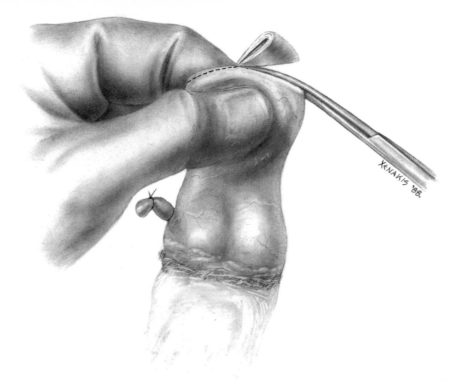

FIGURE 53.3. Slight rounding of the allograft gives more tissue in the area of the stenosis for circumferential expansion.

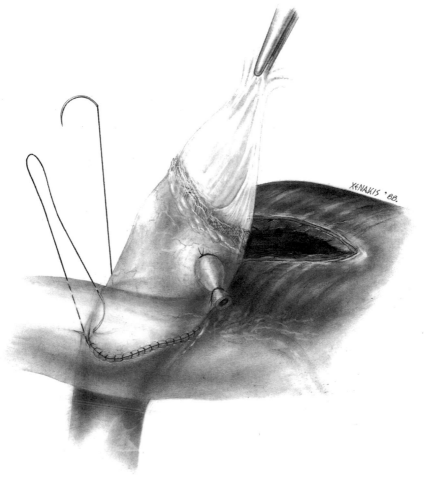

FIGURE 53.4. Distal anastomosis being completed.

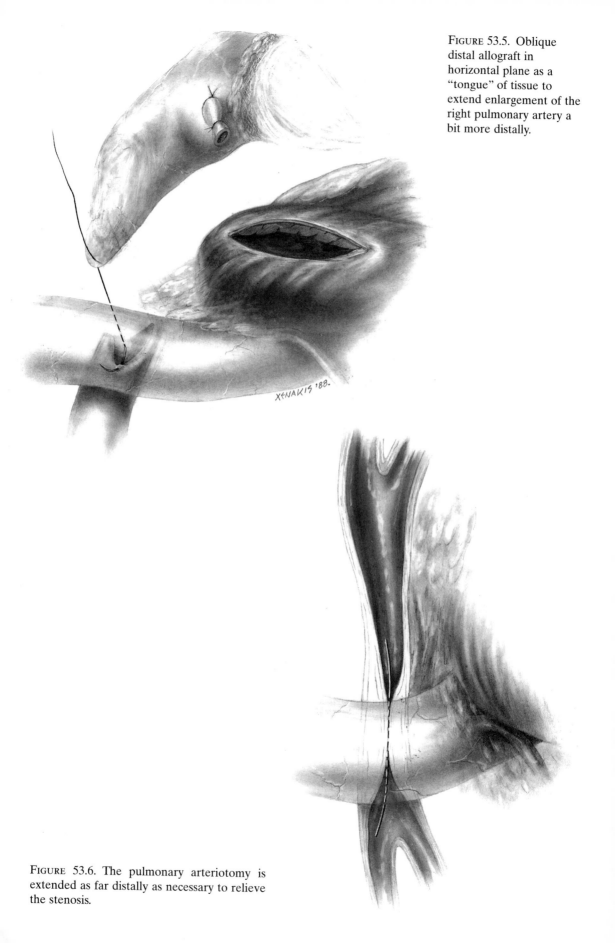

FIGURE 53.5. Oblique distal allograft in horizontal plane as a "tongue" of tissue to extend enlargement of the right pulmonary artery a bit more distally.

FIGURE 53.6. The pulmonary arteriotomy is extended as far distally as necessary to relieve the stenosis.

XENAKIS '88.

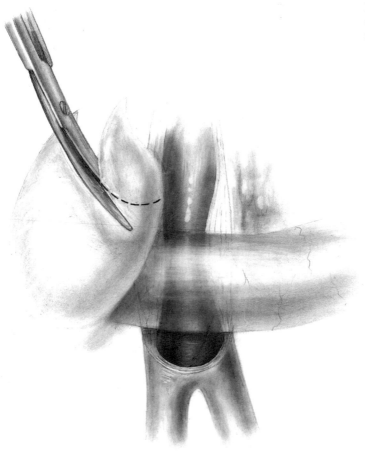

FIGURE 53.7. A hood of pericardium is cut to enlarge the distal right pulmonary artery, sized generously so as to provide height at the medial border. If space is limited behind aorta, the aorta should be divided and extended with a tubular graft insert (see Figure 53.19).

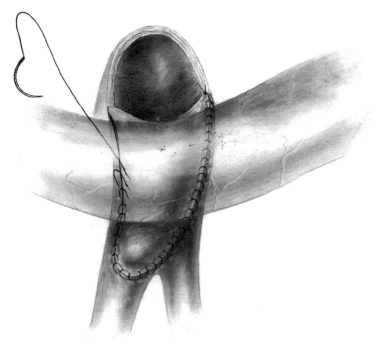

FIGURE 53.8. Pericardial patch sutures are tied. If compression of repair seems likely between aorta and distended PA's, then PTFE should be used for the hood patch as it is a stiffer material.

FIGURE 53.9. The distal allograft is shaped to take advantage of the pericardial enlargement of the pulmonary artery.

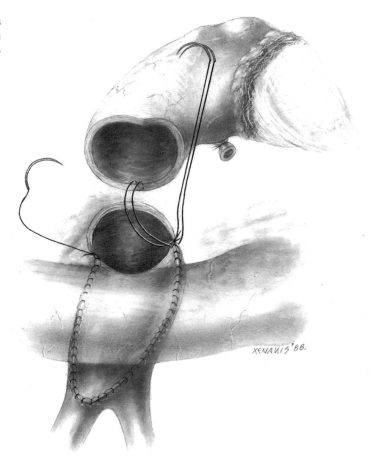

allograft, pericardium, and native pulmonary artery and then running the suture continuously along the inferior border of the anastomosis. A second horizontal mattress suture is placed at the analogous point on the upper border of the anastomosis, and the two suture lines are run to each other and tied (Figure 53.10). Care must be taken with this anastomosis that (as for all other pulmonary artery suture lines) the posterior suture line is particularly well constructed with narrowly placed bites, as it is difficult to suture any leaks later.

The proximal right ventriculotomy to aortic allograft anastomosis is performed in the usual fashion with 4-0 and 5-0 polypropylene set of continuous sutures (Figure 53.11).

Hypoplastic but Confluent Pulmonary Arteries

"Skirt" Technique

With the "skirt" technique an oval piece of pericardium (treated or autologous) that is generously sized is sutured with a continuous suture to a longitudinal pulmonary arteriotomy (Figure 53.12). This method is utilized in

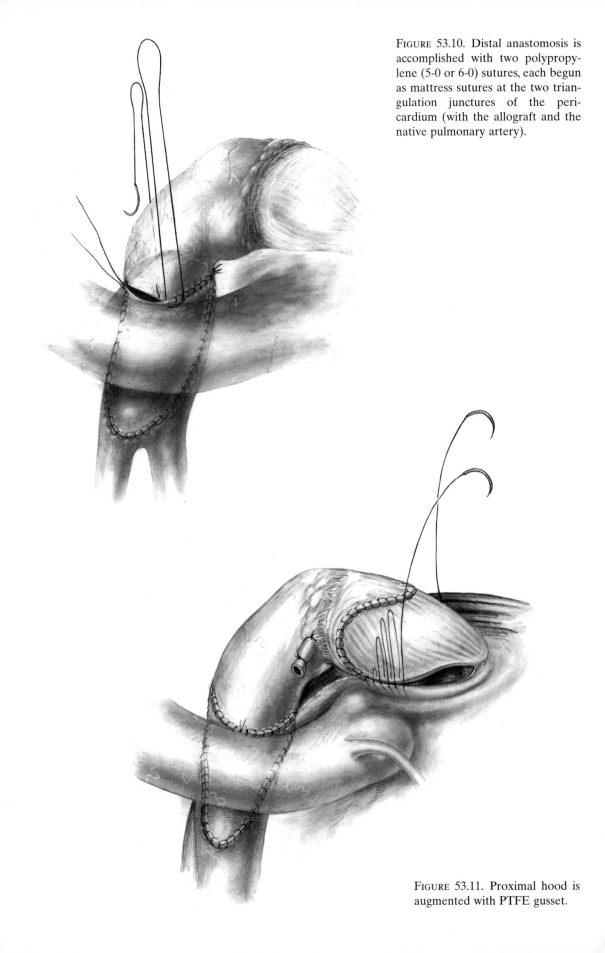

FIGURE 53.10. Distal anastomosis is accomplished with two polypropylene (5-0 or 6-0) sutures, each begun as mattress sutures at the two triangulation junctures of the pericardium (with the allograft and the native pulmonary artery).

FIGURE 53.11. Proximal hood is augmented with PTFE gusset.

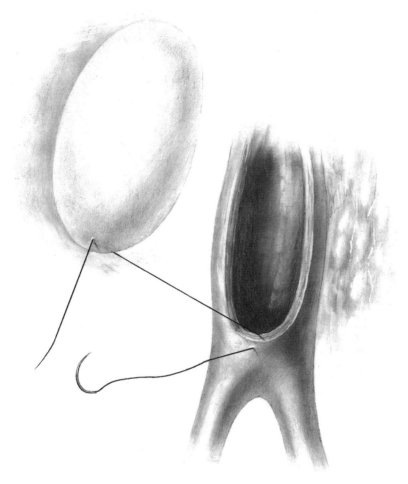

FIGURE 53.12. Incision through the stenotic pulmonary artery confluence and sizing of the oval piece of pericardium for the "skirt" technique.

situations where there is no main pulmonary artery, the confluence is hypoplastic, but the left and right main pulmonary arteries enlarge as they approach the hila. The pulmonary arteriotomy is extended to the more-normal-diameter arteries in the hila. The skirt of pericardium is sutured with a continuous suture to the edges of the arteriotomy (Figure 53.13). The size of the oval pericardium must be generous and actually almost approaches a circle so as to provide "height" to the final reconstruction. It creates an oblong "cone." The concept of restoration of height (surgeon's view) to the pulmonary artery bifurcation is important, as it avoids the recurrence of stenosis at the pulmonary artery origins. Once the suture line is completed, an incision is made in the midportion of the pericardium. A central piece of the pericardium is excised, and this large aperture is then sutured end-to-end to the distal aortic allograft conduit to complete the reconstruction of the pulmonary artery bifurcation (Figure 53.14). The proximal suture line to the right ventriculotomy is completed in the usual fashion (Figure 53.15).

This technique has the advantage of being rapid and geometrically simple. It has the disadvantage that the aortic allograft is not sutured directly to the native human tissue, and an intervening piece of nonviable tissue exists. This situation creates the possibility of calcification and peel formation, which might lead to

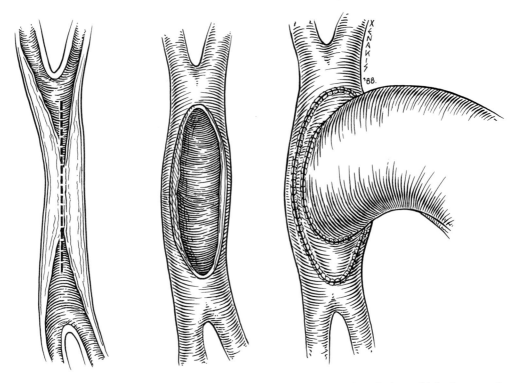

FIGURE 53.13. Enlargement of a stenotic pulmonary artery with a skirt of glutaraldehyde-treated pericardium. Note the circumference added to the pulmonary arterial confluence.

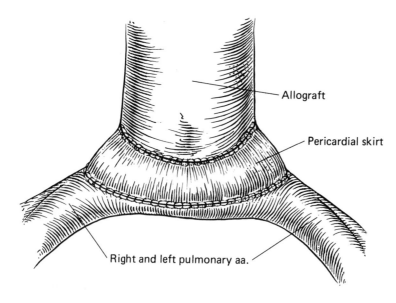

Allograft

Pericardial skirt

Right and left pulmonary aa.

FIGURE 53.14. The pericardial skirt provides height to the bifurcation, enlarging the origins to the right and left pulmonary arteries.

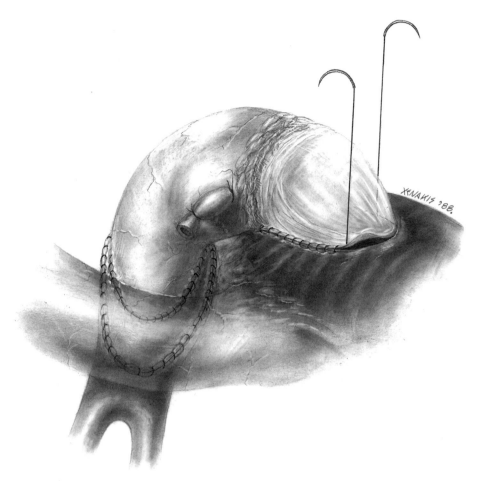

FIGURE 53.15. Completion of the right ventricular outflow tract reconstruction with the proximal anastomosis of allograft to ventriculotomy. Proximal hood is always augmented with PTFE cut from tubular graft as necessary to enlarge outflow (not shown here for clarity).

late obstruction. It often occurs when Dacron is used in this position, but may not be as great a problem with pericardium. Nevertheless, direct suturing of allograft to native tissue is preferred whenever feasible.

Pulmonary Artery Bifurcation Allograft

Another, and to us more satisfying, technique for reconstructing the hypoplastic but confluent pulmonary arteries is to utilize a pulmonary artery allograft with its bifurcation and combine it with a right ventricular outflow reconstruction using an aortic allograft. An adult-sized pulmonary artery allograft, as usually harvested, has a right arterial length of 1.0–2.0cm, a left arterial length of 1.5–3.0cm, and a segment of main pulmonary artery between the sinus ridge (top of the pulmonary valve pillars) attachments and takeoff of the left and right pulmonary arteries of 3–5cm. Although this pulmonary arterial segment is often not long enough to reconstruct the entire conduit from right ventriculotomy to distal pulmonary arteries without the addition of prosthetic material, it can be used to greatly enlarge and reconstruct the patient's pulmonary artery bifurcation. This method has the advantage of joining allograft material directly to human tissue. It also greatly enlarges the pulmonary artery bifurcation and utilizes the "height principle." As we apply the technique, it allows use of an aortic valve allograft as the outlet valve from the ventriculotomy and thus primary closure of allograft material to right ventricular native tissue.

The repair is begun just as for the pericardial "skirt" technique, with dissection of the pulmonary artery confluence to the distal pulmonary arteries where adequate diameters are encountered. An arteriotomy is made anteriorly through the pulmonary artery confluence, leaving the posterior wall intact (Figure 53.16).

The pulmonary bifurcation allograft has been thawed and prepared. The distal right and left main pulmonary arteries are slit with a horizontal incision (Figure 53.17). The filleted allograft is then sutured to the native pulmonary arteriotomy with a running 5-0 polypropylene suture technique (Figure 53.18). This method uses the full circumference of the allograft pulmonary arteries to augment the anterior recipient confluence, thereby enlarging the pulmonary artery bifurcation significantly. If necessary, exposure of the right main pulmonary artery is enhanced by dividing the aorta, which can then be rejoined (Figure 53.19). (This maneuver is particularly helpful when previous scarring, due to Dacron patch enlargement of the right pulmonary artery, makes dissection behind the aorta risky.)

On completion of the distal anastomosis, the aortic cross-clamp can be removed (if cardioplegic arrest was utilized to enhance visibility and decrease blood return in the pulmonary arterial system). Matching the size of the aortic allograft to the pulmonary allograft is not critical, as the anastomosis is oblique, but in general a 1- to 2-mm larger aortic allograft is selected to match the more elastic pulmonary artery bifurcation. The aortic allograft can be chosen to match the ventriculotomy and length requirements from the right ventricle to the pulmonary artery bifurcation so long as it is an adult size for the BSA of the patient. The pulmonary artery bifurcation can then be matched to the native pulmonary arteries and the allograft-to-allograft anastomosis constructed. The thawed aortic allograft is then sutured end-to-end to the pulmonary allograft with a

running 5-0 polypropylene suture technique buttressed with a thin felt strip (Figure 53.20).

The patient is fully rewarmed and the proximal aortic allograft to right ventriculotomy is accomplished in the usual fashion with a running 4-0 polypropylene suture technique (Figure 53.21). The pulmonary valve tissue has been totally excised, and only the pulmonary artery distal to that tissue is utilized for the bifurcation reconstruction.

Nonconfluent Pulmonary Arteries

Pulmonary Artery Bifurcation Allograft

When the pulmonary arteries are nonconfluent, choices exist for reconstruction. First, the pulmonary artery bifurcation can be reconstructed entirely with a pulmonary bifurcation allograft with separate end-to-end anastomoses right and left, as reported by McGrath and colleagues (Figure 53.22), or sewn to an aortic allograft in a manner analogous to the technique just described when the distance is great (Figure 53.23). Second, the absent posterior wall of native pulmonary arterial confluence can be reconstructed primarily or with pieces of allograft pulmonary artery and then end-to-end anastomoses to an allograft pulmonary or aortic valve. Finally, when the right and left pulmonary artery discontinuity extends from hilum to hilum, that lengthy distance can be spanned with a PTFE graft, which is then sutured end-to-side to the allograft. Although this method violates the principle of maximizing allograft to recipient tissue anastomoses, it occasionally is the most feasible reconstruction.

The difficulty with the first method is that the length of allograft spanning the left and right main pulmonary arteries usually available rarely exceeds 5 cm. That method appears to be most applicable in cases of acquired "nonconfluent" pulmonary arteries, resulting from previous shunting procedures, and where at least one of the arteries is relatively centrally located so that the bifurcation can be "cheated" to one side or the other to bridge the gap.

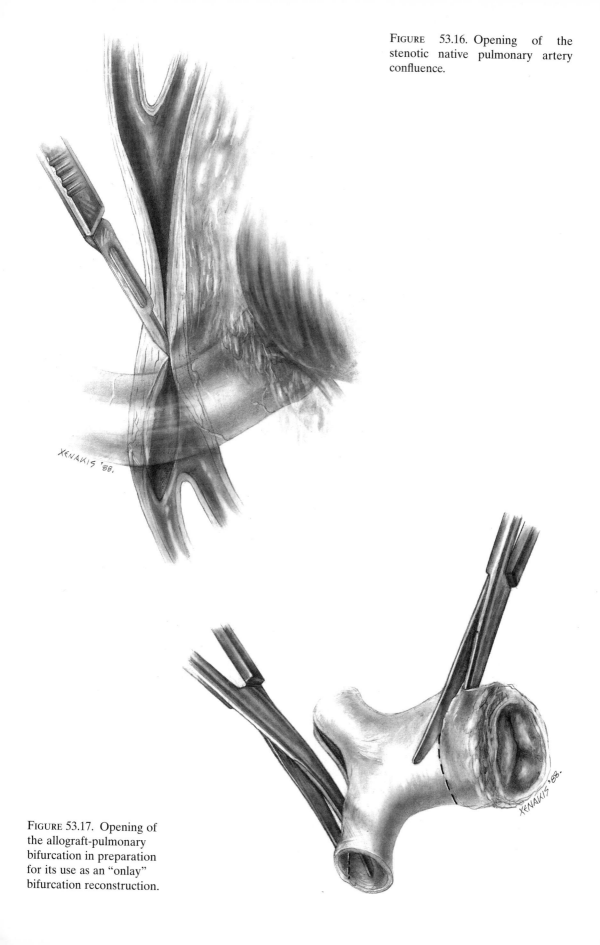

FIGURE 53.16. Opening of the stenotic native pulmonary artery confluence.

FIGURE 53.17. Opening of the allograft-pulmonary bifurcation in preparation for its use as an "onlay" bifurcation reconstruction.

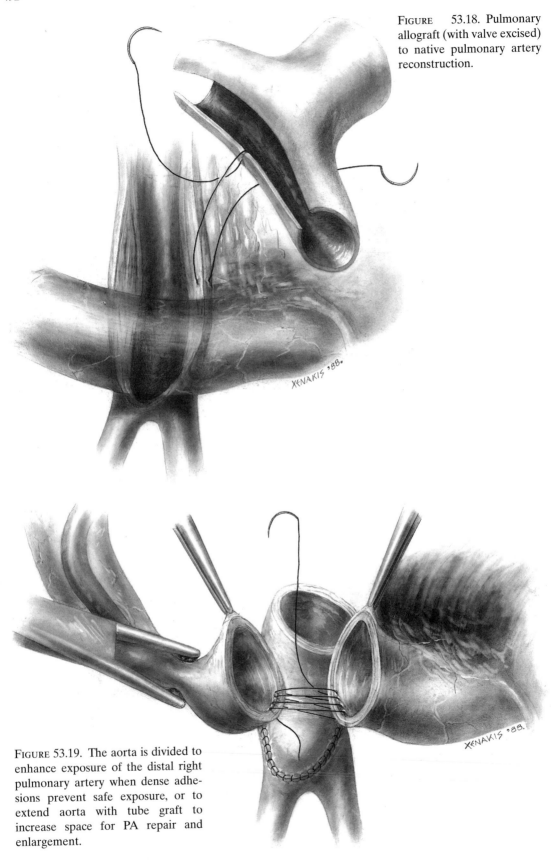

FIGURE 53.18. Pulmonary allograft (with valve excised) to native pulmonary artery reconstruction.

FIGURE 53.19. The aorta is divided to enhance exposure of the distal right pulmonary artery when dense adhesions prevent safe exposure, or to extend aorta with tube graft to increase space for PA repair and enlargement.

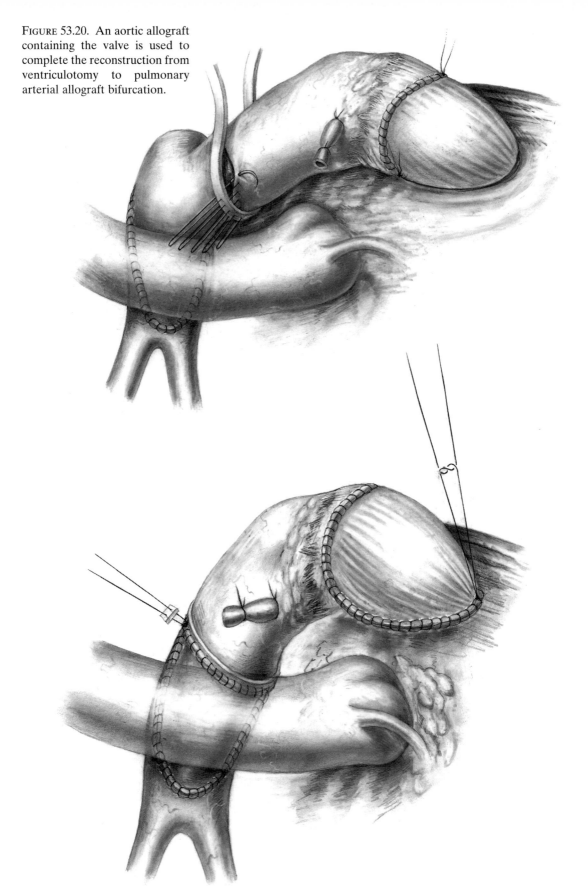

FIGURE 53.20. An aortic allograft containing the valve is used to complete the reconstruction from ventriculotomy to pulmonary arterial allograft bifurcation.

FIGURE 53.21. The proximal suture line with augmentation of ventricular outflow is completed while rewarming the patient.

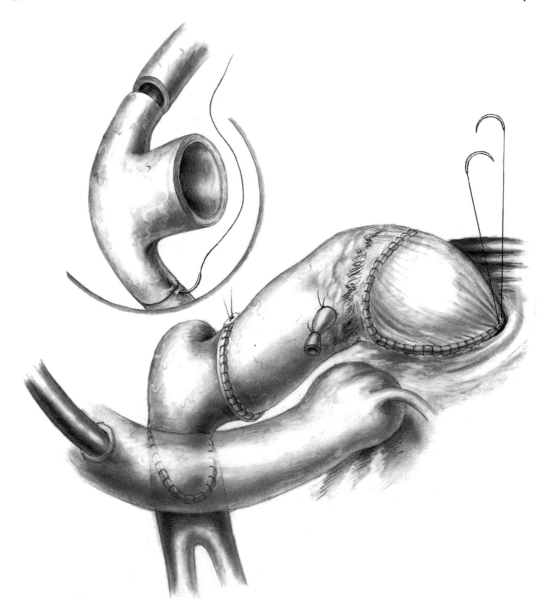

FIGURE 53.22. Pulmonary artery bifurcation graft with end-to-end anastomoses right and left lengthened by adding an aortic homograft. A large gusset of either pericardium or PTFE is shown enlarging the anterior reconstruction from the ventricle. Alternatively, if the distance is short, a pulmonary valved homograft with pulmonary bifurcation left intact can be used similarly with separate left and right pulmonary artery anastomoses which are usually bevelled (main figure) or spatulated (rather than circular end-to-end as depicted in the upper panel) to enlarge and smooth the flow dynamics.

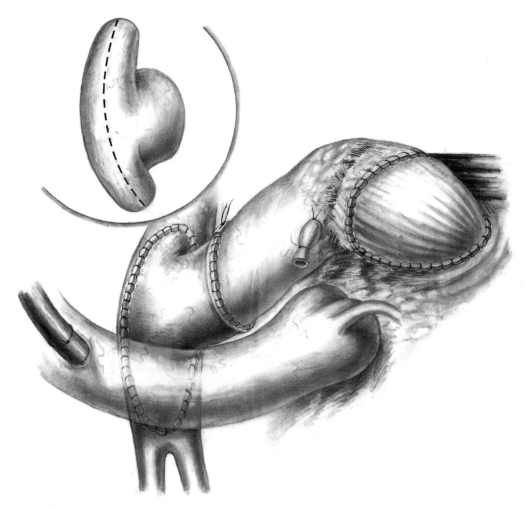

FIGURE 53.23. Valveless pulmonary artery bifurcation graft with split open anastomosis sewn to an aortic valve homograft. These repairs are a spectrum of art and craft and determined by each particular situation including morbility of native pulmonary arteries.

54
Management of Difficult Allograft Alignments: The "Divide and Reapproximate" Principle

Erle H. Austin, III

Occasionally the establishment of pulmonary ventricle to pulmonary artery continuity requires bridging a long curved pathway from the ventriculotomy to a deeply positioned pulmonary artery bifurcation. Such a situation may occur with corrected transposition (atrioventricular discordance and ventriculoarterial discordance) with pulmonary stenosis or atresia in which the ventriculotomy must be positioned near the apex of the anterior ventricle in order to avoid injury to the conduction tissue. Another example is the rare patient with simple transposition (atrioventricular concordance and ventriculoarterial discordance) that requires a left ventricular apex to pulmonary artery conduit to relieve significant left ventricular outflow tract obstruction developing after a Mustard or Senning procedure.[1] A long curved conduit may also be required in some cases of pulmonary atresia with posterior and difficult to mobilize pulmonary arteries. Although the interposition of a synthetic conduit can provide the necessary additional length and curvature, prosthetic material can be avoided by proper implantation of an aortic valve and ascending aortic allograft.

This technique requires harvest and cryopreservation of the ascending aorta and proximal aortic arch along with the allograft aortic valve. The length and curvature of the ascending aorta are utilized to provide an "arching" alignment of the conduit from the ventriculotomy to the pulmonary artery. The aortic allograft is usually cut distally at the level of the innominate artery, but if extra length is necessary the origins of the head vessels can be oversewn. The most straightforward implantation of this "extended" aortic allograft involves anastomosing the distal curved portion of the allograft to the pulmonary bifurcation followed by a proximal anastomosis to the ventriculotomy. Because the plane of the anterior leaflet of the mitral valve is rotated 90 degrees from the plane of the curvature of the ascending aorta (Figure 54.1), the anterior leaflet is usually not in a good position to serve as a "hood" for the proximal anastomosis. As such, to avoid distortion of the valve, it is preferable to excise most of the anterior mitral leaflet and to utilize a piece of pericardium to complete the anastomosis. To take advantage of the anterior leaflet of the mitral valve as well as to assure ideal length and alignment of the "extended aortic allograft, this author has applied a "divide and reapproximate" technique for this reconstruction.

Technique

With this modification the "extended" aortic allograft is cut transversely just above the sinotubular junction (Figure 54.2). The distal portion of the allograft is trimmed and anastomosed to the main pulmonary artery (end-to-side) or pulmonary bifurcation (end-to-end) using a continuous suture of 5-0 polypropylene (Figure 54.3). Once the distal anastomosis is complete, the aortic cross-clamp is removed, the heart de-aired and rewarming is begun. Using the

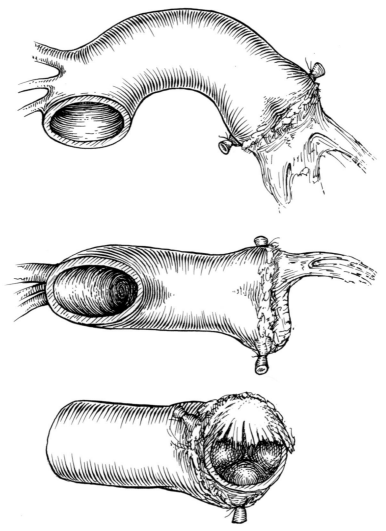

FIGURE 54.1. The plane of curvature of the ascending aorta is rotated approximately 90° from the plane of the anterior leaflet of the mitral valve.

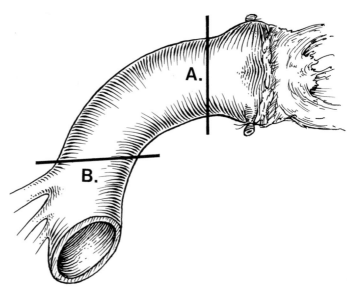

FIGURE 54.2. The aortic allograft is divided just above the sino-tubular junction (A) A distal cut at the base of the innominate artery (B) generally provides adequate length for the distal segment.

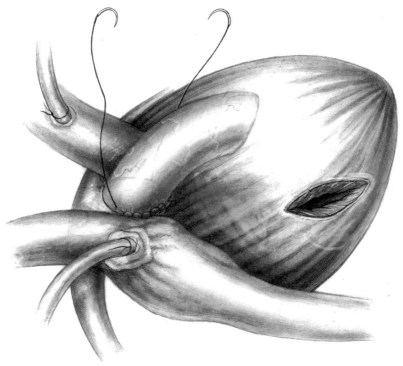

FIGURE 54.3. The distal segment of the divided aortic allograft is anastomosed to the native pulmonary artery in a patient with corrected transposition.

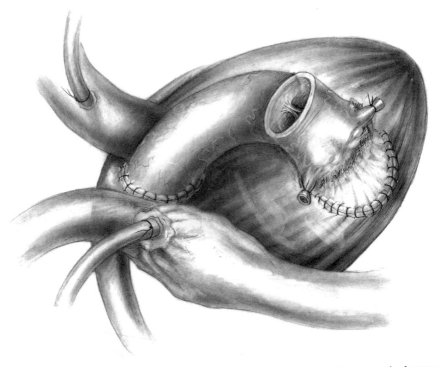

FIGURE 54.4. Anastomosis of proximal segment of divided allograft to ventriculotomy.

proximal portion of the allograft, the proximal anastomosis is performed with running 5-0 polypropylene. Now that the allograft valve has been separated from the curvature of the ascending aorta, the valve can be rotated so that the anterior mitral leaflet can serve as the "hood." The suture line is begun posteriorly making certain that the long axis of the anastomosis is aligned in the direction of the distal segment (Figure 54.4). Once the proximal anastomosis is completed, excess length is trimmed from the distal segment and continuity is re-established with a running 5-0 polypropylene suture (Figure 54.5). With this technique optimal length and alignment can be achieved.

An alternative application of the "divide and reapproximate" principle places the valved segment of the allograft distally with the long curved aortic segment anastomosed to the ventriculotomy (Figure 54.6). The distal portion of the valve may result in less valve distortion than what occurs in the proximal position,[2] particularly when some degree of sternal compression is anticipated. Whichever position is utilized, the "divide and reapproximate" technique facilitates proximal and distal anastomoses, assures optimal length and alignment and allows ideal usage of the natural curvature of the aortic allograft. Accordingly, this principle can also be applied to shorter distances between the ventricle and pulmonary artery.

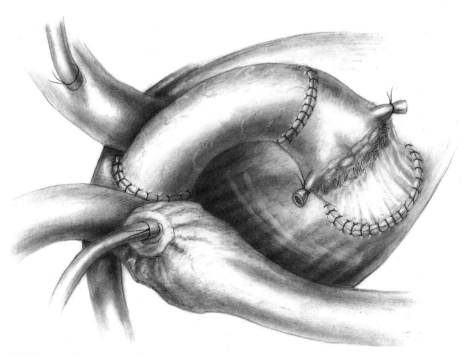

FIGURE 54.5. The distal segment is trimmed and the two allograft segments are reunited in proper orientation.

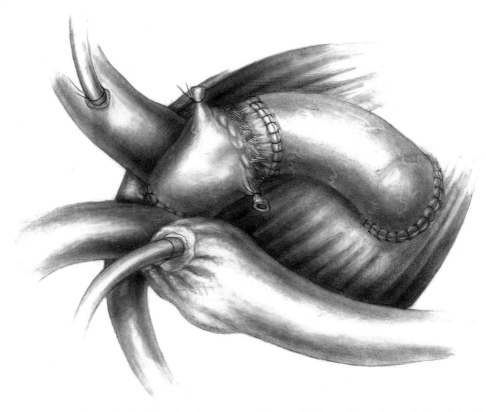

FIGURE 54.6. Alternatively, the valved segment of the aortic allograft can be positioned distally.

References

1. Dasmahapatra H, Freedom R, Moes C, et. al. Surgical experience with left ventricular outflow tract obstruction in patients with complete transposition of the great arteries and essentially intact ventricular septum undergoing the Mustard operation. Eur J Cardio-thorac Surg 1989;3:241–248.

2. Hoots AV, Watson DC, Jr. Construction of an aortic homograft conduit for right ventricle to pulmonary artery continuity. Ann Thorac Surg 1989;48:731–732.

55
Pulmonary Valve Allografts in Children

David R. Clarke and Deborah A. Bishop

Pulmonary valve allografts have been used successfully to reconstruct or repair the right ventricular outflow tract in a variety of pediatric cardiac conditions. One of the most attractive features of pulmonary allografts is their versatility. Allografts are available in a wide variety of sizes and are relatively easy to implant because the tissue is characteristically pliable. Allografts can be placed in critically ill neonates and infants for whom there are limited surgical options but whose congenital defects require surgical attention. Pulmonary allografts are used as a simple valved conduit to replace an existing right ventricular outflow tract as in a pulmonary allograft procedure, or in the presence of pulmonary stenosis, tetralogy of Fallot, or isolated pulmonary valvar atresia. Bifurcated pulmonary allografts can be used to repair stenosis or hypoplasia of the distal main, left and right pulmonary arteries. Complex repairs that involve de novo creation of a functional right ventricular outflow such as with truncus arteriosus, complex pulmonary atresia, transposition of the great arteries, or double outlet right ventricle are also treatable with allograft placement. Pulmonary allografts are hemodynamically more efficient than mechanical prostheses, do not require anticoagulation that can be problematic in an active pediatric patient and are proving more durable than other bioprostheses in most patients.

Right Ventricular Outflow Tract Replacement with the Pulmonary Autograft Procedure

The simplest right ventricular outflow tract procedure that uses a pulmonary allograft is a required consequence of pulmonary autograft replacement of the aortic valve. The technique was first described by Ross in 1967 and includes excision and transplantation of the native pulmonary valve and varied lengths of proximal main pulmonary artery, into the left ventricular outflow tract using one of several techniques.[1-4] Use of the Ross procedure is based on the premise that the best available aortic valve replacement is autologous tissue that is resistant to calcification and degeneration and can likely grow. In theory, allograft implantation into the lower pressure right side of the heart should result in a decreased incidence of degeneration and less severe consequences of failure than with a left sided implant. Originally, Ross described the use of an aortic allograft to reconstruct the right ventricular outflow tract[1] but more recently, a pulmonary allograft valve conduit is preferred.[5]

Indications

The pulmonary autograft is a surgical alternative for children with congenital anomalies of

501

the aortic valve and/or left ventricular outflow tract that are not amenable to balloon valvuloplasty or surgical valvotomy. Recent implementation of the autograft procedure as an aortic root replacement has expanded indications for the procedure to include the presence of endocarditis[6] as well as various aortic root pathologies such as aneurysm, dissection and multiple level obstruction[2,4] that previously were considered contraindications. The pulmonary autograft is not advised in the presence of native pulmonary valve dysfunction, annuloaortic ectasia, Marfan's syndrome, or autoimmune disease.

Perioperative Issues

The appropriate size pulmonary allograft can be determined by patient weight prior to surgery as illustrated in Figure 55.1. In most cases, an acceptable range of sizes is estimated. An allograft oversized by 2mm to 3mm is preferred with the pulmonary autograft procedure. Because the ABO compatibility issue remains unresolved, donor-recipient blood type specificity or compatibility is maintained when

possible. During initial phases of the surgical procedure, the chosen cryopreserved pulmonary allograft is thawed according to processing recommendations. Enclosed in a triple pouch, the allograft valve is submersed in a 37°C to 42°C waterbath until all ice crystals are dissolved. Thawing usually takes 15 to 22 minutes. The outer pouch is dried and cut open with scissors. The second pouch is peeled open to expose the inner pouch that is passed aseptically onto the sterile field. The third pouch is cut open and the allograft is extracted and placed into a sterile basin that contains one liter of 5% dextrose and lactated Ringer's. The allograft is allowed to passively soak for a minimum of five minutes to dilute the dimethylsulfoxide and is then ready for implantation.

Surgical Technique

Right ventricular outflow tract reconstruction with a pulmonary allograft is the final step of the pulmonary autograft procedure. Through a median sternotomy, cardiopulmonary bypass is instituted. The diseased aortic valve is excised, the native pulmonary valve and artery are

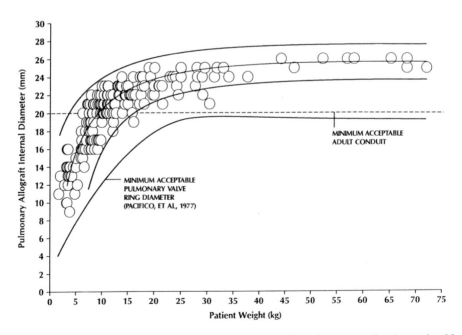

FIGURE 55.1. Before surgery, a range of appropriate pulmonary allograft sizes can be determined by patient weight.

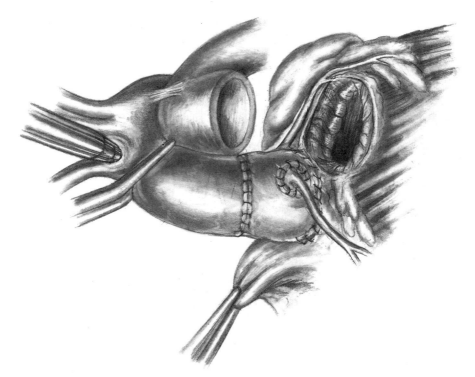

FIGURE 55.2. The diseased pulmonary valve had been excised. The native pulmonary valve and artery have been transplanted from the right to left ventricular outflow tract.

removed from the right ventricular outflow tract and implanted as a root replacement into the left ventricular outflow tract (Figure 55.2). A thawed pulmonary valve allograft is introduced onto the surgical field and used to reconstruct the right sided outflow tract. In general, some or all of this portion of the procedure can be accomplished during rewarming with the cross-clamp off and the heart beating.

Appropriate pulmonary allograft conduit length is determined by positioning the allograft anatomically and transecting excess tissue from the distal end. The pulmonary allograft is tailored to prevent tension or kinking as a result of insufficient or excess conduit length respectively. Distal anastomosis between the allograft and pulmonary artery bifurcation is performed first. Proper orientation of the allograft conduit is achieved by noting its natural curvature which should parallel the curve of the heart and allow the allograft to bend posteriorly and come to rest almost precisely in the anatomic location of the removed autograft.

Using CV-5 polytetrafluoroethylene suture, the distal anastomosis is initiated when a double armed stitch is taken through the left posterior aspect of the native pulmonary artery. This end is tagged and the other needle is passed through the corresponding posterior portion of the allograft. From within the lumen, the latter suture end is used to continue the running anastomosis rightward and posteriorly (Figure 55.3). The allograft conduit then can be rotated and retracted cranially for ectovascular exposure and to facilitate eversion of the vessel wall during the posterior portion of the anastomosis (Figure 55.4). The allograft then is returned to a more anatomic position. The anterior portion of the anastomosis is begun with the previously tagged suture arm and is continued rightward in running fashion (Figure 55.5). The two suture ends are tied where they meet on the rightward anterior surface of the completed anastomosis.

The proximal anastomosis of allograft and pulmonary outflow tract muscle is accomplished with the same suture material. The

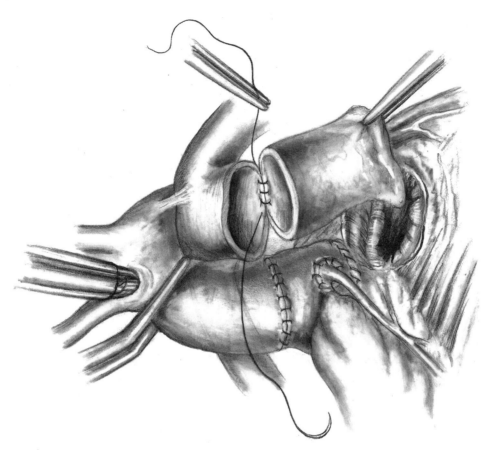

FIGURE 55.3. The distal anastomosis from homograft to native pulmonary artery is performed first. A double armed stitch through the left posterior aspect of the pulmonary artery is tagged. The other needle is passed through the corresponding portion of the allograft and is continued rightward and posteriorly from within the lumen.

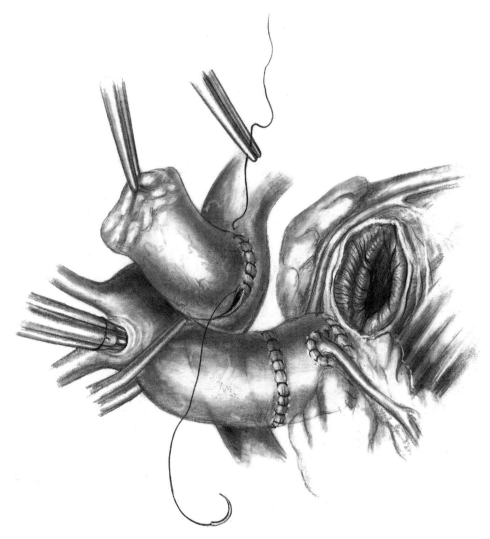

FIGURE 55.4. The allograft is retracted cranially to facilitate exposure and the distal anastomosis is continued posteriorly.

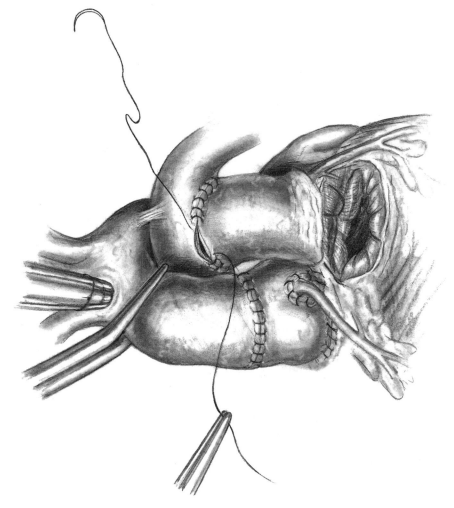

FIGURE 55.5. With the allograft rotated back into anatomic position, the previously tagged suture is used to perform the anterior anastomosis.

initial stitch is placed through the left posterior allograft muscle cuff from inside to outside and tagged. The other suture end is placed in the opposing infundibular muscle and the posterior connection is completed from inside the lumen (Figure 55.6). The former, tagged needle is then used to complete the anterior suture line from outside the lumen (Figure 55.7). The anastomosis is complete when the posterior suture is encountered to the right. The patient is weaned from cardiopulmonary bypass in standard fashion.

Helpful Hints and/or Variations in Technique

— Larger pulmonary allografts than would be chosen for other procedures are useful here.
— Proximal suture bites should include right ventricular endocardium but should be kept shallow to avoid the first septal branch of the left anterior descending coronary artery.
— Knots in the polytetrafluoroethylene suture should be fixed with a clip or separate suture to prevent slippage.

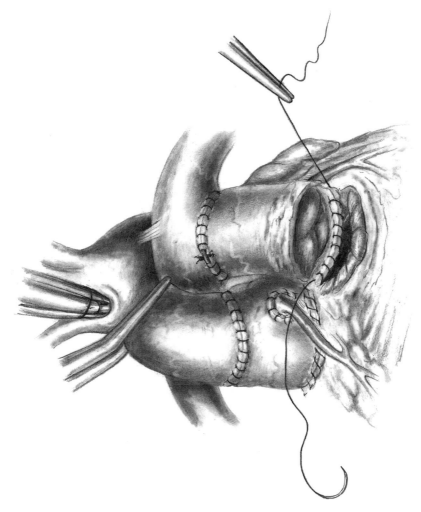

FIGURE 55.6. The proximal anastomosis between allograft and right ventricular outflow tract muscle is performed next. Double armed suture is placed through the left posterior allograft muscle cuff from inside to outside and tagged. The other needle is placed through the opposing infundibular muscle and the anastomosis is completed from within the lumen.

Results with Procedure

The largest series of patients who have undergone the pulmonary autograft procedure are reported by Donald Ross and his colleagues in London and by Ronald Elkins et al. in Oklahoma. Total follow-up in the London series is 24 years with an 80% actuarial survival and 85% freedom from replacement at 20 years postoperative.[7] The Oklahoma series offers shorter follow-up of ten years but confirms Ross' conclusions thus far.[8] There has been little or no residual or recurrent left ventricular outflow tract obstruction, or recurrent or progressive autograft insufficiency. Most importantly, autograft primary tissue failure has not been observed. The right ventricular outflow tract allograft also seems to be relatively durable. Actuarial freedom from reoperation is 80% at 16 years of follow-up.[9]

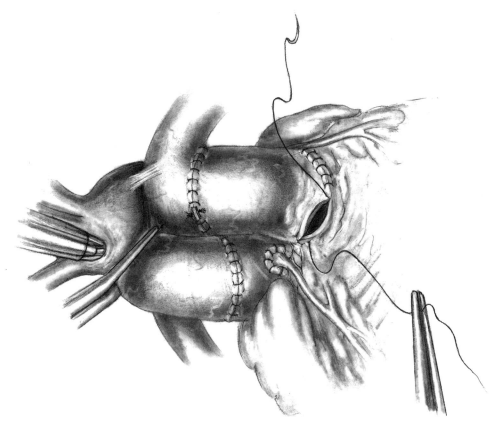

FIGURE 55.7. The suture line is continued anteriorly from outside the lumen using the formerly tagged needle.

Alternative Techniques

Alternatives to the pulmonary autograft procedure include allograft aortic root replacement and aortoventriculoplasty or Konno procedure. These techniques are suitable when the pulmonary valve is significantly abnormal or in the presence of other contraindications to pulmonary autografting.

Repair of Simple Right Ventricular Outflow Tract Anomalies

Pulmonary allograft right ventricular outflow tract reconstruction becomes more complex as cardiac defects such as pulmonary valvar stenosis or atresia and simple tetralogy of Fallot are encountered. In such cases the proximal anastomosis becomes only slightly more complicated thanks to the presence of an outflow tract, but the distal connection can require more extensive reconstruction. Incorporation of some or all of a bifurcated distal pulmonary allograft is sometimes necessary to repair surgically or congenitally distorted or discontinuous branch pulmonary arteries.

Indications

Pulmonary allograft reconstruction of the right ventricular outflow tract is indicated in the presence of obstruction or discontinuity between the right side of the heart and the pulmonary artery system that is sufficient to prohibit relief without creation of excessive pulmonary valve regurgitation. The presence of iatrogenic pulmonary regurgitation is of particular concern when increased distal pulmonary vascular resistance that will accentuate the severity of the insufficiency is anticipated postoperatively. Right ventricular outflow tract reconstruction with a pulmonary allograft often is performed when impending right ventricular failure is secondary to pulmonary regurgitation following a prior surgical procedure.

Perioperative Issues

A median sternotomy is used to open the patient's chest. Total cardiopulmonary bypass with bicaval and ascending aortic cannulation is established. Pulmonary allograft sizing and thawing are accomplished as previously described in the chapter. When distal pulmonary arteries are normal and right ventricular outflow tract reconstruction is an isolated procedure, the aorta is not routinely cross-

clamped and minimal hypothermia is used so that regular cardiac rhythm is maintained. If concomitant intracardiac defects such as atrial and/or ventricular septal defect closure or infundibular muscle resection are required, the aorta is cross-clamped and the aortic root injected with cold blood cardioplegia that is delivered in bolus doses every 20 to 30 minutes.

Surgical Technique

The pulmonary valve and annulus are evaluated and intracardiac repairs accessed through a vertical right ventriculotomy (Figure 55.8). When annular dimensions are deemed inadequate, the incision is extended across the pulmonary annulus and into the main pulmonary artery. The pulmonary artery trunk and distal right and left branches are evaluated and dissected out as necessary. CV-5 polytetrafluo-

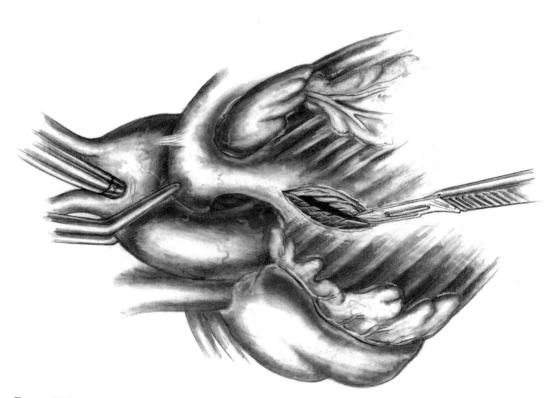

FIGURE 55.8. A vertical right ventriculotomy provides access for repair of more complex cardiac defects such as simple tetralogy of Fallot or pulmonary stenosis or atresia.

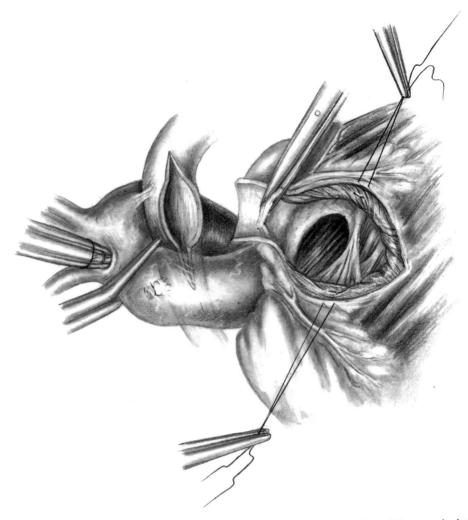

FIGURE 55.9. The right ventriculotomy is extended across the pulmonary annulus when annular dimensions are determined inadequate. Stay sutures are applied to opposing sides of the ventriculotomy and retracted to expose a ventricular septal defect.

roethylene suture is used alone for primary repair of an atrial septal defect and in conjunction with autologous pericardium for patch repair. A ventricular septal defect (Figure 55.9) is closed with a patch and running CV-5 suture, both of polytetrafluoroethylene (Figure 55.10). Final allograft preparations are made by trimming excess muscle from below the valve to minimize suture line bulk. Ideal pulmonary allograft conduit length is approximated and any remaining distal arterial tissue is resected and discarded (Figure 55.11).

The recipient pulmonary artery is transected at the appropriate level and distal anastomosis is performed with one of three surgical options. Two of three variations on the distal anastomosis are completed with continuous running suture of CV-5 polytetrafluoroethylene and are begun posteriorly from within the lumen. If the pulmonary arteries are normal, a circular allograft to native main pulmonary artery connection is accomplished (Figure 55.12B). The first suture is taken through the most posterior, leftward portion of the native and allograft pul-

FIGURE 55.10. If a ventricular septal defect is present, it is closed with a patch.

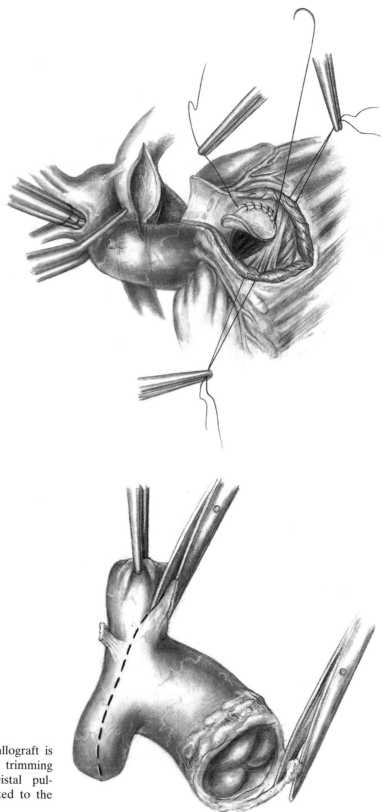

FIGURE 55.11. The pulmonary allograft is prepared for implantation by trimming excess subvalvular muscle. Distal pulmonary artery conduit is resected to the appropriate length.

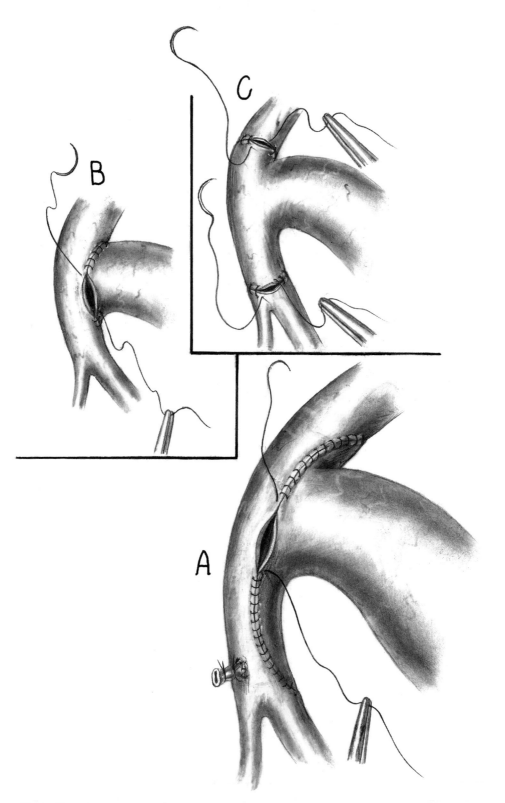

FIGURE 55.12. The distal allograft to pulmonary artery anastomosis is performed with one of three surgical options. (A) In the repair of simple right ventricular outflow tract anomalies, the most common anatomy found is unilateral distal pulmonary artery stenosis. The restrictive area is enlarged with a flap extension of the allograft conduit. (B) In the presence of normal distal pulmonary arteries, a circular allograft to native main pulmonary artery anastomosis is performed. (C) Separate anastomoses to right and left pulmonary arteries is often necessary to establish right ventricle to pulmonary artery continuity in complex right lesions.

monary arteries and is continued bilaterally to the most anterior, rightward aspect of the arteries. A flap extension of the allograft conduit is used to enlarge unilateral distal pulmonary artery stenosis that commonly is resultant of a systemic to pulmonary shunt on the right or an existing stricture caused by remnant ductus arteriosus tissue on the left (Figure 55.12A). Cardiac anatomy that requires distal flap extension is most commonly encountered with simple right ventricular outflow tract anomalies (Figures 55.13A,B). When branch

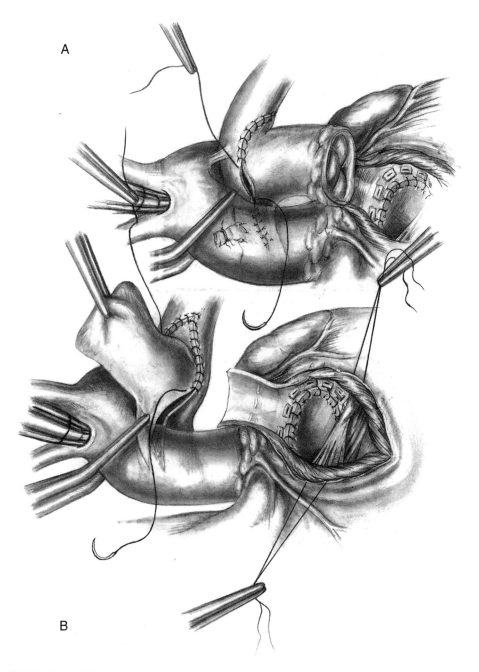

FIGURE 55.13. (A and B) To perform extension of the distal pulmonary arteries, the anastomosis is begun posteriorly from within the lumen and proceeds leftward and rightward to meet anteriorly.

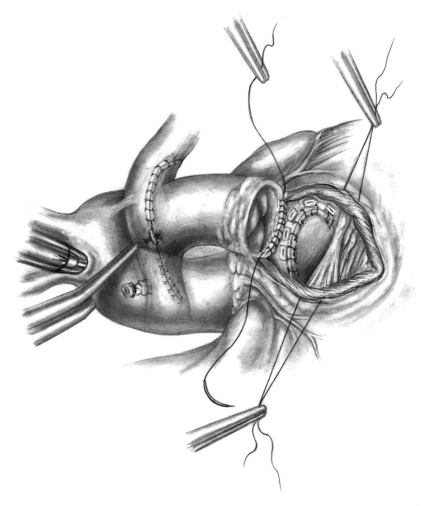

FIGURE 55.14. The proximal anastomosis is initiated by suturing the posterior allograft directly into the recipient pulmonary valve annulus or right ventricular infundibulum proximal to the valve.

pulmonary arteries are discontinuous or severely distorted, a bifurcated pulmonary allograft is anastomosed separately to the right and left branches (Figure 55.12C). In this case, CV-6 polytetrafluoroethylene suture is used for the running anastomosis.

The patient is rewarmed as the proximal connection is begun. If the aorta was clamped, a dose of warm cardioplegia is infused, the clamp is removed and the myocardium is revascularized. The proximal anastomosis is made by suturing the posterior allograft directly into the recipient pulmonary valve annulus or right ventricular infundibulum proximal to the valve (Figure 55.14). A shield shaped patch is constructed of polytetrafluoroethylene and used to form a good from the anterior, lateral allograft to the proximal right ventriculotomy. Initially separate, buttressed, horizontal mattress sutures are taken at each of the two junctions where allograft, patch and ventricular myocardium meet (Figure 55.15). The remaining anterior portion of the allograft is attached to the patch material superiorly (Figure 55.16) and the remainder of the hood is sewn to the edges of the

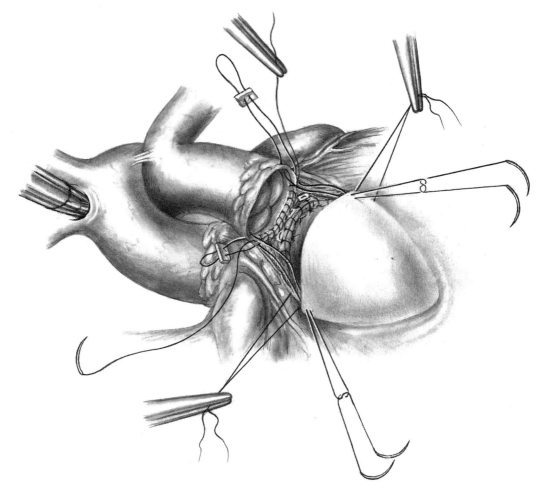

FIGURE 55.15. A shield shaped, polytetrafluoroethylene patch is used to form a hood from the anterior, lateral allograft to the proximal right ventriculotomy.

ventriculotomy (Figures 55.17A, B). After the patient is warmed, cardiopulmonary bypass is withdrawn and decannulation is conducted in standard fashion.

Helpful Hints and/or Variations in Technique

Appropriate sizing of the proximal patch is extremely important. The patch must be large enough both longitudinally and transversely to allow sufficient ballooning to avoid obstruction. However, the length of the patch edge sutured to the proximal allograft must not be excessive

or the annulus will dilate and valve regurgitation result.

Personal Results

From April 1995 through December 1996, 91 children who had a simple right ventricular outflow tract lesion have undergone right sided reconstruction with a pulmonary allograft in Denver. At the time of surgery, the patients were 12 days to 18 years of age (mean age: 5.4 years) and weighed 3.2 to 82.3 kg (mean weight: 18.0 kg). Diagnoses included 74 children with tetralogy of Fallot, with or without absent

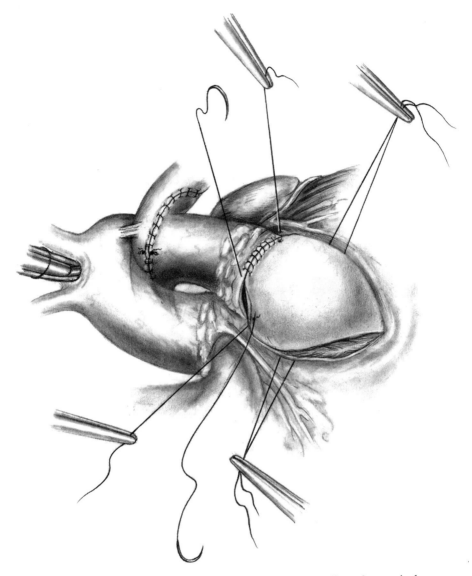

FIGURE 55.16. The patch is attached to the anterior allograft superiorly.

pulmonary valve, 11 with pulmonary stenosis and/or insufficiency and six patients with pulmonary atresia and ventricular septal defect. Nine children suffered hospital deaths (10%) and one child underwent cardiac transplantation two days postoperatively secondary to dilated cardiomyopathy and cardiac failure. Among 81 survivors who were followed for a mean of 5.9 years, there have been seven late deaths (9%). Eight children (10%), all of whom were older than 12 months of age at initial operation, have required pulmonary allograft replacement from 14 months to 10.3 years after implantation.

Alternative Techniques

An alternative to pulmonary allograft conduit repair of the right ventricular outflow tract with an existing pulmonary annulus is transannular

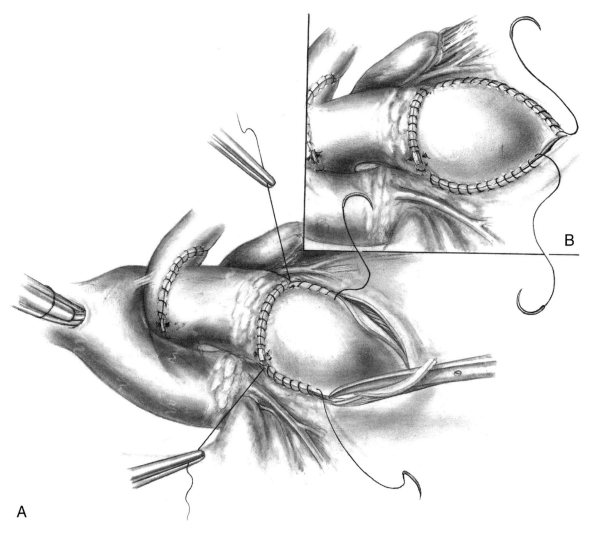

FIGURE 55.17. (A and B) The sides of the hood are sewn to the edges of the ventriculotomy.

patch repair. The technique utilizes synthetic or autologous material to patch enlarge the pulmonary annulus. Transannular patching cannot easily accommodate abnormal distal pulmonary artery anatomy. A patch is not recommended in the presence of elevated pulmonary vascular resistance that increases the obligatory pulmonary regurgitation and thus sacrifices long-term right ventricular function.

Repair of Complex Right Ventricular Outflow Tract Anomalies

From the surgeon's perspective, complex anomalies of the right ventricular outflow tract share two anatomic features; the absence of a connection between the right side of the heart and the pulmonary arteries and the presence of a ventricular septal defect. These features characterize truncus arteriosus, double outlet right ventricle, complex forms of transposition of the great arteries and pulmonary atresia with ventricular septal defect. These cardiac anomalies are managed surgically in a similar fashion. Repair begins with the takedown of previous shunts or pulmonary artery bands if present, followed by ventricular septal defect patching to direct blood from the left ventricle into the aorta. Extra-anatomic continuity is then established between the right side of the heart and pulmonary artery.

Indications

The diagnosis of truncus arteriosus is sufficient indication for surgery. Complete repair is standard procedure soon after the diagnosis is established. Pulmonary atresia with ventricular septal defect often includes the complete absence of a right ventricular outflow tract. With the diagnosis of transposition of the great arteries or Taussig-Bing type double outlet right ventricle, pulmonary allograft reconstruction of the anatomic right side of the heart is indicated if complete repair is anticipated and arterial switch is not possible or desirable. In these cases, right ventricular outflow tract reconstruction would be used in conjunction with a Rastelli,[10] Damus-Kaye-Stansel[11] or Nikaidoh procedure.[12]

Perioperative Issues

There is no defined right ventricular outflow tract in complex anomalies that involve the right ventricle to pulmonary artery reconstruction. Determination of an appropriate sized allograft is therefore more important because the valve usually must sit on top of the right ventricle and might be subject to sternal compression. A range of appropriate allograft sizes is estimated according to age and physical size of the child. An allograft near the small end of this range is then selected. Pulmonary allograft thawing technique is described previously in this section.

Surgical Technique

Truncus arteriosus will be used as the representative lesion to illustrate complex complete repair with a pulmonary allograft. The heart is exposed through a median sternotomy. While the cryopreserved allograft is thawing, the truncal root is mobilized along with its systemic and pulmonary connections. Cardiopulmonary bypass is established with cannulation of the distal ascending aorta above the truncal bifurcation and of superior and inferior vena cavae. Bypass is conducted in a standard fashion using moderate hypothermia. The aorta is cross-clamped and pulmonary arteries are controlled. Cold blood cardioplegia is administered into the aortic root or coronary sinus with reinfusion every 20 to 30 minutes during repair of internal cardiac anomalies. The pulmonary arteries along with surrounding orifice tissue that supplements the distal anastomosis, are detached from the truncal valve. If the pulmonary artery branches arise independently from the main trunk with little or no main pulmonary artery, an increased amount of truncal tissue is excised. The resultant truncal root defect is closed primarily or with a polytetrafluoroethylene or pericardial patch.

The heart is then incised to provide access for intracardiac repairs using a longitudinal right ventriculotomy (Figure 55.18). That is extended proximally onto the free wall to expose the ventricular septal defect adequately (Figure 55.19). The defect is closed with a polytetrafluoroethylene patch and running suture of CV-5 polytetrafluoroethylene to direct left ventricular outflow into the truncus (Figure 55.20). The anterior portion of the ventricular septal defect patch is usually sutured to the edge of the right ventriculotomy. An appropriately sized pulmonary allograft is thawed. The valve conduit is prepared for implantation by cutting a pie shaped wedge from the posterior edge of the subannular muscle to fit the most superior point of the ventriculotomy (Figure 55.21). The right ventricle outflow tract subsequently is constructed using the thawed pulmonary allograft. The distal connection between allograft conduit and native pulmonary trunk or arteries

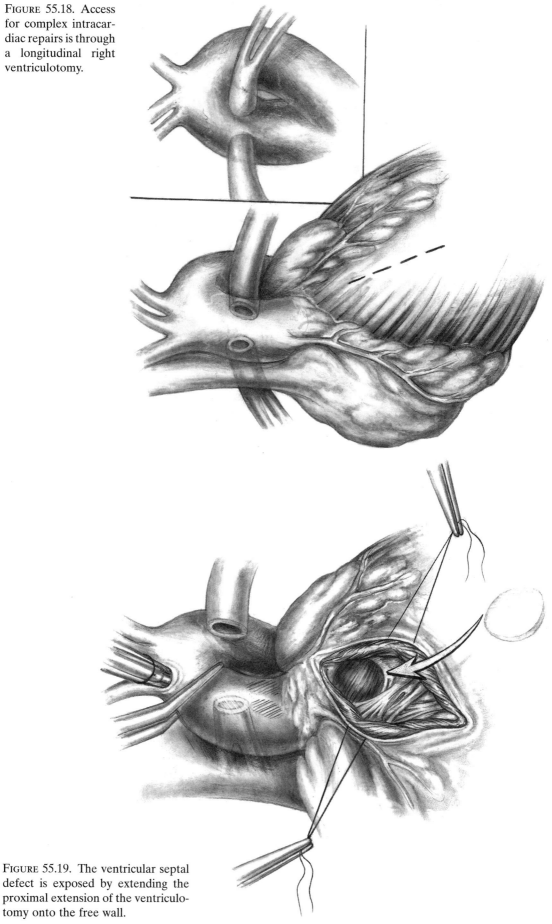

FIGURE 55.18. Access for complex intracardiac repairs is through a longitudinal right ventriculotomy.

FIGURE 55.19. The ventricular septal defect is exposed by extending the proximal extension of the ventriculotomy onto the free wall.

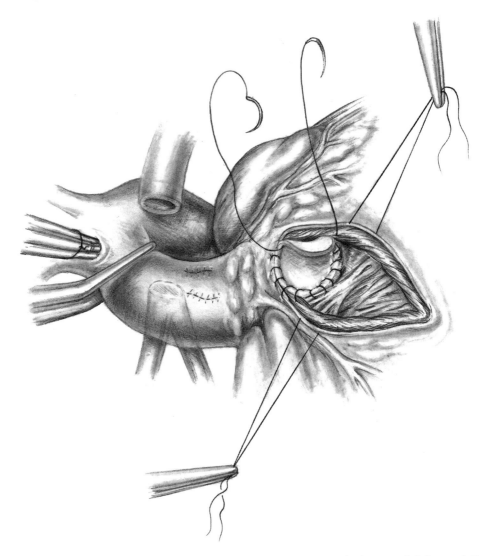

FIGURE 55.20. A polytetrafluoroethylene patch is used to close the ventricular septal defect and direct left ventricular outflow through the truncal valve.

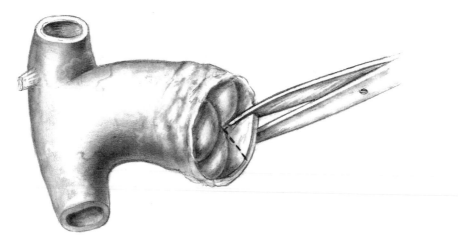

FIGURE 55.21. A pie shaped wedge is cut from the posterior edge of the pulmonary allograft subannular muscle.

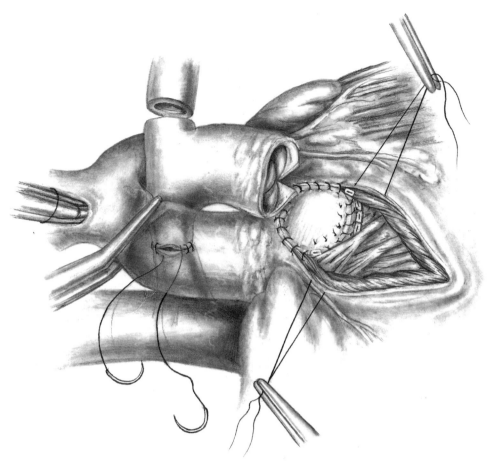

FIGURE 55.22. Beginning with the distal pulmonary allograft to native pulmonary trunk or artery anastomosis, the right ventricular outflow tract is constructed.

is performed first (Figure 55.22). With running, CV-5 or CV-6 polytetrafluoroethylene suture, one of the three techniques described previously is performed (Figure 55.23). Separate anastomoses to each of the left and right pulmonary arteries are most commonly required to establish right ventricle to pulmonary continuity in complex right ventricular outflow lesions (Figure 55.23A). As described previously, the first stitch is placed posteriorly and continued anteriorly and laterally to both sides from within the lumen. From the lateral position, the suture is brought outside the lumen and the most anterior part of the anastomosis is completed (Figure 55.24). The proximal allograft connection is performed directly to the surface of the right ventricle at the apex of the

ventriculotomy incision. The apex of the wedge that was resected from the pulmonary allograft subannular muscle is situated at the most superior point of the ventriculotomy. Care is taken to avoid suture penetration above the allograft annulus that might interfere with pulmonary valve function. The connection is performed using CV-4 or CV-5 polytetrafluoroethylene running suture. Beginning at the apex of the resected annular wedge, the allograft is sewn to the upper edge of the ventriculotomy often including the edge of the ventricular septal defect (Figure 55.25). Anastomosis continues left and right to the lateral aspect of the incision and incorporates approximately 20 to 25 percent of the allograft circumference. At this point, a rounded, kite-shaped patch cut from

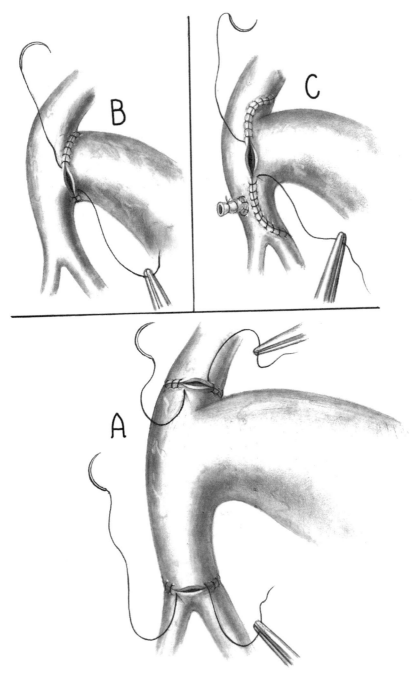

FIGURE 55.23. One of three surgical techniques is used to perform the distal anastomosis. (A) The anatomy most commonly encountered in complex right sided cardiac anomalies includes discontinuous or severely distorted pulmonary arteries. A bifur- cated pulmonary allograft is anastomosed separately to the right and left pulmonary artery branches. (B) Circular anastomosis to the main pulmonary artery or (C) flap extension to relieve unilateral stenosis are other options for distal anastomosis.

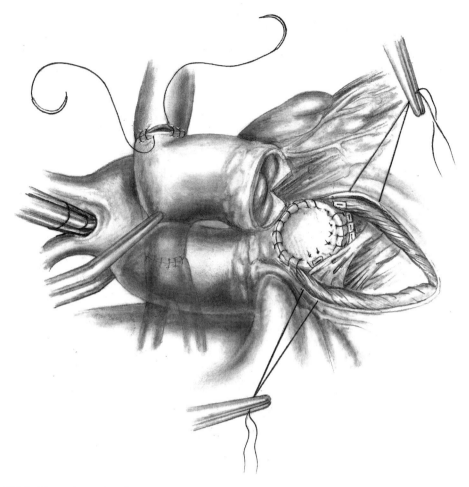

FIGURE 55.24. To perform the distal pulmonary allograft anastomosis, the first stitch is placed posteriorly and continued from within the lumen, laterally and anteriorly to both sides.

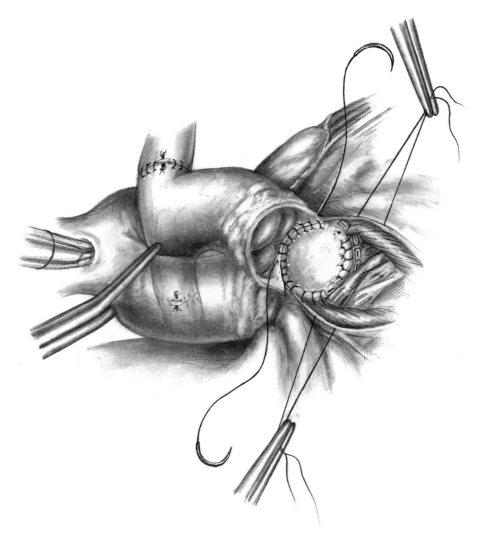

FIGURE 55.25. The wedge that was resected from the pulmonary allograft subannular muscle is fit over the most anterior point of the ventriculotomy. Beginning at the wedge apex, the allograft is anastomosed to the upper edge of the ventriculotomy.

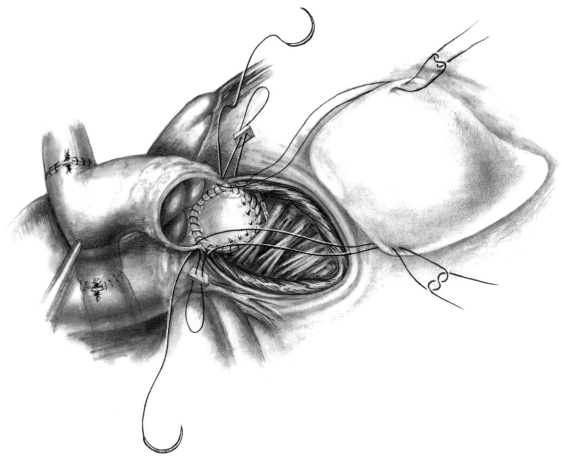

FIGURE 55.26. After the proximal allograft to ventriculotomy suture line has continued right and left to include approximately 30 percent of the allograft circumference, a kite shaped polytetrafluoroethylene patch is incorporated into the anastomosis.

polytetrafluoroethylene material is incorporated into the anastomosis as a hood to complete construction of the right ventricular outflow. Pledgetted sutures are used to initiate and reinforce the points where allograft, ventricle and patch intersect bilaterally (Figure 55.26). The patch allograft anastomosis is completed anteriorly (Figure 55.27) and the patch to right ventricular anastomosis is continued down both sides of the ventriculotomy (Figure 55.28) until they meet at the most inferior point of the ventriculotomy (Figure 55.28) and the suture is tied off. Patch size and shape should be cut generously since both can be modified to fit more exactly during the anastomotic process (Figure 55.29). As the proximal attachment progresses, the patient is rewarmed slowly. Warm blood cardioplegia is injected and the aortic cross-clamp is removed. After rewarming is complete, cardiopulmonary bypass is discontinued and the surgery is concluded in standard manner.

Helpful Hints and/or Variations in Technique

One must note that although the use of pulmonary allografts is recommended for right ventricular outflow reconstruction, aortic allografts occasionally are used if additional conduit length is required or if very high distal pulmonary resistance is anticipated.

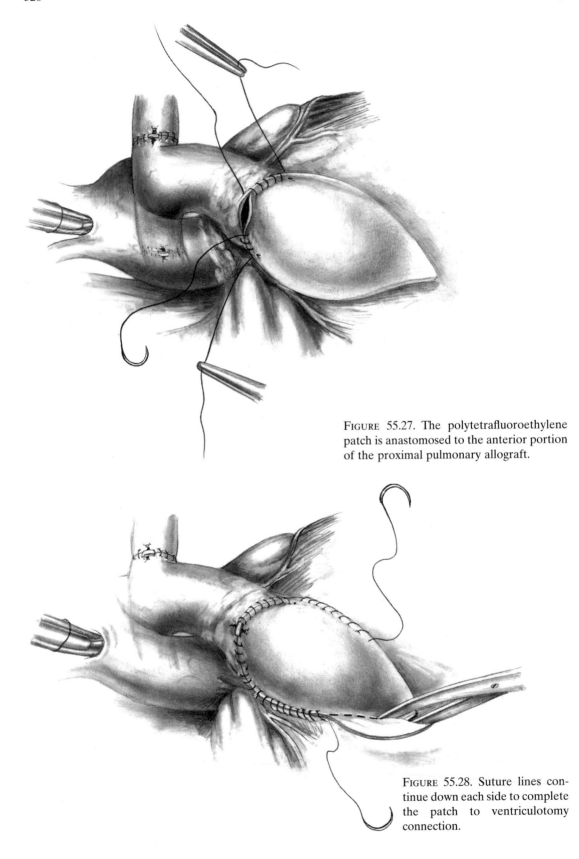

FIGURE 55.27. The polytetrafluoroethylene patch is anastomosed to the anterior portion of the proximal pulmonary allograft.

FIGURE 55.28. Suture lines continue down each side to complete the patch to ventriculotomy connection.

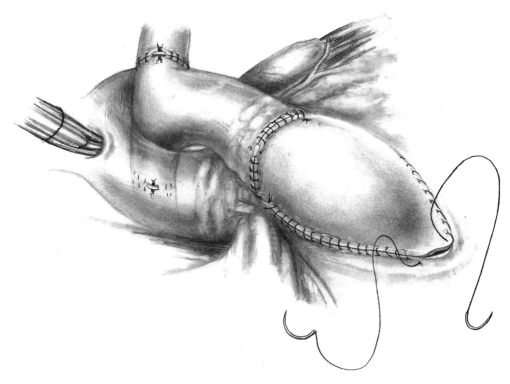

FIGURE 55.29. The suture are tied off where they intersect at the most inferior point of the ventriculotomy.

Personal Results

At the Children's Hospital and the University of Colorado Health Sciences Center in Denver, 122 children have undergone pulmonary allograft reconstruction of complex right ventricular outflow tract anomalies from April 1995 to December 1996. At the time of surgery, patients ranged in age from six days to 17.3 years (mean age: 3.2 years). Preoperative diagnosis was pulmonary atresia with no right sided outflow tract and a ventricular septal defect in 45, truncus arteriosus in 38, transposition of the great arteries in 23, double outlet left or right ventricle in 15 patients and aortic atresia with hypoplastic arch and ventricular septal defect in one child. There were 16 early deaths (13%). One-hundred-and-six operative survivors have been followed a mean of 4.5 years with 14 late deaths (13%) and two cardiac transplants, none of which were allograft related. Eleven children (10%) have required surgery to replace their original cryopreserved pulmonary valve due to allograft fibrocalcification and degeneration. The remaining allograft recipients are clinically well.

Alternative Techniques

If an extracardiac conduit is required to repair a complex anomaly of the right ventricular outflow tract, alternatives to the use of a pulmonary allograft are limited. Aortic allografts continue to be used but pulmonary allografts generally considered more durable in the right ventricular outflow tract because they have proven less prone to calcification and degeneration.[13,14] The use of cryopreserved aortic valves is usually reserved for cases in which a longer conduit is necessary than is available on allografts. Xenograft bioprosthetic valved synthetic conduits are an option for some infants and children. Xenografts in children, however, exhibit early calcification and degeneration, formation of intimal peel within the synthetic conduit, and their rigidity can cause native pulmonary artery distortion and cardiac or coronary compression.[15,16] Stentless xenografts might be useful in reconstruction of the right ventricular outflow tract but to date, they have not been evaluated adequately. Non-valved conduits have been used to provide continuity between the right ventricle and pulmonary artery in neonates.[17] The repair can be disadvantageous in the early postoperative period when elevated neonatal pulmonary vascular resistance can increase pulmonary regurgitation and lead to right ventricular failure.

Conclusion

Pulmonary allograft valve conduits facilitate repair of a variety of right ventricular outflow tract congenital defects from simple to complex. Primary repair of congenital cardiac disease at all levels of complexity in neonates and infants is the generally preferred method of treatment. Early repair reduces detrimental affects on the heart and contributes to more normal development of the lungs[18] and brain.[19]

References

1. Ross DN. Replacement of the aortic and mitral valve with a pulmonary valve autograft. Lancet 1967;2:956–958.
2. Stelzer P, Jones DJ, Elkins RC. Aortic root replacement with pulmonary autograft. Circulation 1989;80:III209–III213.
3. Randolph JD, Toal K, Stelzer P, Elkins RC. Aortic valve and left ventricular outflow tract replacement using allograft and autograft valves: a preliminary report. Ann Thorac Surg 1989;48: 345–349.
4. Angell WW, Pupello DF, Bessone LN, et al. Partial inclusion aortic root replacement with the pulmonary autograft valve. J Heart Valve Dis 1993;2:388–394.
5. Livi U, Abdulla AK, Parker R, Olsen EJ, Ross DN. Viability and morphology of aortic and pulmonary homografts. J Thorac Cardiovasc Surg 1987;93:755–760.
6. Oswalt J. Management of Aortic Infective Endocarditis by Autograft Valve Replacement. J Heart Valve Dis 1994;3:377–379.
7. Ross D, Jackson M, Davies J. Pulmonary Autograft Aortic Valve Replacement: Long-Term Results. J Card Surg 1991;6:529–533.
8. Elkins RC, Knott-Craig CJ, Randolph JD, et al. Medium-term follow-up of pulmonary autograft replacement of aortic valves in children. EJCTS 1994;8:379–383.
9. Gerosa G, McKay R, Ross D. Replacement of the Aortic Valve or Root With a Pulmonary Autograft in Children. The Society of Thoracic Surgeons 1991;51:424–429.
10. Rastelli GC, McGoon DC, Wallace RB. Anatomic correction of transposition of the great arteries with ventricular septal defect and subpulmonary stenosis. J Thorac Cardiovasc Surg 1969;58:545–552.
11. Lin AE, Laks H, Barber G, et al. Subaortic obstruction in complex congenital heart disease: management by proximal pulmonary artery to ascending aorta end to side anastomosis. J Am Coll Cardiol 1986;7:617–624.
12. Nikaidoh H. Aortic translocation and biventricular outflow tract reconstruction: a new surgical repair for transposition of the great arteries associated with ventricular septal defect and pulmonary stenosis. J Thorac Cardiovasc Surg 1984;88:365–372.
13. Albert JD, Bishop DA, Fullerton DA, Campbell DN, Clarke DR. Conduit reconstruction of the right ventricular outflow tract. J Thorac Cardiovasc Surg 1993;106:228–236.
14. Bando K, Danielson GK, Schaff HV. Outcome of pulmonary and aortic homografts for right ventricular outflow tract reconstruction. J Thorac Cardiovasc Surg 1995;109:509–518.
15. Jonas RA, Freed MD, Mayor JE, Castaneda AR. Long term follow-up of patients with synthetic right heart conduits. Circulation 1985;72(Suppll. 2):II77–II83.
16. Reddy VM, Rajasinghe HA, McElhinney DB, et al. Performance of right ventricular to pulmonary artery conduits after repair of truncus arteriosus: a comparison of Dacron-house porcine valves and cryopreserved allografts. Sem in Thor and Card Surg 1995;7:133–138.
17. Peetz DJ, Jr., Spicer RL, Crowley DC, et al. Correction of truncus arteriosus in the neonate using a nonvalved conduit. J Thorac Cardiovasc Surg 1982;83:743–746.
18. Johnson RJ, Haworth SG. Pulmonary vascular and alveolar development in tetralogy of Fallot:

a recommendation for early correction. Thorax 1982;37:893–901.

19. Newburger JW, Silbert AR, Buckley LP, et al. Cognitive function and age at repair of transposition of the great arteries in children. New Eng Journ Med 1984;310:1495–1499.

56
Truncus Arteriosus Repair

Gary K. Lofland

Truncus arteriosus (persistent truncus arteriosus, truncus arteriosus communis, common aorticopulmonary trunk) is a congenital cardiac malformation that involves the ventriculoarterial connection in which a single outlet is present. It is characterized by the presence of a single semilunar valve annulus as the only exit from the heart, a subarterial ventricular septal defect, and the absence or severe deficiency of the aortopulmonary septum. Two related but different malformations are aortopulmonary window and subarterial ventricular septal defect.

Anatomy and Classification

In 1949, Collett and Edwards[1] proposed a classification system based on the arrangement of the origins of the pulmonary arteries from the truncal artery (Figure 56.1). The classification proposed by Van Praagh and Van Praagh[2] also includes cases with a single pulmonary artery and various degrees of development of the ascending aorta and ductus arteriosus. In the Collett and Edwards Type I truncus, the pulmonary arteries arise from a common pulmonary trunk that originates from the truncus. In Type II, the right and left pulmonary arteries arise close together from the dorsal wall of the truncus arteriosus. In Type III, the proximal arteries arise separately from the lateral aspects of the truncus. In Type IV, the proximal pulmonary arteries are absent and pulmonary blood flow originates from the multiple aorticopulmonary collateral vessels.

In practice, the distinction between Types I, II, and III truncus is imprecise, and the actual existence of Type III truncus with lateral origins of the pulmonary arteries is questioned.[3] The Type IV classification of Collett and Edwards should be replaced by the more precise designation, pulmonary atresia with ventricular septal defect. Also the term pseudotruncus should be replaced by the more descriptive designation of a condition characterized by pulmonary atresia and patent ductus arteriosus.[3]

Morphologically, the arterial trunk or truncus is large or larger than a normal aorta and arises as a solitary vessel from the base of the heart. The coronary and pulmonary arteries arise from this truncus. The truncus originates from both ventricles but usually overrides the septum to lie more over the right than over the left ventricle. Although the ventricular septal defect usually is directly subarterial, in our own series we have seen patients with a marked degree of override of the ventricular septal defect, such that the truncal artery emerges predominately from the right ventricle.

In general, the ventricular septal defect associated with truncus arteriosus is in the anterior septum, confluent with the truncus, and the atrioventricular bundle is posterior and unrelated to the rim of the ventricular septal defect. If the ventricular septal defect is related to the membranous septum, the atrioventricular bundle may be close to the ventricular septal defect and susceptible to surgical injury. In truncus, the

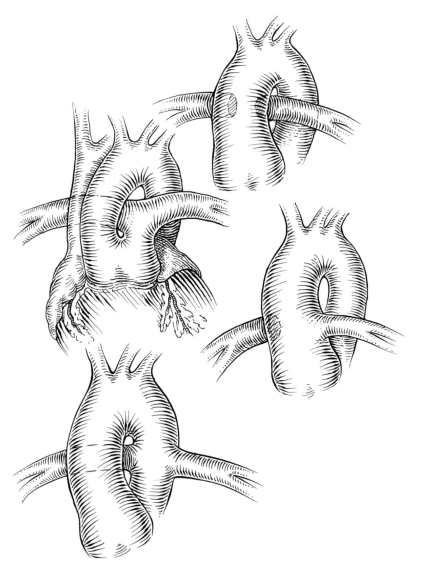

FIGURE 56.1. Anatomic types of truncus arteriosus from Coletti and Edwards' classification, beginning at upper left and continuing clockwise. In Type I truncus the pulmonary arteries arise from a common pulmonary trunk that originates from the truncus. In Type II, the right and left pulmonary arteries arise close together from the dorsal wall of the truncus. In Type III, the pulmonary arteries arise separately from the lateral aspects of the truncus. In Type IV, the proximal pulmonary arteries are absent and pulmonary flow is derived from aortopulmonary collateral vessels.

conduction system varies in its course and is related to the location of the ventricular septal defect and its relationship to the membranous septum.[4] The ventricular septal defect may be close to or related to the membranous septum, and the atrioventricular bundle and the beginning of the bundle branches may be vulnerable to surgical injury.[5]

Although coronary arteries usually arise from orifices in the truncal valve sinuses of Valsalva in a position close to the normal one (left arising posteriorly into the left and right arising anteriorly), variations in coronary anatomy have been reported.[2,6–10]

The pulmonary arteries usually originate just downstream from the truncal valve, on the left posterior lateral aspect of the truncus, although true lateral, true posterior and true anterior origins have been described.[8] There is often a single orifice that soon divides into right and left pulmonary arteries (Type I of Collett and Edwards). Less commonly, the pulmonary arteries have separate orifices (Type II of Collett and Edwards). These 2 types account for 86% of cases in the Barratt-Boyes series.[11] The pulmonary arteries may arise from the ascending aorta, the descending aorta, the innominate artery or the ductus arteriosus.

The morphology of great arteries varies in both pulmonary and aortic pathways, and the pattern of the aortic arch has considerable surgical significance. If the aortic arch is interrupted, it is usually at the level of the isthmus,[12] but sometimes proximal to the origin of the left subclavian artery. In either case, the descending aorta is supplied by the ductus arteriosus, and indeed exists as a continuation of the ductus arteriosus. Truncus arteriosus with aortic arch interruption is found in up to one-fifth of autopsy series.[2,6,7,12] More recently, Bove and associates found interrupted aortic arch in 5 of 46 patients, and Hanley and associates found interrupted aortic arch in 6 of 63 patients.[9,13]

The truncal valve is posterior and inferior in position but still points more anteriorly than the normal aortic valve.[12] There is fibrous continuity between the posterior leaflet and the anterior mitral valve leaflet.[12] The truncal valve usually has three cusps but may have two to six cusps. In one series, truncal valve incompetence was severe in 6%, moderate in 31%, and absent to minimal in 63% of cases.[14] Although dysplastic truncal valves have been seen with some frequency in autopsy series,[15] it was formerly felt that it did not pose a major problem in surgical repair in infancy.[8] More recently, however, one series showed truncal valve regurgitation severe enough to require truncal replacement in 5 of 46 patients, 3 of whom also had significant systolic pressure gradient.[9] In our own series, we have encountered severely dysplastic truncal valves in 2 recent patients, both of whom had interrupted aortic arch concomitantly. The truncal valve gradient in each of these patients was in excess of 100 mmHg.

The pathophysiology of truncus arteriosus is that of a large left to right shunt at a ventricular or great artery level, with a high ratio of pulmonary to systemic blood flow (Q_p/Q_s). Systemic pressures usually exist in the right ventricle and pulmonary arteries. There is increased pulmonary vascular resistance (2 to 4 Wood units/m^2) from birth. Rarely does truncal valve stenosis or a restrictive ventricular septal defect modify this hemodynamic pattern. Through infancy, pulmonary vascular resistance increases progressively with a gradual decrease in arterial oxygen saturation.[4]

The first successful correction of truncus arteriosus was done in 1962, but was not reported until 12 years later.[16] The first report of a successful repair was by McGoon and associates[17] and an additional case was reported was reported by Weldon and Cameron.[18] The first successful conduit repair in an infant was done by Barrett-Boyes in 1971.[19] With some technical modifications, the technique described by McGoon[3] for complete correction is used currently.

Total surgical correction involves closure of the ventricular septal defect and establishment of continuity between the right ventricle and pulmonary artery by using an extracardiac conduit. In the earlier descriptions of total correction, the extracardiac conduit was invariably a tube of synthetic material, with or without interposition of a porcine valve. The pseudoendothelialization of the conduit and the rapid degeneration of the porcine valve became recognizable features of early repair and inevitable replacement of the extracardiac conduit, usually within two years of placement, became a well established component of correction of truncus arteriosus in infancy.[20] The advent of homografts and allografts has largely supplanted the use of Dacron conduits in the early correction of truncus arteriosus.

The operation is done through a median sternotomy incision. After entry into the pericardium and creation of a pericardial cradle, the aorta and pulmonary arteries are dissected. The patient is cannulated for cardiopulmonary

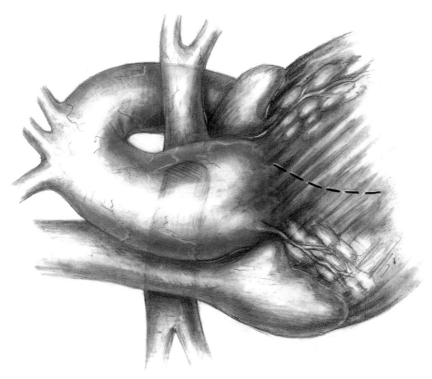

FIGURE 56.2. Upon identifying and obtaining control of the pulmonary arteries, the coronary anatomy is carefully inspected, and a site for the right ventricu- lotomy chosen that will not compromise coronary circulation.

bypass with the aortic cannula placed just prox- imal to the innominate origin. In infants in whom circulatory arrest is anticipated, a single atrial cannula is used. Otherwise, dual caval cannulation with maintenance of cardiopul- monary bypass is preferred. Venting of the left ventricle is desirable to prevent overdistension as the patient is cooled. If ventricular fibrilla- tion has ensued as the patient is cooling, the left ventricle can be vented by simply placing a cannula across the foramen ovale or atrial septal defect. Coronary anatomy is assessed (Figure 56.2).

After bypass has begun, the patient is cooled to a rectal temperature of 20°C which provides latitude for further cooling if circulatory arrest becomes necessary. During cooling, it is desir- able to occlude blood flow to the pulmonary arteries to prevent flooding of the lungs and overdistention of the left atrium and ventricle. It is also necessary to occlude flow to the pul-

monary arteries during instillation of cardio- plegic solution.

After the aorta is cross-clamped, the pul- monary arteries are detached from the truncal artery and the defect in the truncal artery is closed (Figure 56.3). Closure must be done so that distortion of the truncal valve is avoided. Placement of a patch rather than a primary closure may be necessary. It is desirable to leave intact as much proximal length of the truncal artery as possible to prevent distortion of the coronary ostium and possible distortion of the truncal valve.

When the coronary artery pattern over the right and left epicardium has been defined, a longitudinal or transverse incision is made in the right ventricular infundibulum. It is not necessary to excise any right ventricle free wall to accommodate the anastomosis between the right ventricle and the extracardiac conduit. After creation of the ventriculotomy, the

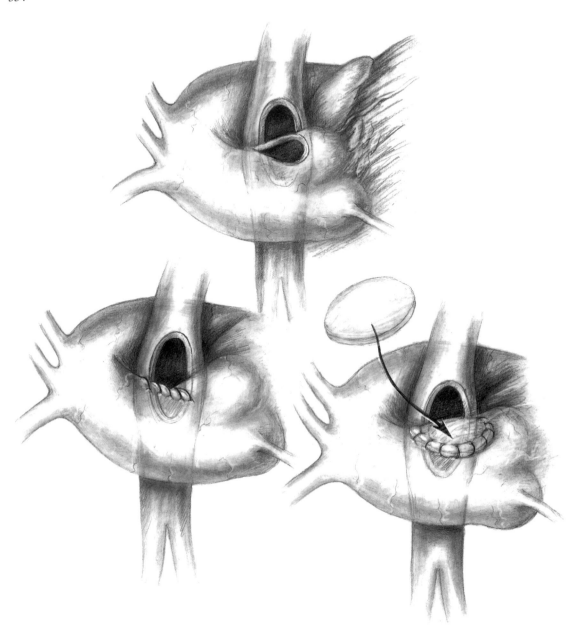

FIGURE 56.3. Immediately following establishment of cardiopulmonary bypass, the pulmonary arteries are occluded. Core cooling is accomplished, and the truncal artery is cross-clamped. Following administration of cardioplegic solution, the pulmonary arteries are then detached from the truncal artery. Occasionally, reconstruction of the pulmonary artery confluence is required. The defect in the truncus created by detaching the pulmonary arteries is then repaired. Previous illustrations have always depicted a primary closure of the defect in the truncal artery. This may result in distortion of the truncal valve or coronary ostia. Consequently, a patch of allograft may be utilized to preserve the three-dimension geometry of truncal artery.

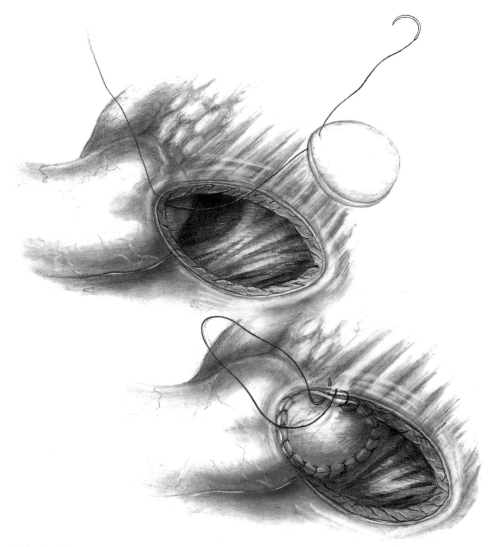

FIGURE 56.4. A right ventriculotomy may be carried up to the annulus of the truncal artery. The ventricular septal defect should be readily visible immediately beneath the truncal valve. Illustrated is a patch closure of the ventricular septal defect utilizing a running continuous suture. Mattress sutures with small Teflon pledgets may also be utilized for this. For the patch, I prefer Dacron Sauvage, the porosity of which gradually diminishes throughout the postoperative period.

ventricular septal defect is usually easily seen, because it involves the infundibular septum. When there is considerable override of the ventricular septal defect and leftward displacement of the ventricular septal defect, it may become necessary to enlarge the ventricular septal defect in order to accommodate unrestricted outflow from the left ventricle into the neoaorta. The ventricular septal defect is closed with a synthetic patch, using either a continuous running or interrupted technique (Figure 56.4). A continuous 4-0, 5-0 or 6-0 polypropylene suture with a tightly curved needle is preferred by the author.

Alternatively, a 5-0 braided polyester suture with small pledgets may be placed in an interrupted horizontal mattress fashion. The suture line should remain on the right ventricular aspect of the ventricular septal defect. The cephalad margin of the suture line may be anchored to the epicardium and myocardium of the cephalad margin of the ventriculotomy.

After closure of the ventricular septal defect, an extracardiac conduit is selected. Because of the increased pulmonary vascular resistance or neonatal pulmonary arterial pressures, a valved conduit usually is necessary, although correction of truncus arteriosus in neonates with non-valved conduits has been reported.[21,22] The valved conduits became commercially available in the 1970s, and are supplied by several manufacturers in sizes ranging from 12 to 30 mm. These conduits usually give an excellent result, but the valve component of the conduit degenerates rapidly and must be replaced within 2 years in approximately 50% of the patients.[20]

Aortic and pulmonary homografts preserved with the various techniques have been used, even before the advent of commercially available conduits. With earlier preservation techniques, homografts tended to calcify, and their use was abandoned in most institutions.[23] Other groups who used homografts have remained enthusiastic about them.[24]

Unlike the disappointing results obtained with synthetic valved conduits in small infants, results have improved considerably with the use of allografts as cryopreservation techniques have been improved. Within the past 5 years there has been a resurgence of interest in cryopreserved human aortic and pulmonary homografts, although the long-term durability of these conduits remains to be seen. In a recent report, small pulmonary allografts (7–9 mm in diameter) were found to last longer than comparable aortic allografts.[25]

The conduit that is selected should be trimmed to an appropriate length by estimating the distance from the ventriculotomy to the transected pulmonary arteries. The length should be such that the conduit is neither redundant nor subject to compression by the sternum. The anastomoses should also be under no tension and should not compress the left coronary artery (Figure 56.5).

The pulmonary anastomoses should be done first. The author uses a continuous suture technique with fine polypropylene suture. The origins of the pulmonary arteries may be enlarged with pericardial patches or by spatulating the pulmonary end of the valve conduit.

The ventricular anastomosis is accomplished by similar technique. Care must be taken to avoid distortion of the conduit, and synthetic conduits may be beveled for this purpose. If an aortic homograft is used, the anterior mitral valve leaflet may be used as a gusset. I have not personally found this to be particularly useful as the tissue is usually fairly thin, somewhat friable, and almost invariably deficient. Alternative materials for proximal augmentation include pericardium or synthetics, usually Dacron or PTFE. Pericardium has the additional disadvantage of being prone to aneurysm formation if there is any downstream resistance in the pulmonary circulation. Dacron is felt by some groups to predispose the allograft to early calcification and degeneration. Whatever material is used, adequate outflow from the right ventricle into the pulmonary circulation is essential. Insufficient augmentation of the proximal portion of the conduit will result in distortion of the pulmonary allograft and compression, which invariably leads to early replacement. The ventricular anastomosis may be done with the aorta still cross-clamped, or may be done during rewarming with the aorta unclamped and heart beating.

A surgical technique for treating the combination of interrupted aortic arch and truncus arteriosus was proposed by Hanley.[13] Because of the need to reconstruct the aortic arch, this procedure should be performed using profound hypothermia and circulatory arrest.

The presence of truncal valve insufficiency complicates the surgical procedure and should be assessed. Mild insufficiency may be tolerated, but the ventricle should be well vented and should not be allowed to overdistend. More severe truncal valve insufficiency may not be amenable to valvuloplasty, and may require valve replacement.[9,26] Good results may nonetheless be achieved with an aggressive approach.

We have recently encountered in our practice several patients with a combination of truncus arteriosus, severe truncal valve stenosis, and interrupted aortic arch. These patients have

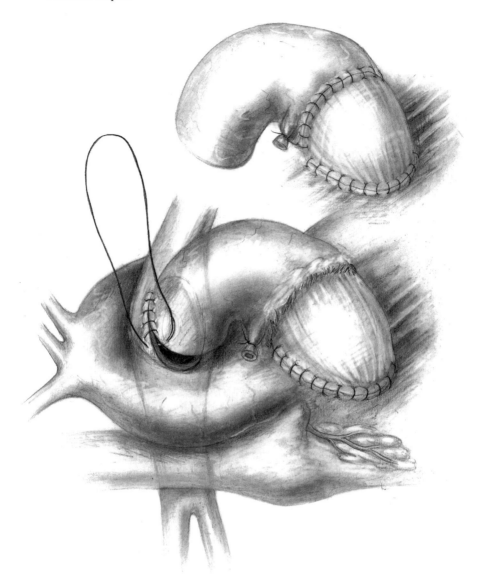

FIGURE 56.5. Following closure of the ventricular septal defect and reconstruction of the truncal artery, right ventricular to pulmonary arterial continuity is established using either an aortic or pulmonary arterial allograft. The lower panel demonstrates use of an aortic allograft in which the anterior mitral valve leaflet has been preserved and is utilized in the anastomosis of allograft to right ventricle. While this is technically an attractive maneuver, utilization of the anterior mitral valve leaflet has been associated with false aneurysm formation if there is downstream obstruction to pulmonary blood flow, from branch pulmonary arterial stenoses. The upper panel demonstrates preservation of the same geometry utilizing a proximal hood of synthetic material. For some time, we have preferred polytetrafluoroethylene (PTFE), as there is some evidence that allograft degeneration is lessened if PTFE, as opposed to Dacron, is utilized for the proximal hood.

been treated with a combination of truncal valve replacement (neo-aortic root replacement), with reattachment of the coronary arteries, anastomosis of the distal end of the allograft to the proximal descending thoracic aorta, and reattachment of the interrupted arch containing the head and neck vessels to the cryopreserved allograft. The remainder of the

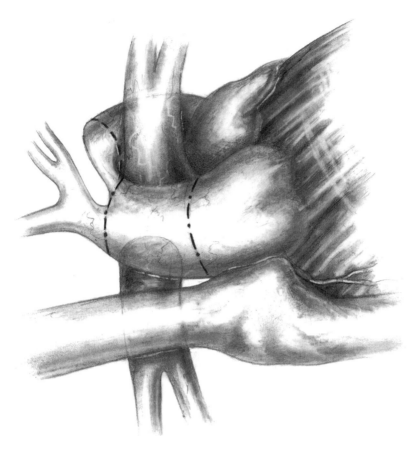

FIGURE 56.6. Interruption of the aortic arch distal to the left subclavian artery is depicted in this illustration. The dotted lines represent possible areas of transection of the truncal artery, proximal aortic arch, and junction between ductus arteriosus and proximal descending thoracic aorta, in preparation for interposition of an allograft as a valveless conduit.

operation is then completed in a usual Rastelli-type manner (Figures 56.6 and 56.7).

One patient with severe truncal valve stenosis and interrupted aortic arch also had what was felt to be a restrictive ventricular septal defect with marked override of the truncal valve, such that there was concern over whether or not the patient would ever be a candidate for a biventricular correction. This patient was treated with replacement of the truncal valve, reattachment of the coronary arteries, enlargement of the ventricular septal defect at the time the valve was replaced, established of continuity between ascending and descending aorta using the cryopreserved allograft, and reattachment of the aortic arch containing the head and neck vessels onto the cryopreserved allograft (Figures 56.8 and 56.9). A patch enlargement of the pulmonary artery confluence was accomplished, and a systemic to pulmonary arterial shunt (modified Blalock-Taussig) performed to both provide for and control pulmonary circulation (Figure 56.10). This patient was later reassessed, and underwent completion of the Rastelli type repair at 11 months of age by closing the ventricular septal defect, and establishing right ventricular to pulmonary arterial continuity, with takedown of the modified Blalock-Taussig shunt. A staged approach was utilized in this patient because of concern over the size and location of the patient's ventricular septal defect. With enlargement of the ven-

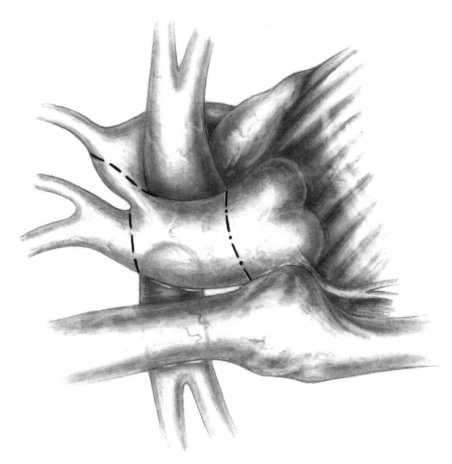

FIGURE 56.7. Interruption of the aortic arch between the left carotid and left subclavian is depicted in this illustration. The dotted lines represent possible areas of transection of the truncal artery, proximal aortic arch, and ductus arteriosus in preparation for interposition of an allograft as a valveless conduit.

tricular septal defect, this proved to be non-restrictive, and a non-restrictive intracardiac conduit could be placed. This procedure is illustrated.

Because truncus arteriosus is relatively rare, few large series of patients have been described. One must be aware of the age of patients included in the series reports as well as the inclusion of patients who have coexistent anomalies or extracardiac valve conduits for other reasons.

A large review of results of surgical repair for truncus arteriosus as a discrete entity was provided by Marceletti and associates at the Mayo Clinic.[27] The initial report of 92 patients was later expanded to 100 patients[28] and then to 167 patients.[14] Marceletti's report described a 25% mortality rate within 30 days of operation, and noted that mortality was correlated with the age of the patient at the time of the repair; patients younger than 2 years had a higher risk. These results have changed dramatically over the years.

A more recent and encouraging experience was described by Ebert and associates[20,29] who reported an 11% mortality rate for repair of truncus arteriosus in 56 infants younger than 6 months of age. They also reported that 50% of the conduits were replaced within 2 years of operation, but note mortality was associated with conduit replacement. The conduits that were used in these patients were commercially

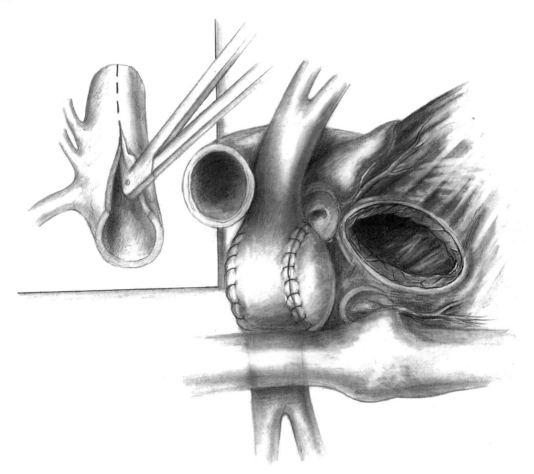

FIGURE 56.8. The dysplastic and stenotic valve has been excised and the coronary arteries have been detached. The proximal truncal artery has been utilized in reconstructing the pulmonary artery confluence. To preserve the geometry of the pulmonary artery confluence and avoid producing a gull-wing deformity, patches have been used to repair the defect created by transection of the truncal artery proximal and distal to the origins of the pulmonary arteries. Pericardium, allograft, or synthetic materials may be used as patches. The insert depicts opening of the aortic arch longitudinally along its entire length.

available synthetic conduits with porcine valves. This series demonstrated the value of early corrective operation. Excellent results have been reported with neonatal correction by two groups.[9,13] Repair should be accomplished once the diagnosis has been established in the neonatal period.

Incremental risk factors identified in the combined experience of the University of Alabama in Birmingham and Green Lane Hospital in Auckland, New Zealand included the following:[11]

1. Poor preoperative clinical status
2. Important truncal valve incompetence
3. A previously placed pulmonary artery band
4. Younger age
5. Pulmonary vascular disease
6. Earlier date of operation
7. Major co-existing cardiac anomalies (this is not supported by multivariate statistical analysis)

In a more recent series, according to both univariate and multivariate techniques, severe

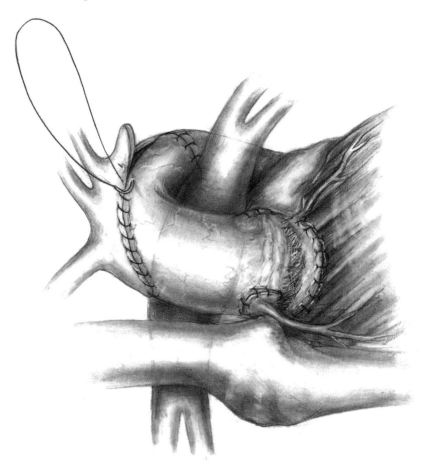

FIGURE 56.9. The distal portion of the aortic allograft has been anastomosed to the proximal descending aorta. 6-0 or 7-0 polypropylene is utilized for this anastomosis. The proximal portion of the allograft has been anastomosed to the truncal valve annulus and the coronary arteries reattached. 5-0 or 6-0 polypropylene is used for the valve anastomosis and 7-0 polypropylene is used to reimplant the coronary arteries. The aortic arch is reattached to a longitudinal arteriotomy in the allograft using 6-0 polypropylene. The reconstructed pulmonary artery confluence is posterior to the allograft.

truncal valve regurgitation, interrupted aortic arch, coronary artery anomalies, and age at repair greater than 100 days were important risk factors for perioperative death. In the 33 patients without these risk factors, early survival was 100%. In the 30 patients with one or more of these risk factors, survival was 63%. Pulmonary hypertensive episodes were fewer, and duration of ventilator dependence and pulmonary artery pressure were significantly less in patients undergoing the operation before 30 days of age. Advances in surgical technique and better understanding of neonatal physiology mean that young age at repair is no longer an incremental risk factor for death. Repair in the early neonatal period clearly reduces the prevalence of postoperative pulmonary vascular morbidity.[13]

The pulmonary vascular structure in a large group of children with various congenital anomalies, including a large group with truncus arteriosus was studied by Juaneda and Haworth[30] by using quantitative morphometric techniques. These studies showed abnormal extension of muscle, increased pulmonary arterial medial thickness, and intimal proliferation

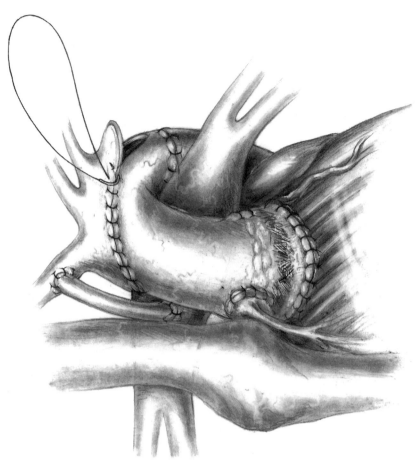

FIGURE 56.10. A shunt of polytetrafluoroethylene has been interposed between innominate and pulmonary artery. This patient was not a candidate for initial biventricular correction because of a restrictive ventricular septal defect. If the ventricular septal defect is of adequate size, this step is not necessary, and the Rastelli type of repair illustrated in Figures 56.4 and 56.5 can be accomplished.

even in infants less than one year of age with truncus arteriosus. Even in the presence of increased pulmonary vascular resistance (>8 woods units/m²), the changes were potentially reversible in infants. These studies strongly support early intracardiac repair.

The natural history of truncus arteriosus is such that only approximately 10% of patients born with truncus survive to 1 year of age without operative intervention. Early definitive correction is clearly the approach of choice. The advent of cryopreserved aortic and pulmonary artery allografts has contributed significantly to the improved survival statistics.

References

1. Collett RW, Edwards JE. Persistent truncus arteriosus: A classification according to anatomic types. Surg Clin North Am 1949;16:1245–1270.
2. Van Praagh R, Van Praagh S. The anatomy of common aorticopulmonary trunk (truncus arteriosus communis) and its embryologic implications: A study of 57 necropsy cases. Am J Cardiol 1965;16:406–425.
3. McGoon DC. Truncus arteriosus. In Sabiston DC, Jr., Spencer FC (eds). Gibbon's Surgery of the Chest. Philadelphia: W.B. Saunders 1983: 1100–1108.

4. Lofland GK. Truncus Arteriosus. In Sabiston DC, Jr., Spencer FC (eds). Surgery of the Chest. Philadelphia: W.B. Sauders 1995:1509–1518.

5. Bharati S, Karp R, Lev M. The conduction system in truncus arteriosus and its surgical significance. J Surg Res 1992;104:954–960.

6. Bharati S, McAllister HA, Jr., Rosenquist GC, Miller RA, Tatooles CJ, Lev M. The surgical anatomy of truncus arteriosus communis. J Thorac Cardiovasc Surg 1974;67:501–510.

7. Crupi G, Macartney FJ, Anderson RH. Persistent truncus arteriosus: A study of 66 autopsy cases with special reference to definition and morphogenesis. Am J Cardiol 1977;40:569–578.

8. Anderson KR, McGoo DC, Lie JT. Surgical significance of the coronary arterial anatomy in truncus arteriosus communis. Am J Cardiol 1978;41:76–81.

9. Bove EL, Lupinetti FM, Pridjian AK, et al. Results of a policy of primary repair of truncus arteriosus in the neonate. J Thorac Cardiovasc Surg 1993;105:1057–1066.

10. Shrivastava S, Edwards JE. Coronary arterial origin in persistent truncus arteriosus. Circulation 1977;55:551–554.

11. Barratt-Boyes BG. Truncus arteriosus. In Kirklin JW, Barratt-Boyes BG (eds). Cardiac Surgery. New York: Churchill-Livingston 1993:1131–1151.

12. Calder L, Van Praagh R, Van Praagh S, et al. Truncus arteriosus communis: Clinical, angiographic, and pathologic findings in 100 patients. Am Heart J 1976;92:23–38.

13. Hanley FL, Heinemann MK, Jonas RA, Mayer JE, Cook NR, Wessel DL, Castaneda AR. Repair of truncus arteriosus in the neonate. Cardiovasc Surg 1993;105:1047–1056.

14. Di Donato RM, Fyfe DA, Puga FJ, et al. Fifteen year experience with surgical repair of truncus arteriosus. J Thorac Cardiovasc Surg 1985;89:414–422.

15. Becker AE, Becker MJ, Edwards JE. Pathology of the semi-lunar valve in persistent truncus arteriosus. J Thorac Cardiovasc Surg 1971;62:16–26.

16. Behrendt DM, Kirsch MM, Stern A, et al. The surgical therapy for pulmonary artery-right ventricular discontinuity. Ann Thorac Surg 1974;18:122–137.

17. McGoon DC, Rastelli GC, Ongley PA. An operation for the correction of truncus arteriosus. JAMA 1968;205:69–73.

18. Weldon CS, Cameron JL. Correction of persistent truncus arteriosus. J Cardiovasc Surg (Torino) 1968;9:463–469.

19. Girinath MR. Case presentation: Truncus arteriosus: repair with homograft reconstruction in infancy. In Barratt-Boyes BG, Neutze JM, Harris EA (eds). Heart Disease in Infancy. Diagnosis and Surgical Treatment. Edinburgh: Churchhill-Livingston 1973:234–241.

20. Ebert PA, Turley K, Stanger P. Surgical treatment of truncus arteriosus in the first six months of life. Ann Surg 1984;200:451–456.

21. Peetz DJ, Jr., Spicer RL, Crowley DC, et al. Correction of truncus arteriosus in the neonate using a nonvalved conduit. J Thorac Cardiovasc Surg 1982;83:743–746.

22. Spicer RL, Behrendt D, Crowley DC, Dick M, Rocchini AP, Uzark K, Rosenthal A, Sloan H. Repair of truncus arteriosus in neonates with the use of a valveless conduit. Circulation 1984;70 (Suppl.I):I-26-I-29.

23. Moodie DS, Mair DD, Fulton RE, Wallace RB, Danielson GK, McGoon DC. Aortic homograft obstruction. J Thorac Cardiovasc Surg 1976;72:553–561.

24. Shabbo FB, Wain WH, Ross DN. Right ventricular outflow reconstructions with aortic homograft: analysis of long-term results. Thorac Cardiovasc Surg 1981;29:21–27.

25. Heinemann MK, Hanley FL, Fenton KN, Jonas RA, Mayer JE, Castaneda AR. Fate of small homograft conduits after early repair in truncus arteriosus. Ann Thorac Surg 1993;55:1409–1412.

26. De Leval MR, McGoon DC, Wallace RB, Danielson GK, Mair DD. Management of truncal valvular regurgitation. Ann Surg 1974;180:427–432.

27. Marcelletti C, McGoon DC, Danielson GK, Wallace RB, Mair DD. Early and late results of surgical repair of truncus arteriosus. Circulation 1977;55:636–641.

28. McGoon DC, Danielson GK, Puga FJ, et al. Late results after extracardiac conduit repair for congenital cardiac defects. Am J Cardiol 1982;49:1741–1749.

29. Walker PG, Kim Y, Muralidharan E, Miyajima Y, Delatore J, Yoganathan AP. Assessment of the accuracy of color Doppler flow mapping by digital image analysis. Echocardiography 1994;11:11–28.

30. Juaneda E, Haworth SG. Pulmonary vascular disease in children with truncus arteriosus. Am J Cardiol 1984;54:1314–1320.

57
Pulmonary Atresia with MAPCAs: Staged Unifocalization Techniques

Richard A. Hopkins and Erle H. Austin, III

The spectrum of pulmonary atresia with ventricular septal defect, nonconfluent or absent central pulmonary arteries with multiple major aortopulmonary collateral arteries (MAPCAs) presents a significant surgical challenge. Complete repair requires unifocalization of all available segmental and lobar pulmonary blood supply so that a central pulmonary ventricle to pulmonary arterial reconstruction can be created. When central pulmonary arteries are not merely nonconfluent but actually absent, there are additional surgical challenges as the central main pulmonary arteries need to be created. When there are central pulmonary arteries, unilateral reconstructions are usually staged with the intention of encouraging pulmonary artery growth as well as eliminating dual blood supplies and the recruitment of segments dependent upon only collateral arteries into the central circulation prior to the final correction. Currently, neonatal unifocalization with complete repair is the approach of choice (See next chapter). Such neonatal corrections are most successful when the number of segments receiving separate multiple aortopulmonary collateral arteries are relatively few and particularly when at least one lung is limited to only one or two MAPCAs. Patients requiring complex unifocalizations sometimes do not present to the surgeon during the neonatal stage of life (as they are often neither in failure or cyanotic), and staged procedures are usually needed in the older children.

We have used cryopreserved valveless pulmonary homografts for hilar reconstructions and unifocalizations as staged procedures prior to completing the central reconstruction with a valved homograft.[1] We have also used PTFE grafts for portions of the repairs and as the conduit of choice for any systemic to pulmonary artery connections.

Technique

In the typical case presented here, the child had three primary MAPCAs supplying the right lung and two primary MAPCAs supplying the right lung and absent central pulmonary arteries. Figure 57.1 shows the anatomy prior to any correction. The first stage operation consists of a left thoracotomy and a valveless pulmonary bifurcation cryopreserved homograft is thawed and sewn into side to arteriotomies in each of the major aortopulmonary collaterals. In this case, the MAPCA was left attached to the aorta with a snare which was later tied at the final operation. Alternatively a PTFE 6 mm tubular graft could have been placed as a modified Blalock to the allograft and ligated at the final operation. This is a long beveled anastomosis utilizing the "legs" of the bifurcation graft trying very hard to extend the anastomosis well out into the hilum into presumably more normal pulmonary arterial wall than just a MAPCA. The main pulmonary artery trunk is positioned (Figure 57.2). The pulmonary valve has been excised from the cryopreserved graft and the main pulmonary artery oversewn. This is tacked to the pericardium anterior to the left

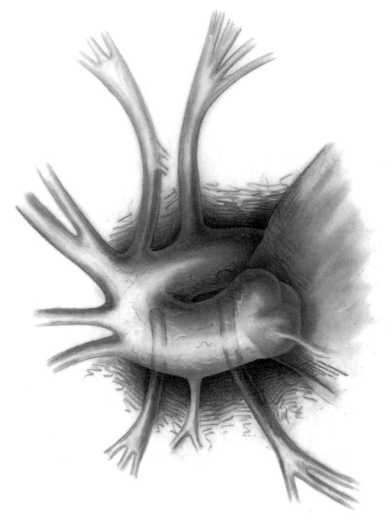

FIGURE 57.1. Anatomy of pulmonary atresia with absent central pulmonary arteries with complete pulmonary blood supply being provided by MAPCAs.

phrenic nerve so the recovery at the final operation is simplified. The second stage is demonstrated in Figure 57.3 which shows the creation of a systemic to pulmonary artery shunt to the right pulmonary artery and the creation of unifocalization with another pulmonary artery bifurcation graft which includes anastomoses to all three MAPCAs and again placing the main pulmonary artery trunk of the unifocalization homograft anterior to the right phrenic nerve and tacked to the pericardium.

Figure 57.4 demonstrates the final correction. There are a number of important features. First, the systemic pulmonary artery blood flow

sources are ligated. The ascending aorta must be divided and lengthened with a Dacron graft to provide space in the retroaortic position for pulmonary arteries. This space does not exist in these patients in the absence of pulmonary arteries because no such space ever developed. Central pulmonary artery tubular reconstruction is best performed with either a homograft tubular graft or with PTFE and this should be at a minimum 14 mm in diameter and preferably 18 mm to approximate an adult size. This tube graft spans from one hilum to the other by attaching to the anteriorly located centralized pulmonary bifurcation grafts on either side.

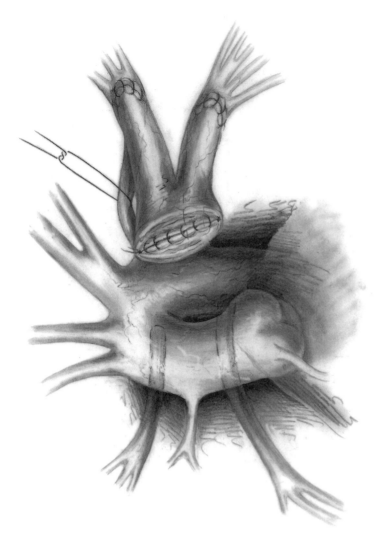

FIGURE 57.2. Left pulmonary arterial reconstruction is performed first. In this case, a staging procedure was performed leaving a MAPCA attached to the aorta with a snare that was later tied. This provided "shunt flow" to maintain patency of the reconstruction. A pulmonary artery bifurcation graft with the valve excised is used to reconstruct the hilar vessels, attaching it to the MAPCAs. It is important to leave the main pulmonary artery of the homograft as far anterior as possible, and tacked to the pericardium so that it can be retrieved without putting the phrenic nerve at risk.

This is then connected to the right ventricular outflow tract with a homograft valve containing conduit with an augmented outflow tract patch utilizing the anterior leaf of the mitral valve and PTFE. If aggressive twists and curves are needed for this midline spanning graft, then we utilize collagen impregnated Dacron tube grafts.

Variations

1. Occasionally it is easier to reconstruct the hilum with PTFE and in this case, the central PTFE graft can be sewn end-to-side to the hilar reconstruction with the PTFE on that side and on the other side to a valveless pulmonary bifurcation graft.

2. Lengthening the aorta is critical and must be adequate to avoid compression to this central spanning graft. Collagen impregnated Dacron is usually the material of choice for aortic lengthening.

3. When done as a staged procedure, it is optimal to perform the first two stages as thoracotomies so as to leave the central mediastinum free of adhesions for the final correction.

4. The valveless pulmonary bifurcation grafts must be anteriorly located as they can be

very difficult to reach and surgery dangerous to the phrenic nerve if they are not tacked to the pericardium.

5. There is a tendency is to use too large a graft for the pulmonary artery bifurcation grafts. A 14mm valveless pulmonary bifurcation graft is the largest necessary. There is also a tendency for these to enlarge a bit for the first year or two after the operation, so therefore, if larger grafts are used, they can become somewhat bulbous. Even smaller grafts in the 10–12mm range (main PA segment, branch PAs 5–7mm) are fully adequate for this reconstruction and simplifies the attachment of the long arms to the segmental or lobar pulmonary arteries.

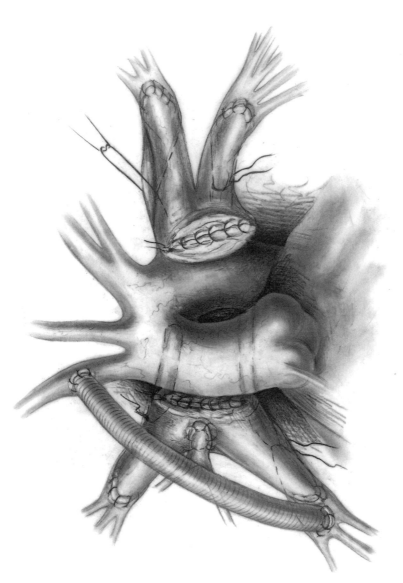

FIGURE 57.3. Second stage consists of reconstructing the right sided arterial supply, separating the MAPCAs from the aorta by ligations, and placing the reconstructed hilar pulmonary arteries on shunt flow which can be easily ligated at the final correction. All three MAPCAs are connected to the pulmonary artery bifurcation graft from which the pulmonary valve has been removed. Again, this graft is fixed anterior to the right phrenic nerve for ease of later retrieval.

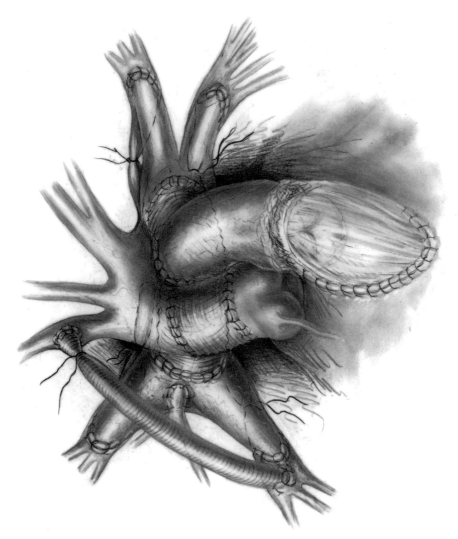

FIGURE 57.4. The final correction in which all systemic pulmonary arterial blood sources are ligated. The ascending aorta must be divided and lengthened so as to provide space in the retroaortic position for the new pulmonary arterial confluence, which is usually best reconstructed with PTFE as this has some resistance to compression than homograft tubular grafts often do not. A homograft valve completes the repair by connecting to the right ventricular outflow tract.

6. These patients are maintained on anticoagulation after each of the first two stages until the centralized reconstruction has been completed to avoid any clot formation in the semiblind pouch. The systemic pulmonary artery supply into the unifocalized allograft reconstruction tends to provide wash-out when the PTFE tube graft is sutured to the top or side of the main pulmonary artery portion of the homograft rather than out into the pulmonary arteries proper.

7. This technique of staged unifocalization is also applicable when MAPCAs supply just one lung (usually the right). The utilization of a shunt is optional, but necessary if the procedure is staged and performed through a right thoracotomy. If performed at one stage, then the shunt is replaced by the anterior recon-

struction as demonstrated in Figures 57.5, 57.6 and 57.7.

A number of groups have published on this topic.[2-10] Other techniques have been used including pericardial tubes, etc. which have been less than ideal because of fibrosis. The advantages of this technique utilizing pulmonary allograft are: 1. facilitates the creation of very distal anastomoses keeping the reconstruction away from the histologic collateral artery 2. results in construction of adult sized hilar pulmonary arteries 3. centralizes and repositions the pulmonary arterial reconstruction more anteriorly which increases accessibility at final repair.

The long-term result of such complete repairs is not yet established. It is possible that many of these patients will ultimately come to heart-lung transplantation. This approach is applicable to the subset of older patients with tetralogy of Fallot accompanied by pulmonary atresia and nonconfluent pulmonary arteries in which more than one aortopulmonary collateral supplies separate lobar segments. It can also be applied to children in whom previous palliative procedures have resulted in complex lobar arterial anatomy constructions which necessitates salvage type procedures in the path towards complete correction.[1,11]

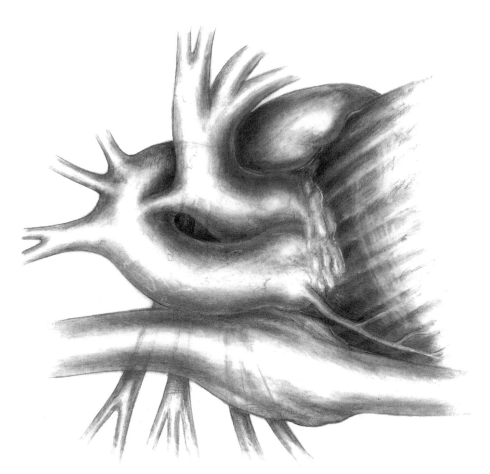

FIGURE 57.5. Anatomy in which right lung is supplied completely by MAPCAs, but left lung has pulmonary arterial origin.

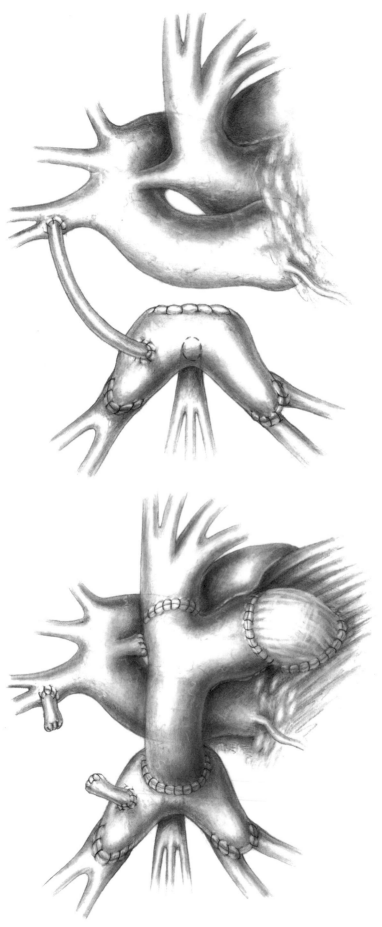

FIGURE 57.6. This demonstrates a first stage unifocalization utilizing the valveless pulmonary artery bifurcation technique with detachment of the MAPCAs from the aorta and reconstruction with anastomoses to various parts of the pulmonary artery bifurcation, which is then positioned anteriorly. The shunt maintains patency and the second stage follows relatively soon (within three months) utilizing a median sternotomy.

FIGURE 57.7. In this case of pulmonary atresia, the right ventricle to pulmonary arterial continuity has been re-established at the final stage, with a pulmonary valve homograft that includes its bifurcation. The reconstruction is positioned anteriorly. The pulmonary homograft hilar reconstruction of the right pulmonary artery is attached to the right limb of a pulmonary homograft that includes the pulmonary arterial bifurcation. The left pulmonary artery is detached from its patent ductus arteriosus blood supply and is sutured end-to-end to the left limb of the pulmonary homograft. The proximal valved end of the homograft is then attached to the ventriculotomy in the right ventricle utilizing a generous hood constructed of PTFE. The shunt is divided.

References

1. Hopkins RA, Imperato DA, Cockerham JT, Shapiro SR. Use of pulmonary arterial unifocalization into cryopreserved homograft pulmonary arterial bifurcation grafts to facilitate complete correction of pulmonary atresia with ventricular septal defect, nonconfluent (absent) central pulmonary arteries and multiple major aortopulmonary collateral arteries. Cardiol Young 1995; 5:217–224.

2. Puga FJ. Unifocalization for pulmonary atresia with ventricular septal defect. Ann Thorac Surg 1991;51:8–9.

3. Puga FJ, McGoon DCJPR, Danielson GK, Mair DD. Complete repair of pulmonary atresia with nonconfluent pulmonary arteries. Ann Thorac Surg 1983;35 (No. 1):36–44.

4. Sullivan ID, Wren C, Stark J, De Leval MR, Macartney FJ, Deanfield JE. Surgical unifocalization in pulmonary atresia and ventricular septal defect. A realistic goal? Circulation 1988; 78 (No. 5 Supp. III):III-5-13.

5. Sawatari K, Imai Y, Kurosawa H, Isomatsu Y, Momma K. Staged operation for pulmonary atresia and ventricular septal defect with major aortopulmonary collateral series. New technique for complete unifocalization. J Thorac Cardiovasc Surg 1989;98:738–50.

6. Barbero-Marcial M, Rizzo A, Lopes AAB, Bittencourt D, Junior JOA, Jatene AD. Correction of pulmonary atresia with ventricular septal defect in the absence of the pulmonary trunk and the central pulmonary arteries (so-called truncus type IV). J Thorac Cardiovasc Surg 1987; 94:911–8.

7. Iyer KS, Mee RBB. Staged repair of pulmonary atresia with ventricular septal defect and major systemic to pulmonary artery collaterals. Ann Thorac Surg 1991;51:65–72.

8. Puga FJ, Leoni FE, Julsrud PR, Mair DD. Complete repair of pulmonary atresia, ventricular septal defect, and severe peripheral arborization abnormalities of the central pulmonary arteries. J Thorac Cardiovasc Surg 1989;98:1018–29.

9. Iyer KS, Varma M, Mee RBB. Use of azygos vein as interposition graft for surgical unifocalization of pulmonary blood supply. Ann Thorac Surg 1989;48:776–8.

10. Shanley CJ, Lupinetti FM, Shah NL, Beekman IRH, Crowley DC, Bove EL. Primary unifocalization for the absence of intrapericardial pulmonary arteries in the neonate. J Thorac Cardiovasc Surg 1993;106:237–247.

11. Tchervenkov CJ, Salasidis G, Cecere R, BEland MJ, Jutras L, Paquet M, Dobell ARC. One-Stage midline unifocalization and complete repair in infancy versus multiple-stage unifocalization followed by repair for complex heart disease with major aortopulmonary collaterals. J Thorac Cardiovasc Surg 1997;114:727–737.

58
Pulmonary Atresia with MAPCAs: Repairs in Neonates and Young Infants

Doff B. McElhinney, V. Mohan Reddy, and Frank L. Hanley

Pulmonary atresia with ventricular septal defect is a spectrum of lesions distinguished by a marked heterogeneity of pulmonary blood supply.[1-3] Perhaps the most challenging subset of patients with this anomaly are those in whom pulmonary blood flow is derived entirely or in large part from aortopulmonary collateral arteries (MAPCAs). These collaterals, which are thought to arise from the embryonic splanchnic plexus, can originate from the aorta, the subclavian or carotid arteries, the coronaries, or the bronchial arteries. Each collateral may supply as little as one lung segment or as much as an entire lung, and may be characterized by extrapulmonary and intraparenchymal stenoses. In such patients, true pulmonary arteries are typically either hypoplastic or absent altogether.[1-6]

A variety of philosophies and therapeutic approaches have been employed in the management of this challenging lesion.[7-19] All of these approaches, whether involving shunts or conduits to the hypoplastic true pulmonary arteries, and/or partial unifocalization of collaterals, entail staged procedures.[7-16,18] It is our opinion that the staged approach is inadequate for the majority of patients, due both to high attrition during infancy and to progressive loss of lung microvascular cross-sectional area because of either underdevelopment, focal pulmonary vascular obstructive disease, or surgical palliation.[10-13,20,21] In order to reduce the morbidity and mortality inherent in the delays associated with the staged method, we have developed a single stage approach for completely unifocalizing and repairing pulmonary atresia with ventricular septal defect and MAPCAs in early infancy.[17,22]

In the single stage approach, allograft tissue is an important material that is used over the full range of patients with pulmonary atresia and MAPCAs. Allograft tissue is employed for three basic purposes: 1) peripheral unifocalization and neo-pulmonary artery reconstruction, 2) central branch pulmonary artery reconstruction, and 3) right ventricular outflow tract reconstruction.

Surgical Techniques

Surgical Exposure and Collateral Mobilization

In patients undergoing single stage unifocalization, our standard approach is through a midline sternotomy. Initially, we attempt to expose and control all collaterals and true pulmonary arteries before resorting to cardiopulmonary bypass, and then ligate the collaterals at the institution of bypass. This is essential to prevent collateral steal, which may be a significant cause of neurologic morbidity in these patients. In order to control and adequately mobilize all collaterals through the midline incision, it is often necessary to dissect through the transverse sinus in order to expose descending aortic collaterals that arise at the level of the carina, and to open the respective pleural sacs and retract the lungs in order to access collaterals arising from other portions of the descending thoracic aorta. Once all collaterals are controlled, cardiopulmonary bypass at moderate hypothermia is instituted and unifocalization is performed with a beating heart.

Peripheral Neo-Pulmonary Artery Reconstruction

Although native tissue to tissue anastomosis is almost always achievable between collaterals and other collaterals or between collaterals and true pulmonary arteries, it is sometimes beneficial to augment the peripheral neo-pulmonary arteries, either to enlarge discreetly hypoplastic or stenotic arterial segments, or to optimize the cross-sectional area of anastomosed collaterals. For this purpose, we prefer to use pulmonary artery allograft, which is more pliable and appropriate to the delicate collateral tissue than aortic allograft. Peripheral pulmonary artery and collateral unifocalization anastomoses are performed with running 7-0 monofilament suture in all infants and most young children. For native tissue to tissue connections, absorbable suture is used, while nonabsorbable suture is used for allograft patch augmentation, primarily because of its better handling properties.

Just as the collateral anatomy is different in every one of these patients, anastomosis and augmentation techniques are highly variable, with an individualized approach in every case. Nevertheless, there are some common types of augmentation. Within reason, we attempt to optimize the cross-sectional area of both the neo-pulmonary arteries and the collateral anastomoses. A technique frequently employed is to fillet open two adjacent parallel collaterals, perform a native tissue side-to-side posterior longitudinal anastomosis to construct the posterior wall of the unifocalized arteries, and then augment the anterior side-to-side anastomosis with allograft tissue. The newly created single vessel will have a larger diameter, and growth potential is maintained since allograft tissue is never placed circumferentially. If necessary, this anterior augmentation can be extended distal to the side-to-side collateral anastomosis onto

branch points with a pantaloon-shaped patch. Similar techniques are frequently used between collateral vessels and true pulmonary arteries. For peripheral anastomoses, we will also frequently enlarge a single dominant collateral over its length (or simply across a discreet stenosis) with a longitudinal anterior arteriotomy and allograft patch reconstruction. Smaller collaterals may be plugged into this dominant collateral posteriorly, with oblique end to side or true side to side anastomosis (Figure 58.1).

Central Pulmonary Artery Reconstruction

In patients with pulmonary atresia and MAPCAs, except those with generous true pulmonary arteries and minor collateral contribution to pulmonary blood flow, it is almost always necessary to augment the central pulmonary arteries. In some cases, the anatomy of collaterals and true pulmonary arteries is conducive to reconstruction of the central pulmonary arteries without the need for nonautologous tissue. But in many cases, it is necessary to reconstruct the central pulmonary arteries using allograft tissue in order to augment the diameter of the left and right branch pulmonary arteries. A segment of pulmonary artery allograft can be fashioned as needed into a single patch that extends from hilum to hilum, as separate patches on the left and right or as a single unilateral patch (Figure 58.1). Sometimes we will use an extension of the right ventricular outflow tract valved allograft conduit for central pulmonary artery augmentation (see below), though there is generally inadequate length to extend such a patch to the hilum, especially on the right side. In the rare situation where there is insufficient pulmonary artery or collateral tissue to create hilum to hilum native tissue continuity, it may be necessary to reconstruct the central pulmonary arteries in their full circumference using an allograft tube (Figure 58.2). In such rare situations we have used nonvalved segments of pulmonary artery allograft. If an appropriately sized conduit is not available,

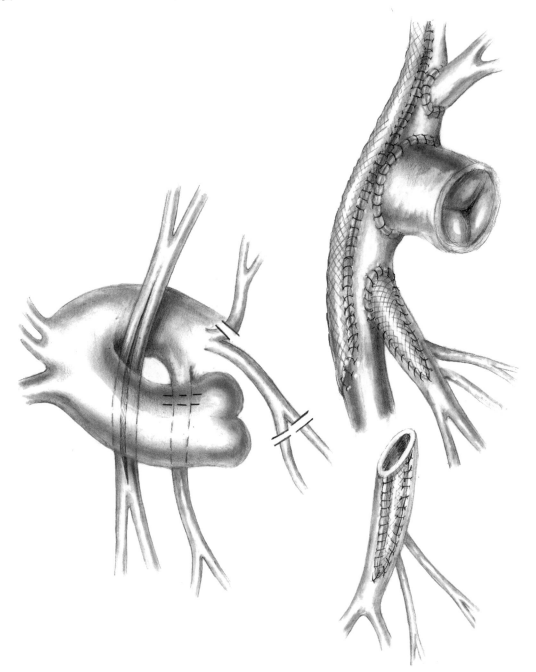

FIGURE 58.1. A large collateral to the right lung is filleted open and augmented with a patch of pulmonary allograft (hatched). Two smaller collaterals are anastomosed end-to-side to the augmented collateral, which is then anastomosed obliquely to the central right pulmonary artery. The small true pulmonary arteries are opened superiorly along most of their length, then augmented with a single patch of pulmonary allograft. A valved pulmonary or aortic allograft conduit is sewn end-to-end to the central pulmonary arteries for reconstruction of the right ventricular outflow tract.

a larger allograft can be downsized and extra tissue used for distal augmentation. As with distal reconstruction, we tend to use running 7-0 monofilament suture for central pulmonary artery repair, with absorbable suture in tissue to tissue anastomoses and nonabsorbable suture when allograft tissue is being sewn.

Right Ventricular Outflow Tract Reconstruction

Conduit reconstruction of the right ventricular outflow tract in pulmonary atresia with MAPCAs is essentially the same as for other lesions requiring right ventricle to pulmonary artery conduit repair. The primary difference is

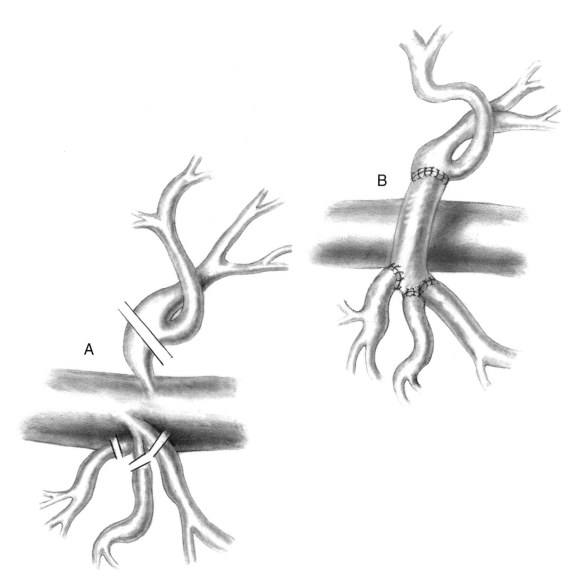

FIGURE 58.2. Four tortuous collaterals to both lungs are divided and sewn to a tube of pulmonary allograft. Blood flow to this unifocalized neo-pulmonary artery will be supplied through either a valved allograft conduit from the right ventricle or a systemic-pulmonary artery shunt.

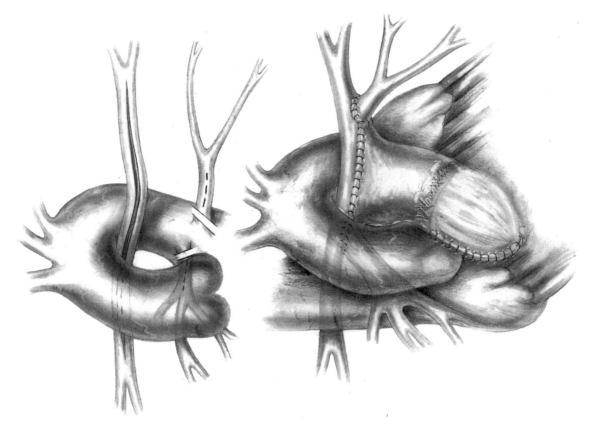

FIGURE 58.3. Moderate sized true pulmonary arteries are opened along their length. Collaterals to each lung are divided from their origin, opened longitudinally, and sewn side to side to the incision in the true left and right pulmonary arteries. A valved right ventricle to pulmonary artery allograft conduit is attached to the unifocalized neo-pulmonary artery, with segments of allograft tissue extended out to augment both central branch pulmonary arteries.

that the distal tissue of the allograft conduit may be employed extensively to augment the left and right pulmonary arteries (Figure 58.3). Also, because pulmonary arterial pressure may be anticipated to be somewhat higher in this lesion than in other defects that require right ventricular outflow tract reconstruction, we tend to utilize aortic valved conduits more often in this patient population.

UCSF Experience

Between July 1992 and May 1997, 42 infants (median: 4.5 months; range 2 weeks to 11 months) with pulmonary atresia, ventricular septal defect, and MAPCAs underwent surgery at UCSF. This represents 70% of all patients (n = 61) who presented during this time period. The median number of collateral arteries in these patients was 4, with a range of 1 to 7. Collaterals supplied a median of 16.5 lung segments (range 4 to 20) and 38% of patients had complete absence of true pulmonary arteries. Complete single stage unifocalization using techniques described above was performed in 93% (n = 39) of patients, while the remaining 3 patients underwent sequential unilateral unifocalization procedures because of multiple peripheral segmental level collateral stenoses or, in one case, because bypass was contraindicated due to severe associated disease.

References

1. Liao PK, Edwards WD, Julsrud PR, et al. Pulmonary blood supply in patients with pulmonary atresia and ventricular septal defect. J Am Coll Cardiol 1985;6:1343–1350.
2. Haworth SG, Macartney FJ. Growth and development of pulmonary circulation in pulmonary atresia with ventricular septal defect and major aortopulmonary collateral arteries. Br Heart J 1980;44:14–24.
3. Rabinovitch M, Herrera-DeLeon V, Castaneda AR, et al. Growth and development of the pulmonary vascular bed in patients with Tetralogy of Fallot with or without pulmonary atresia. Circulation 1981;64:1234–1249.
4. DeRuiter MD, Gittenberger-de Groot AC, Poelmann RE, et al. Development of the pharyngeal arch system related to the pulmonary and bronchial vessels in the avian embryo with a concept on systemic-pulmonary collateral artery formation. Circulation 1993;87:1306–1319.
5. Jefferson KE, Rees S, Somerville J. Systematic arterial supply to the lungs in pulmonary atresia and its relation to pulmonary artery development. Br Heart J 1972;34:418–427.
6. Murphy DA, Sridhara KS, Nanton MA, et al. Surgical correction of pulmonary atresia with multiple large systemic-pulmonary collaterals. Ann Thorac Surg 1979;27:460–464.
7. Haworth SG, Rees P, Taylor JFN, et al. Pulmonary atresia with ventricular septal defect and major aortopulmonary collateral arteries: Effect of systemic pulmonary anastomosis. Br Heart J 1981;45:133–141.
8. Pacifico AD, Allen RH, Colvin EV. Direct reconstruction of pulmonary artery arborization anomaly and intracardiac repair of pulmonary atresia with ventricular septal defect. Am J Cardiol 1985;55:1647–1649.
9. Barbero-Marcial M, Rizzo A, Lopes AAB, Bittencourt D, Junior JOA, Jatene AD. Correction of pulmonary atresia with ventricular septal defect in the absence of the pulmonary trunk and the central pulmonary arteries (so-called truncus type IV). J Thorac Cardiovasc Surg 1987; 94:911–918.
10. Kirklin JW, Blackstone EH, Shimazaki Y, et al. Survival function status, and reoperations after repair of Tetralogy of Fallot with pulmonary atresia. J Thorac Cardiovasc Surg 1987;94:911–914.
11. Puga FJ, Leoni FE, Julsrud PR, Mair DD. Complete repair of pulmonary atresia, ventricular septal defect, and severe peripheral arborization abnormalities of the central pulmonary arteries. J Thorac Cardiovasc Surg 1989;98:1018–1029.
12. Sawatari K, Imai Y, Kurosawa H, Isomatsu Y, Momma K. Staged operation for pulmonary atresia and ventricular septal defect with major aortopulmonary collateral series. New technique for complete unifocalization. J Thorac Cardiovasc Surg 1989;98:738–750.
13. Iyer KS, Mee RBB. Staged repair of pulmonary atresia with ventricular septal defect and major systemic to pulmonary artery collaterals. Ann Thorac Surg 1991;51:65–72.
14. Rome J, Mayer JE, Castaneda AR, et al. Tetralogy of Fallot with pulmonary atresia: rehabilitation of diminutive pulmonary arteries. Circulation 1993;88:1691–1698.
15. Marelli AJ, Perloff JK, Child JS, et al. Pulmonary atresia with ventricular septal defect in adults. Circulation 1994;89:243–251.
16. Dinarevic S, Redington AN, Rigby M, et al. Outcome of pulmonary atresia and ventricular septal defect during infancy. Pediatr Cardiol 1995;16:276–282.
17. Reddy VM, Liddicoat JR, Hanley FL. Midline onestage complete unifocalization and repair of pulmonary atresia with ventricular septal defect and major aortopulmonary collaterals. J Thorac Cardiovasc Surg 1995;109:832–845.
18. Yagihara T, Yamamoto F, Nishigaki K, et al. Unifocalization for pulmonary atresia with ventricular septal defect and major aortopulmonary collateral arteries. J Thorac Cardiovasc Surg 1996;112:392–402.
19. Moritz A, Marx M, Wollenek G, et al. Complete repair of PA-VSD with diminutive or discontinuous pulmonary arteries by transverse thoracosternotomy. Ann Thorac Surg 1996;61: 646–650.
20. Sullivan ID, Wren C, Stark J, De Leval MR, Macartney FJ, Deanfield JE. Surgical unifocalization in pulmonary atresia and ventricular septal defect. A realistic goal? Circulation 1988; 78 (No. 5 Supp. III):III-5–13.
21. Bull K, Somerville J, Ty E, et al. Presentation and attrition in complex pulmonary atresia. J Am Coll Cardiol 1995;25:491–499.
22. Reddy VM, Petrossian E, McElhinney DB, et al. One stage complete unifocalization in infants: When should the ventricular septal defect be closed? J Thorac Cardiovasc Surg 1997;113:858–868.

59
Reoperative Right Ventricular Outflow Tract Reconstructions

Richard A. Hopkins

The issues associated with reoperations with patient with extracardiac valved conduits have been reviewed in depth by one of the true leaders in the field, Professor Jaroslav Stark in Chapter 2 and elsewhere.[1] In essence, if a patient lives long enough, the current generation of homografts need replacement whether in the right or left sided positions. Use of Dacron tube extensions and misplacement of the conduit under the sternum have been the most frequently associated events leading to early replacement. Age of the child at the time of the conduit insertion is clearly important. However, right ventricular outflow tract homograft re-replacements are usually relatively quick and easy operations. In our practice, we have never had a mortality for such a re-replacement for right sided homografts. As the subpulmonary ventricle peak pressure approaches systemic, we prefer to replace so that supra systemic pressures are not reached. Conduit valve incompetence is associated with distal stenoses especially when combined with tricuspid valve regurgitation or especially compelling factors for replacement. Homograft conduit replacement surgery also gives the opportunity to repair any other defects, either residual or acquired such as ventricular septal defect, AV valve regurgitation, multilevel stenoses such as pulmonary artery stenoses, or midchamber muscle bundle development in the right ventricle. Pre-operative assessment must clearly define the areas of obstruction in the conduit as these do occur relatively equivalently at the right ventricular outflow anastomosis, midconduit, homograft leaflet, distal conduit,

distal anastomosis, or pulmonary artery regions. Replacement surgery should include relief of obstruction at all levels. Repair of tricuspid valve when significantly regurgitant should also be accomplished.

Reoperative median sternotomy is the usual approach. If the right ventricle is eroding into the sternum, then we cannulate the femoral artery and vein and place the patient on cardiopulmonary bypass to decompress the heart as sternal entry is accomplished with an oscillating saw. If the homograft is deviated into the left chest and there appears to be a reasonable plane between the anterior ventricle and the sternum, then the femoral vessels are only exposed and reoperative entry is performed in the usual fashion. Aprotinin bleeding prophylaxis protocol is utilized for reoperations. Unless reconstructive procedures are needed on the left side of the heart, aortic cross clamping is not necessary and only mild hypothermia needs to be utilized.

After a sternal entry has been accomplished, dissection of the heart is performed to the point that cannulation can be accomplished and cardiopulmonary bypass initiated. At this point, the conduit is dissected. It is preferable to remove all of the conduit material except the posterior peel on the cardiac structures. If felt or other pledget type materials were used at the original operation, it should be removed as late infections sourced to this material have been described.

All of the homograft is removed and any reconstructions of the pulmonary arteries required are performed in a fashion similar to those described in Chapter 53. Occasionally a nice path exists from the right ventricle to the pulmonary arteries with the posterior peel such that it can be roofed with a patch for a non-valved repair. This is only performed if there are no distal stenoses, no increase in pulmonary vascular resistance, and normal diameter and numbers of pulmonary arteries. In addition, right ventricular function should be normal. There cannot be any significant insufficiency of the tricuspid valve.

While we usually favor a pulmonary homograft, in some RVOT reoperations, the conduit bed insets down into the cardiac structures in such a fashion that an aortic homograft can be sewn into the distal anastomosis and down into the right ventricle in such a fashion that the anterior leaflet of the mitral valve completes the proximal anastomosis along the rim of right ventricular tissue that is stiffened with the previous scar tissue (Figures 59.1 and 59.2). This allows for an all homograft repair without the need for any additional PTFE or Dacron material. Pulmonary arterioplasties are preferentially performed with tongues of homograft or PTFE (*vida supra*).

We have experimented with placement of PTFE artificial pericardium and have come to no firm conclusions about its utility. We have seen patients in whom bovine pericardium has been used previously as an artificial pericardial barrier after reoperation for homograft and would not recommend its use as it increases the difficulty at the next homograft replacement operation. In general, the replacement of a homograft conduit while somewhat challenging to the reconstructive cardiac surgeon, is usually achieved with minimal difficulties and often with surprisingly brief hospital stays.[2-4]

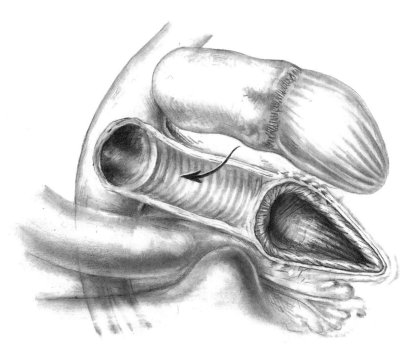

FIGURE 59.1. The aortic homograft can be inset into the gulch created by the previous conduit, thereby reducing the above heart profile, avoiding compression, minimizing need for prosthetic material for the hood and obtaining very laminar flow profiles without excessive curvature of the homograft conduit.

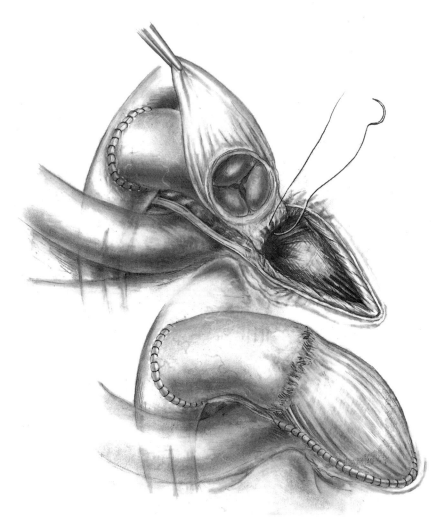

Figure 59.2. Proximal and distal suture lines of continuous polypropylene. Rarely are pledgets needed. The proximal hood is always constructed from PTFE (for pulmonary homograft) usually employed to augment the available mitral valve tissue when aortic homografts are used for this reconstruction. Pulmonary homografts are preferred for RVOT reoperative reconstructions if distance to the native pulmonary artery is short enough.

References

1. Stark J. Reoperations in Patients with Extracardiac Valved Conduits. In Stark J, Pacifico AD (eds). Reoperations in Cardiac Surgery. New York, NY: Springer-Verlag 1989:27–290.
2. Bove EL, Kavey REW, Byrum CJ, et al. Improved right ventricular function following late pulmonary valve replacement for residual pulmonary insufficiency or stenosis. J Thorac Cardiovasc Surg 1985;90:50–55.
3. Bull C, Macartney FJ, Horvath P, et al. Evaluation of long-term results of homograft and heterograft valves and extracardiac conduits. J Thorac Cardiovasc Surg 1987;94:12–19.
4. Merin G, McGoon DC. Reoperation after insertion of aortic homograft-right ventricular outflow tract. Ann Thorac Surg 1973;16:122–126.

60
Proximal and Distal Extensions

Kim F. Duncan

Distal extension of the allograft is seldom required, usually only in cases with nonconfluent central pulmonary arteries or when a long LV-PA conduit is required. The use of proximal extension in all cases of RVOT reconstruction incorporating a valved allograft conduit has been based on the following principles:

1. Placement of the allograft valve cephalad to the native position to reduce sternal compression.
2. Use of a complete cylinder of prosthetic material at the base of the allograft to limit root dilatation.
3. The use of a knitted, collagen-impregnated Dacron tubular prosthesis as the extension.

The need for a competent valve to protect the right ventricle from volume or pressure overload is a fundamental reason for implanting an allograft valve conduit. Insufficiency of the allograft valve can occur early or late postoperatively and is related to either distortion by the sternum, dilatation of the valve root after implantation or leaflet degeneration. Valve obstruction may also result from sternal compression or leaflet degeneration in the early or late postoperative period.

Children requiring a valved allograft will have significant right or biventricular hypertrophy that narrows or obliterates the retrosternal space, most easily recognized on a lateral chest film. When the allograft is sutured directly into the right ventricular outflow tract, the bulk of the muscular base of the allograft and the enlarged heart displace the valve anteriorly, resulting in compression of the allograft by the sternum at the time of chest closure, particularly in infants and small children. The distortion of the natural circular valve structure alters leaflet coaptation, producing insufficiency or reduces the effective cross-sectional area, producing stenosis. These changes can be demonstrated by color Doppler flow imaging. We have observed that sternal compression may produce insufficiency without sufficient compression to cause restriction to antegrade flow. By incorporation a short cylindrical segment of Dacron, the allograft valve will sit cephalad and posterior to the upper end of the right ventriculotomy and will also be angled more toward the distal anastomosis to the native pulmonary artery. The allograft valve will be less susceptible to sternal compression in this position. Additionally, the complete ring of Dacron sewn to the muscular base of the allograft will fix the diameter of the root and reduce early or late dilatation and valve insufficiency. The length of the complete cylinder of Dacron varies, depending on the size of the patient, from 6 to 20mm. The use of the long obliquely cut Dacron extension below the cylindrical portion for anastomosis in the RVOT also removes the trifurcated suture lie and potential sites of troublesome bleeding where the ventricular wall, the base of the allograft and the head meet using the conventional technique.[1]

Early experience with woven Dacron conduit containing a biologic valve was unsatisfactory because of the development of a thick, fibrous, obstructing pseudo-intima immediately proximal to the valve.[2,3] It was inferred that the use of Dacron extensions proximal to an allograft valve conduit would meet a similar fate. Haveric and co-workers in Europe demonstrated that the use of high porosity knitted Dacron allowed fibrous ingrowth and anchoring as well as vascularization of the pseudo-intima,[4] markedly reducing the risk of obstruction. During our early experience in Canada and the United Kingdom, bleeding from the porous knitted Dacron conduit was managed with a commercial form of fibrin glue applied to the conduit immediately prior to use.[5] Unfortunately, the commercial fibrin sealant was unavailable in the United States, and less satisfactory sealant techniques were employed. Since 1990, a collagen-impregnated knitted Dacron vascular graft (Hemashield, Meadox Medicals, Inc., Oakland, NJ) has been used widely with excellent handling characteristics and hemostasis.[2,6] This conduit is now used exclusively in our practice for this procedure.

Technique

1. The pulmonary allograft is intended to lie in its natural orientation with the right and left bronchus aligned appropriately.

2. The muscular base of the allograft is trimmed to 3 or 4mm below the nadir of the valve cusps.

3. The knitted Dacron extension is 1 or 2mm larger than the measured valve diameter and is sutured end-to-end to the base of the allograft with 4-0 polypropylene, taking care to avoid injury to the valve cusps.

4. The allograft is positioned to lie cephalad and posterior to the top of the surgical defect in the right ventricular outflow tract. It is usually possible to locate the allograft valve such that the cylindrical portion of the Dacron extension is at least 3 or 4mm long in infants, and up to 20mm long in larger patients.

5. The distal end of the allograft is then trimmed as close as necessary to the top of the valve commissures, leaving adequate allograft tissue to augment the PA confluence as necessary.

6. With the distal end of the allograft held against the native PA confluence, the posterior wall of the cylindrical portion of the Dacron extension is then marked where it meets the upper end of the defect in the RVOT. The Dacron extension is tailored obliquely from this point to a length 5–8mm longer than the right ventriculotomy.

7. The distal anastomosis between pulmonary artery confluence and allograft conduit is completed with running 4-0 polypropylene suture. The proximal anastomosis between the hooded Dacron extension and right ventricle is then completed with a running 4-0 polypropylene suture and appropriate tailoring of Dacron to fit the defect.

Results with a Cylindrical Dacron Proximal Extension

Between July 1988 and June 1996, 43 patients underwent reconstruction of the right ventricular outflow tract incorporating an allograft valve conduit with a sealed knitted Dacron extension. Ages ranged from five days to 14 years with a mean of 2.1 years. Diagnostic categories included tetralogy of Fallot with hypoplastic pulmonary arteries, pulmonary atresia with ventricular septal defect, pulmonary atresia with ventricular septum, absent pulmonary valve syndrome, transposition of the great arteries with subpulmonary stenosis, complete AV canal with pulmonary artery band, and pulmonary artery band with mycotic aneurysm of the PA. There were three early deaths from viral pneumonia, inadequate pulmonary blood flow and myocardial failure. There were three late deaths, two in patients with pulmonary atresia and respiratory failure; the third died from cardiac tamponade secondary to endocarditis and dehiscence of the Dacron-allograft suture lie. Gram positive cocci were present on histological section at the site of rupture. The patient was two months postoperative without a positive history of perioperative infection.

Editor's Note

In general, as the reader will note in other chapters of this book, the editor tries to avoid using Dacron conduit extensions. As noted in the contribution by Dr. Duncan, there is a history of peel formation. However, anatomical constraints as described by Dr. Duncan sometimes occur and therefore these techniques are included so that the surgeon reader will have available some options for alternative reconstructions. In general, while controversial, the editor of this book would recommend use of material other than Dacron, such as PTFE, autologous or bovine pericardium (for applications where shrinkage is not a problem), etc. for reconstructions in the right ventricular outflow tract and pulmonary arteries. However, Dacron extensions have been used by many surgeons in many complex situations with good results. The Dacron material preferred by Dr. Duncan does not bleed, has excellent handling characteristics and is especially useful in situations where the conduit needs to bend sequentially in different planes—i.e. needs to be both flexible but rigid enough to resist compression by surrounding structures and scar tissue.

References

1. Kirklin JW, Barratt-Boyes B. Tetralogy of Fallot. In Kirklin JW, Barratt-Boyes BG (eds). Cardiac Surgery. New York: Churchill-Livingstone, Inc. 1993:953–956.
2. Jonas RA, Freed MD, Mayor JE, Castaneda AR. Long term follow-up of patients with synthetic right heart conduits. Circulation 1985;72 (Suppll. 2):II77–II83.
3. Fiore A, Peigh P, Brown J, et al. Valved and non-valved right ventricular-pulmonary arterial extracardiac conduits. J Thorac Cardiovasc Surg 1993;86:490–494.
4. Haverich A, Oelert H, Maatz W, et al. Histopathological evaluation of woven and knitted Dacron grafts for right ventricular conduits: A comparative experimental study. Ann Thorac Surg 1984; 37:404–409.
5. Haverich A, Walterbusch G, Borst H. The use of Fibron glue for sealing vascular prostheses of high porosity. Thorac Cardiovasc Surg 1981;29: 252–257.
6. Sano S, Karl TR, Mee RB. Extracardiac valved conduits in the pulmonary circuit. Ann Thorac Surg 1991;52:285–290.

61
Reconstruction with Nonvalved Cryopreserved Cardiovascular Tissues

John L. Myers

Hypoplastic Left Heart Syndrome

The first stage of palliation for hypoplastic left heart syndrome requires reconstruction of the entire aortic arch by augmenting the often diminutive ascending aorta, transverse aortic arch and region of the excised ductus arteriosus.[1-4] The proximal main pulmonary artery is anastomosed to the newly constructed ascending aorta.

PFTE and glutaraldehyde fixed autologous pericardium were used initially as the material to augment the aortic arch. PTFE and pericardium are "sheets" that can be rolled in one dimension to develop a tubular patch, however, reconstruction of the entire aortic arch requires that this tubular graft have a secondary curvature of 180° as it extends from the ascending aorta around the transverse arch to the descending aorta. Pericardium and PTFE are inelastic and cannot develop a curvature in two different planes at 90° to one another without developing ridges or buckles. This results in obstruction within the aortic arch. Also the PTFE suture line frequently bleeds excessively.

The introduction of cryopreserved allograft pulmonary artery for the repair of hypoplastic left heart syndrome alleviated many of these problems. The patch of pulmonary allograft is cut from the curvature between one of the branch arteries (usually the left) and the main pulmonary artery.

Operative Technique

A median sternotomy incision is made. Cardiopulmonary bypass is established by a venous cannula placed in the right arterial appendage and arterial return via an arterial cannula placed in the main pulmonary artery. As soon as bypass has commenced, the branch pulmonary arteries are occluded with tourniquets. Arterial inflow into the main pulmonary artery perfuses the systemic circulation through the patent ductus arteriosus. Core cooling is continued for 20–25 minutes until a nasopharyngeal temperature and rectal temperature of 16–18° has been reached. Circulatory arrest is established and the branches of the aortic arch are occluded with tourniquets. Cold blood cardioplegia is delivered. With the circulation arrested, the atrial cannula is removed. Through the atrial appendage cannulation site, the atrial septum is identified and excised. The main pulmonary artery is transected just proximal to the bifurcation which is usually several millimeters distal to the commissural posts of the pulmonary valve (Figure 61.1, dashed line 1). The ductus arteriosus is ligated close to the pulmonary artery confluence. The ascending aorta is incised and this incision is carried distally through the aortic arch to the opened ductus arteriosus (Figure 61.1, dashed line 2). All of the ductal tissue is excised and the incision is carried distally onto the descending aorta for a distance of about 1 cm (Figure 61.2). The patch of pulmonary allograft used to reconstruct the arch is taken from one of

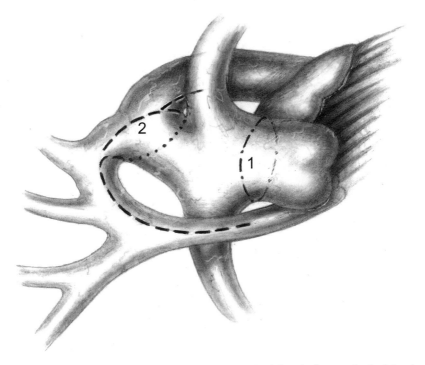

FIGURE 61.1. Hypoplastic left heart syndrome.
1. Dashed line indicates the level of transection of
the proximal main pulmonary artery

2. Dashed line indicates the incision in the ascending aorta extending around the aortic arch and past
the ductal orifice for a distance of 1 cm.

the branch pulmonary arteries and extends
onto the main pulmonary artery segment of
the allograft (Figure 61.2 inset). This patch
has a tubular shape with an additional curvature to allow this tubular patch to extend from
the descending aorta to the ascending aorta
leaving a normal curvature to the underside of
the newly reconstructed aortic arch. It is important to keep the homograft slightly taut as
it is being sewn into place. If redundancy is left
in the allograft patch, then the allograft will
develop a bulge when the arch is exposed
to systemic output and pressure (Figure 61.3).
It is important to trim the patch so that the
patch has a nice radius of curvature on the
underside of the arch to direct flow around
the arch in a normal fashion (Figure 61.4). If
the midportion of the patch is too large, the
transverse arch becomes quite large which can
compress the left pulmonary artery and/or the
left mainstem bronchus as they pass under the

reconstructed arch and result in poor growth of
these two structures. In addition, the distended
allograft can result in a ledge-like deformity
at the suture line on the descending aorta
(Figure 61.3).

The incision in the ascending aorta is carried
proximally to the point that corresponds with
the level of the adjacent transected main pulmonary artery (Figure 61.5). Six to seven interrupted sutures of 7-0 Prolene are placed to
approximate the often tiny ascending aorta
to the proximal transected main pulmonary
artery. Any compromise in this anastomosis
may result in coronary insufficiency. This may
be immediately apparent when coming off
bypass or may lead to sudden cardiovascular
collapse in the postoperative period. The
remaining portion of the main pulmonary
artery is sewn to the proximal part of the reconstructed aortic arch (Figure 61.4). The heart is
filled with saline solution to displace any air.

The neo-ascending aorta and right atrial appendage are recannulated and cardiopulmonary bypass is resumed. Complete rewarming is begun. The first stage palliation is completed by construction of a right modified Blalock-Taussig shunt between the innominate artery and right pulmonary artery. The distal main pulmonary artery is either closed primarily if adequate tissue is present or, more often, with a small circular patch of pulmonary allograft.

The pulmonary allograft, when properly tailored, conforms more naturally to the curvature of the reconstructed aortic arch and the suture lines are more hemostatic. During the second and third stages of the palliation for hypoplastic left heart syndrome, reoperation involves recannulation of the reconstructed aortic arch. The pulmonary allograft, in general, can be cannulated the same as native aorta. Pursestring sutures are easily placed and cannulation can be accomplished in the normal fashion.

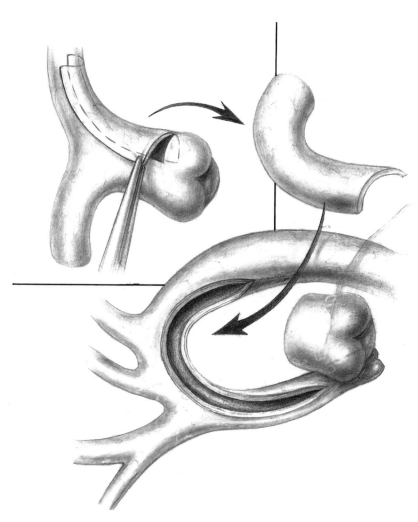

FIGURE 61.2. The hypoplastic aortic arch is augmented with a piece of pulmonary allograft taken from the main and branch portion of the pulmonary allograft (inset). The augmentation patch is sewn into the aortic arch starting in the descending aorta. The suture line is continued around the aortic arch onto the ascending aorta.

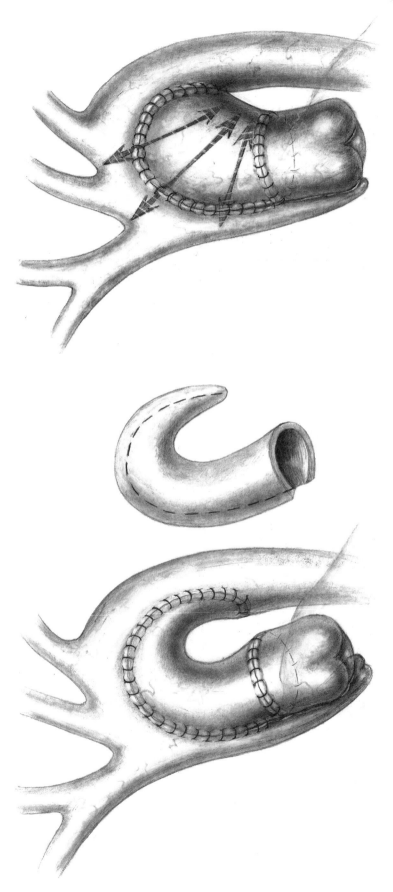

FIGURE 61.3. This figure depicts reconstruction of a hypoplastic aortic arch with a patch of pulmonary allograft which is too large. This large piece of allograft bulges out when under systemic pressure causing a pseudocoarctation at the distal suture line as well as compression of the left mainstem bronchus and left branch pulmonary arteries.

FIGURE 61.4. The correctly tailored piece of pulmonary allograft (inset) will restore a normal size and shape to the aortic arch.

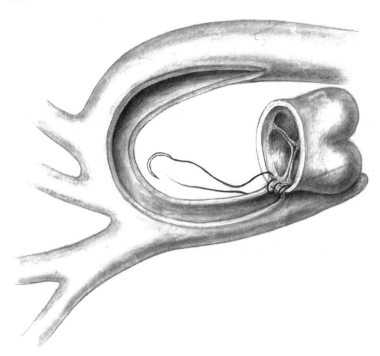

FIGURE 61.5. The proximal main pulmonary artery is attached to the proximal ascending aorta with multiple interrupted sutures of 7.0 Prolene. These interrupted sutures are necessary to avoid narrowing of the orifice into the proximal ascending aorta which is the pathway for all coronary blood flow.

L-Transposition of the Great Arteries with Outflow Chamber and Aortic Arch Hypoplasia

The patients with L-transposition of the great arteries with an outflow chamber and hypoplastic aortic arch present a technical challenge for reconstruction of the aortic arch.[5,6] The aorta is positioned anterior and leftward and the main pulmonary artery is rightward and posterior (Figure 61.6). One option for repair of the aortic arch and association of the proximal main pulmonary artery into the aortic arch is accomplished by augmenting the aortic arch in the same fashion as described above for typical hypoplastic left heart syndrome.[5] Following the arch reconstruction, an additional hood of allograft is used to associate the main pulmonary artery to the rightward aspect of the reconstructed aortic arch. This is similar to the technique of Damus-Kaye-Stanzel anastomosis.

Another technique, which we prefer, involves transection of the ascending aorta (Figure 61.7). The aortic arch is opened longitudinally from the divided ascending aorta all the way around to the ductus arteriosus. The ductus arteriosus is completely excised and the incision is extended onto the descending aorta for a distance of about 1 cm. All of this is accomplished utilizing deep hypothermia and circulatory arrest. A piece of pulmonary allograft is then sewn into place to reconstruct the entire aortic arch and ascending aorta (Figure 61.8). This reconstructed aortic arch is then anastomosed in an end-to-end fashion to the divided mail pulmonary artery (Figure 61.9). The proximal end of the divided ascending aorta is then incorporated into the suture line. The location of this anastomosis is determined by bringing the divided proximal ascending aorta over against the suture line. An ellipse of either pulmonary allograft or proximal main pulmonary artery or both, is taken to create a nice defect in which to anastomose the proximal ascending aorta (Figure 61.9 inset). The small ascending aorta functions primarily as a large single coronary artery with some antegrade flow possible depending upon the degree of subaortic obstruction. This technique, I believe, gives a more anatomic outflow tract from the single ventricle into the reconstructed aortic arch. The distal main pulmonary artery is closed with a circular patch of pulmonary allograft and the

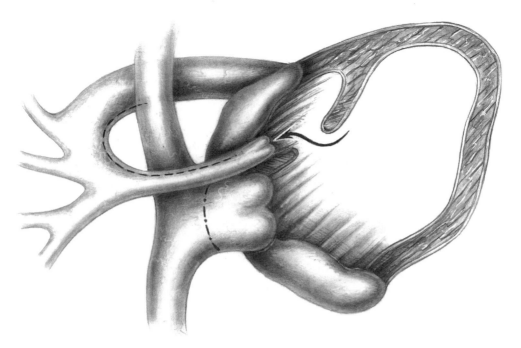

FIGURE 61.6. This depicts the anatomy of L-transposition of the great arteries with hypoplasia of the ascending aorta and a potentially restrictive bulboventricular foramen.

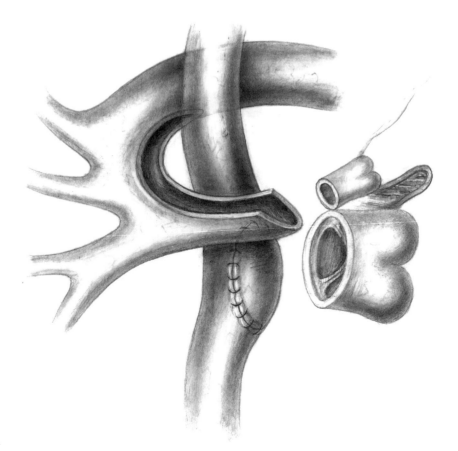

FIGURE 61.7. The main pulmonary artery is divided. The distal pulmonary artery is closed with a patch of allograft material. The ascending aorta is divided about 5 mm distal to the level of the pulmonary artery transection. The aorta is incised from the ascending aorta, around the aortic arch and into the descending aorta.

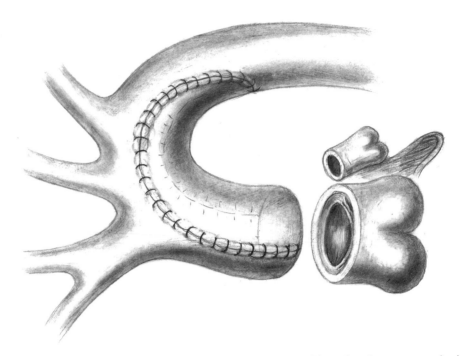

FIGURE 61.8. A piece of pulmonary allograft taken from the main and branch pulmonary arteries is used to reconstruct the entire aortic arch.

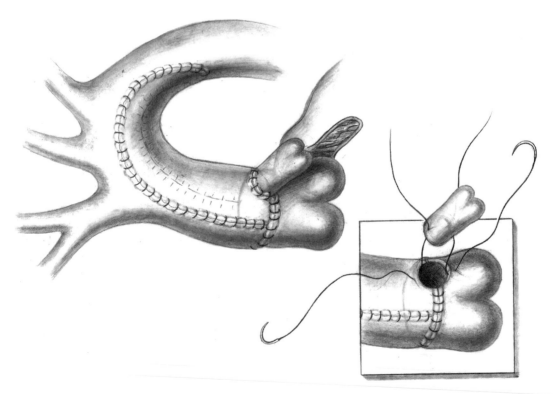

FIGURE 61.9. The reconstructed aortic arch is anastomosed to the proximal main pulmonary artery arising from the dominant ventricular chamber. An ellipse is taken from either side of the suture line to create an opening for anastomosis of the proximal aorta into the suture line (inset).

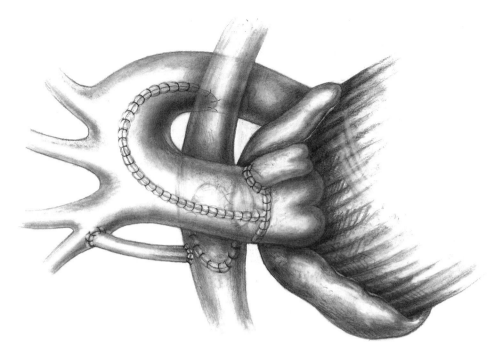

FIGURE 61.10. The complete procedure showing the reconstructed aortic arch and inclusion of the proximal ascending aorta into the suture line. The distal pulmonary artery is closed with a patch of allograft material and pulmonary blood flow is obtained by a modified Blalock-Taussig shunt.

operation completed by placing a 3.5 to 4.0 Gore-Tex shunt between the innominate artery and the right pulmonary artery (Figure 61.10).

Interrupted Aortic Arch (Isolated or Associated with Ventricular Septal Defect, Truncus Arteriosus or Transposition of the Great Arteries)

Interrupted aortic arch can occur in isolation or in association with ventricular septal defect, truncus arteriosus or transposition of the great arteries. When the operation is performed through a median sternotomy incision, deep hypothermia and circulatory arrest are employed to facilitate the repair. Arterial cannulae are placed in both the ascending aorta as well as the main pulmonary artery. Venous return is accomplished through a cannula in the right atrial appendage. Once cardiopulmonary bypass is commenced, the branch pulmonary arteries are occluded tourniquets. The aortic arch, ductus arteriosus and descending aorta are mobilized during core cooling. Following the establishment of circulatory arrest, the head vessels are occluded with tourniquets. The ductus arteriosus is ligated and all ductal tissue is excised. Usually the distal aorta can be mobilized enough and brought superior and anterior to allow a direct anastomosis to the side of the ascending aorta with extension of the incision into the most distal branch of the ascending aorta (Figure 61.11). However, sometimes undue tension on the anastomosis may result in anastomotic stenosis. In addition, a very taut anastomosis can cause compression of the left mainstem bronchus. In those situations, several techniques can be utilized to augment the aortic anastomosis by incorporating pulmonary allograft into the repair. In the first technique, usually involving a Type B interruption, the

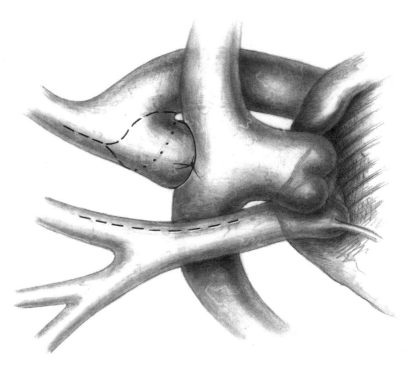

FIGURE 61.11. Interrupted aortic arch. The ductus arteriosus is ligated and the ductal tissue is excised. The incision is extended proximally onto the left sub-clavian artery. An incision in the ascending aorta is extended up onto the left carotid artery.

superior aspect of the anastomosis is begun and the upper half of the circumference of the anastomosis is made directly with a running suture (Figure 61.12).[5] The remaining portion of the anastomosis is made utilizing a gusset of pulmonary allograft to bridge the distance and permit an anastomosis without undue tension particularly in the inferior aspect of the anastomosis (Figure 61.13). The complete repair (Figure 61.14).

Another technique involves sewing the entire back wall of the anastomosis first. An incision on the left lateral aspect of the aorta is carried down further on the descending aorta and another incision is carried onto the proximal ascending aorta (Figure 61.15). An elliptical portion of pulmonary allograft is then sewn into this defect to augment the aortic arch anastomosis (Figure 61.16). This technique does allow extension of the incision down into the proximal ascending aorta to augment a small ascending aorta when an adequate size aortic valve is present.

Some patients with interrupted aortic arch and ventricular septal defect have severe posterior malalignment of the infundibular septum which results in severe left ventricular outflow tract obstruction. In these patients the divided proximal main pulmonary artery is incorporated into the aortic arch reconstruction.[5] The distal main pulmonary artery is closed with a patch of allograft and a modified Blalock-Taussig shunt is placed.

Tubular Hypoplasia of the Transverse Aortic Arch with or without Coarctation

When coarctation is associated with a diffusely hypoplastic transverse aortic arch, coarctation repair alone may not relieve the aortic obstruction because of residual obstruction across the hypoplastic transverse arch. These patients may have an associated ventricular septal

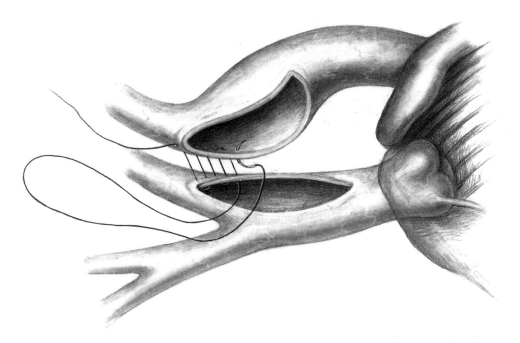

FIGURE 61.12. The upper one-half of the anastomosis, both anteriorly and posteriorly, is made with a running suture.

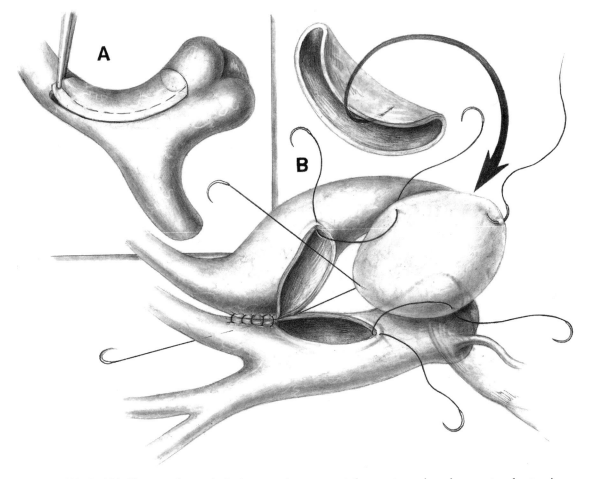

FIGURE 61.13. (A) Homograft patch is harvested from the inner curve of pulmonary artery bifurcation. (B) The allograft patch is sewn in place to augment the anastomosis and prevent undue tension in the lower half of the suture line between the descending aorta and the proximal ascending aorta.

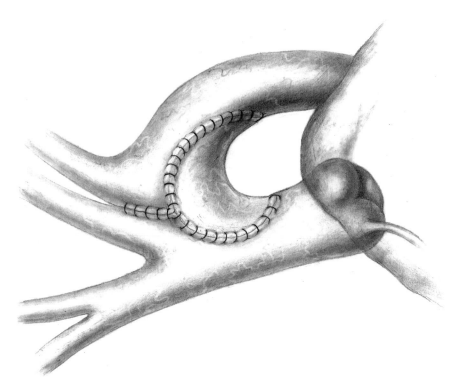

FIGURE 61.14. The completed repair showing a widely patent anastomosis with autologous tissue making up one-half of the circumference of the aortic arch and the pulmonary allograft making up the underside of the aortic arch.

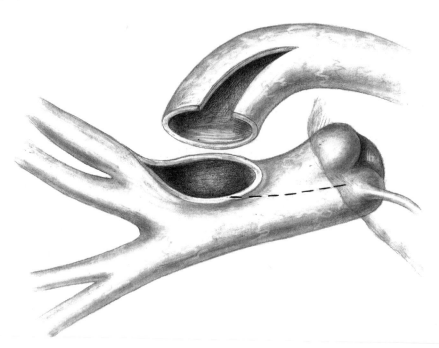

FIGURE 61.15. The mobilized and divided descending aorta with an additional left lateral incision. The posterior suture line is completed by direct anastomosis. An incision is extended into the descending aorta and into the proximal ascending aorta.

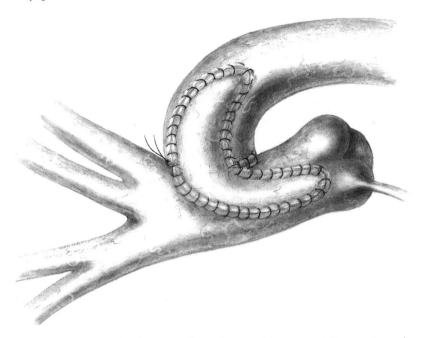

FIGURE 61.16. An elliptical piece of pulmonary allograft is used to augment the anastomosis as well as the proximal ascending aorta and descending aorta.

defect which can be repaired at the same time. During core cooling for deep hypothermia and circulatory arrest, the entire aortic arch is mobilized. Following establishment of circulatory arrest, the ductus arteriosus is ligated and all of the ductal tissue is excised. An incision (dotted line) is carried from the proximal ascending aorta around the hypoplastic transverse aortic arch to the orifice of the ductus arteriosus (Figure 61.17). All of the ductal tissue is excised. A piece of pulmonary allograft is cut from the inner curvature between the left or right branch pulmonary artery and main pulmonary artery. This patch is sewn into place (Figure 61.18). It is important not to make this patch too large as this will result in bulging of the allograft posteriorly and inferiorly into the pulmonary artery. The allograft should be kept taut during the anastomosis. A properly cut patch will result in a reconstructed aortic arch which appears normal in size and shape (Figure 61.19).

Damus/Kaye/Stanzel Anastomosis with or without Aortic Arch Augmentation

Those patients with subaortic obstruction and who are destined to a single ventricle repair (Fontan) and who have a normal pulmonary valve, can frequently undergo a Damus/Kaye/Stanzel anastomosis.[7,8] This involves association of the divided proximal main pulmonary artery with the aortic arch so that the unobstructed outflow tract to the pulmonary valve an be utilized for systemic outflow to the aorta (Figure 61.20). Depending upon the anatomy and relationship of the great vessels and whether there is an associated aortic arch hypoplasia will determine whether the allograft needs to extend just onto the proximal aortic arch or whether it will need to be extended around the entire aortic arch onto the descending aorta similar to a Norwood type of repair. In most

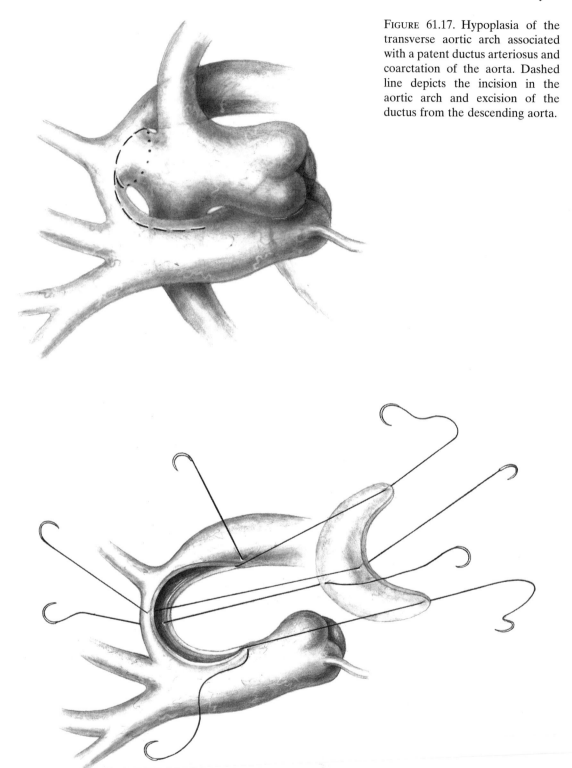

FIGURE 61.17. Hypoplasia of the transverse aortic arch associated with a patent ductus arteriosus and coarctation of the aorta. Dashed line depicts the incision in the aortic arch and excision of the ductus from the descending aorta.

FIGURE 61.18. The ductus arteriosus tissue has been excised from the descending aorta. A patch of pulmonary allograft is cut and sewn into the underside of the aortic arch.

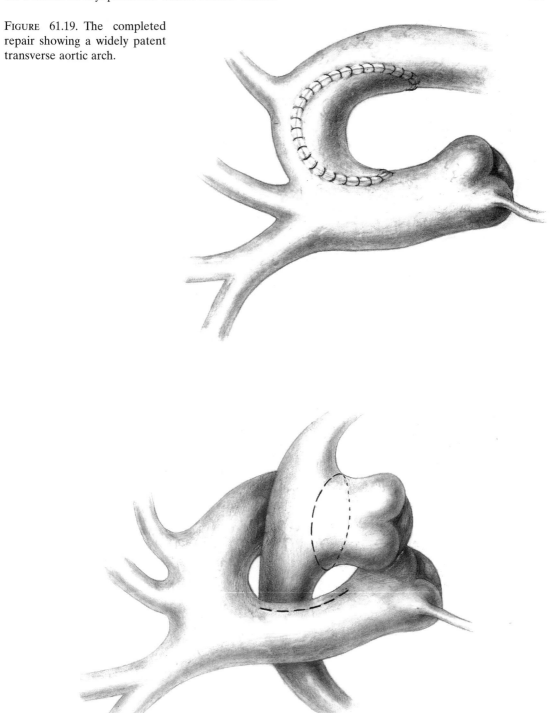

FIGURE 61.20. In patients who have subaortic obstruction and require a Damus-Kaye-Stanzel anastomosis, the proximal main pulmonary artery is divided (dashed line). An incision is made in the ascending aorta (dashed line).

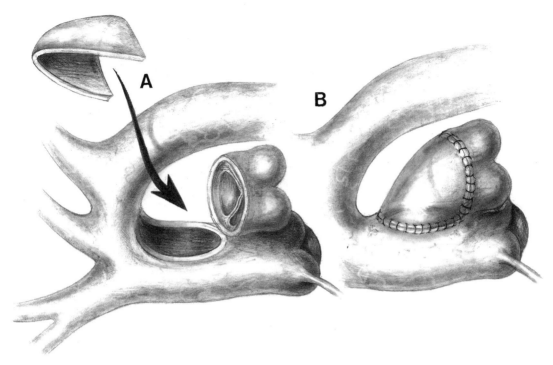

FIGURE 61.21. The proximal mail pulmonary artery is attached for a distance of about 1 cm to the ascending aorta. The remainder of the anastomosis is made by using a hood of pulmonary allograft to direct flow from the proximal pulmonary artery into the ascending aorta. (A) A piece of pulmonary allograft is fashioned so as to direct blood flow into the ascending aorta with out distorting the pulmonary valve. (B) Completed repair.

instances, if the proximal main pulmonary artery is just sewn to an incision in the aortic arch, distortion of the pulmonary valve will occur with the development of pulmonary insufficiency. It is usually necessary to use a hood of pulmonary allograft to fashion a pathway from the divided proximal main pulmonary artery into the aorta so that no distortion of the pulmonary root or aortic root will occur. When the aortic arch is normal, the pulmonary allograft hood can be attached just to the ascending aorta (Figure 61.21A, B). This can be performed under continuous cardiopulmonary bypass. When the arch is hypoplastic and the entire arch needs to be augmented, deep hypothermia and circulatory arrest is required. A Norwood operation is then undertaken (Figure 61.22).

When the relationship of the great arteries is a posterior and rightward pulmonary artery and an anterior and leftward aorta, the technique depicted in Figures 61.22 and 61.23 A and B is used. The main pulmonary artery is divided and the distal end closed primarily or with a patch of pulmonary allograft. An "L" incision is made in the ascending aorta to create a flap of aorta which will make up part of the posterior wall of the connection between the proximal main pulmonary allograft and the ascending aorta (Figure 61.23 A and B). A hood of pulmonary allograft is used to complete the anastomosis. The repair is completed by making a systemic artery to pulmonary artery shunt. Usually this is a 3.5mm or 4mm PTFE graft from the innominate or subclavian artery to the pulmonary artery.

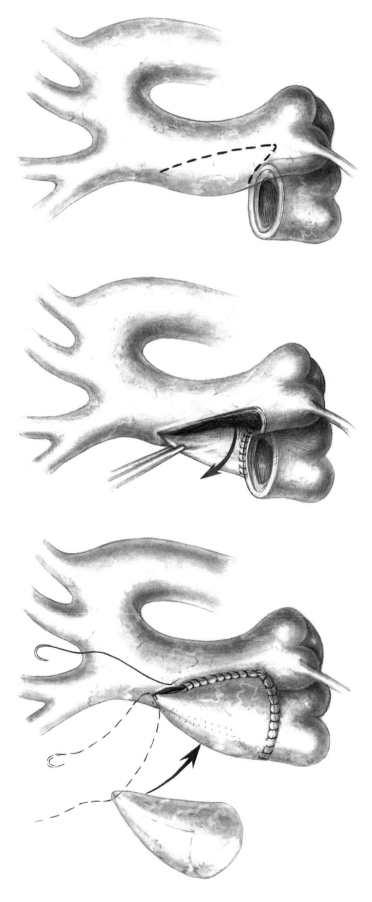

FIGURE 61.22. When the pulmonary artery is posterior and rightward, an L-shaped incision is made in the ascending aorta creating a posteriorly based flap. This flap makes up a portion of the posterior wall of the hood to direct flow from the proximal main pulmonary artery into the aorta.

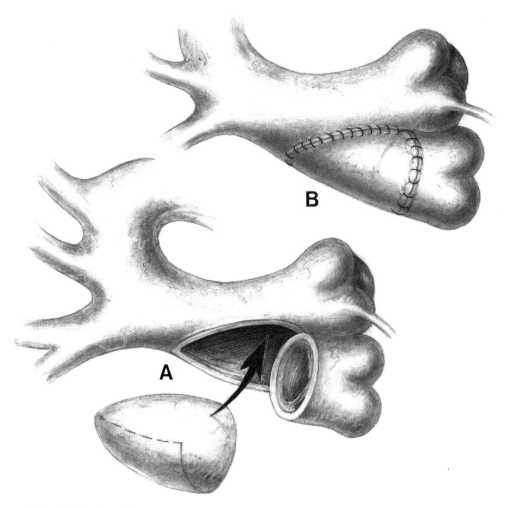

FIGURE 61.23. (A) A piece of pulmonary allograft is tailored to direct the blood flow from the proximal pulmonary artery into the ascending aorta. (B) It is important not to distort the pulmonary valve as this will likely result in pulmonary insufficiency.

Pulmonary Artery Reconstruction during the Fontan Operation

Often times patients who are candidates for a Fontan operation for terminal palliation have some pulmonary distortion or need augmentation of their central pulmonary arteries. This is most frequently seen in patients following a Norwood operation where the central pulmonary artery confluence may sometimes be narrowed. Whether the patient is to undergo a total cavopulmonary connection or a hemi-Fontan, the superior cavopulmonary connection can be accomplished in the same fashion. following commencement of cardiopulmonary bypass, an incision is made in the right pulmonary artery and extended as far leftward as necessary to augment the pulmonary arteries (Figure 61.24). The incision is extended rightward to a point just past the posterior aspect of the superior vena cava. This incision in the main pulmonary artery is T'd off for a few millimeters transversely. An additional incision is made in the superior vena cava in a transverse manner. The medial one-half of the superior vena cava is incised. A small ellipse of cava is

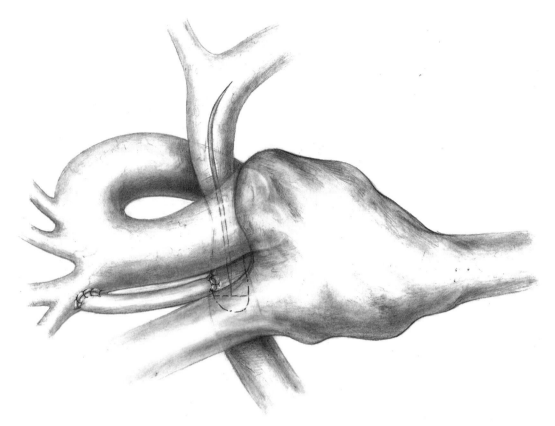

FIGURE 61.24. This depicts a patient status post a Norwood procedure and prior to a hemi-Fontan or Fontan operation. There is frequently hypoplasia of the central pulmonary arteries. An incision is made in the right pulmonary artery and extended all the way to the left pulmonary artery at the pericardial reflection. The incision is T'd off at the rightward most aspect of the incision in the right pulmonary artery.

cut away from each edge of the incision. The posterior aspect of the superior vena cava is anastomosed with a fine monofilament suture to the anterior aspect of the right pulmonary artery. A piece of pulmonary allograft is cut in a fashion so that the one end will taper into the left pulmonary artery and the proximal end will be incorporated into the medial aspect of the vena cava and right pulmonary artery (Figure 61.25). This creates a good sized, streamlined anastomosis between the superior vena cava and the pulmonary artery. For those patients undergoing a hemi-Fontan, a small circular piece of Gore-Tex is sewn into the atrial side of the superior caval orifice to prevent superior caval flow from entering the right atrium (Figure 61.26).

At the time of subsequent completion Fontan, this piece of Gore-Tex occluding the orifice to the superior vena cava is excised and a fenestrated baffle is placed between the inferior vena cava and the superior caval orifice. For those patients undergoing a primary Fontan, a fenestrated baffle is placed between the inferior vena caval orifice and the superior caval orifice from within the atrium (Figure 61.27). This directs all of the inferior caval blood flow into the cavopulmonary anastomosis.

Another technique for completing the Fontan circulation is to utilize a tube of pulmonary or aortic allograft to connect the divided inferior vena cava to the pulmonary arteries (Figure 61.28). A standard bidirectional Glenn anastomosis is used to connect the

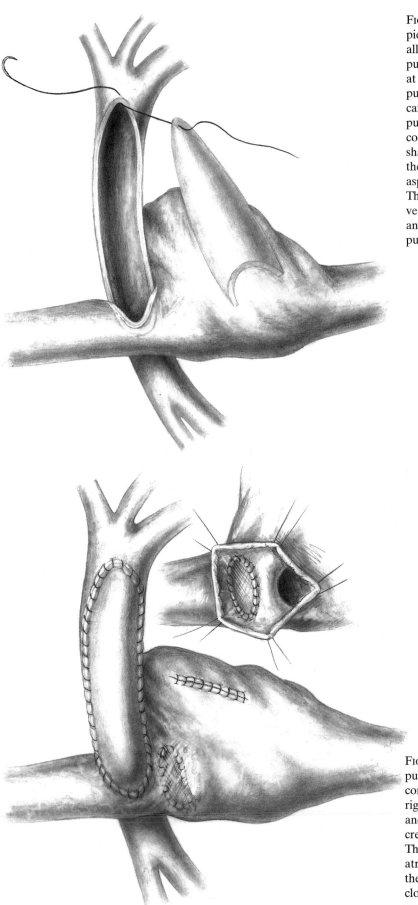

FIGURE 61.25. A long piece of pulmonary allograft is sewn into the pulmonary artery starting at the distal left pulmonary artery and carried across the entire pulmonary artery confluence. An oval shaped defect is created in the posterior and medial aspect of the vena cava. The posterior aspect of the vena cava is sutured to the anterior aspect of the right pulmonary artery.

FIGURE 61.26. The pulmonary allograft is continued across onto the right pulmonary artery and superior vena cava to create a large anastomosis. Through a limited right atriotomy, the orifice to the superior vena cava is closed with a circular patch of Gore-Tex.

FIGURE 61.27. When a full Fontan is performed, a fenestrated baffle of Gore-Tex is placed from the inferior vena cava to the superior vena caval orifice. When the patient has had a previous hemi-Fontan, the circular piece of Gore-Tex occluding the orifice of the superior vena cava is excised and a fenestrated piece of Gore-Tex is used to baffle the inferior vena caval drainage to the superior vena cava.

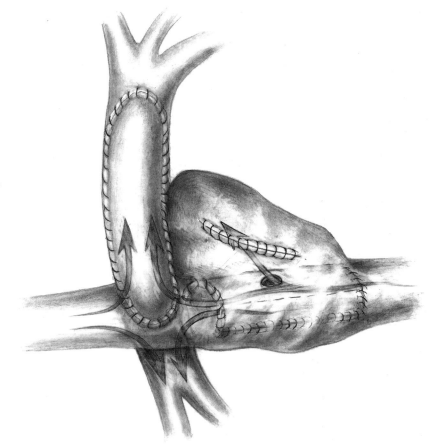

FIGURE 61.28. To avoid intra-atrial conduits, a connection can be made between the inferior vena cava and the pulmonary arteries with a tube graft of pulmonary or aortic allograft. The inferior and superior vena cavae are divided and the cardiac ends oversewn. The superior vena cava is anastomosed directly into the right pulmonary artery as standard bidirectional Glenn anastomosis. A tube graft of aorta or pulmonary allograft is used to connect between the divided inferior vena cava and the right pulmonary artery.

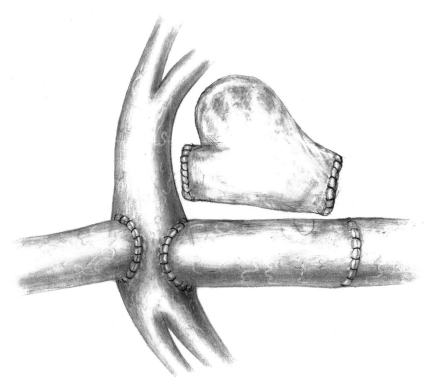

superior vena cava to the pulmonary artery either previously or at the time of the full Fontan.

References

1. Piggott JD, Murphy JD, Barber G, Norwood WI. Palliative reconstructive surgery for hypoplastic left heart syndrome. Ann Thorac Surg 1988;45: 122–128.
2. Norwood WI. Hypoplastic left heart syndrome. Ann Thorac Surg 1991;52:688–695.
3. Iannettoni MD, Bove EL, Mosca RS, Lupinetti FM, Dorostkar PC, Ludomirsky A, Crowley DC, Kulik TJ, Rosenthal A. Improving results with first-stage palliation for hypoplastic left heart syndrome. J Thorac Cardiovasc Surg 1994;107:934–940.
4. Weldner PW, Myers JL, Gleason MM, Cyran SE, Weber HS, White MG, Baylen BG. The Norwood operation and subsequent Fontan operation in infants with complex congenital heart disease. J Thorac Cardiovasc Surg 1995;109:654–662.
5. Jacobs ML, Rychik J, Murphy JD, Nicholson SC, Steven JM, Norwood WI. Results of Norwood's operation for lesions other than hypoplastic left heart syndrome. J Thorac Cardiovasc Surg 1995; 110:1555–1562.
6. van Son JAM, Reddy VM, Haas GS, Hanley FL. Modified surgical techniques for relief of aortic obstruction in [S,L,L] hearts with rudimentary right ventricle and restrictive bulboventricular foramen. J Thorac Cardiovasc Surg 1995;110: 909–915.
7. Carter TL, Mainwaring RD, Lamberti JJ. Damus-Kaye-Stansel procedure: midterm follow-up and technical considerations. Ann Thorac Surg 1994; 58:1603–1608.
8. Laks H, Gates RN, Elami A, Pearl JM. Damus-Stansel-Kaye procedure: Technical modifications. Ann Thorac Surg 1992;54:169–172.

62
Extracardiac Fontan Operation

Ed Petrossian, V. Mohan Reddy, and Frank L. Hanley

Introduction

Despite steady advances, persistent morbidity and mortality among patients with single ventricle physiology continued to stimulate congenital heart surgeons to devise new techniques and strategies to improve event-free survival. In the absence of a true anatomic repair, cure for these patients is unfortunately not an option. Physiologic repair, based on the Fontan principle of right heart bypass originally described in 1971,[1] consists of converting the parallel circulation to one that is series, with the single ventricle as the only power source. This approach provides the best long-term palliation for selected. Over the years numerous modifications of the Fontan operation have been proposed with the ultimate goal of improving functional results.[2-7] To our knowledge the extracardiac Fontan was originally described independently by Humes et al. and Nawa et al. in 1988.[8,9] Since 1992 we have used this operation as the technique of choice for physiologic correction of patients with single ventricle physiology.

Preoperative Strategy

An essential component of the extracardiac conduit Fontan circulation is a bidirectional superior cavopulmonary shunt. We prefer to perform this procedure prior to completion of the extracardiac conduit Fontan, as either a primary palliative procedure between 2 and 4 months of age,[10] or between 3 and 6 months following neonatal palliation with a systemic to pulmonary artery shunt or pulmonary artery banding.[11] In toddlers and older children who have been palliated earlier in life, we create a bidirectional cavopulmonary shunt prior to completion of the extracardiac Fontan in the majority of cases, though on occasion we will perform the cavopulmonary shunt during the same operation as Fontan construction.

After bidirectional superior cavopulmonary shunt, the patient is managed medically until he or she reaches a minimum weight of 15 kg (usually about 3 years of age). At this weight, the patient is large enough that an adult size conduit measuring 20 to 22 mm can be used for the extracardiac conduit without difficulty, thereby eliminating the need for reoperation as the patient grows by the time the patient is scheduled to undergo the extracardiac Fontan operation, every effort has been made to prepare the patient so the Fontan operation is limited simply to placement of the extracardiac conduit without additional procedures. The objective of this strategy is to minimize operative and cardiopulmonary bypass time, allowing for maximum preservation of pulmonary vascular and ventricular function in order to lower the potential for postoperative Fontan failure. This requires that other procedures (such as atrioventricular valve repair, relief of residual outflow tract arch obstruction, extensive pulmonary artery reconstruction or enlargement of an atrial septal defect) be performed prior to the extracardiac Fontan. In our experience, these can usually be conveniently performed at the time of the bidirectional Glenn shunt.

Operative Procedure

The operative plan for extracardiac Fontan centers on preservation of ventricular and pulmonary vascular function. Aortic cross-clamping and cardioplegic arrest are avoided. No active cooling is used and the operation is performed on a warm beating heart. The pump priming solution is supplemented with calcium to optimize cardiac function. Whenever possible, partial cardiopulmonary bypass with continued ventilation is used to maintain perfusion of the pulmonary circulation via the bidirectional Glenn shunt.

Through a standard median sternotomy, the ascending aorta, main and branch pulmonary arteries and superior and inferior venae cavae are dissected free using electrocautery to minimize postoperative bleeding. The diameter of the inferior vena cava is inspected and an aortic allograft conduit or non-ringed polytetrafluoroethylene tube of approximate size is selected. If a descending aortic allograft is to be used, care is taken to ensure that all intercostal arteries are ligated securely.

Following heparinization, the aorta and inferior and superior cavae are cannulated (Figure 62.1). To improve operative exposure, the inferior venous cannula is positioned as low as pos-

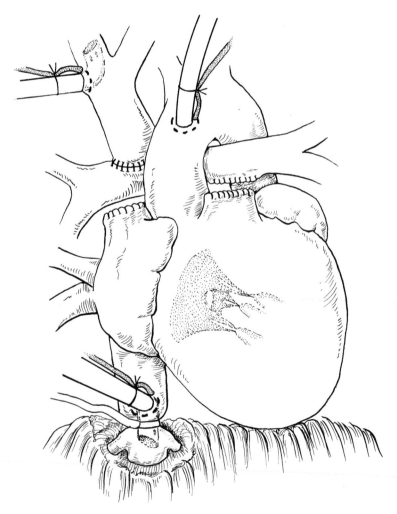

FIGURE 62.1. Extracardiac Fontan operation. Aorta and the inferior and superior venae cavae are cannulated. The inferior venous cannula is positioned as low as possible.

sible. To gain additional length on the inferior vena cava below the level of the diaphragm, we usually take down the pericardial reflection of the inferior vena cava using electrocautery and dissect the vessel to the level of the hepatic veins. A pursestring suture is placed immediately above the hepatic veins (Figure 62.1 inset). When cannulation of the superior vena cava is required, the cannula is placed as cephalad as possible at the junction of the innominate veins, or alternatively in the left innominate vein (Figure 62.1).

The patient is then placed on normothermic cardiopulmonary bypass. The superior vena cava is not connected to the circuit at this stage, allowing the superior cavopulmonary shunt to continue to perfuse the lungs. Mild to moder-

ate ventilation is maintained, allowing adequate operative exposure. The main pulmonary artery (if present) is divided and both ends are oversewn with running polypropylene suture. Two straight vascular clamps are placed across the inferior vena cava, one at the cavopulmonary junction, taking care to avoid injury to the coronary sinus and the right coronary artery (Figure 62.2), and the other just above the inferior caval cannula. The inferior vena cava is divided between the clamp and the cannula leaving sufficient length on the caudal segment to facilitate the subsequent anastomosis. The vessel is divided with a moderate bevel to allow for a non-stenotic anastomotic lumen. The cardiac stump of the inferior cava is oversewn in two layers with running polypropylene

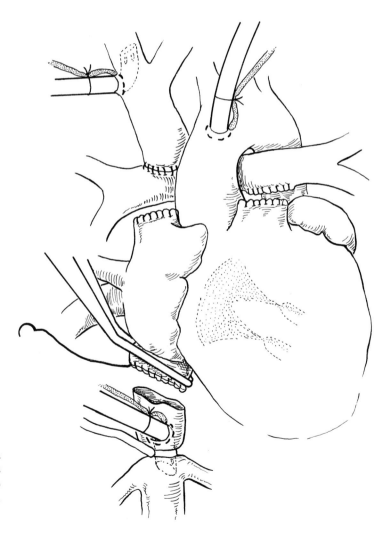

FIGURE 62.2. The inferior vena cava is divided above the venous return cannula. Care is taken to avoid injury to the coronary sinus and the right coronary artery.

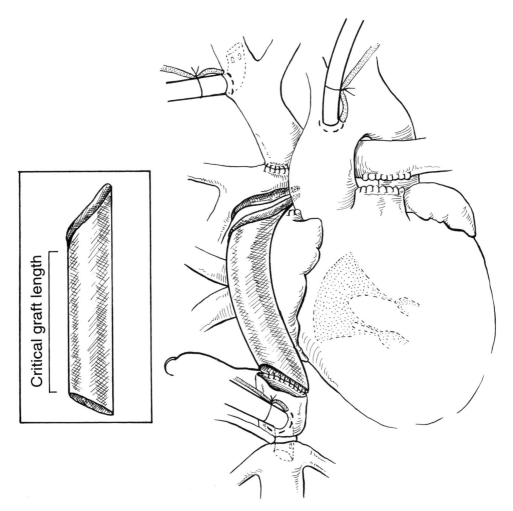

FIGURE 62.3. The incision in the pulmonary artery is made as long as possible, which allows for some offset of the superior and inferior cavopulmonary connections.

suture. The graft is cut with a similar bevel and anastomosed to the inferior vena cava with a single continuous polypropylene suture (Figure 62.3).

Following completion of the inferior vena caval anastomosis, the superior caval cannula is connected to the circuit, the patient is placed on full bypass, and the superior vena cava is clamped just below the cannula. A longitudinal incision is then made on the antero-inferior aspect of the right pulmonary artery. This incision is made as long as possible to allow unobstructed flow of inferior vena caval blood to both pulmonary arteries. It is started from a point just below the takeoff of the right upper lobe artery and carried centrally to the medial aspect of the superior cavopulmonary anastomosis (Figure 62.3). This arrangement allows for the superior and inferior cavopulmonary connections to be offset from one another, which has been shown to minimize flow turbulence and energy loss and to direct the larger inferior caval flow to the larger right lung (Figure 62.4).[12,13]

In selected patients, we have performed the inferior cavopulmonary anastomosis on partial cardiopulmonary bypass, without superior caval cannulation. With this technique, a large side-biting vascular clamp is placed on the undersurface of the right pulmonary artery,

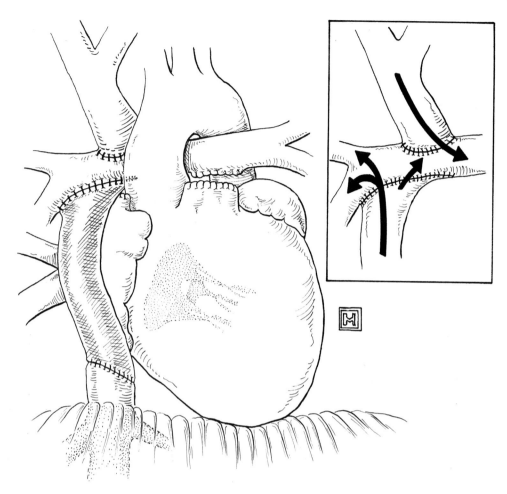

FIGURE 62.4. Completed suture lines for extracardiac Fontan.

allowing flow from the superior cavopulmonary anastomosis to continue unimpeded into the left pulmonary artery. This approach requires adequately large pulmonary arteries that the clamp can be placed without occluding the superior vena cava. In addition, superior caval cannulation is required if central or left pulmonary artery augmentation is required.

In the event that significant stenosis exists in the proximal right pulmonary artery, the pulmonary artery incision can be extended centrally under the aorta to include the stenotic area. This technique expedites the operation by avoiding the need for separate patch enlargement of stenotic areas. The graft is carefully measured and then cut with a long medial taper to accommodate the large right pulmonary artery incision. The length of the lateral aspect of the graft is most critical since it joins the right pulmonary artery nearly at a right angle and it is at risk of distorting the lateral corner of the anastomosis if the graft is not cut to just the right length (Figure 62.3 inset). The graft is also cut and positioned in such a fashion so as to give it a slight anterior and lateral curvature in order to avoid compression of the pulmonary venous drainage. The graft-right pulmonary artery anastomosis is then carried out in a similar fashion using a single circumferential suture line (Figure 62.4).

Before completion of the proximal anastomosis, the graft is de-aired by loosening the inferior vena caval snare. The position of the graft is carefully inspected with special attention to possible pulmonary artery distortion or pulmonary vein compression. Prior to discontinuation of bypass, catheters for monitoring pressure are placed in the extracardiac conduit via the inferior vena cava and in the common atrium via the right atrial appendage. The patient is then weaned from bypass on low dose dopamine.

If the systemic venous pressure following bypass is ≤18 mmHg with a transpulmonary gradient ≤10 mmHg, the patient is decannulated. If those pressure guidelines are not met, consideration is given to placing a fenestration between the conduit and the right atrial free wall. This can be performed without return to cardiopulmonary bypass by anastomosing the extracardiac conduit to the right atrium in a side to side fashion with the aid of partial occlusion vascular clamps. Alternatively, a 4–5 mm polytetrafluoroethylene tube graft can be anastomosed between the right atrium and the conduit,[14] and an adjustable snare can be used to occlude the shunt postoperatively in a manner similar to the method described by Laks.[7]

UCSF Experience

Between October 1990 and October 1996, 59 patients underwent an extracardiac conduit Fontan operation. Median age was 5.7 years (1.5 to 44 years) and median weight was 17 kg (10–70 kg). Eight of the 59 patients had previously undergone an atriopulmonary or atrioventricular Fontan at an outside institution and subsequently presented 8 to 20 years later with complications related to the original operation.[15] In these patients, the previous Fontan connection was taken down and replaced with an extracardiac conduit.

In the majority of the patients (83%), a non-ringed polytetrafluoroethylene graft was used to complete the extracardiac Fontan. In 8 patients, a cryopreserved descending aortic allograft was used, and direct anastomosis between the main pulmonary artery and the inferior vena cava was performed in 2 patients with L-transposition of the great arteries. The median conduit size was 20 mm (range 16–

25 mm) and was similar among patients with synthetic and allograft conduits. The smallest allograft conduit used was 18 mm and the largest was 25 mm.

There was one early death and another five months after surgery. The early death was a patient who underwent revision of a failing atriopulmonary Fontan. Follow-up was available at a median of 2 years postoperatively, with 92% of patients in New York Heart Association functional class I (70%) or II (22%). Five patients (12%) had new persistent early postoperative arrhythmia or conduction block and four patients (10%) had transient abnormalities. Fontan failure occurred in one patient, in whom the Fontan was taken down to a cavopulmonary shunt.

Comparison to Other Fontan Techniques

A persistent source of postoperative morbidity and mortality following the Fontan operation has been supraventricular arrhythmias. The reported overall incidence of early and late postoperative atrial tachyarrhythmias following various Fontan techniques has ranged from 5–32%.[16–20] Four primary factors are important potential contributors to atrial arrhythmias and sinus node dysfunction: 1) exposure of the right atrium to the elevated post-Fontan systemic venous pressure with subsequent atrial dilatation and hypertrophy, 2) extensive atrial incisions and suture lines, 3) surgery in the vicinity of the sinus node, and 4) poor ventricular function. In contrast to the lateral tunnel Fontan, the extracardiac Fontan operation excludes the right atrium from the systemic venous circulation entirely and is only exposed to the low pressure pulmonary venous circulation. In the absence of ventricular dysfunction or valvar regurgitation, elevated atrial pressures are avoided. The extracardiac Fontan also has the advantage of completely avoiding atrial suture lines and surgery in the vicinity of the sinus node. Finally, the extracardiac conduit Fontan operation is performed on a warm beating heart so that ischemic arrest and its deleterious effects on ventricular function are avoided. We believe that the combination of these factors contributes to the low incidence of postoperative arrhythmias in our experience.

In a modification of the lateral tunnel technique, an intra-atrial conduit Fontan has also been described.[8] This requires reduced atrial suturing relative to the lateral tunnel technique, as it requires anastomotic suture lines only around the orifices of the inferior and superior venae cavae. However, this is still a significant suture load, and it also requires an atriotomy incision and cardiac ischemic arrest. Another recent modification of the lateral wall technique involves placement of an incomplete conduit in an epicardial location to connect the inferior vena cava to the pulmonary artery.[21] This is essentially the mirror image of the lateral wall technique with the "baffle" on the outer aspect of the atrium. While an atriotomy incision is avoided, this operation involves extensive atrial suture lines, albeit epicardial in location, with some of the suture lines in the vicinity of the sinus node. Aside from its growth potential advantage, the main feature of this operation that is shared by the extracardiac Fontan is that it can be accomplished without arresting the heart.

Potential disadvantages of the extracardiac Fontan operation include the lack of growth potential, the risk of conduit obstruction secondary to neointimal peel formation, and the risk of thromboembolism. Lack of growth potential of the conduit theoretically puts the patient at risk for reoperation as the patient's increasing cardiac output outstrips the conduit diameter. By performing the extracardiac conduit Fontan when the patient is ≥15 kg in weight, it is possible to use a conduit measuring 20–22 mm in diameter. A conduit of this size should accommodate the patient's future growth and exercise demands. In our experience with the extracardiac Fontan there have been no cases of conduit obstruction. However, we do recommend close monitoring of these patients with frequent echocardiography or magnetic resonance imaging, especially in symptomatic patients. We believe that the use of allografts or expanded polytetrafluoroethylene tubes, rather than Dacron, will reduce or eliminate progressive conduit obstruction due to pseudointimal peel formation.

The risk of postoperative thromboembolism has been reported to be 18–20% in patients undergoing various types of Fontan operation. The high incidence of thromboembolic events, regardless of technique, points to the possibility of an underlying hypercoagulable state in the post-Fontan circulation. In view of this elevated incidence of thromboembolic complications, our patients are currently discharged from the hospital on chronic acetylsalicylic acid and a three month course on warfarin. With this management strategy, there have been no cases of thromboembolism among our patients and no significant complications from anticoagulation or antiplatelet therapy. Until more is known about the post-Fontan hypercoagulable state, it seems prudent to us to recommend this regimen.

References

1. Fontan F, Baudet E. Surgical repair of tricuspid atresia. Thorax 1971;26:240–246.
2. Kirklin JW, Barratt-Boyes BG. Tricuspid atresia and the Fontan operation. In New York: Churchill Livingstone 1993:1055–1104.
3. Kreutzer GO, Galindez E, Bono H, et al. An operation for the correction of tricuspid atresia. J Thorac Cardiovasc Surg 1973;66:613–621.
4. Fontan F, Kirklin JW, Fernandez D, et al. Outcome after a "perfect" Fontan operation. Circulation 1990;81:1520–1536.
5. Driscoll DJ, Offord KP, Feldt RH, et al. Five to fifteen year follow up after Fontan operation. Circulation 1992;85:469–496.
6. De Leval MR, Kilner P, Gewillig M, et al. Total cavopulmonary connection: a logical alternative to atriopulmonary connection for complex Fontan operations. J Thorac Cardiovasc Surg 1988;96:682–695.
7. Laks H, Pearl JM, Haas GS, et al. Partial Fontan: advantages of an adjustable interatrial communication. Ann Thorac Surg 1991;52:1084–1095.
8. Humes RA, Feldt RH, Porter CJ, et al. The modified Fontan operation for asplenia and polysplenia syndromes. J Thorac Cardiovasc Surg 1988;96:212–218.
9. Nawa S, Teramoto S. New extension of the fontan principle: inferior vena cava-pulmonary

artery bridge operation. Thorax 1988;43:1022–1023.

10. Reddy VM, Liddicoat JR, Hanley FL. Primary bidirectional superior cavopulmonary shunt in infants between 1 and 4 months of age. Ann Thorac Surg 1995;59:1120–1126.

11. Reddy VM, McElhinney DB, Moore P, Haas GS, Hanley FL. Outcomes after bidirectional cavopulmonary shunt in infants less than 6 months old. J Am Coll Cardiol 1997;29:1365–1370.

12. Van Haesdonck J, Mertens L, Sizaire R, et al. Comparison by computerized numeric modeling of energy losses in different Fontan connections. Circulation 1995;92 [suppl II]:II-322–II-326.

13. Barratt-Boyes BG. Clinical experience with the zero-pressure-fixed Medtronic Intact bioprosthetic valve. EJCTS 1992;6:s79–281.

14. Black MD, van Son JAM, Haas GS. Extracardiac Fontan operation with adjustable communication. Ann Thorac Surg 1995;60:716–718.

15. McElhinney DB, Reddy VM, Moore P, et al. Revision of previous Fontan connections to extracardiac or intra-atrial conduit cavopulmonary anastomosis. Ann Thorac Surg 1996;62:1276–1283.

16. Balaji S, Gewillig M, Bull C, et al. Arryhthmias after Fontan prodecure: comparison of total cavopulmonary connection and atriopulmonary connection. Circulation 1991;84 [suppl III]:III-162–III-167.

17. Peters NS, Somerville J. Arrhthmias after the Fontan procedure. Br Heart J 1992;68:199–204.

18. Kurer CC, Tanner CS, Vetter VA. Electrophysiologic findings after Fontan repair of functional single ventricle. J Am Coll Cardiol 1991;17:174–181.

19. Cromme-Dijkhuis AH, Hess J, Hahlen K, et al. Specific sequelae after Fontan operations at mid and long term follow-up. J Thorac Cardiovasc Surg 1993;106:1126–1132.

20. Gelatt M, Hamilton RM, McCrindle BW, et al. Risk factors for atrial tachyarrhythmias after the Fontan operation. J Am Coll Cardiol 1994;24:1735–1741.

21. Laschinger JC, Ringel RE, Brenner JI, et al. The extracardiac total cavopulmonary connection for definitive conversion to the Fontan circulation: a summary of early experience and results. J Card Surg 1993;8:524–533.

Section XIII
Future Directions

63
FDA Regulatory Policy

Scott Bottenfield and Margaret Deuel

Advances in medical research in recent years have led to the use of human allograft tissue for the replacement or repair of diseased or injured tissues. Tissue banks exist for the purpose of facilitating this process and are an integral part of providing this health care service. A tissue bank is defined as an organization that recovers, processes, stores, and/or distributes tissues for clinical transplantation.[1] Tissue banking encompasses a wide array of tissues, and the scope of activities pursued by various tissue banking organizations is broad and varied. As the field of tissue banking grows, the need for adequate oversight of the activities of tissue banking has emerged.

Until recently, tissue banking was performed without the oversight of the federal government. Although voluntary compliance with national standards-setting organizations like the American Association of Tissue Banks (AATB) has been encouraged, and pursued by the allograft heart valve banking community, federal regulations have been imposed on allografts which are similar to medical devices used for comparable purposes. This review addresses the current status of federal oversight for human allograft tissue heart valves, and reviews the historical developments of such regulations.

A Brief History of Tissue Banking

Although tissue transplantation has been described as early as the 17th century,[2] the establishment of the United States Navy Tissue Bank in Bethesda, Maryland in 1949 marked the emergence of the modern tissue bank. The formation of the U.S. Navy Tissue Bank was a result of the need to recover and preserve tissues to be used both at the battle front, and at home to facilitate the recovery of traumatically injured servicemen. Furthermore, the Navy Tissue Bank sought to advance the science of tissue banking through ambitious research programs. These programs, pioneered by noted researchers and clinicians, have added a significant amount of knowledge to the field and have led many to accept tissue transplantation as a legitimate treatment method.

The initial clinical use of human heart valve allografts for reconstruction of ventricular outflow tracts was reported in the early 1960s.[3] Since then, technological advances and the emergence of cryopreservation techniques have led to the use of allografts as a superior alternative to the use of xenografts or mechanical prostheses for certain surgical repairs of defective or diseased hearts. The advantages of human valve allografts are well known, and include a superior record of mortality and morbidity in children, optimal hydraulic function resulting in minimal pressure gradients and central non-obstructive flow, as well as freedom from thromboembolism and hemolysis.[4,5]

As the use of allograft tissue as an accepted treatment modality gained popularity, the demand for such tissue has increased. This increased demand has been the impetus for the formation and evolution of tissue banking organizations. Today, tissue banks differ in size, scope, and service area, ranging from hospital-based services to large, regional organ and multi-tissue banking organizations.[6]

Regional tissue banks are usually established as nonprofit organizations, whether part of a hospital, university, or as an independent organization, to satisfy the need for allograft tissue, as well as to provide a mechanism for the donation of cadaveric human tissues. Large regional tissue banks may be part of the local organ procurement organization (OPO) or they may work in close cooperation with the local OPO, relying primarily on tissue donations from the next-of-kin of cadaveric donors. These tissue banks usually supply many different types of allograft tissues to local and regional health care institutions, and practitioners. The banking methodologies employed by large regional tissue banks are diverse and complex. Many different types of preservation techniques are utilized, based on the tissues being preserved as well as the needs of the clinicians within the tissue bank's service area.

Recently, the tissue banking/transplant community has witnessed the establishment of commercial tissue banking organizations. Although the National Organ Transplantation Act of 1984 (PL 98-507) prohibits the sale of human organs and tissues, tissue banks are allowed to charge for the services they render. It is generally held that the performance of tissue banking activities is a service intended not for the benefit of the organizations or personnel performing the task, but rather for the benefit of both the donating individual and the recipients of the graft material.

American Association of Tissue Banks

The American Association of Tissue Banks is a scientific, not-for-profit, peer group organization founded in 1976 to facilitate the provision of transplantable tissues of uniform high quality in quantities sufficient to meet national needs. AATB publishes the **Standards for Tissue Banking**[1] to ensure that the conduct of tissue banking meets acceptable norms of technical and ethical performance. The American Association of Tissue Banks established these Standards in 1984. Although voluntary, compliance with the **Standards for Tissue Banking** ensures all activities related to the collection, processing, storage, and distribution of human tissues are carried out in a safe and professional manner.

Among the Association's accomplishments in its continued evolution, is the establishment of a constructive dialogue with the U.S. Food and Drug Administration (FDA), and the formal training and certification of tissue bank technical specialists. In addition, AATB carries out a program of inspection and accreditation, established in 1986, to ensure that tissue banking activities are being performed in a professional manner consistent with the Standards of the Association. Based upon the Standards and procedures developed by the Association, desiring tissue banks may receive accreditation for retrieval, processing, storage, and distribution of tissues, following a rigorous inspection of operations.

A Brief History of Federal Regulatory Efforts

The Medical Device Amendments of 1976, with broad sweeping implications for all medical devices manufactured and sold in the U.S., were not written with allograft tissue in mind. However, these regulations have come to affect several types of allograft tissue currently banked in this country, including cryopreserved allograft heart valves. Although the U.S. Food and Drug Administration has involved itself in the tissue banking community for many years, this involvement was limited to one of monitoring the activities of tissue banking, and engaging in dialogue with the tissue banking community.

This passive role changed when the FDA's Center for Devices and Radiological Health (CDRH), announced a meeting to be held in June, 1990 for the purpose of engaging the tissue banks in dialogue related to the regulation of heart valve allografts as a medical device. This meeting, attended by heart valve processors, FDA staffers, and AATB representatives, established the fact that the FDA would require the processors of allograft heart valves to submit substantial data intended to support the continued distribution and use of allograft heart valves. Two documents were discussed during this meeting. The first, dated May 1, 1990, is entitled "Replacement Heart Valves-Guidance for Data to be Submitted to the Food and Drug Administration in Support of Applications for Premarket Approval (Draft Version)." It presents requirements for the types of data to be submitted for premarket approval for mechanical or biological heart valves introduced into interstate commerce after the enactment of the 1976 Medical Device Amendments to the Food, Drug and Cosmetic Act. The second document, an outline guidance for human heart valve allografts, was written for the purpose of developing a comprehensive guidance concerning the information necessary to submit to the FDA for the market clearance of allograft heart valves. The unique nature of heart valve allografts was discussed, and the difficulties in comparing human origin heart valves to manufactured mechanical or biological heart valves was brought to light. By meeting's end, it was apparent that allograft processors would be required to submit data, substantially equivalent to a Premarket Approval Application (PMA), including clinical data, in order to continue to distribute allograft heart valves for patient use. It also became apparent during the summer of 1990 that the FDA intended to regulate allograft heart valves in the same manner that the agency regulates all other replacement heart valves; as Class III medical devices.

The FDA held a subsequent meeting to discuss the regulation of allograft heart valves on August 20, 1990 with the convening of the FDA's Circulatory System Devices Panel. The purpose of this meeting was to further discussions regarding proposed regulation, as well as to review a draft guidance document for this regulation, entitled "Preliminary Draft Guidance for the Submission of PMA Applications to FDA for Heart Valve Allografts" (Dated August 8, 1990). This document explains and supplements the requirements of the regulation "Premarket Approval of Medical Devices".[7] During the panel meeting, several experienced and prominent cardiothoracic surgeons presented data related to allograft use. The allograft's unique niche in valve replacement and outflow tract repair was emphasized, as well as the fact that allografts had been successfully used for over twenty years in the absence of federal regulation. Regardless of these presentations, it was apparent that the FDA had made its decision to regulate allograft heart valves within the strictest medical device category.

The FDA classifies medical devices according to the attendant risk associated with their use. A Class III medical device is a designation given by the FDA to indicate medical devices that are considered to carry with them, the highest risk to the patient, should they fail. Mechanical and bioprosthetic heart valves fall into this category, as determined by regulations promulgated by the FDA during the 1980s.[8,9] Under the regulatory scheme of a Class III device, a manufacturer is expected to submit data to the FDA indicating that the device is both safe and effective for the mitigation or treatment of disease. Normally, data is generated from preclinical *in vitro* studies as well as clinical trial data generated from the use of the device under an Investigational Device Exemption (IDE). Clinical studies conducted under IDEs are usually carried out by a limited number of centers over several years to accumulate enough data to support the claim of safety and effectiveness. Investigational Device Exemption applications include all aspects of manufacturing, labeling, distribution, preclinical data and clinical study design. Once approved by the FDA, the manufacturer is free to distribute the investigational device under the auspices of the protocol outlined in the IDE application. This regulatory scheme posed many unique challenges to the allograft heart valve processors, including the enormous financial burden required to successfully comply with the regulations.

In preparation to bear the burden of the regulatory pressures, six nonprofit heart valve processors, LifeNet, American Red Cross, University of Chicago Cryolab, Oregon Tissue Bank, Alabama Tissue Center at the University of Alabama, Birmingham, and Northwest Tissue Center, formed a consortium in the fall of 1990. The purpose of this consortium was to seek legal and regulatory advice concerning compliance, and to navigate the unknown waters of FDA regulation. In September, 1990, the nonprofit heart valve consortium met with a representative of the FDA to begin the process of education with regard to the many issues of federal regulatory compliance.

Shortly after the issue of a final draft guidance document for heart valve allografts in June, 1991, the FDA issued a "Notice of Applicability of a Final Rule" (NAFR),[10] informing tissue banks that allograft heart valves were indeed subject to the regulations issued in the 1980s governing all replacement heart valves. In order for allograft heart valve processors to continue distributing heart valves, they were required to have an approved PMA application by August 26, 1991. Since none of the processors had sufficient data to submit a PMA application, all were expected to support an IDE application within the allotted time. Through the assistance of legal counsel and some Congressional support, several requests for filing extensions were granted, postponing the final required submission date until June, 30, 1992. These extensions allowed the nonprofit heart valve consortium time to compile the lengthy IDE submission in order to fulfill regulatory requirements. The nonprofit heart valve consortium, with advice and consent of the FDA, filed a joint IDE application (IDE# G910145P). This necessitated an intense examination of the intricacies of each members' tissue procurement and processing methods, and cooperation to develop identical procedures needed to

compare data generated following the implantation of each members' valves. Once received and approved by the FDA's Office of Device Evaluation, the clinical study outlined in the consortium's Investigational Device Exemption application began in earnest on September 18, 1992. Although the consortium made every effort to comply with federal regulations, the statutory authority to regulate allograft heart valves, as well as the timing and administrative procedures in imposing these regulations on allograft heart valve processors continued to be questioned by the consortium.

Litigation

On July 25, 1991, at the same time the tissue banks were preparing for the rigors of an IDE application and the resultant clinical trial, the consortium filed a petition in the United States Court of Appeals for the Seventh Circuit seeking review of the NAFR published in the Federal Register on June 26, 1991.[10] While awaiting the Seventh Circuit Court's decision, the heart valve processors simultaneously filed suit in the United States District Court, again challenging the NAFR for reasons similar to those presented in the Court of Appeals. On that same day, the tissue banks also filed a motion with the Court of Appeals seeking an order to stay any action by the FDA pending the court's decision on their petition. On November 12, 1991, the Court of Appeals denied the motion to stay FDA action, concluding that the NAFR was a permissible interpretation of the regulations. But, on December 12, 1991, the District Court granted the request to stay pending resolution of the action before the Court of Appeals.

Following dismissal of the petition in the Seventh Circuit Court, the consortium pursued their suit in the District Court.[9] They claimed: 1) the FDA did not have the authority to regulate the distribution of human heart valves under the Food, Drug and Cosmetic Act; 2) the FDA's attempt to require premarket approval of allografts under the 1980 and 1987 regulations violated the procedural requirements of the Food, Drug and Cosmetic Act; and 3) the

FDA denied the banks the opportunity to comment on the 1980 and 1987 regulations, which was in violation of the Administrative Procedures Act and the Food, Drug and Cosmetic Act. Nothing in the regulations or administrative record provided notice that the regulations would apply to allograft heart valves. These claims were subsequently dismissed in the District Court. Two of the tissue banks in the consortium appealed the decision. The other banks decided to forge ahead and collect the required PMA data in an effort to obtain valuable clinical information for all parties involved.

As a result of the appeal, The United States District Court for the Northern District of Illinois accepted a settlement of this litigation, in which the FDA agreed to rescind its premarket approval requirements for allograft heart valves. On October 14, 1994, approximately two years after the IDE went into effect, the FDA published its rescission of the NAFR in the Federal Register.[11] Their intent was to begin initiating procedures for the purpose of placing these valves into a Class II device category with the establishment of "special controls" to ensure safety and effectiveness.

Federal Oversight of Tissue Banking

Until late 1993, the federal regulatory efforts aimed at human tissue only incorporated a small amount of the total tissue donated and distributed in the country. With the publication of what is called the "Interim Rule for Banked Human Tissue" in December of 1993, FDA made its most ambitious foray into the transplant community. The stated intention of this rule is to ". . . require certain infectious disease testing, donor screening, and record keeping to help prevent the transmission of AIDS and hepatitis through human tissue used in transplantation."[12] This regulation became effective December 14, 1993, and while it encompasses all human tissue, it specifically exempts tissues currently regulated under other regulatory schemes, including allograft heart valves. This regulation was promulgated under the author-

ity granted by section 361 of the Public Health Service Act (42 U.S.C. 264), which authorizes the Secretary of Health and Human Services to make and enforce such regulations as are deemed necessary to prevent the spread of communicable disease. The invocation of section 361 is usually reserved for crisis situations, where the spread of communicable disease is imminent. Allograft tissues have enjoyed a remarkably safe use for decades, with the rate of disease transmission far less than that of blood transfusions. However, the FDA discovered through undercover investigations, that human tissue was being made available from sources outside the U.S., that did not meet minimal screening standards for the transmission of infectious agents. Although the FDA admitted that these instances did not represent the practices of most tissue banks in this country, it felt it was necessary to promulgate these regulations.

Following the publication of the interim rule, several guidance documents have been circulated giving interpretative guidance to FDA compliance officers and the tissue banking community. The FDA published its "Final Rule for Human Tissue Intended for Transplantation" on July 29, 1997, which amends CFR part 1270, clarifies sections originally published in the 1993 publication, and provides additional guidance for industry.[13] This "Final Rule" became effective for human tissues procured on or after January 26, 1998. A new guidance document accompanied the "Final Rule" entitled "Guidance for Industry; Screening and Testing of Donors of Human Tissue Intended for Transplantation." This, the Agency's most ambitious and complete guidance document is the product of more than three years of interface and communication with the tissue banking community.

The FDA established a special office, the Human Tissue Program within the Office for Blood Research and Review of the Center for Biologics Evaluation and Research (CBER) to monitor tissue banking activities. CBER is one of the FDA centers responsible for regulating biologic products such as therapeutics, vaccines, blood, and blood products. The mission of the Human Tissue Program, established in 1995, is to develop and coordinate policy, and to provide scientific review of issues and findings to assure that tissue of human origin meets all requirements as defined in the regulations for banked human tissue.

Although the human tissue regulations and accompanying guidance documents do not specifically apply to allograft heart valves, it is quite difficult to separate the donor screening, testing, and record keeping requirements from other human tissue in programs that bank multiple tissues. In fact, all of the nonprofit heart valve processors also bank other tissues, such as musculoskeletal tissues. Since many donors of heart valves are also donors of other tissues, the application of different regulatory requirements for each tissue has resulted in an untenable system for most tissue banks. The result has been an awkward regulatory scheme for allograft heart valves, which encompasses both medical device law and the regulations for banked human tissue.

The Future of Regulation

The future of federal regulatory oversight of heart valve allografts is uncertain at this writing. Since the Federal Register publication of October 14, 1994, rescinding the enforcement of the IDE, little progress has been made to resolve issues regarding the regulation of allograft heart valves. A meeting of the Circulatory System Devices Panel scheduled for August, 1995 for the purpose of classifying allograft heart valves, has been indefinitely postponed. In October, 1995, a FDA conference was held to discuss the development of "special controls" under Class II medical device regulations which may be appropriate for allograft heart valves, should they be placed in Class II. It is interesting to note that the FDA's proposed special controls include issues traditionally out of the scope of medical device regulation, including adherence to the interim rule for banked human tissue, and infectious disease screening criteria found in blood banking regulations.

On February 28, 1997, the FDA published a proposed regulatory scheme for human tissue, entitled "A Proposed Approach to the Regulation of Cellular and Tissue-Based Products."[13] The new regulatory framework as proposed in this document, is intended to provide a unified approach to the regulation of both traditional and new products. In addition, this proposed approach would provide only the degree of government oversight thought necessary to protect the public health. It is interesting to note that this proposal calls for the reclassification of allograft heart valves, moving them from the medical device regulations to those of traditional banked human tissue. The implementation of this regulatory scheme is currently underway and anticipated to be fully implemented by early in the twenty-first century. The first steps in the proposed regulatory approach were carried out when the FDA published three proposed rules, covering establishment registration in 1998,[14] donor suitability in 1999,[15] and good tissue practices in 2001.[16] To-date, only the registration rule[17] has been finalized.

Summary

Presently, heart valve allografts, and the processors and distributors of these medical products are subject to the general controls applicable to all medical devices, including the requirements of premarket notification, quality systems regulations, and FDA inspection. The regulatory fate ought to be consistent with the regulation of other allograft tissue. Regardless of all of the activity in CDRH, the speculation that allograft heart valves may be moved to CBER, and regulated under the auspices of the Human Tissue Program is encouraging. In the interim, allograft heart valves, having survived the initial onslaught of federal regulatory pressure, continue to be made available for patients in need. Although the experience of the past ten years has at times been overwhelming for the providers of these needed medical products, and has no doubt contributed to the elimination of some tissue banking programs, the education gained from the experience has enabled the remaining tissue banks to successfully face the impact of future regulatory efforts.

References

1. American Association of Tissue Banks. Standards for Tissue Banking. 2001. Arlington, Virginia, AATB.
2. Burchardt H, Enneking WF. Transplantation of bone. Surg Clin North Am 1978;58:403–427.
3. Ross DN. Homograft replacement of the aortic valve. Lancet 1962;2:487.
4. Lefrak EA, Starr A. Aortic valve homograft. In Cardiac Valve Prosthesis. New York: Appleton-Century-Crofts 1979:283–300.
5. Villani M, Bianchi T, Vanini V, et al. Bioprosthetic valve replacement in children. In Cohn L, Gallucci V (eds). Cardiac Bioprostheses. New York: Yorke Medical Books 1982:248–255.
6. Friedlaendar GE. Bone banking in support of reconstructive surgery of the hip. Clin Orthop 1987;225:17–21.
7. 51 Federal Register. Code of Federal Regulations. Title 21, Parts 16 and 814. 1986. 26364.
8. 45 Federal Register. Code of Federal Regulations. Title 21, Part 870. 1980. 7948.
9. Alabama Tissue Center of the University of Alabama Health Services Foundation, PC et al. versus Louis Sullivan, Secretary of the United States Department of Health and Human Services et al. [Docket # 91 C 6515]. 2003. District Court for Northern District of Illinois, Eastern Division.
10. 56 Federal Register. Code of Federal Regulations. Title 21, Part 812. 1991. 29177.
11. 59 Federal Register. Code of Federal Regulations. Title 21, Part 812. 1994. 52078.
12. 58 Federal Register. Code of Federal Regulations. Title 21, Parts 16 and 1270. 1993. 65514.
13. 62 Federal Register. Code of Federal Regulations. Title 21. 1997. 9721.
14. 63 Federal Register. Code of Federal Regulations. Title 21, Parts 207, 807 and 1271. 1998. 26744.
15. 64 Federal Register. Code of Federal Regulations. Title 21, Part 210, 211, 829 and 1271. 1999. 52696.
16. 66 Federal Register. Code of Federal Regulations. Title 21, Part 1271. 2001. 1508.
17. 66 Federal Register. Code of Federal Regulations. Title 21, Parts 207, 807 and 1271. 2001. 5447.

64
The Biological Valve Spectrum and a Rationale for Prosthetic Valve Choice

Richard A. Hopkins, R. Eric Lilly, and James St. Louis

There is a broad spectrum of biological valves available for use in patients. These valves offer the advantage of decreased need for anticoagulation, decreased incidence of thromboembolism and with variable hemodynamic performance. The spectrum ranges from porcine prostheses, modified orifice porcine prostheses, bovine pericardial valves, fresh and cryopreserved homografts, and stentless xenografts. All of these have been discussed in previous chapters, but a synopsis of each currently available prosthesis and their characteristics are defined below.

Choice of Valvular Prosthesis

Since the initial placement of a prosthetic device by Hufnagel in 1953,[1] a wide variety of valvular prostheses have become available for native valve replacement. The evolution of valvular surgery, from the original Starr-Edwards mechanical prosthesis to the commonly used St. Jude Medical and Carpentier-Edwards Pericardial bioprosthesis, has produced a plethora of technology. Valvular reconstruction and auto-replacement has become exceedingly popular over the last decade, but prosthetic valve replacement still remains the most reliable and only alternative to severely diseased cardiac valves. The choice of which valve prosthesis to employ requires individualization to specific patient needs and limitations. Particular characteristics which must be considered include patient age, activity status, ability to self medicate, geographical area, opportunity for follow-up, social situation, life expectancy, and contraindication to anticoagulation. Specific valve characteristics to be considered include durability, thrombogenicity, hemodynamics, performance, availability, failure modes and cost.

Valvular prostheses can be broadly classified into either mechanical or biological. Mechanical prostheses generally have a greater longevity than biological prostheses, but have the disadvantage of requiring long-term anticoagulation. Warfarin therapy is commonly employed, with a goal of prothrombin ratio of 1.5 to 2.0 (INR 2.0 to 2.5) times normal for aortic position. Anticoagulation with warfarin carries a mortality rate of 0.2% per patient-year and a 2–3% per patient-year of anticoagulant-related hemorrhage. Bioprosthetic valves have the advantage of not requiring anticoagulation, although their are inferior long-term durability makes them a poor choice in certain populations.

Randomized studies over the last two decades have chronicled the disadvantages and advantages of mechanical and biological valve prostheses. The Veterans Affairs Cooperative Study reported no difference between mechanical and biological prostheses in patient survival or in the incidence of thromboembolic events at 11 years.[2] Mechanical valves had a higher incidence of hemorrhage whereas biological valves had a higher incidence of reoperation. The purpose of the present review is to summarize selected *in vitro* studies and provide an overview of certain valve characteristics.

Mechanical Valve Prostheses

Starr-Edwards Valve

St. Jude Valve

Medtronic-Hall Valve

The Medtronic-Hall valve is a pyrolytic carbon and metal single tilting disk prosthesis first implanted in 1977 and now available in 20mm to 31mm sizes.[3] The valve has a unique design with the disk centrally positioned resulting in an enlarged orifice. This enlargement reduces the stagnation and turbulence of blood in this area. Ten year data reveals a low incidence of thromboembolic events and a 100% freedom from prosthetic dysfunction.[4-6]

Björk-Shiley Valve

The Björk-Shiley valve is a single tilting disk mechanical prosthesis first implanted in the aortic position in 1969.[7] Since then, it is estimated that nearly 24,000 of these valves were implanted in patients worldwide, with as many as 7,000 presently living with the valve in place.[8] This valve was removed from the market in 1986 because of reports of strut fracture in certain models. A review of the valve's performance in 785 patients over a 15 year period revealed no structural deterioration, but valve thrombosis was observed at a rate of 0.36% per patient-year.[9,10] Prophylactic valve replacement is only indicated in certain models released in Europe only.[11]

Carbomedics Valve

The Carbomedics valve is a pyrolytic carbon bileaflet valve which was first marketed in 1986. Its design allows rotation of the valve within the sewing ring for optimal orientation of the prosthesis during implantation. The design also protects against deformity of the sewing ring which can result in leaflet binding. Early data reveals 100% freedom from prosthetic failure and 92% freedom from thromboembolic events.[12]

Omniscience and Omnicarbon Valve

The Omniscience valve is constructed of a pyrolytic carbon tilting disk seated in a metal housing. This valve became available in 1978 in 19mm and 31mm sizes. Freedom from structural dysfunction of the Omniscience has been reported as 100% at 9 years.[13] Reports of somewhat higher rates of thromboembolic events at five year follow-up led to the development of the Omnicarbon valve.[14] The Omnicarbon is an improved version of the Omniscience valve, modified with the purpose of improving antithrombotic characteristics by changing the housing material to pyrolytic carbon and shortening the pivot to form a low profile. Four year follow-up with this valve reports a freedom from thromboembolic complications of 96%.[13]

Biological Valve Prostheses

Carpentier-Edwards Porcine Valve

The standard Carpentier-Edwards model 2625 porcine valve became available in 1975[15] and was followed in 1982 by the supra-annular model, which incorporated low pressure fixation and slight modification of the sewing ring and stent.[16] The second generation CE porcine bioprosthesis provides improved tissue preservation and reduced failure from structural valve deterioration.[17] The porcine tissue of the second generation prosthesis is fixed with glutaraldehyde at 2mm HQ and treated with polysorbate 80, an antimineralization surfactant. Although significant advances have occurred over that last two decades, but long-term durability continues to be the main disadvantage.[18-20] In a review of 2,444 patients receiving a second generation CE porcine valve, freedom from structural valve deterioration at 10 years was $90 \pm 2\%$ but fell to $82 \pm 6\%$ at 12 years.[21] First generation CE porcine valves have an overall freedom from valve deterioration of 29% at 17 years.[16] Multiple long-term studies have shown that age and valve position play a significant role in valve durability.[22,23] Jamieson showed that freedom from valve deterioration at 10 years in the age group between 36 to 50 years was 85 ± 6%, but increased to 99 ± 1% in the group 70 years and older.[21]

Hancock II Porcine Valve

The Hancock II bioprosthesis is a second generation porcine aortic valve manufactured by Medtronic. The valve is fixed in glutaraldehyde at low pressure and chemically treated with sodium dodecyl sulfate to retard calcification. It mounted on a low profile Delrin stent and designed for supra-annular implantation. A review of 843 patients over a 10 year period reveal a freedom from valve failure of 92%, but the freedom from thromboembolic complications was only 80% in the aortic position.[24]

Medtronic Intact Porcine Valve

The Medtronic Intact porcine xenograft was introduced into the market in 1984 and is the first zero-pressure glutaraldehyde-fixed valve.[25] The prosthesis is treated with the anticalcification agents toluidine blue and has an intra-annular configuration similar to that of the first-generation porcine bioprosthesis. Reported data at seven years reveals a freedom from structural valve deterioration of 97%.[26,27] Long-term durability remains to be defined.

Carpentier-Edwards Pericardial Valve

The Carpentier-Edwards pericardial valve was introduced into clinical use in 1981 to overcome the complications and failures associated with previous pericardial valve substitutes.[28] Long-term follow-up suggest that durability in the aortic position of the CE pericardial valve may be superior to existing porcine bioprosthesis, with freedom from prosthetic dysfunction being 100% and 83% at 12 and 13 years, respectively.[29] The initial mitral version of the CE pericardial valve was rapidly withdrawn from the market because of excessive flexibility of the stent, but was reintroduced for clinical implantation in 1984. Freedom from primary valve dysfunction in the mitral position in all age groups was 79% at 8 years.[30] Age adjusted freedom from valve dysfunction in the mitral position was 100% among patients 70 years and older, 91% ± 9% in the 60 to 69 year age group, and 64% ± 17% in the less than 60 year age group (Table 64.1 and 64.2).[31]

In vitro Hydraulic Performance Data for the Available Prostheses

It is very difficult to compare hydraulic performance of prostheses to the next *in vivo*. While measurements can be obtained by

TABLE 64.1. Age Adjusted Aortic Valve Performance.

Valve Aortic Position	Freedom from Structural Deterioration	Freedom From Thromboembolic Event	Freedom From Hemorrhage	Freedom From Reoperation	Freedom From Endocarditis
Starr-Edwards[361]	100%	75%	75%	80%	93%
St. Jude[372]	100%	90% ± 4%	81% ± 11%	94% ± 3%	NA
Metronic-Hall[53]	100%	87% ± 4%	80% ± 8%	97% ± 2%	96% ± 2%
Carbomedics[124]	100%	94% ± 1%	87% ± 1%	95% ± 1%	98% ± 1%
Omniscience[135]	100%	89% ± 4%	98% ± 1%	95% ± 2%	95% ± 2%
Omnicarbon[136]	100%	95% ± 3%	100%	97% ± 2%	97% ± 1%
CE Porcine[217] First generation	39% ± 8%	76% ± 3%	98% ± 1%	37% ± 8%	93% ± 1%
CE Porcine[208] Second generation	82% ± 6%	85% ± 2%	96% ± 1%	80% ± 6%	96% ± 1%
Hancock II[233]	92% ± 3%	80% ± 4%	96% ± 3%	89% ± 2%	95% ± 1%
Medtronic Intact Porcine[259]	97% ± 1%	94% ± 1%	98% ± 1%	94% ± 2%	95% ± 1%
CE Pericardial[2810]	100%	95% ± 3%	95% ± 2%	100%	98% ± 1%

[1]: 20 Years; [2]: 16 years; [3]: 10 years; [4]: 5 years; [5]: 9 years; [6]: 4 years; [7]: 17 years; [8]: 12 years; [9]: 7 years; [10]: 8 years.

TABLE 64.2. Age Adjusted Mitral Valve Performance.

Valve Mitral Position	Freedom from Structural Deterioration	Freedom From Thromboembolic Event	Freedom From Hemorrhage	Freedom From Reoperation	Freedom From Endocarditis
St. Jude[372]	100%	86% ± 7%	90% ± 7%	93% ± 3%	NA
Metronic-Hall[53]	100%	91% ± 3%	86% ± 5%	88% ± 4%	88% ± 4%
Carbomedics[124]	100%	89% ± 2%	87% ± 1%	95% ± 3%	98% ± 1%
CE Porcine[167]	14% ± 4%	79% ± 3%	83% ± 6%	10% ± 5%	93% ± 1%
CE Porcine[218] Second generation	82% ± 6%	76% ± 10%	96% ± 1%	40% ± 8%	92% ± 2%
Hancock II[243] Porcine	81% ± 6%	88% ± 3%	97% ± 3%	81% ± 6%	96% ± 1%
Medtronic Intact[9] Porcine[26]	97% ± 2%	94% ± 1%	98% ± 2%	94% ± 2%	95% ± 1%
CE Pericardial[3010]	79% ± 13%	92% ± 3%	98% ± 2%	66% ± 11%	95% ± 3%

[1]: 20 Years; [2]: 16 years; [3]: 10 years; [4]: 5 years; [5]: 9 years; [6]: 4 years; [7]: 17 years; [8]: 12 years; [9]: 7 years; [10]: 8 years.

echocardiography, the characteristics of valves do change over time and the best evaluation is done with serial echocardiographic studies over many years. Explant studies also define the fact that the hydraulic and hemodynamic performance of a given prosthesis at the time of implantation changes and evolves over time. However, it is helpful to have *in vitro* hydraulic performance data for the comparison of various valves as a starting point for selection, and as an estimate of relative performance early after implantation (Table 64.3).

Rationale for Valve Choice in Atrioventricular and Ventricular Outflow Tract Reconstructions

Choosing an **AV valve replacement** from the available options is relatively straightforward. For the mitral position, all patients under the age of 65 or who have more than a 12 year expected survival should receive a mechanical prosthesis, unless there is a specific and significant contraindication to anticoagulation.[32] While multiple styles have been used and are available, the double tilting disc valve made of pyrolytic carbon currently offers the best combination of low thromboembolic potential, durability, low profile and hydraulic performance. For patients over the age of 65, bioprosthetic valves in the mitral position have functioned well with infrequent need for re-replacement and the advantage of anticoagula-

tion flexibility. Thus, in patients who are in atrial fibrillation, the tendency would be to place a mechanical valve since there is already a need for anticoagulation. However, elderly patients do develop additional illnesses which can be complicated by anticoagulation, and thus the placement of a bioprosthesis leaves at least the option for discontinuing anticoagulation as necessary in the future, simplifying other kinds of medical care, such as orthopedic or genitourinary operations. Many elderly patients become so frail and unstable that falls while on anticoagulation become quite risky. Similarly, younger patients who are mentally retarded or otherwise might have difficulty with anticoagulation can also be appropriately managed with a bioprosthetic mitral valve. Selection depends upon profile, surgeon's familiarity, acute hydraulic and hemodynamic performance, durability expectations related to manufacturing processes aimed at reducing the rate of calcification, and cost.

For the tricuspid valve position, multiple studies have reaffirmed the bioprosthesis as the valve replacement of choice when valve repair cannot be accomplished. First choice is always repair. Since the tricuspid valve prosthetic replacement is always extraordinarily large, hemodynamic performance becomes less of an issue and choice depends upon the surgeon's belief about durability claims made by the manufacturers for their specific processing methodologies.

TABLE 64.3. In Vitro Data.

Valve Label	EOA	Internal Diameter (mm)	External Diameter (mm)	Mean Gradient (mmHg)	Open Angle (Deg)	Closed Angle (Deg)
Mechanical Aortic Valve Replacements						
St. Jude Medical (Standard)						
19	1.63	14.7	19	22.3	85	30
21	2.06	16.7	21	13.3	85	30
23	2.55	18.5	23	8.2	85	30
25	3.09	20.4	25	3.6	85	30
27	3.67	22.3	27	2	85	25
29	4.41	24.1	29	>1	85	25
31	5.18	26	31	>1	85	25
St. Jude Medical HP						
17	1.63	14.7	17	22.3	85	30
19	2.06	16.7	19	13.3	85	30
21	2.55	18.5	21	8.2	85	30
23	3.09	20.4	23	3.6	NA	NA
25	3.67	22.3	25	2.5	NA	NA
27	4.41	24.1	27	>1	NA	NA
Carbomedics (Standard)						
19	1.59	14.7	19.8	35	78	25
21	2.07	16.7	21.8	15	78	25
23	2.56	18.5	23.8	12	78	25
25	3.16	20.5	25.8	8	78	25
27	3.84	22.5	27.8	4	78	25
29	4.44	24.2	29.8	2	78	25
31	4.44	24.2	31.8	NA	78	25
Carbomedics (TopHat Supra-Annular)						
19	1.59	14.7	23.7	45	NA	NA
21	2.07	16.7	26.1	20	NA	NA
23	2.56	18.5	28.3	15	NA	NA
25	3.16	20.5	31.1	8	NA	NA
27	3.84	22.5	33.5	4	NA	NA
Carbomedics (Reduced)						
19	1.59	14.7	18.8	45	78	25
21	2.07	16.7	20.8	20	78	25
23	2.56	18.5	22.6	15	78	25
25	3.16	20.5	25	8	78	25
27	3.84	22.5	27	4	78	25
29	4.44	24.2	29	2	78	25
Medtronic Hall Mechanical Valve						
20	1.74	16	20	14.4	75	0
21	1.74	16	21	14.4	75	0
22	2.26	18	22	8.4	75	0
23	2.26	18	23	8.4	75	0
24	3.07	20	24	4.6	75	0
25	3.07	20	25	4.6	75	0
27	3.64	22	27	3	75	0
29	5.45	24	29	1.4	75	0
31	5.45	24	31	1.4	75	0
Omniscience						
19	1.63	14.4	19	47	80	12
21	2.11	16.4	21	31	80	12
23	2.55	18	23	15	80	12
25	3.14	20	25	8	80	12
27	3.8	22	27	NA	80	12
29	3.8	22	29	3	80	12
31	4.52	24	31	>1	80	12

TABLE 64.3. *Continued*

Valve Label	EOA	Internal Diameter (mm)	External Diameter (mm)	Mean Gradient (mmHg)	Open Angle (Deg)	Closed Angle (Deg)
Sorin Monostrut						
17	1.1	12	17	95	70	0
19	1.5	14	19	50	70	0
21	2	16	21	28	70	0
23	2.5	18	23	20	70	0
25	3.1	20	25	10	70	0
27	3.8	22	27	4	70	0
29	4.6	24	29	>1	70	0
31	4.6	24	31	NA	70	0
Starr-Edwards						
21	1.41	13	21	39	NA	NA
23	1.67	15	23	28	NA	NA
24	1.79	15	24	22	NA	NA
26	1.94	16	26	18	NA	NA
27	2.16	17	27	15	NA	NA
29	2.57	18	29	11	NA	NA
31	2.89	19	31	10	NA	NA
Bioprosthetic Aortic Valve Replacements						
Carpentier-Edwards Porcine Valve				(Standard)		
19	0.9	17	19	32.7		
21	1.2	19	21	21.3		
23	1.1	21	23	30.2		
25	1.5	23	25	19.4		
27	2.4	25	27	11		
29	2.7	27	29	18.3		
31	1.6	29	31	29.3		
Carpentier-Edwards Pericardial Valve				(supra-annular)		
Model 2700 Perimount						
19	2.54	18	28	26.3		
21	3.14	20	31	22.6		
23	3.79	22	33	14.4		
25	4.52	24	35	NA		
27	5.31	26	38	NA		
29	6.15	28	40	NA		
Carpentier-Edwards Pericardial Valve				(supra-annular)		
Model 2800 Perimount						
19	2.54	18	26	NA		
21	3.14	20	28	NA		
23	3.79	22	31	NA		
25	4.52	24	32	NA		
27	5.31	26	35	NA		
29	6.15	28	37	NA		
Medtronic Intact Porcine Valve						
19	1.01	16.6	25	32.35		
21	1.37	18.5	27	17.55		
23	1.56	20.3	30	13.8		
25	1.85	22.1	33	9.75		
27	2.11	23.7	35	7.33		
29	2.51	25.5	38	5.13		
Hancock Standard Porcine Valve						
23	1.74	20	28.5	10.9		
25	1.94	21.8	31.5	8.63		
27	2.14	22.3	34.25	7.03		
29	2.71	24.1	36.5	4.53		
31	2.85	26	40	3.98		

Continued

TABLE 64.3. *Continued*

Valve Label	EOA	Internal Diameter (mm)	External Diameter (mm)	Mean Gradient (mmHg)	Open Angle (Deg)	Closed Angle (Deg)
Hancock II Porcine Valve						
21	1.46	21	18.5	15.45		
23	1.8	23	20.5	10.08		
25	2.06	25	22.5	7.7		
27	2.36	27	24	5.73		
29	2.93	29	26	3.8		
Hancock MO Porcine Valve						
19	1.21	16	23.5	23.3		
21	1.43	18	26	16.5		
23	1.94	20	29.25	9		
25	2.16	21.8	32.5	7.15		
Stentless Freestyle Aortic Root Bioprosthesis (Medtronic)						
19	1.84	16	19	9.83		
21	2.17	18	21	6.98		
23	2.69	20	23	4.43		
25	3.41	21.5	25	2.8		
27	3.75	23.5	27	2.3		

EOA: Effective Orifice Area (cm2); Mean Gradients (400 ml/sec).

In the **ventricular outflow tract positions**, except for endocarditis, when the homograft is always preferred, choices become a little more complex. Repairs are generally preferred to sacrifice of the native valve when applicable. For right sided positions, the cryopreserved homograft appears currently to be the best option for most patients. There are occasional anatomic constraints where a more rigid tube and bioprosthesis combination are advantageous but a mechanical valve in the pulmonary position is to be discouraged.

For the systemic, aortic outflow tract reconstruction, there are various factors which control selection. In general, a mechanical valve is chosen for the adult patient under 60 years of age without specific contraindications to anticoagulation as in most cases, this provides the best durability and hemodynamic performance. If necessary, annulus enlargement techniques can be used to ensure adequate size prosthesis. Over the age of 70, pericardial or porcine bioprostheses offer excellent choices for durability and hemodynamic performance and again, annulus enlargement techniques can be used as required. Anticoagulation can be used as driven by other factors, but the bioprostheses allow Coumadin or aspirin to be discontinued when other medical conditions complicate the picture.

The stentless xenograft prostheses in their various formats are useful for the small aortic root in patients over 55, particularly those with left ventricular hypertrophy (LVH) and thus the need for optimal hydraulic performance. Homografts can be used but offer no specific advantage in the elderly patient except for the rare (in this age) complex multilevel outflow reconstructions. There is evidence that the superb hydraulics of stentless and allograft valves result in very very low gradients (e.g., 2 to 6 mmHg) and impedence to total flow which in turn results in better ventricular remodeling and regression of LVH[33–35] that may only be captured with stented valves when aggressive upsizing with annulus enlargement is performed. Durability for stentless valves and stentless root xenografts will likely be as good or better than stented pericardial valves and homografts. This makes them an attractive option for the patient who can't have a Ross, especially those that fall in the "between" age group of 50 to 65 years.

For patients who have other indications for anticoagulation (e.g., atrial fibrillation, history of stroke, peripheral vascular disease, low ejection fraction, history of thromboembolism, etc.), a mechanical valve in the aortic position is a routine choice. For those patients with relative or absolute contraindications to anticoagulation who are under the age of 55, there are a number of choices. The first choice is the Ross autograft procedure as it achieves the aortic reconstruction with the procedure durability of a homograft in right sided position as opposed to the left sided position. A homograft is a good choice for the left sided position, but will require replacement in most patients between 10 and 25 years after transplantation and cannot grow. Xenograft prostheses can be selected for ease of insertion, but recognizing that a patient will require re-replacement. Xenografts can be a useful strategy for certain subgroups of patients such as young women entering the child bearing years who do not wish to have a homograft or for whom the autograft procedure is not applicable because of deformity of their own pulmonary valve. In this case, a strategy based upon lifetime goals would be reasonably defined by placing a homograft, pericardial or porcine prosthesis in the aortic position, recognizing that re-replacement would be required in 10 to 15 years, during which time the pregnancies could be accomplished. After that, the implant could be a mechanical valve or a Ross procedure with the goal of achieving lifelong durability.

Complex multilevel outflow tract disease is often easier to reconstruct with homografts or autografts even when adding other outflow reconstructions (e.g., subaortic resections, etc. See Chapter 8). Aortic valve SBE is statistically best treated with homografts (See Chapter 9). Small aortic roots or severe LVH favors choosing either autograft/homografts or stentless valves except with severe hypertrophic cardiomyopathy (IHSS) when either a stented valve may prevent LVOT collapse in systole or a Morrow type operation is concomitantly performed.

Whatever valve prosthesis chosen, patients are best served when the surgeon is capable of conceptualizing the operation as a "ventricular outflow tract reconstruction" contrasted with a "prosthesis insertion." Then the best operation can be devised for each patient by repairing or replacing the subvalvular, valvular and supravalvular components of outflow as necessary to achieve the best functional hemodynamic and hydraulic performance using materials with specific properties chosen with the characteristics optimized for the individual patient to lower, not only operative risk, but lifelong morbidity and mortality.[35,36]

References

1. Hufnagel CA, Harvey WP. The surgical correction of aortic regurgitation: Preliminary report. Bulletin of Georgetown Univ Med Cntr 1953; 60.
2. Hammermeister KE, Sethi GK, Henderson WG, Oprian C, Kim T, Rahimtoola SH. A comparison of outcomes in men 11 years after heart valve replacement with a mechanical or bioprosthesis. Veterans Affairs Cooperative Study on Valvular Heart Disease. New Eng Journ Med 1993; 328(18):1289–1296.
3. Hall KV, Kaster RL, Wolfe WG. An improved pivotal disc-type prosthesis heart valve. Oslo City J Hosp 1979;29:3–21.
4. Nitter-Hauge S, Abdelnoor M. Ten-year experience with the Medtronic Hall valvular prosthesis. Circulation 1989;80(Suppl):43–48.
5. Akins C. Long-term results with the Medtronic-Hall valvular prosthesis. Ann Thorac Surg 1996; 61:806–813.
6. Obadia JF, Martelloni YA, Bastien OH, Durant de Gevigney GM, et al. Long-term follow-up of small (20 and 21) Medtronic-Hall aortic valve prosthesis. Ann Thorac Surg 1997;64:421–425.
7. Bjork VO. A new tilting disc valve prosthesis. Scand J Thorac Cardiovasc Surg 1969;4:1–10.
8. Wieting DW. The Bjork-Shiley Delrin tilting disc heart valve: historical perspective, design and need for scientific analysis after 25 years. J Heart Valve Dis 1996;5(Suppl):S157–S168.
9. Mikaeloff P, Jegaden O, Ferrinin M, Coll-Mazzei J, et al. Prospective randomized study of St. Jude Medical versus Bjork-Shiley or Starr-Edwards 6120 valve prostheses in the mitral position. J Cardiovasc Surg 1989;30:966–975.
10. Flemma R, Mullen D, Kleinman L. Survival and event-free analysis of 785 patients with Bjork-Shiley spherical-disc valves at 10 to 16 years. Ann Thorac Surg 1988;45:258–265.

11. Birkmeyer J, Marrin C, O'Conner G. Should patients with Bjork-Shiley valves undergo prophylactic replacement? Lancet 1992;340:520.

12. Rodler SM, Moritz A, Schreiner W, End A, Dubsky P, Wolner E. Five-year follow-up after valve replacement with the Carbomedics bileaflet prosthesis. Ann Thorac Surg 1997;63: 1018–1025.

13. Kazui T, Yamada O, Yamagishi M, Watanabe N, Komatsu S. Aortic valve replacement with Omniscience and Omnicarbon valves. Ann Thorac Surg 1991;52:236–244.

14. Kazui T, Komatsu S, Inoue N. Clinical evaluation of the Omniscience aortic disc valve prosthesis. Scand J Thorac Cardiovasc Surg 1987;21:173–188.

15. Jamieson W, Allen P, Miyagishima RT. Carpentier-Edwards standard porcine bioprosthesis: A first generation tissue valve with excellent long-term clinical performance. J Thorac Cardiovasc Surg 1990;99:543–561.

16. Jamieson WRE, Munro AI, Miyagishima RT, et al. Carpentier-Edwards standard porcine bioprosthesis: Clinical performance to seventeen years. Ann Thorac Surg 1995;60:999–1007.

17. Carpentier A, Dubost C, Lane E et al. Continuing improvements in valvular bioprostheses. J Thorac Cardiovasc Surg 1982;83:27–42.

18. Jones E, Weintraub W, Craver J. Ten-year experience with the porcine bioprosthetic valve: interrelationship of valve survival and patient survival in 1,050 valve replacements. Ann Thorac Surg 1990;49:370–384.

19. Aberdeen J, Corr L, Milner P, Lincoln J, Burnstock G. Marked Increases in Calcitonin Gene-Related Peptide-containing Nerves in the Developing Rat Following Long-term Sympathectomy with Guanethidine. Neuroscience 1990;35(1):175–184.

20. Hartz R, Fisher B, Finkelmeier B, et al. An eight year experience with porcine prosthetic cardiac valves. J Thorac Cardiovasc Surg 1986;91:910–917.

21. Jamieson W, Burr LH, Tyers GF, Miyagishima RT, Janusz MT, et al. Carpentier-Edwards Supraannular Porcine Bioprosthesis: Clincal Performance to Twelve Years. Ann Thorac Surg 1995; 60:S235–S240.

22. Glower DD, White W, Hattan A, et al. Determinants of reoperation after 960 valve replacements with Carpentier-Edwards prostheses. J Thorac Cardiovasc Surg 1994;107: 381–393.

23. Geha AS, Laks H, Stensel HC et al. Late failure of porcine valve heterografts in children. J Thorac Cardiovasc Surg 1979;78:351–364.

24. David T, Armstrong S, Sun Z. The Hancock II bioprosthesis at ten years. Ann Thorac Surg 1995;60:S229–S234.

25. Barratt-Boyes BG, Jaffe WM, Hong Ko P, Whitlock RML. The Zero Pressure Fixed Medtronic Intact Porcine Valve: An 8.5 Year Review. J Heart Valve Dis 1993;2:604–611.

26. Lemieux MD, Jamieson W, Landymore RW, Dumesnil JG, Metras J, Munro AI, et al. Medtronic Intact Porcine bioprosthesis: clinical performance to seven years. Ann Thorac Surg 1995;60:S258–S263.

27. O'Brien MF, Stafford EG, Gardner MA, Pohlner PG, Tesar P, et al. The Medtronic Intact Xenograft: an analysis of 342 patients over a seven year follow-up period. Ann Thorac Surg 1995;60: S253–S257.

28. Cosgrove DM, Lytle BW, Williams WG. Hemodynamic performance of the Carpentier-Edwards pericardial valve in the aortic position in vivo. Circulation 1985;72(Suppl):146.

29. Pellerin M, Mihaileanu S, Couetil JP, Relland J, Deloche A, et al. Carpentier-Edwards Pericardial bioprosthesis in aortic position: long term follow-up 1980 to 1994. Ann Thorac Surg 1995; 60:S292–S296.

30. Pelletier LC, Carrier MC, Leclerc Y, Dyrda I. The Carpentier-Edwards Pericardial bioprosthesis: clinical experience with 600 patients. Ann Thorac Surg 1995;60:S297–S302.

31. Vitale N, Giannolo B, Nappi G, DeLuca L, Piazza L, Scardone M, Cotrufo M. Long term follow up of different models of mechanical and biological mitral prostheses. EJCTS 1995;9:181–189.

32. Committee on Management of Patients with Valvular Disease, Robert O.Bonow MC. ACC/AHA Practice Guidelines: Guidelines for the Management of Patients with Valvular Disease. Circulation 1998;98:1949–1984.

33. Jin XY, Zhang Z, Gibson DG, Yacoub MH, Pepper JR. Effects of valve substitute on changes in left ventricular function and hypertrophy after aortic valve replacement. Ann Thorac Surg 1996;62:683–690.

34. Del Rizzo DF, Goldman BS, Christakis GT, Powell AF, David TE. Hemodynamic Benefits of the Toronto Stentless valve. J Thorac Cardiovasc Surg 1996;112:1431–1446.

35. Walther T, Weigl C, Falk V, Deigler A, Shilling L, Autschbach R, Mohr FW. Impact of stentless in

comparison to conventional aortic valves on postoperative left ventricular remodeling. European Heart Journal 1997.

36. Orszulak TA, Schaff HV, Puga FJ, Danielson GK, Mullany CJ, et al. Event status of the Starr-Edwards Aortic Valve to 20 years: A benchmark for comparison. Ann Thorac Surg 1997;63:620–626.

37. Baudet E, Puel V, McBride J, Grimaud J, Roques R, et al. Long-term results of valve replacement with the St. Jude Medical Prosthesis. J Thorac Cardiovasc Surg 1995;109:858–870.

65
Tissue Engineered Heart Valves: The Next Challenge

Stephen L. Hilbert and Richard A. Hopkins

The safety and effectiveness of the current generation of mechanical and bioprosthetic replacement heart valves (HVs) have been clearly demonstrated, although attention must be given to specific anatomic and patient-related factors before a particular valve design is selected for use.[1] In infants and children requiring ventricular outflow tract reconstructions, the availability of a suitable valve conduit is quite restricted.[2] Cryopreserved allograft (homograft) heart valves remain an attractive option for ventricular outflow tract reconstruction in infants, children and young adults as discussed in the preceding chapters of this book. Although the long-term safety and clinical performance of cryopreserved allografts is encouraging,[3] their use is limited in children due to the reduced availability of small diameter allografts and the lack of allograft HV somatic growth. The application of emerging tissue engineering (TE) concepts may provide a solution to this current limitation, through the development of a TE valve conduit that remains viable for the life of the patient as well as undergoes somatic growth as the child grows.

The development of the ideal replacement heart valve continues to be elusive. An ideal replacement HV should having the following characteristics: 1) elicit no inflammatory or foreign body response; 2) be non-immunogenic; 3) be viable having long-term durability and the capability to repair degenerated components; 4) be available in unlimited supply; 5) non-thrombogenic; 6) be capable of somatic growth; and 7) have design features which uniquely satisfy individual patient requirements.[4] The design and fabrication of previous generations of replacement heart valves (i.e., mechanical, bioprosthetic and polymeric) have been limited by a combination of restrictions placed on design features constrained by manufacturing capabilities and the availability of suitable biomaterials possessing the requisite materials properties to satisfy the demands made by the design requirements. In addition to limitations imposed by fabrication and the selection of biomaterials, semilunar and atrioventricular (AV) valves differ anatomically as well as function in differing physiologic settings.[5] Historically, replacement HVs have been designed to respond passively to changes in pressure initiating forward blood flow and valve opening replicating semilunar valve physiologic mechanisms. The valve apparatus (i.e., chordea tendinae and papillary muscles), a unique anatomic feature of native AV valves, has not been incorporated into tricuspid and mitral valve designs; although, a stentless pericardial valve currently undergoing limited clinical trial does include segments of pericardium joining the four leaflets to papillary muscle attachment sites.[6] Whether or not the incorporation of mitral valve apparatus anatomic features intended to replicate native AV valve structure-function will improve mitral valve replacement HV safety and durability remains to be demonstrated. However, it is encouraging to note that anatomic and physiologic differences between semilunar and AV valves are being considered as design features.

This chapter will discuss the current "state of the art" in the development of tissue engineered (TE) HVs highlighting areas of success as well as identifying important lessons learned from these initial experiences by various research teams. Although the initial research goals of developing a viable TE HV capable of somatic growth, renewal of cell populations, regeneration of extracellular matrix components and adequate hemodynamic performance for the lifetime of the patient has not been met, the need for continuing basic research in cell and molecular biology and engineering have been identified by this initial experience. Areas of future research will also be discussed with the hope that other investigators will be both encouraged concerning the rapid advances that have been made thus far[6–20] as well as stimulate interest in conducting fundamental research which is expected to provide solutions to deficiencies that are impeding the development of next generation of TE HVs.

Two TE HV approaches are being explored which are based on the use of either biodegradable polymeric materials[7–13] or decellularized valve conduits (e.g., pulmonary and aortic valve allografts; composite porcine aortic valve xenograft)[14–20] intended to replicate the anatomic, histologic and biomechanical characteristics of semilunar HVs. Current TE HV designs are based on the use of a three dimensional structure (referred to as a scaffold) consisting of either a biodegradable polymer (e.g., polyglycolic acid, polylactic acid, polyhydroxyoctanoate) or a tissue-derived biomaterial (e.g., decellularized pulmonary and aortic valves). In addition to the use of polymeric and decellularized tissues, fibrin gel, gelatin, folded cell sheets (myofibroblasts; collagen) and elastin-collagen composite scaffolds are also being designed.[21–23] All of these TE HV designs are based on the expectation that the scaffold material will be recellularized by the patient's autologous cells either before implantation (e.g., in vitro cell seeding) or after implantation. The recellularized scaffold would than be capable of renewing valvular cellular and extracellular matrix (ECM) components resulting in a viable replacement HV satisfying the requirements of an ideal HV.

A summary of polymeric and ECM scaffold TE and preclinical animal model experience gained with each will next be reviewed.

Polymeric Scaffolds

The initial efforts to develop a biodegradable polymeric scaffold for use in the construction of a TE HV consisted of the evaluation of polyglycolic acid (PGA) alone or in combination with polylactic acid (PLA) fabricated into the shape of a single pulmonary valve cusp.* The PGA-PLA leaflet was than seeded with autologous vascular cells (mixed cell population-endothelial cells, fibroblasts, smooth muscle cells) and implanted in lambs.[7–9] The in vivo preclinical evaluation of PGA-PLA single pulmonary leaflet replacements were encouraging; however, attempts to replace the pulmonary valve with a trileaflet PGA-PLA valve were not successful due to the limitations imposed by the materials properties of the biodegradable polymer. Although rapid PGA-PLA degradation was observed (e.g., within 6 weeks), the investigators felt that this leaflet design was limited by the rigid materials properties of PGA which stimulated a search for a more flexible biodegradable polymer.

Polyhydroxyoctanoate (PHO) was next identified as a possible leaflet material. PHO is a member of a family of polymers know as polyhydroxyalkanoates (PHA). PHAs are linear polyester thermoplastics that are biosynthesized by various microorganisms as well as by fermentation commercially. PHAs have the advantage of being quite flexible (e.g., % elongation, 1000) as compared to PGA and PLA (% elongation < 5%). In addition to favorable materials properties, PHO can be made porous (potentially increasing cell adhesion and tissue ingrowth) by using a salt leaching technique.[10] Valve conduits have been fabricated from PHO and evaluated following implantation as a pulmonary artery interposition grafts in sheep.

---

* Nomenclature clarification: semilunar valve-cusp; atrioventricular valve-leaflet; heart valve synthetic materials-leaflet.

After 24 weeks of implantation hemodynamic performance was noted to be adequate with mild regurgitation observed. Histologically fibrous encapsulation and ingrowth were observed in the conduit wall; however, PHO was still present in the leaflets after 6 months of implantation.[11] Although the materials properties of PHO were better suited for the fabrication of HV leaflets, the long *in vivo* biodegradation time exceeding 6 months is problematic. The presence of residual PHO may impede the recellularization of the valve and conduit as well as stimulate a long term chronic inflammatory and fibrotic response. The long-term fibrotic response would be expected to increase the TE HV mechanical strength as well as the long-term durability; however, progressive leaflet thickening (fibrotic response) may continue as long as the polymer was present. Leaflet thickening may then continue to progress to the extent that valvular function is impaired.

The ideal biodegradable polymeric scaffold material has not yet been identified. Efforts are continuing to discover novel materials possessing the requisite materials properties suitable for the construction of a flexible leaflet TE HV which are resorbed within four to six weeks of implantation but yet provide a scaffold for the *in vivo* formation of a leaflet histologically and functionally resembling a native semilunar valve cusp.

ECM Scaffolds

The development of an ECM scaffold has been occurring in parallel with the research activities focusing of biodegradable polymers. As discussed above, the limitations imposed by synthetic biodegradable materials such as the polymer degradation rate and biomaterials properties, may be circumvented by the selection of a tissue-derived biomaterial capable of accommodating the biomechanical requirements of a HV. Decellularized (also referred to as acellular or devitalized) aortic and pulmonary valve tissues have emerged as the tissue of choice for the creation of a TE HV scaffold. Various approaches have been reported to

effectively remove the cellular components from semilunar valve tissue while retaining the majority of the ECM components (primarily collagens, elastin and the less water soluble proteoglycans). The following decellularization methods effectively remove endothelial cells and cuspal interstitial cells; however, cardiac myocytes and arterial wall smooth muscle cells are variably present after processing: 1) anionic detergents; 2) non-ionic detergents; 3) trypsin/EDTA and 4) deionized water. These agents are frequently used in combination with protease inhibitors. In addition to removing the cellular components, residual nucleic acids are also removed from the tissue by DNase and RNase digestion. The tissues are then further rinsed to facilitate removal of cellular remnants and tissue processing reagents. The various decellularization processes may also reduce the immunogencity of allograft and xenograft tissues; however, this belief has not been substantiated by extensive studies assessing systemic cellular and humoral responses to decellularized tissue.

Explant pathology findings have been described for the following three distinctly different pulmonary and aortic valve decellularization methods: 1) sodium dodecyl sulfate, anionic detergent; 2) trypsin/EDTA, serine protease/divalent cation chelation; and 3) deionized water. The first two methods were used to decellularize canine and sheep allograft valves, respectively. The third method (deionized water) has been used to decellularize a composite porcine aortic valve xenograft bioprosthesis which was then cryopreserved and gamma irradiated. This unique composite bioprosthesis consisted of three non-coronary cusps, their corresponding arterial wall segments and anterior mitral valve leaflets. A combination of decellularization (deionized water) and cryopreservation has also been used to process human pulmonary allograft heart valves.[15] These decellularized heart valve ECM scaffolds were implanted as pulmonary artery interposition grafts in canine and sheep models or humans (adjunct to Ross aortic valve replacement or replacement of dysfunctional pulmonary allografts).[14–18] We have also investigated the use of either an anionic detergent

(N-lauroyl sarconsinate) or the combination of two non-ionic detergents (Triton X-100 and n-octyl glucopyrinoside) as a means of removing pulmonary and aortic valve cellular components. These decellularized allografts were implanted (pulmonary artery interposition grafts for 20 weeks) in juvenile sheep.

The explant pathology findings reported in the literature[14–18] as well as those observed in our studies are quite similar despite the markedly different decellularization methods used. The following observations summarize our histopathology findings and are comparable to those reported in the literature. Nuclei and cellular remnants were not present in the unimplanted decellularized cusps; however, arterial wall smooth muscle cells and subvalvular cardiac myocytes remnants were variably present. The typical trilaminar histologic architecture of the semilunar cusps (i.e., ventricularis, spongiosa, fibrosa) was preserved, although small circular voids were present in the fibrosa and, to a lesser extent, in the ventricularis. These voids in the fibrosa may represent the previous sites of interstitial cells removed by the decellularization process. Polarized light microscopy demonstrated the retention of collagen crimp (waviness) within the fibrosa similar to the repeating birefringent pattern seen in native semilunar cusps; however, very small microscopic kinks or bends were observed. Whether these regions visualized by polarized light represent sites previously occupied by interstitial cells or reflect changes in biomechanical properties remains to be determined.

Fibrous sheath formation was present on the luminal surface of the conduit and extended over the cuspal surfaces (inflow side > outflow side) to a variable distance (approximately 20% to 30% of the length of the inflow cusp; 10% or less of the outflow cusp length). The thickness of the fibrous sheath decreased as it progressed from the base of the cusp toward the free edge. The fibrous sheath was predominantly covered by a continuous layer of endothelial cells; however, a focal endothelial cell distribution was observed on the cuspal surfaces not covered by fibrous sheathing. It is noteworthy that a similar pattern of fibrous sheathing has previously been observed covering the surface of explanted cryopreserved allograft valves that became acellular after implantation in both sheep and humans.[24,25] Recellularization was variably present in the conduit wall and limited to the basal region of the cusp. Microscopically, autologous cells migrated through both of the anastomotic sites and the adventitial side of the graft. The repopulation of the basal region of the cusp histologically appears to be an extension of the tissue ingrowth occurring at the proximal anastomosis. Cuspal recellularization occurred as the result of tissue ingrowth into the spongiosa, the middle histologic layer of cusp which is composed of loose connective tissue rich in proteoglycans. Autologous cells migrate into the wide spongiosa present in the base of the cusp, but are not seen in the thin spongiosal layer which continues toward the free edge of the cusp. Similarly, recellularization of the cusp does not progress into either the fibrosa or ventricularis. The ventricularis and fibrosa may in fact be anatomic barriers preventing the complete recellularization of the cusp (e.g., fibrosa-dense circumferentially oriented collagen bundles; ventricularis-dense radially oriented elastic fibers). The cells repopulating the decellularized conduit wall and the basal region of the cusp are predominately myofibroblasts and fibroblasts within an ECM consisting of primarily collagen and proteoglycans.

As described in our explant pathology findings, recellularization of the cuspal tissue was limited to the basal region of the cusp, while fibrous sheathing extended a variable distance over the cuspal surface. Similar observations have been reported by others investigators describing the recellularization of decellularized allografts.[14–18] However, the pattern and extent of cuspal recellularization is notably different for decellularized xenograft valvular tissue.

Cuspal and conduit wall components in decellularized allograft tissue do not elicit an inflammatory response with the exception of the presence of inflammatory cells surrounding cardiac myocytes remnants present in the subvalvular region of a decellularized allograft valve. In contrast to the decellularized allograft findings, a mixed cell population (i.e., inflammatory cells and fibroblasts) in the mid-portion of the cusp has been reported in decellularized xenograft tissues, although no observations were reported concerning the inflammatory cell response to smooth muscle or cardiac myocytes remnants which may be present in these decellularized xenografts.[17] The investigators hypothesize that revascularization and "adaptive remodeling" (initiated in the mid-portion of the cusp where activated mononuclear cells are localized) resulted in the repopulation of the cusp by mature cuspal interstitial cells.[17] These observations suggest that different mechanisms are involved in the recellularization of allograft and xenograft valvular tissues. Additional studies are needed to clarify these differences.

Calcification of decellularized allograft and xenograft cusps has not been observed following chronic implantation as pulmonary interposition grafts in juvenile sheep[16-19]. All of the various methods previously described (detergents, deionized water, trypsin/EDTA) effectively prevent cuspal calcification, indicating calcification nucleation sites such as cellular membrane remnants, have been removed or inhibited. Although published reports clearly demonstrate the lack of decellularized cuspal tissue calcification, there is a paucity of data (e.g., radiographic and histologic) describing the extent of calcification occurring in smooth muscle cell remnants present in the conduit wall smooth muscle cells, subvalvular cardiac myocytes or extracellular matrix components. In our study, no calcification of the cuspal tissue was observed; however, variable amounts of calcification occurred in the conduit wall (elastic fibers and smooth muscle cell remnants) and subvalvular cardiac myocytes remnants as demonstrated in radiographic and histologic sections (von Kossa stain).

We have also observed a marked thinning of the conduit wall following implantation in the RVOT in our series of explants. In fact, a saccular dilation was present in the wall of the sinus of Valsalva in one explanted valve. This observation raises a concern that the biomechanical properties of the arterial wall are significantly altered by detergent decellularization

methods. Histologic sections in which the smooth muscle cells are essentially removed resulted in a compressive thinning of the conduit after implantation in the RVOT. In regions where removal of smooth muscle cells was incomplete, thinning of the conduit wall was less apparent. This observation implies that aggressive decellularization may compromise valve conduit safety (e.g., aneurysm formation) and performance (e.g., saccular dilation resulting in loss of valve coaptation). These observations clearly indicate that comparative mechanical testing studies of native and decellularized cusps (pre- and postimplantation) and the conduit wall tissues need to be undertaken. In addition to conduit wall thinning secondary to detergent decellularization, intracuspal hematoma formation and collagen fraying were also observed in explanted cusps.

Of the published findings describing decellularized allograft valve recellularization, a most promising method involves the treatment of valvular tissue with trypsin/EDTA and the static seeding of the upper surface of the valve with autologous myofibroblasts (6 days) followed by endothelial cells (2 days) before implantation in sheep (pulmonary artery interposition graft). This method resulted in complete cuspal recellularization and the formation of a confluence endothelial cell layer on the surface of the cusp, while partial degeneration was observed in the unseeded decellularized valves without evidence of cuspal interstitial cell repopulation.[18] Remnants of subvalvular cardiac myocytes initiated an inflammatory cell response as well as calcification. In contrast, no inflammatory cells or calcification was observed in conduit wall or cuspal tissues; however, descriptive findings concerning arterial wall thinning were not mentioned.

The studies summarized above demonstrate the ability of a variety of decellularization methods to effectively remove cuspal interstitial cells from valvular tissue; however, their ability to decellularize subvalvular cardiac myocytes and conduit wall smooth muscle cells is less certain. It is noteworthy that methods which effectively remove conduit wall smooth muscle cells also result in arterial wall thinning and intracuspal hematoma formation indicating that the potential for significant structural deterioration must be considered. In addition to biomechanical and long-term durability concerns, these investigations also highlight the need for additional research addressing optimal methods to facilitate the complete and consistent recellularization of decellularized allograft valve tissues. Although the initial decellularized xenograft bioprosthesis findings suggest that the initial inflammatory cell response may stimulate recellularization, additional studies will be required to fully elucidate this mechanism of recellularization. In addition, safety studies characterizing the systemic cellular and humoral immune response to decellularized xenograft and allograft cuspal and conduit wall tissues should be addressed, since the immune response to allograft tissue has been implicated in the failure of cryopreserved allograft heart valves in children.[26,27] The interesting findings concerning the use of *in vitro* cell seeding of a decellularized (trypsin/EDTA) allograft valve prior to implantation[18] have encouraged us to further explore the effectiveness of this approach in our laboratory. In addition, based on the experience gained in the development a pulsatile flow bioreactor for the preconditioning of an *in vitro* cell seeded biodegradable polymer scaffold[12] we have been further encouraged to investigate the *in vitro* effects of mechanical factors on cuspal interstitial cell, vascular smooth muscle cell and endothelial cell proliferation, differentiation, ECM protein synthesis and mechanisms of cuspal and conduit wall recellularization.

Future Research

Tissue Processing: Decellularization, Sterilization and Storage

The currently available decellularization methods effectively remove cuspal endothelial cells and interstitial cells; however, incomplete removal of conduit wall smooth muscle cells and subvalvular cardiac myocytes remain problematic. An inflammatory cell infiltrate is typi-

cally observed surrounding remnants of cardiac myocytes. In addition to triggering an inflammatory response, muscle cell remnants (e.g., disrupted plasma membranes) serve as nucleation sites for calcification. Further research is needed to develop a decellularization process which will completely remove all of the smooth muscle cell and cardiac myocyte cellular components, while still retaining the biomechanical properties of the native valve conduit.

Sterilization of the decellularized tissue is highly recommended rather than the routinely used cryopreserved allograft valve disinfection methods. Again, the selection of the appropriate sterilization method must be based on the retention of the biomechanical properties of the native valve conduit. Electron beam or gamma irradiation may prove to be acceptable sterilization methods.

After the decellularized valve conduit is sterilized, a storage method will have to be developed which will maintain sterility as well as preserve the biomechanical properties of the valve conduit. Cryopreserved and vitrified decellularized allograft valves are currently being evaluated as RVOT reconstructions in our chronic sheep model.

In Vitro Cell Seeding

The following fundamental and practical questions are being addressed in our laboratory as well as by other investigators concerning the *in vitro* cell seeding of TE HV scaffolds:

1. What quantity of tissue is required initially and how many passages will provide an adequate number of cells for *in vitro* seeding?
2. Is there a safe tissue source and practical method to harvest autologous vascular and valvular tissues? and;
3. Does the anatomic source of autologous cells affect *in vivo* recellularization?

Studies are currently ongoing in our laboratory to determine the optimal media and culture conditions for smooth muscle cells, endothelial cells and interstitial leaflet cells. Comparative studies have also been undertaken to identify differences between arterial versus venous sources of smooth muscle cells and endothelial cells. We have investigated the suitability of using tricuspid valve leaflet tissue obtained by biopsy as a way of harvesting interstitial leaflet cells.[28] Our initial findings indicate that this technique is feasible in sheep without causing clinically significant valvular dysfunction, morbidity or mortality. Interstitial leaflet cells were successfully isolated and propagated using standard cell culture methods. Carotid artery and jugular vein tissues are also being studied as a source of vascular smooth muscle cells and endothelial cells. Although our findings are encouraging, we are concerned, as are others, that clinical sources of autologous valvular and vascular tissue which can be used as cell sources for in vitro seeding of TE scaffolds are for all practical purposes limited to venous blood vessels (e.g., saphenous vein). Other sources of myofibroblasts, smooth muscle cells and endothelial cells will have to be explored.

Dermal fibroblasts have been considered as an alternative cell source for seeding biodegradable polymeric scaffolds; however, after 8–10 weeks of implantation (replacement of the pulmonary valve right posterior cusp) the leaflet was thickened and contracted.[13] At this time valvular and vascular tissue potential tissue sources suitable for in vitro autologous cell seeding of TE scaffolds; however, the use of autologous bone marrow mesenchymal stem cells is currently being investigated.

Preconditioning: Mechanical Factors

Another approach may be to expose fibroblasts or smooth muscle cells to extracellular proteins or to mechanical forces in vitro which may trigger a change in phenotypic expression (e.g., fibroblast to myofibroblast; smooth muscle cell to myofibroblast). This avenue of investigation has only recently been pursued. Alterations in extracellular adhesion proteins have been reported to change the phenotypic expression of smooth muscle cells.[29] The presence of laminin and collagen IV were observed to change the morphology of smooth muscle cells

to a cell type in which peripherally located cytoplasmic filaments were present resembling myofibroblasts histologically. The following mechanical factors have been reported to alter intracellular cytoskeletal features, protein synthesis and proliferation: hydrostatic pressure, shear stress and stretch.[19–36] These individual observations, when viewed collectively, suggest that the development of a bioreactor (i.e., culture chamber in which in vitro cell seeded TE scaffolds are exposed to mechanical factors) may provide a practical way to precondition autologous cell seeded TE scaffolds by replicating in vivo mechanical factors before implantation. The questions being addressed concerning preconditioning are focused on the identification of mechanical factors which will effect differentiation, proliferation, protein synthesis, cell adhesion and the in vivo recellularization of the TE scaffold. Fundamental studies identifying mechanical factors which trigger specific cell signaling mechanisms need to be pursued and the findings applied to the development of the next generation of bioreactors.

Conclusion

As reviewed in this chapter, remarkable progress has been made in a relatively short period of time in the development of TE HV degradable polymeric scaffolds and decellularized ECM scaffolds. Many challenges remain before the next generation of TE HVs will be ready for initial in vivo animal studies. Foremost among these will be the development of optimal decellularization, sterilization and storage processes that retain the biomechanical properties of the native valve conduit. While these methods are being developed, basic studies will have to be completed to identify appropriate clinical sources of autologous vascular tissue for harvesting. Optimal culture media and conditions will have to be further defined as well as the identification of specific mechanical factors which will effectively precondition autologous seeded EMC scaffolds. Chronic sheep studies will have to be conducted to assess the safety and effectiveness of the next generation of decellularized TE HVs.

Lastly, extensive safety studies, as defined by the FDA and other international regulatory bodies, will need to be undertaken, before a limited clinical trial will be initiated. Realistically, it may take a decade of challenging biological, engineering and surgical research before a limited TE HV clinical trial is feasible. However, the investment of time and resources may result in the development of the ideal replacement heart valve for patients of all ages.

References

1. Schoen FJ, Levy RJ. Tissue Heart Valves: Current Challenges and Future Research Perspectives. J Biomed Mat Res 1999;47:439–465.
2. Mayer JE Jr. Uses of homograft conduits for right ventricle to pulmonary artery connections in the neonatal period. Seminars in Thoracic and Cardiovascular Surgery 1995;7:130–132.
3. Yacoub M, Rasmi NRH, Sundt TM, Lund O et al. Fourteen-year experience with homovital homografts for aortic valve replacement. J Thorac Cardiovasc Surg 1995;110:186–194.
4. Harken DW, Curtis LE. Heart surgery: legend and a long look. American Journal of Cardiology 1967;9:393–400.
5. Gross L, Kugel MA. Topographic anatomy and histology of the valves in the human heart. Am J Pathol 1931;7:445–473.
6. Lazarous DF, Shou M, Stiber JA, Dadhania DM, Thirumurti V, Hodge E, Unger EF. Pharmacodynamics of basic fibroblast growth factor: route of administration determines myocardial and systemic distribution. Cardiovascular Research 1997;36:78–85.
7. Shinoka T, Breuer CK, Tanel RE, et al. Tissue engineering heart valves: valve leaflet replacement study in a lamb model. Ann Thorac Surg 1995;S513–S516.
8. Shinoka T, Shum-Tim D, Ma PX, Tanel RE, Isogai N, Langer R, Vacanti JP, Mayer JE Jr. Creation of viable pulmonary artery autografts through tissue engineering. The Journal of Thoracic and Cardiovascular Surgery 1998;115:536–546.
9. Stock U, Nagashima M, Khalil PN, Nollert GD, Herden T, Sperling JS, Moran A, Schoen FJ, Vacanti JP, Mayer JE. Tissue-Engineered valve conduits in the pulmonary circulation. J Thorac Cardiovasc Surg 2000;119:732–740.
10. Shum-Tim D, Stock U, Harkach J, Shinoka T, Lien J, Moses MA, Stamp A, Taylor G, Moran A, Landis W, Langer R, Vacanti JP, Mayer JE. Tissue Engineering of autologous aorta using a new biodegradable polymer. Ann Thorac Surg 1999; 68:2298–2304.
11. Hoerstrup SP, Sodian R, Daebritz S, Wang J, Backa EA, Martin DP, Moran AM, Guleserian KJ, Sperling JS, Kaushal S, Vacanti JP, Schoen FJ, Mayer JE. Functional Living Trileaflet Heart Valves Grown In Vitro. Circulation 2000;102 (suppl):III-44–III-49.
12. Hoerstrup SP, Sodian R, Sperling JS, Vacanti JP, Mayer JE. New Pulsatile Bioreactor for *In Vitro* Formation of Tissue Engineered Heart Valves. Tissue Engineering 2000;6:75–79.
13. Shinoka T, Shum-Tim D, Ma PX, Tanel RE, Langer R, Vacanti JP, Mayer JE Jr. Tissue-engineered heart valve leaflets: does cell origin affect outcome? Circulation 1997;96:II-102–II-107.
14. Wilson GJ, Courtman DW, Klement P, Lee JM, Yeger H. Accellular Matrix: A biomaterials approach for coronary artery bypass and heart valve replacement. Ann Thorac Surg 1995;60: S353–S358.
15. Elkins RC, Dawson PE, Goldstein S, Walsh SP, Black KS. Decellularized Human Valve Allografts. Ann Thorac Surg 2001;71:S428–S432.
16. O'Brien M, Goldstein S, Walsh S, et al. The SynerGraft recellularization: first studies before clinical implantation. Seminars in Thoracic and Cardiovascular Surgery 1999;13:87–92.
17. Elkins RC, Goldstein S, Hewitt CW, Walsh SP, Dawson PE, Ollerenshaw JD, Black KS, Clarke DR, O'Brien MF. Recellularization of heart valve grafts by a process of adaptive remodeling. Sem in Thor and Card Surg 2001;13:87–92.
18. Steinhoff G, Stock U, Karim N, Mertsching H, Timke A, Meliss RR, Pethig K, Haverich A, Bader A. Tissue engineering of pulmonary heart valves on allogenic acellular matrix conduits: *in vivo* restoration of valve tissue. Circulation 2000;102:III-50–III-55.
19. Booth C, Korossis SA, Wilcox HE, Watterson K, Kearney JN, Fisher J, Ingham E. Tissue engineering of cardiac valve prostheses I: Development and histological characterization of an acellular porcine scaffold. The Journal of Heart Valve Disease 2002;11:457–462.
20. Korossis SA, Booth C, Wilcox HE, Watterson K, Kearney JN, Fisher J, Ingham E. Tissue engineering of cardiac valve prostheses II: bio-

mechanical characterization of decellularized porcine aortic heart valves. The Journal of Heart Valve Disease 2002;11:463–471.

21. Jockenhoevel S, Zund G, Hoerstrup SP, et al. Fibrin gel-advantages of a new scaffold in cardivascular tissue engineering. European Journal of Cardio-Thoracic Surgery 2001;19:424–430.

22. Sakai T, Li RK, Weisel RD, Mickle DAG, Kim ET, Jia ZQ, Yau TM. The fate of tissue-engineered cardiac graft in the right ventricular outflow tract of the rat. J Thorac Cardiovasc Surg 2001;121:932–942.

23. Shi Y, Ramanurthi A, Vesley I. Towards tissue engineering of a composite aortic valve. Biomedical Sciences Instrumentation 2002;38:35–40.

24. Hilbert SL, Luna RE, Zhang J, Wang Y, Hopkins RA, Yu ZX, Ferrans VJ. Allograft heart valves: the role of apoptosis-mediated cell loss. J Thorac Cardiovasc Surg 1999;117:454–462.

25. Mitchell RN, Jonas RA, Schoen FJ. Pathology of explanted cryopreserved allograft heart valves: comparison with aortic valves from orthotopic heart transplants. J Thorac Cardiovasc Surg 1998;115:118–127.

26. Hopkins RA, Reyes A, Imperato DA, et al. Ventricular outflow tract reconstructions with cryopreserved cardiac valve homografts: a single surgeon's 10 year experience. Ann Surg 1996; 223:544–553.

27. Clarke D, Campbell D, Hayward A, et al. Degeneration of aortic valve allografts in young recipients. J Thorac Cardiovasc Surg 1993;105:934–942.

28. Maish MS, Hoffman-Kim D, Krueger PM, Souza JM, Harper JJ, Hopkins RA. Tricuspid Valve Biopsy—A potential source of cardiac myofibroblast cells for tissue engineered cardiac valves. J Heart Valve Dis 2002; In press.

29. Hayward IP, Bridle KR, Campbell GR, et al. Effect of extracellular matrix proteins on vascular smooth muscle cell phenotype. Cell Biology International 1995;19:727–734.

30. Sutherland FWH, Perry TE, Masuda Y, Sherwood MC, Mayer JE Jr. Stem cell engineered heart valves: short term follow-up. Engineered Tissues 2003;26.

31. Weston MW, Yoganathan A. Biosynthetic activity in heart valve leaflets in resopnse to in vitro flow environments. Annals of Biomedical Engineering 2001;29:752–763.

32. Vouyouka AG, Powell RJ, Ricotta J, et al. Ambient pulsatile pressure modulates endothelial cell proliferation. Journal of Molecular and Cellular Cardiology 1998;30:609–615.

33. Predel HG, Yang Z, von Segesser, et al. Implications of pulsatile stretch on growth of saphenous vein and mammary artery smooth muscle. Lancet 1992;340:878–879.

34. Juliano RL, Haskill S. Signal transduction from the extracellular matrix. The Journal of Cell Biology 1993;120:577–585.

35. Salwen SA, Szarowski DH, Turner JN, et al. Three-dimensional changes of the cytoskeleton of vascular endothelial cells exposed to sustained hydrostatic pressure. Medical and Biological Engineering and Computing 1998;36:520–527.

36. Hayward IP, Bridle KR, Campbell GR, et al. Effect of extracellular matrix proteins on vascular smooth muscle cell phenotype. Cell Biology International 1995;19:727–734.

Appendix: Valve Diameters

Table A1 lists mean "normal valve diameters: the first column for each valve comes from the data measured by Rowlatt and associates. The Great Ormond Street (GOS) group have found that these valve measurements tend to underestimate the true *in vivo* sizes. The data from Rowlatt and coworkers (RRL data) were derived from a large series of normal hearts examined at autopsy. The Great Ormond Street group noted that there was a shrinkage factor due to formalin. Their angiographic estimates were correlated to fresh autopsy material and

TABLE A1. Mean Cardiac Valve Diameters (mm) Normalized to Body Surface Area.

BSA	Mitral Valve		Tricuspid Valve		Aortic Valve		Pulmonary Valve	
	RRL[a]	GOS[b]	RRL	GOS	RRL	GOS	RRL	GOS
0.25	11.2	16.0	13.4	19.2	7.2	10.3	8.4	12.0
0.30	12.6	18.0	14.9	21.3	8.1	11.6	9.3	13.3
0.35	13.6	19.4	16.2	23.2	8.9	12.7	10.1	14.4
0.40	14.4	20.6	17.3	24.7	9.5	13.6	10.7	15.3
0.45	15.2	21.7	18.2	26.0	10.1	14.4	11.3	16.2
0.50	15.8	22.6	19.2	27.5	10.7	15.3	11.9	17.0
0.60	16.9	24.2	20.7	29.6	11.5	16.4	12.8	18.3
0.70	17.9	25.6	21.9	31.3	12.3	17.6	13.5	19.3
0.80	18.8	26.9	23.0	32.9	13.0	18.6	14.2	20.3
0.90	19.7	28.2	24.0	34.3	13.4	19.2	14.8	21.2
1.0	20.2	28.9	24.9	35.6	14.0	20.0	15.3	21.9
1.2	21.4	30.6	26.2	37.5	14.8	21.2	16.2	23.2
1.4	22.3	31.9	27.7	39.6	15.5	22.2	17.0	24.3
1.5	23.1	33.0	28.9	41.3	16.1	23.0	17.6	25.2
1.8	23.8	34.0	29.1	41.6	16.6	23.6	18.0	25.7
2.0	24.2	34.6	30.0	42.9	17.2	24.6	18.2	26.0

Standard Deviations

Mitral Valve	BSA < 0.3 = ±1.9	To convert to approximate predicted manufactured rigid
	BSA > 0.3 = ±1.6	prosthetic valve sizes, add 3–4 mm to measurement.
Tricuspid Valve	BSA < 1.0 = ±1.7	
	BSA > 1.0 = ±1.5	
Aortic Valve	All BSA ± 1.0	
Pulmonary Valve	All BSA ± 1.2	BSA = m^2

[a] RRL: data derived from Rowlatt and associates. [b] GOS = Great Ormond Street "normalized" diameters. Adapted from de Leval.

suggested that the atrioventricular valves were certainly under-estimated by the earlier techniques. The London (GOS) workers suggested that the RRL measurements should be multiplied by a factor of 1.43 to equal their fresh measurements (C. Bull, personal communication). Thus this table includes both the original data of Rowlatt and coworkers and the larger estimates of "normal."

The way we use this table relative to ventricular outflow valves is to consider the RRL valve diameters as the minimun acceptable diameter for a given body surface area and the GOS diameters as the mean to upper limits of achievable valve transplants. From a practical standpoint it means that we would try to place, for an "adult" sized freehand aortic valve implant, an allograft of 20 mm (internal diameter) for an individual with a body surface area (BSA) of $1 m^2$ and a valve as large as 24.6 mm for a $2 m^2$ individual. Once a patient reaches approximately 20 kg in weight, an aortic valve of 17 mm or larger is usually implantable in the aortic position with the techniques described in the foregoing chapters, which is within the acceptable range.

The pulmonary outflow tract is optimally reconstructed with a 22 mm pulmonary valve for a $1 m^2$ individual and could be as large as a 26 mm for a $2 m^2$ individual adult. In most patients a valve between the upper and lower sizes is almost always achievable. On the right ventricular outflow tract side, a 14 mm (internal diameter) aortic valve can usually be place in a 5 kg child; once the child weighs more than 10 kg, a right ventricular allograft conduit of 16 mm or larger is implantable; and in children above 20 kg, it is almost always possible to place a 20 mm or larger conduit in the right ventricular outflow tract position. Mercer has argued that a more than 50% reduction in pulmonary valve orifice size is required before significant gradients occur. However, right-sided *conduits* have length as well as diameter, thus sizes below the RRL values are not recommended.

With use, we have found that this table has been best at predicting the aortic and pulmonary valve diameters. It is important to remember that the diameters in these tables refer to the internal diameters, not the external diameters.

TABLE A2. AV Valve Ring Diameter for Reconstruction.

BSA (m²)	Mitral Valve (mm)	Tricuspid Valve (mm)
1.0	26	32
1.2	28	34
1.4	29	36
1.5	30	37
1.8	31	38

The aortic and pulmonary valve columns are immediately translatable to homograft sizes which are also measured in internal diameter. For manufactured valves, at least 2–4 mm needs to be added to correlate with the external sewing ring diameter as usually listed for rigid stented valves. Thus, a mechanical mitral valve choice for a $2.0 m^2$ BSA individual, would be preferably a size 27. For the aortic position, the smallest aortic prosthesis one would ever consider for a $2.0 m^2$ individual would be 17.2 plus 4.0 mm which equals a 21, but the GOS value gives the preferred size of 25.

Manufactured valve sizes do not necessarily reflect either the predicted internal diameter of a natural valve for the patient or, in fact, even the measured external diameter of the prosthesis, but in fact are an approximation of those two values based upon manufacturing requirements. The mean diameters listed in Table I are actual internal diameters as would be measured by echocardiography from the hinge point of the base of the leaflets across the orifice of each valve. Thus they reflect the target values for reconstructions. They do not directly represent the prosthetic sewing ring valve size as is normally tabulated for manufactured valves. The mitral and tricuspid valve measurements have been correlated with empiric use of valve ring diameters used in reconstructions for patients between 1.0 and 2.0 BSA. These are listed in Table A2.

These "ring" estimates are target values based on BSA normalized valve measurements. They must be modified by specific measurements at surgery of available leaflet tissue for orifice coverage and the specific type and configuration of ring being used. We do not use rigid rings in smaller children to allow for growth.

Index